Digital Mental Health

Davor Mucić • Donald M. Hilty
Editors

Digital Mental Health

The Future is Now

Second Edition

Springer

Editors
Davor Mucić
The Little Prince Psychiatric Centre
Copenhagen, Denmark

Donald M. Hilty
Department of Psychiatry and Behavioral Sciences
Keck School of Medicine University of Southern California
Los Angeles, CA, USA

ISBN 978-3-031-59938-5 ISBN 978-3-031-59936-1 (eBook)
https://doi.org/10.1007/978-3-031-59936-1

This Springer imprint is published by the registered company Springer Nature Switzerland AG
The registered company address is: Gewerbestrasse 11, 6330 Cham, Switzerland

Foreword

The advent of digitalization is poised to fundamentally redefine the landscape of psychiatry. Using digital tools, such as telepsychiatry, in everyday practice is starting a new chapter in mental health care. This change means we need to train healthcare workers who are not yet used to these technologies. It is important they learn how to use these digital tools effectively to improve their work in psychiatry.

Today, we are seeing more mental health issues, but fewer professionals in psychiatry. This calls for new, creative solutions. Technology can help us, but it is not a complete solution in itself. The success of these digital tools depends a lot on how skilled and experienced the psychiatrists using them are. Unfortunately, medical training for students and young doctors has not really focused enough on using technology in psychiatry. There is a global shortage of experts who know how to apply technology in this field. This shows how much we need better international cooperation to share what we know and learn from each other.

Organizations like the World Psychiatric Association, the European Psychiatric Association, or the American Psychiatric Association need to work together more to create common rules and share expertise internationally. They play a crucial role in shaping the future of psychiatry.

With careful planning and managing risks wisely, digital mental health (DMH), particularly telepsychiatry, can become a key part of mental health care, making it easier for more people to get the help they need. This book represents a pivotal opportunity to deepen our understanding of the synergy between traditional psychiatric services and modern digital methodologies. It charts a course for the development of integrated models that leverage digital technologies to revolutionize mental health care.

Additionally, this book has the potential to serve as a foundational resource for educating medical students and training young doctors in the fundamental skills associated with DMH. It offers an opportunity to integrate digital psychiatry into the core of medical education, ensuring that future healthcare professionals are well-equipped to utilize these emerging technologies effectively in their practice.

Institute of Psychiatric Phenomics and Genomics (IPPG) Thomas G. Schulze
University Hospital, LMU Munich
Munich, Bavaria

Department of Psychiatry and Behavioral
Medicine, Norton College of Medicine
SUNY Upstate Medical University
Syracuse, New York

Department of Psychiatry and Behavioral Medicine
Johns Hopkins University
Baltimore, Maryland

World Psychiatric Association
Geneva

Contents

Part I Introduction

1 Technology, Health, and Contemporary Practice: How Does Digital Mental Health Fit It and What Does It Offer? . . . 3
Davor Mucić and Donald M. Hilty

2 Entangled in the Web: Unexpected Events with New Technologies—Safety Issues, Addiction, and Consequences on Communication . . . 35
Agnes Wrobel and Janusz Wrobel

3 Information Technology for Behavioral Health: Global Perspectives on Access, Services, and Stigmatization . . . 51
Donald M. Hilty, Shalini Ahuja, John A. Naslund, Allison Crawford, and Norman Sartorius

4 Detection, Evaluation, and Best Practices for Technology-Based Fatigue to Promote Well-Being . . . 89
Donald M. Hilty, Christina M. Armstrong, Shawna D. Wright, Shelby A. Smout, Kenneth P. Drude, Marlene M. Maheu, and Elizabeth A. Krupinski

Part II Access, Evaluation, User Design

5 Designing New Technology for Neurodevelopmental Disorders and the Importance of Involving Users (Not Only Robots) . . . 117
Thomas Gargot, Arzu Guneysu, Carlos Cifuentes, and Silvia Orlandi

6 Digital Mental Health Improves Access to Care, Facilitates Early Intervention, and Provides Evidence-Based Treatments at a Distance . . . 141
Donald M. Hilty, Alice Zhang, Annaleis K. Giovanetti, Dorothy Stubbe, and Eve-Lynn Nelson

7 How to Build, Evaluate, and Improve Your Telemental Health Program . . . 155
Donald M. Hilty and Jay Shore

8 Digital Mental Health Toward Cross-cultural Populations Worldwide ... 175
Davor Mucić, Donald M. Hilty, and Peter M. Yellowlees

Part III Integrating Technology Into the Clinical Practice

9 Telepsychiatry: From "Telepathy" to the Mainstream ... 215
Davor Mucić, Donald M. Hilty, and Jay Shore

10 How Digital Mental Health Adds to Traditional Outpatient and Newer Models of Integrated Care for Patients, Providers, and Systems ... 255
Robert M. McCarron, Donald M. Hilty, and Krzysztof Krysta

11 Social Media and Clinical Practice: What Stays the Same, What Changes, and How to Plan Ahead? ... 275
Donald M. Hilty, Myo Thwin Myint, Kristoffer Calvert Strauss, Pamela E. Hoffman, and Dorothy Stubbe

Part IV Updates on Patient Centered Digital Mental Health Treatments

12 Web-and Internet-Based Services: Education, Support, Self-Care, Formal, and Hybrid Treatment Approaches ... 299
Davor Mucić, Donald M. Hilty, Peter M. Yellowlees, and Marek Krzystanek

13 Artificial Intelligence and Predictive Modeling in Mental Health ... 323
Donald M. Hilty, Yang Cheng, and David D. Luxton

14 Cognitive Behavioral Therapy, and Cognitive Bias Modification in Internet-Based Interventions for Mood, Anxiety, and Substance Use Disorders ... 351
Matthijs Blankers, Elske Salemink, and Reinout W. Wiers

15 Internet-Delivered Psychodynamic Therapy in Psychiatric Disorders ... 379
Jakob Mechler and Karin Lindqvist

16 Psychiatric Apps: Patient Self-Assessment, Communication, and Potential Treatment Interventions ... 397
Nanik Ram, Aditya Vaidyam, Amrik Eadara, Carsten Langholm, and John Torous

Part V Perspectives on Technology, Healthcare and Life

17 Advancing Mental Health Care: Global Perspectives on Digital and Telepsychiatry Solutions 409
Davor Mucić, Donald M. Hilty, and Peter M. Yellowlees

18 How Does the Internet Influence the Doctor–Patient Relationship? 437
Mark Agius, Michaela Agius, Rashid Zaman, and Helen Stangeland

19 Lessons Learned or Forgotten? Future Direction of Global Digital Mental Health Care 459
Davor Mucić, Jay Shore, Donald M. Hilty, Marek Krzystanek, and Krzysztof Krysta

About the Editors

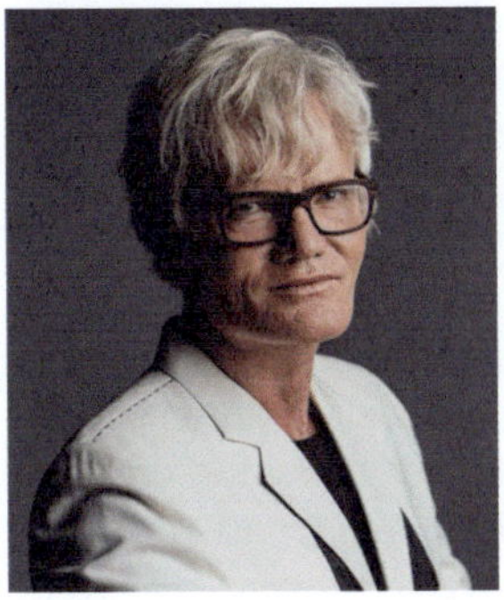

Davor Mucić is a distinguished medical doctor, educated in Rijeka, Croatia, with specialized training in psychiatry obtained in Denmark. He has a profound interest in leveraging technology to enhance mental health care, particularly in the field of e-Mental Health.

In 2000, he founded the Little Prince Psychiatric Centre in Copenhagen, where he pioneered the development of telepsychiatry. In 2011, he launched the Telemental Health Section within the European Psychiatric Association (EPA) and currently serves as the chair of the WPA's Digital Mental Health Section. Prof. Mucić serves as the Editor-in-Chief of the *Edorium Journal of Psychiatry* and actively contributes as a reviewer for the *Egyptian Journal of Psychiatry*, as well as a member of the Editorial Advisory Board for the *Journal of Pakistan Psychiatric Society*.

He has authored numerous scientific articles on telepsychiatry, including foundational work on the first international and cross-cultural telepsychiatry services, which were established in 2004. Additionally, he has explored various e-mental health applications in the edited book, *e-Mental Health*, published by Springer in 2016.

In response to the mental health challenges posed by the COVID-19 pandemic, he coordinated the WPA's "Expert Group on e-Mental Health" in 2020. He is also the main author of the recently published WPA Global Telepsychiatry Guidelines. For his significant contributions to the field, Prof. Mucić was honored with WPA Honorary Membership in 2020 and successfully defended the first doctoral dissertation on telepsychiatry in the EU in May 2022.

https://davormucic.com/

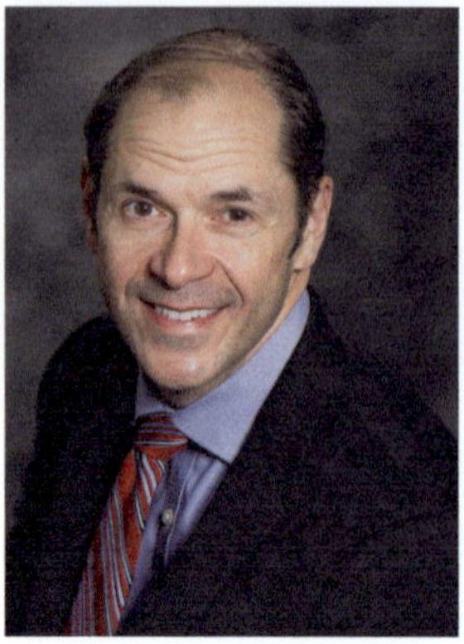

Donald M. Hilty is a scholar in psychiatric and medical education, health services, and telemedicine. He serves as a Professor of Psychiatry at the UC Davis School of Medicine and as the Chief Medical Officer (CMO) of United Health Services and Heritage Oaks Hospital. Additionally, he acts as a liaison to professional organizations and the Veterans Health Administration to implement technology. As CMO, he has overseen the development of COVID-19 psychiatric and medical-psychiatric units and The Joint Commission accreditations. He speaks internationally and has obtained approximately 20 federal and state grants for models of care, health services, mood disorders, health economic outcomes, and the implementation of technology (e.g., video, mobile health, wearable sensors, and artificial intelligence). Dr. Hilty's current research focuses on the implementation and evaluation of video, social media, mobile health, and asynchronous technologies, with an emphasis on user-centered design, workflow, technology fatigue, clinical competencies for clinicians, and institutional competencies for organizations. He facilitates collaborations with teams worldwide through his service to the American, European, and World Psychiatric Associations (APA; WPA).

Dr. Hilty is actively involved in pedagogy, professional and faculty development, and publishing. Dr. Hilty serves as the Editor of the *Journal of Technology in Behavioral Science* (*JTIBS*) and the Editor of the Innovation in Technology Column for *Academic Psychiatry*. He is also a member of many editorial boards. He has led or co-led ten special editions related to video and mobile health technology, clinical care, and professional development. These include: "The WPA Global Digital Mental Health Care: Evidence, Implementation, Guidelines and Policy" in *JTIBS,* "Professional Development in Psychiatry and Medicine" in *Psychiatric Clinics of North America*, and "Digital Interventions for Mental Health" in *Frontiers in Psychiatry*. He has written over 180 journal articles, more than 100 chapters, and numerous publications, including to the APA-Institute of Medicine and APA-American Telemedicine Association Guideline Writing Groups. Dr. Hilty led a team in publishing *Virtual Mental Health for Rural, Underserved and Diverse Settings* in 2023, and Dr. Mucić and he are doing a second edition of *Digital Mental Health* in 2024, both by Springer Nature Publishing.

Part I

Introduction

When Springer proposed an updated edition of the 2016 book E-Mental Health, we anticipated new developments. Back in 2013, while preparing the first edition, we believed that the future of digital mental health had already arrived—or was at least just around the corner. However, we were mistaken. Until the COVID-19 pandemic, that future remained distant. The pandemic experience unlocked the potential of digital technologies, accelerating their integration into clinical practice. Digital health tools have immense potential to expand access to care (C6), enhance diagnostic precision, and extend mental health services across national borders (C3,8,17). To fully harness these benefits, it is crucial to raise awareness of available technologies, evaluate existing services (C7), and establish best practices (C1,4). In this edition, telepsychiatry remains at the forefront as the cornerstone of digital mental health care. Additionally, we introduce entirely new chapters on designing technology for neurodevelopmental disorders and integrating digital mental health into outpatient and broader healthcare systems (C5,10). Other key topics include social media (C11), mental health apps (C16), online therapy, digital support, education (C12,14,15), and the evolving impact of the internet on patient interactions and professional collaboration (C2,18). Digital technologies are reshaping mental health care, shifting from the traditional in-person gold standard to a hybrid model that blends face-to-face and remote therapy. Experienced telepsychiatrists no longer use the term face-to-face, as high-quality video conferencing enables both direct interaction and the ability to read body language from a distance. Today, the distinction is between in-person and remote care—provided that it is delivered using appropriate technology and by professionals trained in its use. A dedicated chapter on telepsychiatry (C9) explores videoconferencing beyond standard Zoom meetings, while lessons learned from COVID-19 offer insights that may shape the future of global digital mental health care (C19). Lastly, the transformative role of artificial intelligence in mental health diagnosis, treatment, and service delivery (C13) is examined in depth. Yet, digital technology alone is not enough to drive meaningful innovation—it must be effectively understood and implemented. A state-of-the-art Rolls Royce is useless if the driver lacks a license. Likewise, if political correctness outweighs competence, conformity stifles innovation, and bureaucracy obstructs common sense and good clinical practice, progress in digital mental health will remain slow. This is why the role of international associations and educational institutions is vital—not only to embrace technological advancements but to ensure their seamless integration into mental health institutions and everyday clinical practice. This book underscores the importance of integrating digital health technologies into clinical practice—not as replacements for traditional methods, but as complementary tools that enhance, streamline, and revolutionize mental health care.

1 Technology, Health, and Contemporary Practice: How Does Digital Mental Health Fit It and What Does It Offer?

Davor Mucić and Donald M. Hilty

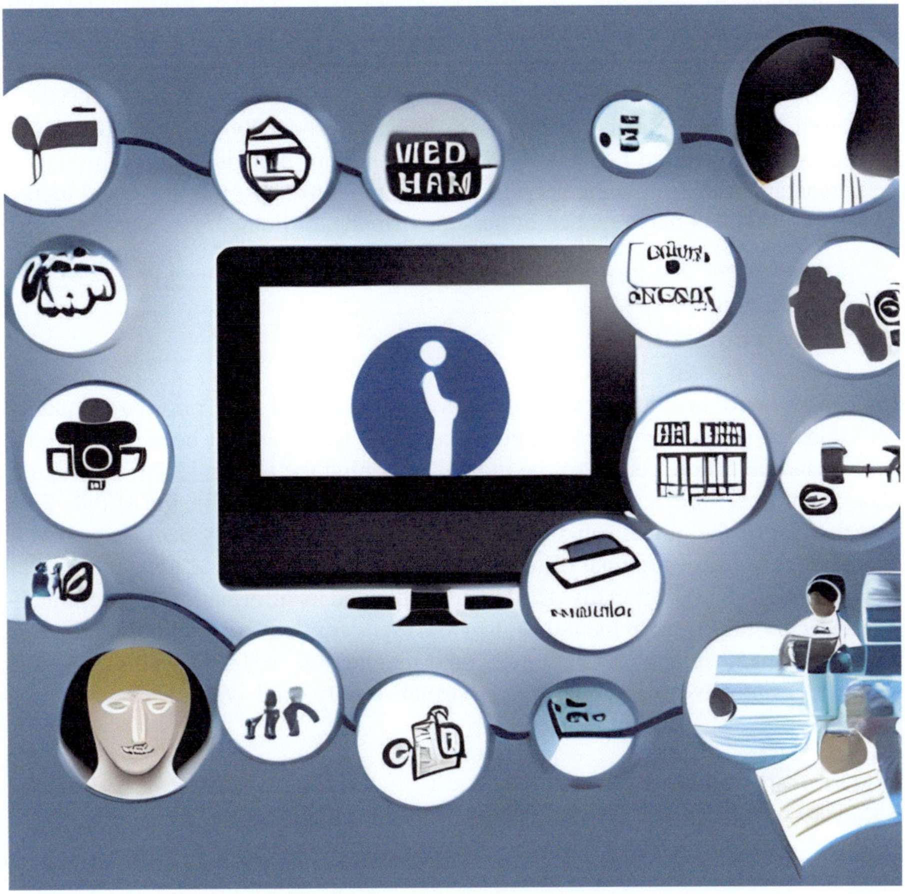

D. Mucić, D. M. Hilty (eds.), *Digital Mental Health*,
https://doi.org/10.1007/978-3-031-59936-1_1

Abstract

Patient- or person-centered healthcare poses questions on delivering quality, affordable, and timely care in diverse settings. The international history of medicine, patient-centered care models, healthcare financing, and technology utilization shape the development, implementation, and positive impact of Digital Mental Health (DMH). The coronavirus disease-2019 (COVID-19) pandemic has significantly influenced the adoption of DMH worldwide, further accelerating the shift toward digital care. Care models and patient-centered approaches drive DMH services forward, transitioning from in-person to videoconferencing and online formats—technology complements traditional medical approaches. Telemedicine empowers patients, personalizes care, increases administrative efficiency, and ensures expertise reaches patients wherever they are. Telepsychiatry, as the earliest DMH application, is effective, well accepted, and comparable to in-person care. As technology is employed, maintaining high-quality clinical care and professional standards while being sensitive to participant differences is crucial. Good care requires evaluation and addressing clinical, legal, and reimbursement concerns along with technological issues. DMH is poised to reshape healthcare service delivery, especially since telepsychiatry seems more suitable for certain disorders and care models than traditional in-person approaches. Online services will continue to boost this shift, and mental health providers may practice in-person, virtually, or both.

1.1 Introduction

Patient-centered healthcare, proposed as early as 2001 [1], prioritizes quality, affordability, and timely care [2]. Person-centered healthcare has been revitalized to understand the whole person or the individual behind the patient [3, 4]. The regulatory disparities, for example, between the USA, Europe, Australia, the Middle East, and the rest of the globe, can slow down the pace of regulatory decisions. Due to this, there are major regional differences in the development and uptake of digital mental health (DMH) globally. DMH can be defined as information and communication technology used in mental health (MH) services delivered or boosted through the Internet and related technologies, smartphone and wearable technologies, as well as immersive solutions (e.g., virtual reality and video games). It is

D. Mucić (✉)
The Little Prince Psychiatric Centre, Copenhagen, Denmark
e-mail: davor@denlilleprins.org

D. M. Hilty
Department of Psychiatry and Behavioral Sciences, Keck School of Medicine University of Southern California, Los Angeles, CA, USA
e-mail: donald.hilty@uhsinc.com; hilty@med.usc.edu

predominantly used as self-help services or with the assistance of a (para-)professional and/or artificial intelligence for the provision of mental health promotion as well as mental ill-health identification, prevention, and intervention.

Over time, a number of social, political, and scientific variables have affected the way that we understand DMH. Social science, the germ theory of disease, the metaphor of healthcare as a battlefield, the market metaphor, the social justice model of Health for All, and evidence-based medicine can all be used to track this development [5]. We can reframe health and healthcare as interconnected experiences that span individual, community, and societal domains by putting people and their needs at the center of our approach, as stressed by the International Classification of Functioning, Disability, and Health framework of the World Health Organization and the European Society of Person-Centered Healthcare.

Two of the significant trends are in the USA and Europe, though the World Health Organization, too: surveying on telemedicine opportunities and developments in member states [6]. The patient-centered medical home (PCMH) is one such specific movement—along with the Affordable Care Act (ObamaCare; ACA) in the USA—which involves a deceptively simple set of key structural practice features that have been proposed to result in enhanced access for routine primary care, improved delivery of preventive services, high-quality chronic disease management, and reduced emergency department and hospital utilization [7, 8]. The approaches or tools for the changing environment are PCMH, collaborative or integrated care, stepped care, and still more innovative models. The European Commission's ROAMER initiative aims to identify gaps in care and mental health service needs in Europe. To support clinicians in selecting appropriate treatment modalities, blended Digital Health/mental health decision aids and guidance tools have been proposed, with the potential to increase treatment efficacy and impact [9].

Across the globe, there are various funding models for healthcare, ranging from tax-funded national health systems to national insurance systems with competing regulated private health insurance plans, some operating through health insurance marketplaces or their equivalents [10]. The level of attention given to the most vulnerable populations in terms of benefit design, cost-sharing thresholds and exemptions, and subsidies varies among nations. A critical characteristic of these many healthcare systems is a skewed distribution of healthcare utilization across the population (e.g., about 25% of all medical care is consumed by 1% of the patient population and nearly half by just 5%) [11]. DMH—or more broadly e-service delivery—is in the thick of things due to its versatility and leveraging of essential resources [12, 13] at multiple points of service [13, 14]. Indeed, DMH providers' input to the primary care provider has improved patient care, is convenient, and is less costly with desk-mounted video systems [12, 15, 16]. DMH also leverages interdisciplinary team members' clinical, administrative, and other care coordination expertise [17].

DMH, encompassing a broad definition for online services, is at the forefront for several reasons. First, it enhances our capabilities by offering numerous new communication options (Chap. 2), improving access to the best treatments (Chap. 6), and disseminating culturally sensitive care (Chap. 8). Second, DMH provides clinicians with more virtual options via the Internet or web (Chaps. 12, 14, and 15). Designing new technology is an ongoing process, but technology is not a goal in itself, i.e., user involvement is equally important (Chap. 5). Further, DMH is improving access, quality, and sustainability of remote treatment (Chap. 6). Are the expectations of artificial intelligence to improve the quality of care and increase the efficiency of doctors unrealistic? (Chap. 13). New technologies are great, but we must not forget the basics related to the oldest DMH, i.e., telepsychiatry, which we rediscovered due to the coronavirus disease-2019 (COVID-19) pandemic (Chap. 9). While they are adapting, many feel that DMH is transforming their clinical practice (Chap. 16). Newer generations embrace these changes but must also learn the fundamentals of the doctor–patient relationship and how DMH impacts it (Chap. 18). Third, clinicians and administrators require an approach to develop and evaluate mental health care program (Chap. 7), detect best technology-based practices (Chap. 4), and apply it to patient-centered and integrated care movements (Chap. 10). Having a plan beforehand is essential not only for its own sake but also to guide others on pressing topics like online psychotherapy options (Chaps. 14 and 15) and managing social media in patient care (Chap. 11). Clinicians and patients understandably question how the future of service delivery will be in the future (Chap. 19) and how biased the global trends look like (Chap. 17). Finally, the lessons learned during the great COVID-19 pandemic must not be forgotten (Chap. 19) because those who forget risk repeating history.

The integration of technology and the Internet with traditional mental health care has led to user-friendly, more accessible, and personalized additional care. This has resulted in a broader range of services available for patients, with a more diverse process of accessing care. With better knowledge of patients' preferences for help-seeking, education, and treatment, mental health (MH) providers need to address the challenges and requirements to fulfill care-related demands. As informal or self-directed services expand, the question arises whether a professional should oversee a patient's care when engaged in such services, and if so, how. While options have grown, there is the concern of whether the patient can navigate to the best service for them. In comparison, the banking industry transitioned to ATMs for simple tasks, and tellers were only used as needed. Therefore, the question remains: Is mental health as straightforward?

This chapter aims to help readers: (1) Understand the history of telemedicine and DMH; (2) Examine how DMH, technology, and online options have become part of and shaped current healthcare trends in the USA and globally; and (3) Apply telehealth to realize the benefits of new technology for patients (access to care, innovative treatment), providers, systems, and global communities (e.g., empowerment, more versatile approaches to care, and "better" care).

1.2 Current Healthcare Trends: A Historical Perspective and the Platform of Technology with Focus on Digital Mental Health

In recent years, healthcare systems worldwide have undergone significant changes. As a consequence of technological advancements in medical practice, DMH has been instrumental in these changes. This paper examines healthcare trends in the

USA and around the world with an emphasis on DMH. It also offers a historical perspective on how technology has impacted the medical sector.

We might begin by examining how medicine and DMH are framed, conceptually, and in other dimensions. To "frame" is to select certain aspects of a perceived reality and make them more salient in a communicating text, promoting a specific problem definition, causal interpretation, moral evaluation, and/or treatment recommendation for the item described [18]. These frames focus on causal, instrumental, political/economic, or social aspects. Although all remain relevant, merely recycling individual past frames in response to current problems will not achieve the desired outcomes. Frames "organize everyday reality by providing meaning to an unfolding strip of events and promoting particular definitions and interpretations" [19]. Notably, framing the same issue through positive or negative reference points [20] offers different contexts that influence our perception and decision-making, leading to different cognitive and motivational consequences [21].

The history of telemental health, telepsychiatry, and other technology shows a remarkable evolution and shift over time (Table 1.1). Key things like the analog wave radio and predictive modeling —now catching hold in health care —began pre-1950. The 1950s brought telephone, ultrasound, artificial intelligence, machine learning, and nanotechnology. The 1960s brought video at speeds 32–56 kilobits per second (KBPS), the electronic health record (EHR), prototypes of the Internet, the Transmission System 1 line (T1), the autonomous virtual human, the chatbot (ELIZA), natural language processing, and augmented reality—again, the substantial impact of these has come decades later.

Australia has been progressive in the use of DMH and digital platforms, particularly for rural and remote communities to improve access to specialists, quality care, decision support/supervision, and therapies [22–24]. Telepsychiatry is proving successful through various programs servicing rural Australian regions (e.g., Wagga Wagga, Dubbo, Western Australia, and South Australia) across different psychiatric services. The Mental Health Emergency Care-Rural Access Program, a telehealth solution, has provided specialist emergency mental health care to rural and remote communities across western NSW, Australia, since 2008, offering timely information and support, emergency telephone triage assessments, and video assessments. Benchmarks for efficient service delivery and information about the development of similar telehealth programs are needed both in Australia and internationally [25]. Due to accessibility, the telephone has become a standard tool for Australian psychiatrists in scheduling, consultation, payment, and crisis management.

The most popular current "frame" for taking action in healthcare appears to be the Patient Centered Mental Health (PCMH) and a hybrid of patient-centered, stepped, and/or collaborative care worldwide. The PCMH is based on the absence of adequate treatment or access to it in primary care [26]. It is believed to be efficient in a high-performing, cost-effective healthcare system [7]—though other models, approaches, or tools may function better in that context. Integrated care and stepped care models provide efficient expertise at the point of service. The core characteristics of integrated care are (1) responsibility, decision-making, and oversight of patient care; (2) co-location of services, both literally and virtually, applying to both inpatient and

Table 1.1 Telemental health, telepsychiatry, and other technology history: evolution, key events, and shifts

Decade	Technologies	Event(s)
Pre-1950s	Analog wave radio Predictive modeling	Communication (military, ship)
1950s	Telephone Ultrasound Artificial intelligence Machine learning Nanotechnology	1st Programs: Nebraska, Other UK, 1956 USA, 1956 USA, 1959 USA, 1959
1960s	Video 32–56 KBPS[a] Electronic health record (EHR) Prototypes Internet Transmission System 1 (T1) Autonomous virtual human Chatbot (ELIZA) Natural language processing Augmented reality	Plain old telephone service (POTS) USA, 1960s US military, 1960 US Bell System, 1962 USA, 1964 Germany, 1964 USA, Massachusetts Institute of Technology USA, University of Salt Lake City
1970s	128 KBPS Computer tomography Magnetic resonance imaging (MRI) Hand held phone Automated network	UK, 1972 UK, 1972 USA, Motorola, 1973 Japan, 1979
1980s	Handheld on market Facsimile/fax 1G network ISDN[b] Modern Internet Virtual reality	DynaTAC8000x, Motorola Mid -1980s Ditto Ditto Ditto; USA, Europe, and others USA, 1984
1990–1994	2G network SIM card SMS (short message service) texting	Finland, 1991 Germany, 1991 Finland, 1993
1995–1999	18–384 KBPS Mixed reality Social media (e.g., six degrees) Human behavior modeling	Mid-1990s USA, 1994 USA, 1997 USA, 1999
2000–2004	Brain–computer interface (BCI) 3G network	USA, 2000 2001
2005–2009	Internet paid media content iPhone STP[c] ATP[d] 4G networks	2006 USA, 2007 USA, comparable to in-person USA, 2008 2008
2010–2014	*Digital phenotyping* e-consult	USA, 2011 USA, 2012
2015–2019	Fibertronics Wearable health trackers 5G networks	USA, 2015 USA, 2015 2018

(continued)

Table 1.1 (continued)

Decade	Technologies	Event(s)
2020s?		
2030s?		
2040s?		

[a]*KBPS* kilobits per second
[b]*ISDN* Integrated Services for Digital Network
[c]*STP* synchronous telepsychiatry
[d]*ATP* asynchronous telepsychiatry (or store and forward telepsychiatry)

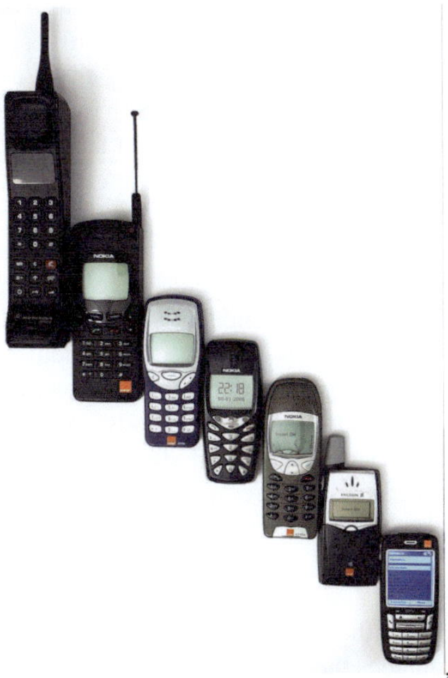

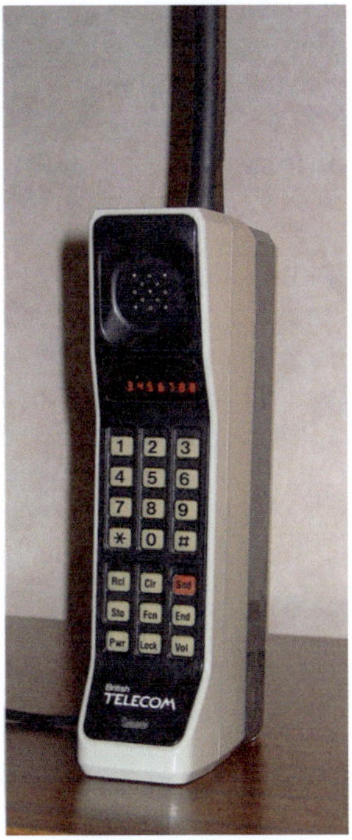

outpatient sector care; (3)–(5) integrated funding, evaluation, and outcome measurement; (6) a digital platform; and (7) reimbursement, preferably aligned (e.g., a capitated or sole "Medicare" population) rather than unaligned (i.e., mixed populations). Stepped care models may be the most cost-effective models in a health system where the effectiveness of the intervention is maximized by making the best use of resources adequately available at the right time [27, 28].

Digital platforms have traditionally distributed academic networks of like-minded researchers and clinicians into regional health information organizations (RHIOs) [29]. These RHIOs empower consumers and clinicians in day-to-day healthcare delivery by improving access to evidence-based information at the point of care; facilitating the delivery of a wider range of health services, particularly to primary and community care; providing accurate data to support research and clinical policy and governance arrangements; and ensuring a sustainable, secure, reliable electronic environment, underpinned by strong, policy-driven privacy protection [29]. Previously, the single most important technical innovation was broadband distribution, which enabled high-quality videoconferencing, multimedia-based applications, and other options, particularly at the doctor's desk.

The contemporary digital platform adds the electronic medical record (EMR), integration of in-person and DMH care administration (i.e., scheduling, documentation, payment, and others), enhanced patient to doctor or system engagement/communication (e.g., HIPAA[1] compliant email "into" the EMR [e.g., Relay Health]), and leveraging the expertise at a distance (phone, email, video, asynchronous and other methods).

Another trend is participatory medicine and patient-centered care, embodied in the personal health record (PHR). Participatory medicine can be defined as a movement where networked patients transition from being mere passengers to responsible drivers of their health, with providers encouraging and valuing them as full partners [30]. This movement may also encompass patient-driven research [31]. The patient-centered PHR (PCPHR) is progressing, but its adoption has been limited, partly due to patient factors such as comorbid illness, culture/ethnicity, and age [32].

Involving patients in personal healthcare decisions can employ decision aids that facilitate shared decision-making between patients and clinicians. These aids present relevant scientific information in balanced, understandable ways, help clarify patients' goals, and guide the decision-making process. International standards dictate that both patients and clinicians should participate in decision-aid development [33]. Patient-reported outcomes (PROs) are standardized methods for gauging patients' perspectives on their health status. An international study demonstrated that experts in clinical practice and performance measurement supported the integrated collection of PRO data for use in both clinical care and performance measurement [34].

A broader theme related to the PCPHR is shared medical decision-making. Complex situations necessitate partnerships with patients or learners to achieve the best outcomes. Shared decision-making balances the information and power dynamics between doctors and patients, with both parties sharing information and reaching a consensus on decisions [35]. Psychiatry serves as a good model for early and contemporary shared decision-making. Patients more frequently selected psychotherapy over pharmacotherapy when offered the choice between various treatment choices for depression as opposed to being randomly assigned to treatment groups, with no appreciable difference in patient satisfaction or outcomes. In a research on the continuation or discontinuation of antipsychotic depot medication in schizophrenia patients, 87% of 96 patients—a noticeably high rate—continued their medication [35]. DMH plays a significant role in these efforts, as it facilitates the

[1] HIPAA is the US Federal Health Insurance Portability and Accountability Act of 1996. The primary goal of the law is to make it easier for people to keep health insurance, protect the confidentiality and security of healthcare information, and help the healthcare industry control administrative costs.

provision of integrated and collaborative care. The collaborative care model (CoCM) is a well-established system of behavioral health care in primary care settings. There is potential for digital and mobile technology to augment the CoCM to improve access, scalability, efficiency, and clinical outcomes. The use of digital and mobile health technologies in CoCM is unfortunately still limited [36].

1.3 History of Technology, Telemedicine, and DMH

1.3.1 What We Know So Far: An Overview on DMH

The integration of technology into healthcare has led to significant advancements in the delivery of mental health services. DMH has played a critical role in shaping current healthcare trends. An overview on DMH's worldwide trends is shown in Table 1.2.

The oldest and best-documented DMH application, that aims to provide real-time remote assessment and/or treatment of mentally ill people, is telepsychiatry (videoconferencing in real time). The American Telemedicine Association (ATA) Videoconferencing Guidelines [114] review organizations' technical responsibilities to ensure the equipment readiness, safety, effectiveness, security of data, connectivity, and compliance with legal/regulatory guidelines. The WPA Telepsychiatry Global Guidelines cover a wide range of essential elements, such as clinical practice, ethical considerations, technological challenges, education and training, research, and specific populations and settings, with an emphasis on international and cross-cultural dimensions [115].

Evaluation of telepsychiatry has gone through three phases [12]. First, it was found to be effective in terms of increasing access to care, acceptance, and good educational outcomes [12]. Second, it was noted to be valid and reliable as compared to in-person services [114]. In addition to comparison (or "as good as") studies, telepsychiatric outcomes are not inferior to in-person care (i.e., non-inferiority studies). Third, frameworks are being used to approach complex themes like costs and models [114, 116, 117].

Globally, healthcare trends vary significantly due to differences in funding models, regulatory environments, and cultural factors. However, some common trends include the push for universal healthcare coverage, the integration of DMH into mental health service delivery, and the development of innovative care models, such as stepped care and blended care [14]. DMH models of clinical care and education have pros and cons [12, 17, 117, 118] including their level of overall intensity, cost, feasibility, and depth of the relationship between the DMH provider, the PCP, and the patient. *Low-intensity* models include tele-education, formal case review, and in-person, telephone, or email doctor-to-doctor "curbside" consultations. A systematic approach was a multispecialty phone and email teleconsultation system for adults and children with developmental disabilities [119]. *Moderate-intensity* models include an integrated program of mental health screening, therapy on site, and telepsychiatric consultation (phone, email, or video), with continuing medical

Table 1.2 TMH worldwide trends

Country	Description	Comment(s)/planning
Australia	Australia has been progressive in the use of DMH and e-platforms, particularly for rural and remote communities, to improve access to specialists, quality care, decision support/supervision, and therapies [22–24]. Telepsychiatry is proving successful through a number of programs to service rural Australian regions (e.g., Wagga Wagga, Dubbo, Western Australia, and South Australia) across different psychiatric services. Benchmarks for efficient service delivery and information about the development of similar telehealth programs are needed both in Australia and overseas [25]. The Mental Health Emergency Care-Rural Access Program (MHEC-RAP), which is a telehealth solution, provides specialist emergency mental health care to rural and remote communities across western NSW, Australia, since 2008, and provides timely information and support, emergency telephone triage assessments, and video assessments	Due to accessibility, the telephone has become a standard tool for Australian psychiatrists in scheduling, consultation, payment, and crisis management [37]. The telephone has also been widely used for psychotherapy (e.g., free, confidential, and anonymous telephone counseling service for young people aged between 5 and 25). Counselors respond to more than 10,000 phone calls each week about issues ranging from relationship breakdown and bullying to sexual abuse, homelessness, suicidal thoughts, and drug and alcohol usage. Since 1991, there have been more than 5.2 million telephone and online chat sessions (audio and visual) [38]
Canada	Telemental Healthcare has been widely adopted in Canada, particularly outside of Ontario, near Alberta, and for Native American (e.g., Nunavut), geriatric, and child and adolescent populations [39–42]	Canada has led in terms of some education models in child and adolescent psychiatry, as well as the call for objectives, goals, and curricula [43, 44]
Middle East	The middle east (ME) and DMH use may be a good example of some of the main struggles of programs across the world. The ME is a heterogeneous part of the world with certain variations in mental health services. The spectrum includes countries that have very good (e.g., Israel), fair (e.g., Turkey, Iran, Saudi Arabia), or poor (e.g., Iraq, Syria) services. Given the disparities, there is a need to implement DMH in the ME, but there are only three reports of randomized controlled trials related to eMH, which were done in Turkey, Israel, and Iraq, which focus on effectiveness, psychoeducation, and the doctor–patient working alliance [45–47]. As telemedicine is not an integrated part of health systems in the ME, there are no regulations or legislations that guide such practices. Fear of political persecution is a threat unique to, and commonly seen in, the ME, and it may also impact patients' acceptance to DMH [48, 49]	Four main barriers to implement DMH in the ME are frequently observed: cultural, technical, financial, and regulatory barriers. The process of building an eMH in the ME would require a parallel reconstruction of the medico-legal system to allow for more considerate approach to sensitive ethical concepts such as confidentiality, informed consent, and liability. Countries in the ME also vary in their readiness to adopt the technology and built DMH systems

European Union (EU)	The EU has supported the project MasterMind [50], which treats depression in the home in Southern Denmark so that developing the methods for treatment can be continued and the experiences can be shared with other EU countries. The MasterMind consortium consists of 23 partners from different European countries (Denmark, Greenland, Scotland, Wales, The Netherlands, Germany, Estonia, Belgium, Spain, Italy, Turkey, and Norway) eMEN ("e-mental health innovation and transnational implementation platform, North-West Europe") project is a collaborative effort across Europe aimed to develop and implement digital mental health services [51]. The project partners from Belgium, France, Germany, Ireland, the Netherlands, and the U K carry out a unique combination of activities in research, product development, policy guidance development, and communications, and initiate a transnational cooperation platform for DMH stakeholders	Similar situation is with other European countries where the use of videoconference in assessment and/ or treatment has not been grounded yet while internet-based approaches have One of the key outcomes of the project is the development of a transnational policy, which outlines the framework for the implementation and scaling up of digital mental health services in different countries [52]
Denmark	The Treatment Centre Little Prince in Copenhagen [53] augmented individual efforts in development and promotion of various telepsychiatry services since 2004. Clinicians from the Centre have conducted several pilot projects supported by the Ministry of Health, Ministry of Internal Affairs, and private grants (e.g., Egmont Foundation) Center for Digital Psychiatry in Odense was launched in 2013. It is a development and research center with expertise in the use of digital solutions for mental health promotion and psychiatric treatment [54]	Cross-cultural service, shared care within general practice service, and finally international telepsychiatry service are some of the most important projects launched by The Treatment Centre Little Prince, which helped pave the way for today's DMH expansion in Denmark [55–57]
Spain	The Canary Islands telepsychiatry program in Spain provides psychiatric service to rural regions. From the same program in the Canary Islands, a randomized controlled trial demonstrated that telepsychiatry treatment has equivalent efficacy to face-to-face consultation in psychiatric treatment [58]	
UK	The use of videoconferencing has proved its potential to enhance psychiatric services within the UK, especially for those patients who live in rural areas [59]. The integration of an eMH service into rural primary medical care is an obvious way to improve assessment and treatment of mild mental health. UK psychiatrists have achieved more than the rest of Europe within this task, followed by the development of forensic telepsychiatry [59–62]	Unfortunately, lack of training and experience, inadequate access to equipment, and insufficient technical support have all limited the take-up of this technology in the UK [63]

(continued)

Table 1.2 (continued)

Country	Description	Comment(s)/planning
Sweden	Sweden is one of Scandinavian countries that invested in equipment in the 1990s but has not used it on a large scale. Few telepsychiatry projects have been done, but videoconferencing is used for staff communications in northern part of the country. Internet- based cognitive behavioral therapy (ICBT) has been well accepted and adopted by both patients and professionals [64]	
France	In France, eMH is still not widely developed, but applications are of supportive character, i.e., staff meetings via videoconference while patient-centered service is described within the autistic spectrum [65]	
Netherlands	In Netherlands there are a number of DMH-related activities, primarily web–/mobile-based applications, where cognitive therapy in different settings leads [66, 67]	
Romania	Guided ICBT as a promising treatment approach [68, 69]	
Non-EU		
China	China initiated telemedicine in the late 1980s. In 2018, China's telemedicine network has covered more than 3000 hospitals across the country [70] Teleconsultation and telediagnosis were the core charging services [71] In 2020, some hospitals in China launched online visual contact events with the support of live-stream platforms [72] However, the usage of telemedicine is relatively insufficient despite the fact that most health care professionals have fairly positive opinions toward telemedicine [73] DMH applications were effective in the treatment of trauma victims [74] Technology-based mental health intervention (ICBT) [75]	
Russia	Study on the mental health app for subjective well-being prediction in a Russian-speaking population, and the first to combine language, social network, and phone app usage features in well-being research [76, 77]	Despite the great needs and potentials, DMH is still in its infancy
Other	Developing countries are far behind despite a numbers of clinical, economical, and other benefits DMH offers. Despite promising activities outlined below, progress in DMH service development has been slow in most low- and middle-income countries	

India	The Society for Administration of Telemedicine and Healthcare Informatics (SATHI) offered telepsychiatry services to tsunami-affected persons in Nagapattinam district in the state of Tamil Nadu [78] SMS text-messaging for promoting positive mental health among young women living in urban slums [79, 80]	
Pakistan	Training and education of existing staff in Pakistan from a distance [81] Culturally adapted low-intensity CBT for depression and psychosis has been developed and tested in both primary and the secondary care in Pakistan [82–84]	
Sri Lanka	The combination of SMS text-message reminders and supportive telephone calls significantly reduced suicidal ideation and depression among individuals after a suicide attempt [85]	
Thailand	Telephone motivational interviews showed promise in being effective in reducing the frequency and amount of drinking for non-treatment-seeking primary care patients who abuse alcohol [86]	
Malaysia	Psychoeducation or cognitive behavioral therapy programs adapted for delivery through online platforms to treat depression or anxiety disorders [87]	
South Africa	A pilot project within forensic telepsychiatry [88, 89] Weekly telephone lifestyle coaching sessions in reducing antipsychotic-induced weight gain in individuals diagnosed with serious mental illness [90–92]	
Nigeria	Randomized controlled trials from Nigeria have shown that SMS text-message reminders were effective in promoting attendance at clinical appointments among individuals with serious mental illness [93, 94]	
Somaliland	e-Learning demonstrates potential benefits to students in contrasting locations of brief, focused, online peer-to-peer education partnerships, expanding the scope of health links to the medical professionals of the future [95, 96]	
Ethiopia	The USAID-funded Digital Health Activity (DHA) is a 5-year project that supports Ethiopia in improving the quality and availability of healthcare services through the deployment of data-driven and patient-centered digital tools [97]: https://dha.jsi.com/. Most frequently reported barriers to the implementation of telemedicine were primarily related to infrastructure, costs, and staff resistance [98]	

(continued)

Table 1.2 (continued)

Country	Description	Comment(s)/planning
Brazil	Telephone support or online self-help programs targeting alcohol use and other substance misuse [99] e-learning was highly appreciated as a learning tool [100, 101] A web-based intervention to reduce alcohol use and related problems [102–105]	
Columbia	The asynchronous model is the most cost-effective model of telepsychiatry care for patients with depression admitted to a detention center, according to the results of clinical effectiveness, cost measurement, and patient satisfaction [106]	
Uruguay	Web-based substance use preventive intervention supported by periodic reminders via email and short message service (SMS) text-messages had a positive impact on participation [107]	
Mexico	Psychoeducation or cognitive behavioral therapy programs adapted for delivery through online platforms to treat depression or anxiety disorders [108–110]	
Chile	Online video game for supporting depression treatment among adolescents [111] An online program for symptom monitoring in patients receiving treatment for major depression [112] A telephone-based monitoring in promoting treatment adherence. The intervention involved non-professional providers who offered education and reinforced adherence and treatment goals to patients, leading to a reduction in symptoms [113]	

education (CME) and training on screening questionnaires [120] or asynchronous telepsychiatry (ATP) to primary care in English- and Spanish-speaking patients in primary care [121]. In India, asynchronous telepsychiatry's viability in primary care was also proven [122]. *High-intensity* models are typically the ones previously mentioned involving collaborative care [17, 123–125].

The traditional models of care have been in-person, synchronous telepsychiatry (STP), and more recently ATP—that is really only the beginning, and emerging models are sprouting quickly. On general, it is how technology affects basic clinical practice. Its impact on clinical boundaries, communication, and engagement has been under review [126]. The American Psychiatric Association (APA) has a guideline on e-prescribing [127]. The effect on professionalism and education/training of the next generations has been explored [128]. Telepsychiatry can extend beyond videoconferencing modalities to other mechanisms: (1) New digital communication from one user to another user using standard protocols: email, SMS text-messaging, MMS messaging, and instant messaging; (2) New digital communication from one user to another user using proprietary networks: Twitter direct messages, Facebook Messenger, Epic MyChart electronic medical record messaging, and My HealtheVet electronic medical record messaging; (3) New social media communication platforms that transmit from one to many users: Internet forums, Facebook pages and profiles, and Twitter streams.

Depending on the socioeconomic situation of various locations and countries around the world, the extent of the use of digital communication in mental health care varies.

A randomized trial from Iran [129] found that daily SMS text-messages encouraging the use of a paper booklet for depression treatment among individuals from rural areas did not result in a significant reduction in depressive symptoms compared with using the paper booklet alone. However, in Sri Lanka, the combination of SMS text-message reminders and supportive telephone calls significantly reduced suicidal ideation and depression among individuals after a suicide attempt [85].

Two pilot studies from Chile indicate the potential of digital technology in treating depression. The first study involved an online video game for supporting depression treatment among adolescents [111], while the second study focused on an online program for symptom monitoring in patients receiving treatment for major depression [112]. Both studies showed promising results, demonstrating the acceptability and feasibility of using online platforms to support depression treatment. Moreover, a telephone-based monitoring intervention was found to be effective in promoting treatment adherence and positive clinical outcomes for depression in Chile. The intervention involved non-professional providers who offered education and reinforced adherence and treatment goals to patients, leading to a reduction in symptoms [113].

In an exploratory study conducted in Bangalore, India, SMS text-messaging was found to be a feasible and acceptable means for promoting positive mental health among young women living in urban slums [79].

Randomized controlled trials from Nigeria and China have shown that SMS text-message reminders were effective in promoting attendance at clinical appointments among individuals with serious mental illness [93, 94, 130, 131]. A study conducted in South Africa [90] demonstrated that weekly telephone lifestyle coaching sessions were effective in reducing antipsychotic-induced weight gain in individuals diagnosed with serious mental illness.

A pilot study [91] examined evidence-based psychoeducation or cognitive behavioral therapy (CBT) programs adapted for delivery through online platforms to treat depression or anxiety disorders among individuals in various countries, including Mexico [108–110], Romania [68, 69], China, and Russian-speaking populations [76].

Digital technology makes it possible to support the provision of mental health care in clinical settings and to give health workers basic mental health education. Examples are described in Pakistan [81], Somaliland [95, 96], South Africa [92], India [80], and Brazil [100, 101].

With regard to clinical outcomes, patient satisfaction, therapeutic relationship, treatment adherence, and medication compliance, Home-telepsychiatry experiences from Brazil demonstrate that this DMH application is feasible and equally effective as standard care, i.e., in-person treatment, for depressed outpatients.

The use of digital technology has the potential to aid in reaching individuals affected by trauma in conflict zones or areas that are difficult to access. An online intervention was found to be a promising approach for supporting traumatized individuals in Iraq [132, 133]. A survey of Syrian refugees in Turkey found that nearly half were interested in receiving mental health services through telepsychiatry [49], and, lately, efforts have focused on the use of technology to reach Syrian refugees in Jordan [134].

DMH applications were effective in the treatment of trauma victims in China. Studies have shown that these programs were effective in improving the mental health outcomes of those who had experienced trauma, with one study documenting a marked decrease in posttraumatic stress disorder (PTSD) symptoms [26] and another emphasizing the efficiency of the programs in enhancing coping mechanisms [74].

An example of technology-based mental health intervention for Chinese-speaking populations involved an online program designed to identify individuals at risk of suicide or depression, deliver suicide prevention content, and provide support for coping [87].

Telephone support or online self-help programs targeting alcohol use and other substance misuse have been described. Telephone-based brief motivational interventions were effective for reducing alcohol consumption compared with standard print materials in Brazil [99] and Thailand [86]. In Brazil, an online self-help program was effective for reducing alcohol consumption among harmful or hazardous users and users with suggested dependence, although program adherence was low [102]. Online motivational interventions launched in Brazil for preventing general substance misuse w as effective at reducing use of alcohol, cannabis, and other drugs as an in-person version of the same intervention [103, 107].

Mental health services are made more effective and accessible to a variety of population groups by leveraging opportunities offered by technology and digital platforms. Instead of merely facilitating change in the delivery of mental health care in low- and middle-income nations, technology use may actually be driving it. It may not be possible to establish expensive psychiatric care practices and inpatient services in such environments, where healthcare systems are often fragmented and mental health care is not distributed equally. Direct-to-consumer mental health care programs provided via mobile devices may be a better option, eliminating the need for costly infrastructure while improving access to care for millions of people. Furthermore, this approach could improve access to highly skilled specialists in mental health care. It could ultimately enhance the general delivery and standard of those services.

The COVID-19 pandemic has played a significant role in the rapid adoption of DMH worldwide [135]. The need for social distancing and remote healthcare services during the pandemic has led to an unprecedented demand for telehealth and digital mental health services. Governments, healthcare systems, and insurance providers have responded by revising regulations and reimbursement policies, enabling healthcare providers to quickly adopt and integrate DMH into their practices [136]. These changes have not only increased the accessibility of mental health services but also highlighted the potential benefits of DMH in addressing pre-existing disparities and barriers to care [137, 138].

DMH offers the potential to transform mental health services by providing greater accessibility, flexibility, and cost-effectiveness. However, the rapid expansion of DMH also raises concerns about maintaining high-quality clinical care and professional standards, addressing privacy and security issues, and ensuring equitable access to digital mental health services across diverse populations.

1.4 Digital Communication: Email, Messaging Services, and Online Options

Digital information has become a crucial resource for online users. As of January 2014, 90% of adults possessed a cell phone, and 58% owned a smartphone [139]. In the public health domain, 35% of US adults used the Internet to research health information and learn from others' experiences [140]. People aged 13–54 in the USA primarily use their smartphones to socialize, manage personal aspects like health, and gather information [141].

These trends have significant consequences for psychiatrists. Firstly, online messaging is mandatory for providers treating Medicare and Medicaid patients, as per federal electronic medical record guidelines and meaningful use stage 2 by 2014 [142]. The government's financial incentives and penalties program necessitates that over 5% of unique patients send secure messages to clinicians, promoting messaging use. While the general public might utilize email, SMS, and MMS, these do not inherently offer HIPAA-compliant encryption. Surprisingly, patient-centered Googling (PTG) and other Internet searches are now employed to address emergencies and assist in forensic psychiatric evaluations [143]. Providers need to balance the value and risk of treatment [144], always prioritizing the patient's best interests.

Digital mental health services can be divided into several groups: (1) Online health resources; (2) Community involvement or support groups focusing on all or a specific subject; (3) Formal materials for patients (psychoeducation) and providers (professional education); (4) Tools for self-evaluation and healthy lifestyle promotion; and (5) Decision-making regarding illness management, one-time medical guidance, professional-led group advice, self-directed formal treatment, and mental health services with professionals, such as Internet-based CBT (ICBT). For people facing particular challenges, such as those who live far from services, have special needs (such as autism spectrum, sensory, and motor disabilities), are housebound (due to physical or mental health issues like panic disorder or phobias), or belong to certain age groups, the Internet can provide resources, connections, and worthwhile activities (e.g., teenagers).

These changes have an impact on how psychiatrists and other mental health specialists modify their procedures and use technology to better service their patients. Providers can reach a larger audience, provide customized support, and eventually help better the mental health outcomes for people across various demographic groups by embracing the potential of digital resources and online services. Psychiatrists and other mental health workers need to keep up with the newest trends and best practices for integrating technology into their practice as the digital landscape continues to change. This entails getting acquainted with the various web resources, support networks, and technological tools that are accessible to both patients and providers.

It is crucial for providers to modify their services to meet the particular needs and preferences of digital natives as they represent a bigger proportion of the population seeking mental health care. Mental health professionals can contribute to the de-stigmatization of mental health problems and give accessible, individualized support that fits with the way people naturally interact with technology by providing a variety of technology-based resources and treatment options.

In conclusion, the growing prevalence of digital information and online resources presents both opportunities and challenges for mental health professionals. By staying informed about the latest trends, utilizing technology effectively, and addressing ethical and legal considerations, providers can better serve their patients and contribute to improved mental health outcomes in an increasingly connected world.

1.5 Social Media Communication

Social media offers several advantages, including spreading health information and connecting healthcare providers with the general public. Digital natives, particularly children and adolescents, are more skilled at using social media, which may help de-stigmatize mental health issues. Users seek trustworthy and personalized information that respects their anonymity and confidentiality. An increasing number of treatments are being conducted via mobile phones [145]. Social networks also foster social connections among cancer survivors [146], new mothers [147], and older adults and their families and friends [148]. Additionally, social networks can serve as an entry point for those hesitant to seek help in person. For example, 33% of soldiers who were unwilling to consult with an in-person counselor were open to using technology-based social networks for mental healthcare [149]. Among young college students, 68% reported a willingness to use the Internet for mental health support, and 94% of participants with mental illnesses used social networking sites [150].

However, caution is necessary when using social media. A patient's expression of suicidal intent could go unnoticed if posted on a provider's "wall" or in an email inbox. Though the literature is limited, preliminary guidelines address concerns about patient privacy, confidentiality, and expectations, as well as providers' professionalism [126, 151–155]. Both the timing and style of communication should be carefully considered [126].

International and US guidelines have been established for using social media. The American College of Physicians published a comprehensive overview of physician online professionalism, offering recommendations [107] that focus on patient communication, information gathering, online education, and other areas. In general, providers should maintain professionalism, adhere to institutional policies, assume all exchanged information is public, enhance informed consent, pay attention to user interactions, and support and empower others [156].

1.6 Program and Administration Approaches to Evaluation, Legal Issues, and Reimbursement Issues

In today's healthcare landscape, organizational leadership and program evaluation have become increasingly important to ensure high-quality care that meets the needs of patients, providers, and regulatory requirements. This includes considerations such as accreditation by organizations like the Joint Commission, reimbursement, and the implementation of best practices. Evaluations typically encompass various factors including satisfaction, technology, cost, clinical measures, and care processes, with continuous feedback loops for quality improvement.

It is important for healthcare programs in countries with similar economies to address fundamental issues such as credentialing, licensing, confidentiality, privacy, malpractice, and reimbursement. Financial viability is also critical, especially in countries with socialized or capitalized healthcare systems, and those with an electronic platform. Feasibility is often assessed based on factors such as technical costs, patient volume, appointment adherence, payment models, patient complexity, payer mix, and other factors. Current studies employ economic modeling, clinical encounter costing, data sets, healthcare reform, healthcare costs related to changing health risks among employers of all sizes, and prototypes of existing health systems, such as the Veterans Affairs system. The Veterans Health Administration (VA) is the largest integrated healthcare system in the USA. On average, the VA serves more than nine million veterans annually across 171 medical centers and more than 1112 ambulatory care centers and community-based clinics [157]. The VA's continuous culture of innovation makes implementation research and practice accessible, applicable, and impactful. Innovations are embedded in clinical work, and successful, effective program implementation efforts can be applied iteratively to scale up and disseminate practices across many medical centers in diverse regions across the USA [158].

In contrary to the above mentioned, the Middle East (ME) faces significant challenges in implementing DMH programs. This region has diverse mental health services ranging from excellent in countries like Israel to fair or poor in countries like Turkey, Iran, Saudi Arabia, Iraq, and Syria. Despite these disparities, there is a pressing need for DMH in the ME. However, the number of randomized controlled trials related to DMH in the ME is limited, with only three reports so far, conducted in Turkey, Israel, and Iraq. These studies have focused on various aspects of DMH, including its effectiveness, psychoeducation, and the doctor–patient working alliance [45–47]. To overcome the difficulties related to implementing DMH programs tailored to the specific requirements and cultural contexts of each nation, a collaboration between governments, health organizations, and mental health providers is essential.

1.7 Access, Versatility, and Empowerment: Benefits of DMH for Patients, Providers, and Systems of Care

1.7.1 Patient Benefits

DMH has had four primary impacts for patients: (1) better access (many sites including home and primary care); (2) evidence-based psychosocial treatments per their preference; (3) empowerment, in the form of choice, access, and incentive to participate; and (4) ability to engage providers, clinics, or systems more directly (e.g., web-based, texting, Relay Health). Especially for people living in remote or underserved areas, DMH enables greater patient empowerment, individualized care, and better access to mental health resources [159, 160]. Service points are theoretically limitless: clinics, emergency rooms, patients' homes, nursing homes, homeless shelters, hospices, schools, forensic facilities, and at the battlefront. For example, one significant advantage of telepsychiatry has been improved access to psychiatric care in rural, suburban, and urban areas [118]. Indeed, DMH sometimes is better than in-person care as previously mentioned [13]. Child and adolescent [161] and other populations have been greatly served, including with asynchronous telepsychiatry [162].

Important questions remain—some of these are acutely sensitive to MH issues. While the buffet of informal or self-directed services is increasing, one question is: "If the person or patient is in care, should this be overseen by a professional, and if so, how?" "Can we assume the person or patient will plug in and get where they need to go or find the best service for them?" For persons with MH issues, symptoms, and disorders, a key question is, "What if someone's awareness/perspective is diminished or 'lost' (in formal psychiatric wording, capacity; in legal wording, competence) such that insight on the what, how, when, and why components of decision-making suggests additional informal (i.e., family, Internet) or formal (i.e., primary care or MH clinician) advice and direction?"

1.7.2 Provider Benefits

Access to telepsychiatrists, via phone, email, texting, or consultation by store-and-forward telemedicine (STP) or real-time audio–video telemedicine (ATP), has improved the competencies of primary care providers enabling them to make more correct diagnoses and accordingly offer suitable treatment [118]. Additionally, telemedicine has been shown to improve provider knowledge and skills over time —if consulting psychiatrists have adequate skills to teach [163], especially the rural primary care providers [164, 165], it has a direct impact on the patients they see and an indirect impact on the population they serve. Telemedicine also offers formal training opportunities, such as guided laryngoscopic evaluations with a specialist at a distance, as well as on-the-fly clinical procedural assistance, such as a pediatric intensivist assisting a rural provider with a code when transfer by helicopter is not feasible. A review of effectiveness of video-based tele-education showed high satisfaction and that it is equivalent or better than in-person education, in terms of knowledge acquisition and integration [166]. Coaching via telehealth [167] and clinical procedural assistance is on the rise [168].

Medical and nursing education continues to evolve in terms of skills, competencies, attitude, and other foci in addition to knowledge [118, 169]. Aside from the "core" nursing training, there may be a need for additional training in technology, teamwork, healthcare systems, and changing roles/"hats," depending on what is "needed." Technology is already a target area for skill development—both by using it and being a leader in implementation—using simulated patients at a distance to teach general nursing skills, how to work as part of a team, how to gain experience in work settings previously unfamiliar to them, and how to get on the same page across disciplines (i.e., how to develop shared mental models) for the care of a patient [168]. This reduces potential misunderstanding among large teams and creates a shared mental model of expectation, roles, and out comes [170]. Shared mental models will also enhance team performance by their organizing knowledge structures, concepts, and associations around education [171].

The healthcare industry may be reaching a tipping point in two areas. Firstly, a hybrid model of in-person, Internet-based, and other virtual care is emerging [172], particularly if care for depression and attention deficit/hyperactivity disorder [125, 173] is better at a distance than usual care. Secondly, there may be a new standard of practice. Patients are increasingly accessing health information, utilizing support groups, undergoing formal training, using tools for care, self-managing their conditions, and receiving Internet- or application-based treatment. However, with the growing array of services, it raises questions on whether a professional should oversee the care of a person or patient engaged in such services and, if so, how? This would require new terminology that takes into account the patient's central contextualization of disease and traditional healthcare services. While terms like PCMH, mobile health, and connected care may apply in part, they do not fully capture the emerging hybrid care model.

1.7.3 Healthcare Systems and Administration

Healthcare is facing challenges in providing quality, affordable, and timely care to patients in various settings [174]. Enhancing clinical operating efficiency enables clinicians with expertise to reach the point of service and emphasizes teamwork for clinical, administrative, and informal care coordination. This requires various disciplines to work at the "top of one's license." In psychiatry, this is facilitated by having non-MD MH professionals manage less complex cases, while reserving the psychiatrist's direct clinical time for more complicated cases or providing clinical oversight and review of cases seen by others.

DMH may soon reshape healthcare service delivery, particularly as telepsychiatry appears better for some disorders and models of care are better than traditional in-person or usual care approaches (e.g., depression and attention deficit/hyperactivity disorder) [125, 173]. Clinicians are adapting to "hybrid" models of care that incorporate both in-person and virtual assessments and treatments [172, 175]. New "hybrid care models" use both in-person and technology-based care [172, 175], which can include various levels of technological complexity, ranging from low-intensity email and phone to high-intensity videoconferencing.

1.8 Discussion and Conclusion

Telemedicine has transformed healthcare by improving administrative effectiveness, expanding patient access to treatment, and giving patients more control over their own health. Comparable to in-person therapy, telepsychiatry is turning into a highly effective and accepted type of care. To remain sensitive to patient ethnic differences while maintaining the highest levels of clinical and professional standards is necessary as technology continues to influence how healthcare is delivered. Evaluation of DMH programs should encompass clinical, legal, reimbursement, and technological factors. Innovative models of care and patient-centered approaches, supported by digital platforms, are steering DMH services toward more diverse and flexible forms of engagement. Online tools and resources are facilitating traditional treatments while also creating new opportunities for patient education and treatment.

The speed and extent of the development and adoption of DMH around the world are influenced by regulatory differences among countries, such as those between the USA, Europe, Australia, and the Middle East. These differences have resulted in various barriers to implementation, including cultural, technical, financial, and regulatory factors. In some countries, the lack of regulations and legislation governing DMH practices, combined with concerns about political persecution, can pose a threat to patient acceptance. Building a robust DMH infrastructure would require addressing these regulatory issues, along with a reconstruction of the medico-legal system to ensure sensitive ethical concepts such as confidentiality, informed consent, and liability are adequately addressed.

Sharing best practices and lessons learned is essential for advancing DMH globally. It may help nations in preventing potential pitfalls and maximize the advantages of DMH interventions, which will eventually improve mental health outcomes and people's access to care worldwide. To make sure that these interventions are successful and long-lasting, DMH programs must be continuously evaluated and modified based on research that is supported by proof. We can handle the mental health issues affecting our communities today by cooperating and establishing a global network of DMH providers, researchers, and policymakers. To scale up DMH services worldwide, it is necessary to have flexible policies, enough funding, effective inter-professional communication, evidence-based training, and an assessment strategy that compares results to predetermined benchmarks.

References

1. Institute of Medicine. http://www.iom.edu/~/media/Files/Report%20Files/2001/Crossing-the-Quality-Chasm/Quality%20Chasm%202001%20%20report%20brief.pdf. Accessed 28 Feb 2015.
2. Council LS, Geffken D, Valeras AB, et al. A medical home: changing the way patients and teams relate through patient-centered care plans. Fam Syst Health. 2012;30:190–8.
3. Miles A, Mezzich J. The care of the patient and the soul of the clinic: person-centered medicine as an emergent model of modern clinical practice. Int J Pers Cent Med. 2011;1(2):207–22.
4. Ekman I, Swedberg K, Taft C, et al. Person-centered care—ready for prime time. Eur J Cardiovasc Nurs. 2011;10(4):248–51.
5. Sturmberg JP, et al. Health care frames—from Virchow to Obama and beyond: the changing frames in health care and their implications for patient care. J Eval Clin Pract. 2014;20(6):1036–44.
6. World Health Organization. Telemedicine opportunities and developments in member states. Results of the second global survey on eHealth. Geneva: WHO Press; 2011.
7. Crabtree BF, Nutting PA, Miller WL, et al. Summary of the National Demonstration Project and recommendations for the patient-centered medical home. Ann Fam Med. 2010;8(Suppl 1):80–90.
8. Jackson GL, Powers BJ, Chatterjee R, et al. The patient-centered medical home: a systematic review. Ann Intern Med. 2013;158(3):169–78.
9. Elfeddali I, van der Feltz-Cornelis CM, van Os J, et al. Horizon 2020 priorities in clinical mental health research: results of a consensus-based ROAMER expert survey. Int J Environ Res Public Health. 2014;11(10):115–39.
10. Osborn R, et al. International survey of older adults finds shortcomings in access, coordination, and patient-centered care. Health Aff (Millwood). 2014;33(12):2247–55.
11. Cohen S, Yu W. The concentration and persistence in the level of health expenditures over time: estimates for the US population. Agency for Healthcare Research and Quality, 2008–2009 [Statistical Brief No. 354]. http://meps.ahrq.gov/mepsweb/data_files/publications/st354/stat354.pdf. Accessed 28 Feb 2015.
12. Hilty DM, Ferrer D, Callahan EJ, et al. The effectiveness of telemental health: a 2013 review. Telemed J E Health. 2013;19(6):444–54.
13. Hilty DM, Yellowlees PM, Chan S, et al. Telepsychiatry: effective, evidence-based and at a tipping point in healthcare delivery. Psych Clin N Am. 2015;38(3):559–92.
14. Davis MH, Everett A, Kathol R, et al. American Psychiatric Association ad hoc work group report on the integration of psychiatry and primary care. 2011. https://naapimha.org/wordpress/media/Integration-of-Psychiatry-and-Primary-Care.pdf. Accessed 28 Feb 2015.

15. Hollingsworth JM, et al. Specialty care and the patient-centered medical home. Med Care. 2011;49(1):4–9.
16. Cluver JS, Schuyler D, Frueh BC, et al. Remote psychotherapy for terminally ill cancer patients. J Telemed Telecare. 2005;11:157–9.
17. Hilty DM, Rabinowitz T, McCarron RM, et al. An update on Telepsychiatry and how it can leverage collaborative, stepped, and integrated services to primary care. Psychosomatics. 2018;59(3):227–50. https://doi.org/10.1016/j.psym.2017.12.005.
18. Entman RM. Framing: toward clarification of a fractured paradigm. J Commun. 1993;43(4):51–8.
19. Chong D, Druckman JN. Framing theory. Ann Rev Polit Sci. 2007;10:103–26.
20. Tversky A, Kahneman D. Loss aversion in riskless choice: a reference-dependent model. Q J Econ. 1991;106(4):1039–61.
21. Levin IP, Schneider SL, Gaeth GJ. All frames are not created equal: a typology and critical analysis of framing effects. Organ Behav Hum Decis Process. 1998;76(2):149–88.
22. Rajkumar S, Hoolahan B. Remoteness and issues in mental health care: experiences from rural Australia. Epidemiol Psichiatr Soc. 2004;13:78–82.
23. Moffatt JJ, Eley DS. The reported benefits of telehealth for rural Australians. Aust Health Rev. 2010;34:276–81.
24. Griffiths L, Blignault I, Yellowlees P. Telemedicine as a means of delivering cognitive-behavioural therapy to rural and remote mental health clients. J Telemed Telecare. 2006;12(3):136–40.
25. Saurman E, et al. Assessing program efficiency: a time and motion study of the mental health emergency care—rural access program in NSW Australia. Int J Environ Res Public Health. 2014;11(8):78–89.
26. Rosenthal TC. The medical home: growing evidence to support a new approach to primary care. J Am Board Fam Med. 2008;21(5):427–40.
27. Haaga DA. Introduction to the special section on stepped care models in psychotherapy. J Consult Clin Psychol. 2000;68:547–8.
28. van't Veer-Tazelaar N, van Marwijk H, van Oppen P, et al. Prevention of anxiety and depression in the age group of 75 years and over: a randomized controlled trial testing the feasibility and effectiveness of a generic stepped care program among elderly community residents at high risk of developing anxiety and depression versus usual care. BMC Public Health. 2006;1:186.
29. Yellowlees PM, Hogarth MA, Hilty DM. The development of distributed academic networks in America. Acad Psychiatry. 2006;30(6):451–5.
30. Frydman GJ. Patient-driven research: rich opportunities and real risks. J Participat med. 2009;1(1):e12. http://ojs.jopm.org/index.php/jpm/article/view/28/18. Accessed 28 Feb 2015.
31. Frydman GJ. A patient-centric definition of participatory medicine. 2010. http://e-patients.net/archives/2010/04/a-patient-centric-definition-of-participatory-medicine.html. Accessed 28 Feb 2015.
32. Krist AH, et al. Engaging primary care patients to use a patient-centered personal health record. Ann Fam Med. 2014;12(5):418–26.
33. Whitteman HO, et al. User-centered design and the development of patient decision aids: protocol for a systematic review. Syst Rev. 2015;4(1):11.
34. Der Wees V, et al. Integrating the use of patient-reported outcomes for both clinical practice and performance measurement: views of experts from 3 countries. Milbank Q. 2014;92(4):754–75.
35. Hamann J, Leucht S, Kissling W. Shared decision making in psychiatry. Acta Psychiatr Scand. 2003;107(6):403–9.
36. Moon K, Sobolev M, Kane JM. Digital and Mobile Health Technology in collaborative behavioral health care: scoping review. JMIR Ment Health. 2022;9(2):e30810.
37. Mallen JM, Vogel DL, Rochlen AB, et al. Online counseling: reviewing the literature from a counseling psychology framework. Couns Psychol. 2005;33(6):819–71. https://www.researchgate.net/...Counseling/.../00b7d53c017b765594000000.pdf.

38. Kids Help Line. 1-800-551-1800, Mass Media Studio, Australia. https://www.kidshelp.com.au. Accessed 28 Feb 2015.
39. Urness D, Wass M, Gordon A, et al. Client acceptability and quality of life–telepsychiatry compared to in-person consultation. J Telemed Telecare. 2006;12(5):251–4.
40. Simms DC, Gibson K, O'Donnell S. To use or not to use: clinicians' perceptions of telemental health. Can Psychol. 2011;52(1):41–51.
41. Volpe T, Boydell KM, Pignatiello A. Mental health services for Nunavut children and youth: evaluating a telepsychiatry pilot project. Rural Remote Health. 2014;14(2):2673.
42. Statistics Canada. Mortality rates among children and teenagers living in Inuit Nunangat, 1994 to 2008. http://www.statcan.gc.ca/pub/82-003-x/2012003/article/11695-eng.htm. Accessed 28 Feb 2015.
43. Pignatiello A, Boydell KM, Teshima J, et al. Transforming child and youth mental health via innovative technical solutions. Healthc Q. 2011;14(2):92–102.
44. Sunderji N, Crawford A, Jovanovic M. Telepsychiatry in graduate medical education: a narrative review. Acad Psychiatry. 2015;39(1):55–62.
45. Modai I, Jabarin M, Kurs R, et al. Cost effectiveness, safety, and satisfaction with video telepsychiatry versus face-to-face care in ambulatory settings. Telemed J E Health. 2006;12:515–20.
46. Ozkan B, et al. Effect of psychoeducation and telepsychiatric follow up given to the caregiver of the schizophrenic patient on family burden, depression and expression of emotion. Pak J Med Sci. 2013;29:1122–7.
47. Wagner B, Brand J, Schulz W, et al. Online working alliance predicts treatment outcome for posttraumatic stress symptoms in Arab war-traumatized patients. Depress Anxiety. 2012;29:646–51.
48. Jefee-Bahloul H. Telemental health in the Middle East: overcoming the barriers. Front Public Health. 2014;2:86.
49. Jefee-Bahloul H, et al. Pilot assessment and survey of Syrian refugees' psychological stress and openness to referral for telepsychiatry (PASSPORT study). Telemed J E Health. 2014;20(10):977–9.
50. Mastermind. http://www.southdenmark.com/showcases/terapi-hjemme-i-dagligstuen.aspx/. Accessed 28 Feb 2015.
51. www.nweurope.eu/emen.
52. Gaebel W, Trost N, Diekmann S, et al. Transnational policy for e-mental health: a guidance document for European policymakers and stakeholders. Interreg North-West Europe; 2020.
53. www.denlilleprins.org.
54. https://psykiatrienisyddanmark.dk/.
55. Mucic D. Telepsychiatry in Denmark: mental health care in rural and remote areas. J E Health Technol Appl. 2007;5(3):426. https://doi.org/10.1016/j.eurpsy.2007.01.1163.
56. Mucic D. International telepsychiatry: a study of patient acceptability. J Telemed Telecare. 2008;14:241–3.
57. Mucic D, Jokumsen M. Telepsychiatry—prevention and treatment in the outskirt areas, a shared-care model within a Danish context. J Intensive Crit Care. 2017;3:2.
58. De Las CC, Arredondo MT, Cabrera MF, et al. Randomized clinical trial of telepsychiatry through videoconference versus face-to-face conventional psychiatric treatment. Telemed J E Health. 2006;12(3):341–50.
59. Norman S. The use of telemedicine in psychiatry. J Psychiatr Ment Health Nurs. 2006;13(6):771–7.
60. Bose U, McLaren P, Riley A, et al. The use of telepsychiatry in the brief counselling of non-psychotic patients from an inner-London general practice. J Telemed Telecare. 2001;7(Suppl 1):8–10.
61. McLaren P, Ahlbom J, Riley A, et al. The north Lewisham telepsychiatry project: beyond the pilot phase. J Telemed Telecare. 2002;8(Suppl 2):98–100.
62. Harley J. Economic evaluation of a tertiary telepsychiatry service to an Island. J Telemed Telecare. 2006;12(7):354–7.

63. Saleem Y, Taylor MH, Khalifa N. Forensic telepsychiatry in the United Kingdom. Behav Sci Law. 2008;226(3):333–44.
64. Andersson G, Hesser H, Veilord A, et al. Randomised controlled non-inferiority trial with 3-year follow-up of internet-delivered versus face-to-face group cognitive behavioural therapy for depression. J Affect Disord. 2013;151(3):986–94.
65. Saint-Andre S, Neira Zalentein W, Robin D, et al. La telepsychiatrie au service de l'autisme (Telepsychiatry at the service of autism). L'Encéphale. 2011;37(1):18–24.
66. Kok G, Bockting C, Burger H, et al. Mobile cognitive therapy: adherence and acceptability of an online intervention in remitted recurrently depressed patients. Internet Interv. 2014;1(2):65–73.
67. Riper H, Blankers M, Hadiwijaya H, et al. Effectiveness of guided and unguided low-intensity internet interventions for adult alcohol misuse: a meta-analysis. PLoS One. 2014;9(6):e99912. https://doi.org/10.1371/journal.pone.0099912.
68. Mogoase C, Brailean A, David D. Can concreteness training alone reduce depressive symptoms? A randomized pilot study using an internet-delivered protocol. Cognit Ther Res. 2013;37:704–12.
69. Tulbure BT, Szentagotai A, David O, Ştefan S, Månsson KN, David D, Andersson G. Internet-delivered cognitive-behavioral therapy for social anxiety disorder in Romania: a randomized controlled trial. PLoS One. 2015;10(5):e0123997.
70. Gao J, Fan C, Chen B, Fan Z, Li L, Wang L, Ma Q, He X, Zhai Y, Zhao J. Telemedicine is becoming an increasingly popular way to resolve the unequal distribution of healthcare resources: evidence from China. Front. Public Health. 2022;10:916303.
71. Cui F, Ma Q, He X, Zhai Y, Zhao J, Chen B, Sun D, Shi J, Cao M, Wang Z. Implementation and application of telemedicine in China: cross-sectional study. JMIR Mhealth Uhealth. 2020;8(10):e18426.
72. Chen R, Jiang Q. Evolution of telemedicine in China during COVID-19 pandemic: from 2020 to 2022. J Public Health Pol. 2022;43:469–72.
73. Ma Q, Sun D, Tan Z, Li C, He X, Zhai Y, Wang L, Cui F, Li M, Gao J, Wang L, Zhao J. Usage and perceptions of telemedicine among health care professionals in China. Int J Med Inform. 2022;166:104856.
74. Xu W, Wang J, Wang Z, et al. Web-based intervention improves social acknowledgement and disclosure of trauma, leading to a reduction in posttraumatic stress disorder symptoms. J Health Psychol. 2015;21:2695.
75. Kishimoto T, Krieger T, Berger T, Qian M, Chen H, Yang Y. Internet-based cognitive behavioral therapy for social anxiety with and without guidance compared to a wait list in China: a propensity score study. Psychother Psychosom. 2016;85:317–9.
76. Moritz S, Russu R. Further evidence for the efficacy of association splitting in obsessive-compulsive disorder. An internet study in a Russian-speaking sample. J Obsessive Compuls Relat Disord. 2013;2:91–8.
77. Panicheva P, Mararitsa L, Sorokin S, et al. Predicting subjective Well-being in a high-risk sample of Russian mental health app users. EPJ Data Sci. 2022;11:21.
78. Majumdar AK. Advances in telemedicine and its usage in India. In: 15th International Conference on advanced computing and communications. Piscataway, NJ: IEEE; 2007. http://ieeexplore.ieee.org/xpl/articleDetails.jsp?reload=true&arnumber=4425958. Accessed 28 Feb 2015.
79. Chandra PS, Sowmya HR, Mehrotra S, Duggal M. 'SMS' for mental health—feasibility and acceptability of using text messages for mental health promotion among young women from urban low income settings in India. Asian J Psychiatr. 2014;11:59–64.
80. Kale N, Jacob I, Laux T, Kataria R, Jain Y, Gogia P. Managing major psychiatric illnesses through tele-consultation in a secondary care setting in rural India. Ann Glob Health. 2016;82:323–4.
81. Rahman A. E-mental health in Pakistan: a pilot study of training and supervision in child psychiatry using the internet. Psychiatr Bull. 2006;30:149–52.
82. Naeem F, Gul M, Irfan M, et al. Brief culturally adapted CBT (CaCBT) for depression: a randomized controlled trial from Pakistan. J Affect Disord. 2015;177:101–7.

83. Naeem F, Phiri P, Munshi T, et al. Using cognitive behaviour therapy with south Asian Muslims: findings from the culturally sensitive CBT project. Int Rev Psychiatry. 2015;27:233–46.
84. Naeem F, Saeed S, Irfan M, et al. Brief culturally adapted CBT for psychosis (CaCBTp): a randomized controlled trial from a low income country. Schizophr Res. 2015;164:143–8.
85. Marasinghe RB, Edirippulige S, Kavanagh D, Smith A, Jiffry MT. Effect of mobile phone-based psychotherapy in suicide prevention: a randomized controlled trial in Sri Lanka. J Telemed Telecare. 2012;18:151–5.
86. Wongpakaran T, Petcharaj K, Wongpakaran N, et al. The effect of telephone-based intervention (TBI) in alcohol abusers: a pilot study. J Med Assoc Thail. 2011;94:849–56.
87. Liu NH, Contreras O, Muñoz RF, Leykin Y. Assessing suicide attempts and depression among Chinese speakers over the internet. Crisis. 2015;35:322–9.
88. Mars M, Ramlall S, Kaliski S. Forensic telepsychiatry: a possible solution for South Africa? Afr J Psychiatry. 2012;15:244–7.
89. Wynchank S, Fortuin J. Telepsychiatry in South Africa—present and future. S Afr J Psychiatry. 2010;16(1):16–9.
90. Temmingh H, Claassen A, van Zyl S, et al. The evaluation of a telephonic wellness coaching intervention for weight reduction and wellness improvement in a community-based cohort of persons with serious mental illness. J Nerv Ment Dis. 2013;201:977–86.
91. Burton C, Szentagotai Tatar A, McKinstry B, et al. Pilot randomised controlled trial of Help4Mood, an embodied virtual agent-based system to support treatment of depression. J Telemed Telecare. 2016;22:348–55.
92. Chipps J, Ramlall S, Madigoe T, King H, Mars M. Developing telepsychiatry services in KwaZulu-Natal—an action research study. Afr J Psychiatry. 2012;15:255–63.
93. Maiga DD. Intérêt de l'utilisation du téléphone mobile dans la réponse aux rendez-vous des patients atteints de psychoses aiguës fonctionnelles au service de psychiatrie de l'Hôpital national de Niamey. Inf Psychiatr. 2011;87:127–32.
94. Thomas IF, Lawani AO, James BO. Effect of short message service reminders on clinic attendance among outpatients with psychosis at a psychiatric hospital in Nigeria. Psychiatr Serv. 2017;68:75–80.
95. Keynejad R, Garratt E, Adem G, Finlayson A, Whitwell S, Sheriff RS. Improved attitudes to psychiatry: a global mental health peer-to-peer E-learning partnership. Acad Psychiatry. 2016 Aug;40(4):659–66.
96. Abdi YA, Elmi JY. Internet based telepsychiatry: a pilot case in Somaliland. Med Confl Surviv. 2011;27:145–50.
97. https://dha.jsi.com/.
98. Sagaro GG, Battineni G, Amenta F. Barriers to sustainable telemedicine implementation in Ethiopia: a systematic review. Telemed Rep. 2020;1(1):8–15.
99. Signor L, Pierozan PS, Ferigolo M, Fernandes S, Mazoni CG, Barros HMT. Efficacy of the telephone-based brief motivational intervention for alcohol problems in Brazil. Rev Bras Psiquiatr. 2013;35:254–6.
100. Pereira CA, Wen CL, Tavares H. Alcohol abuse management in primary care: an e-learning course. Telemed J E Health. 2015;21:200–6.
101. Lowenthal R, Wen CL, Paula CS. Child mental health training for primary care providers in Brazil by telemedicine. Neuropsychiatr Enfance Adolesc. 2012;60:S30–1.
102. Andrade AL, de Lacerda RB, Gomide HP, et al. Web-based self-help intervention reduces alcohol consumption in both heavy-drinking and dependent alcohol users: a pilot study. Addict Behav. 2016;63:63–7.
103. Christoff ADO, Boerngen-Lacerda R. Reducing substance involvement in college students: a three-arm parallel-group randomized controlled trial of a computer-based intervention. Addict Behav. 2015;45:164–7.
104. Novaes MA, Machiavelli JL, Verde FCV, Campos Filho AS, Rodrigues TRC. Tele-educação para educação continuada das equipes de saúde da família em saúde mental: a experiência de Pernambuco, Brasil. Interface—Comunicação, Saúde, Educação. 2012;16:1095–106.

105. Pereira CA, Wen CL, Miguel EC, Polanczyk GV. A randomised controlled trial of a web-based educational program in child mental health for schoolteachers. Eur Child Adolesc Psychiatry. 2015;24:931–4.
106. Barrera-Valencia C, Benito-Devia AV, Vélez-Álvarez C, Figueroa-Barrera M, Franco-Idárraga SM. Costo-efectividad de telepsiquiatría sincrónica frente a asincrónica Para personas con depresión privadas de la Libertad [cost-effectiveness of synchronous vs. asynchronous Telepsychiatry in prison inmates with depression]. Rev Colomb Psiquiatr. 2017;46(2):65–73.
107. Balsa AI, Gandelman N, Lamé D. Lessons from participation in a web-based substance use preventive program in Uruguay. J Child Adolesc Subst Abuse. 2014;23:91–100.
108. Lara MA, Tiburcio M, Aguilar Abrego A, Sanchez-Solis A. A four-year experience with a web-based self-help intervention for depressive symptoms in Mexico. Rev Panam Salud Publica. 2014;35:399–406.
109. Plata LAF, López GC, Baca XD, Gómez AR. Psicoterapia vía Internet: aplicación de un programa de intervención cognitivo-conductual para pacientes con depresión. Psicología Iberoamericana. 2014;22:7–15.
110. López GC, Arbona CB, Castellano SQ, Gómez Adl R, Rivera RMB. Programa de telepsicología para el tratamiento de la fobia a hablar en público en pobláció Mexicana. Psicología Iberoamericana. 2014;22:45–54.
111. Carrasco ÁE. Acceptability of an adventure video game in the treatment of female adolescents with symptoms of depression. Res Psychother Psychopathol Process Outcome. 2016;19:10–8.
112. Espinosa HD, Carrasco A, Moessner M, et al. Acceptability study of "Ascenso": an online program for monitoring and supporting patients with depression in Chile. Telemed J E Health. 2016;22:577–83.
113. Fritsch R, Araya R, Solís J, Montt E, Pilowsky D, Rojas G. Un ensayo clínico aleatorizado de farmacoterapia con monitorización telefónica para mejorar el tratamiento de la depresión en la atención primaria en Santiago, Chile. Rev Med Chile. 2007;135:587–95.
114. Yellowlees PM, Shore JH, Roberts L, et al. Practice guidelines for videoconferencing-based telemental health. Telemed J E Health. 2010;16(10):1074–89.
115. World Psychiatric Association. WPA Telepsychiatry Global Guidelines. Geneva: World Psychiatric Association; 2021.
116. Shore JH, Mishkind MC, Bernard J, et al. A lexicon of assessment and outcome measures for telemental health. Telemed J E Health. 2013;3:282–92.
117. Hilty DM, Serhal E, Crawford A. A telehealth and telepsychiatry economic cost analysis framework: scoping review. Telemed J E Health. 2023;29(1):23–37. https://doi.org/10.1089/tmj.2022.0016.
118. Hilty DM, Torous J, Parish MB, et al. A literature review comparing clinicians' approaches and skills to in-person, synchronous, and asynchronous care: moving toward competencies to ensure quality care. Telemed J E Health. 2021;27(4):356–73. https://doi.org/10.1089/tmj.2020.0054.
119. Hilty DM, Ingraham RL, Yang RP, et al. Multispecialty phone and email consultation to primary care providers for patients with developmental disabilities in rural California. Telemed J E Health. 2004;10:413–21.
120. Yellowlees PM, Marks SL, Hilty DM, et al. Using e-health to enable culturally appropriate mental health care in rural areas. Telemed J E Health. 2008;14(5):486–92.
121. Yellowlees PM, Odor A, Iosif A, et al. Transcultural psychiatry made simple: asynchronous telepsychiatry as an approach to providing culturally relevant care. Telemed J E Health. 2013;19(4):1–6.
122. Balasinorwala VP, Shah NB, Chatterjee SD, Kale VP, Matcheswalla YA. Asynchronous telepsychiatry in Maharashtra, India: study of feasibility and referral pattern. Indian J Psychol Med. 2014;36:299–301.
123. Fortney JC, Pyne JM, Mouden SP, et al. Practice-based versus telemedicine-based collaborative care for depression in rural federally qualified health centers: a pragmatic randomized comparative effectiveness trial. Am J Psychiatry. 2013;170(4):414–25.

124. Richardson L, McCauley E, Katon W. Collaborative care for adolescent depression: a pilot study. Gen Hosp Psychiatr. 2009;31:36–45.
125. Myers KM, van der Stoep A, Zhou C, et al. Effectiveness of a telehealth service delivery model for treating attention-deficit hyperactivity disorder: results of a community-based randomized controlled trial. J Am Acad Child Adolesc Psychiatry. 2015;54(4):263–74.
126. Hilty DM, Belitsky R, Cohen MB, et al. Impact of the information age residency training: the impact of the generation gap. Acad Psychiatry. 2015;39(1):104–7.
127. APA e-Prescribing (e-RX). https://www.psychiatry.org/psychiatrists/practice/practice-management/health-informationtechnology/e-prescribing?utm_source=chatgpt.com
128. DeJong SM, Benjamin S, Anzia JA, et al. Professionalism and the internet in psychiatry: what to teach and how to teach it. Acad Psychiatry. 2012;36(5):356–62.
129. Taleban R, Zamani A, Moafi M, Jiryaee N, Khadivi R. Applications of text messaging, and bibliotherapy for treatment of patients affected by depressive symptoms. Int J Prev Med. 2016;7:46.
130. Fang C-x, Ye M-j, Yang Y-f, Chen S-l. Effects of daily short message reminder for preventing schizophrenia recrudescence. Nurs J Chin PLA. 2011;7:74–6.
131. Chen L, Li Z, Chen Y. Comparative study of relapse prevention in schizophrenia by network. J Clin Psychol Med. 2007;17:234–6.
132. Knaevelsrud C, Brand J, Lange A, Ruwaard J, Wagner B. Web-based psychotherapy for posttraumatic stress disorder in war-traumatized Arab patients: randomized controlled trial. J Med Internet Res. 2015;17:e71.
133. Wagner B, Schulz W, Knaevelsrud C. Efficacy of an internet-based intervention for posttraumatic stress disorder in Iraq: a pilot study. Psychiatry Res. 2012;195:85–8.
134. Jefee-Bahloul H. Use of telepsychiatry in areas of conflict: the Syrian refugee crisis as an example. J Telemed Telecare. 2014;20:167–8.
135. Hollander JE, Carr BG. Virtually perfect? Telemedicine for Covid-19. N Engl J Med. 2020;382(18):1679–81.
136. Keesara S, Jonas A, Schulman K. Covid-19 and health care's digital revolution. N Engl J Med. 2020;382(23):e82. https://doi.org/10.1056/nejmp2005835.
137. Torous J, Wykes T. Opportunities from the coronavirus disease 2019 pandemic for transforming psychiatric care with telehealth. JAMA Psychiatry. 2020;77(12):1205–6.
138. Moreno C, Wykes T, Galderisi S, et al. How mental health care should change as a consequence of the COVID-19 pandemic. Lancet Psychiatry. 2020;7(9):813–24. Epub 2020 Jul 16. Erratum in: Lancet Psychiatry. 2021 Jul;8(7):e16. https://doi.org/10.1016/S2215-0366(20)30307-2.
139. Pew Research Center. 2013. At (Internet survey): http://www.pewinternet.org/~/media//Files/Reports/PIP_HealthOnline.pdf (or smart phone). Accessed 28 Feb 2015.
140. Fox S, Maeve D. Health online. 2013. https://www.evernote.com/shard/s277/nl/36107944/281a93a5-fc31-4de9-a1df-76cfc7d2d33f/. Accessed 28 Feb 2015.
141. How people really use mobile. Harvard Bus Rev. 2013;91(1):30–31.
142. HealthIT.gov. Meaningful use definition & objectives. EHR incentives & certification. 2015. http://www.healthit.gov/providers-professionals/meaningful-use-definition-objectives.
143. Mossman D, Farrell HM. Facebook: social networking meets professional duty. Curr Psychiatry. 2012;11(3):34–7. http://www.currentpsychiatry.com/index.php?id=22661&tx_ttnews[tt_news]=176674. Accessed 28 Feb 2015.
144. Clinton BK, Silverman BC, Brendel DH. Patient-targeted googling: the ethics of searching online for patient information. Harv Rev Psychiatry. 2010;18(2):103–12.
145. Seko Y, Kidd S, Wiljer D, et al. Youth mental health interventions via mobile phones: a scoping review. Cyberpsychol Behav Soc Netw. 2014;17(9):591–602.
146. McLaughlin M, Nam Y, Gould J, et al. A videosharing social networking intervention for young adult cancer survivors. Comput Hum Behav. 2012;28(2):631–41.
147. McDaniel BT, et al. New mothers and media use: associations between blogging, social networking, and maternal well-being. Matern Child Health J. 2012;16(7):1509–17.

148. Sundar SS, Oeldorf-Hirsch A, Nussbaum J, et al. Retirees on Facebook: can online social networking enhance their health and wellness? In: CHI'11 extended abstracts on human factors in computing systems. New York, NY: ACM; 2011. p. 2287–92.
149. Wilson JA, Onorati K, Mishkind M, et al. Soldier attitudes about technology-based approaches to mental health care. Cyberpsychol Behav. 2008;11(6):767–9.
150. Horgan A, Sweeney J. Young students' use of the internet for mental health information and support. J Psychiatr Ment Health Nurs. 2010;17(2):117–23.
151. Silk KR, Yager J. Suggested guidelines for E-mail communication in psychiatric practice. J Clin Psychiatry. 2003;64(7):799–806.
152. Frankish K, Ryan C, Harris A. Psychiatry and online social media: potential, pitfalls and ethical guidelines for psychiatrists and trainees. Australas Psychiatry. 2012;20:181–7.
153. Kane B, Sands DZ. Guidelines for the clinical use of electronic mail with patients. J Am Med Inform Assoc. 1998;5(1):104–11.
154. Koh S, Cattell GM, Cochran DM, et al. Psychiatrists' use of electronic communication and social media and a proposed framework for future guidelines. J Psychiatr Pract. 2013;19(3):254–63.
155. Farnan JM, Snyder Sulmasy L, et al. Online medical professionalism: patient and public relationships: policy statement from the American College of Physicians and the Federation of State Medical Boards. Ann Intern Med. 2013;158(8):620–7.
156. Grajales FJ, Sheps S, Ho K, et al. Social media: a review and tutorial of applications in medicine and health care. J Med Internet Res. 2014;16(2):e13.
157. Veterans Health Administration. https://www.va.gov/health/aboutvha.asp.
158. Sullivan JL, Hughes JM. The Veterans Health Administration: opportunities and considerations for implementing innovations in a National, Integrated Health Care System. Public Policy Aging Rep. 2022;32(1):19–24.
159. Schueller SM, Hunter JF, Figueroa C, et al. Use of digital mental health for marginalized and underserved populations. Curr Treat Options Psych. 2019;6:243–55.
160. Porche MV, Folk JB, Tolou-Shams M, Fortuna LR. Researchers' perspectives on digital mental health intervention co-design with marginalized community stakeholder youth and families. Front Psych. 2022;13:867460.
161. Myers KM, Vander Stoep A, McCarty CA, et al. Child and adolescent telepsychiatry: variations in utilization, referral patterns and practice trends. J Telemed Telecare. 2010;16:128–33.
162. Yellowlees PM, Odor A, Patrice K, et al. PsychVACS: a system for asynchronous telepsychiatry. Telemed J E Health. 2011;17(4):299–303.
163. Srinivasan M, Li ST, Meyers FJ, et al. "Teaching as a competency": competencies for medical educators. Acad Med. 2011;86(10):1211–20. https://doi.org/10.1097/ACM.0b013e31822c5b9a.
164. Hilty DM, Yellowlees PM, Nesbitt TS. Evolution of telepsychiatry to rural sites: change over time in types of referral and PCP knowledge, skill, and satisfaction. Gen Hosp Psychiatry. 2006;28(5):367–73.
165. Hilty DM, Nesbitt TS, Kuenneth TA, et al. Telepsychiatric consultation to primary care: rural vs. suburban needs, utilization and provider satisfaction. J Rural Health. 2007;23(2):163–5.
166. Chipps J, et al. A systematic review of the effectiveness of videoconference-based tele-education for medical and nursing education. Worldviews Evid Based Nurs. 2012;9(2):78–87.
167. Young H, et al. Sustained effects of a nurse coaching intervention via telehealth to improve health behavior change in diabetes. Telemed J E Health. 2014;20(9):828–34.
168. Rutledge CM, Haney T, Bordelon M, et al. Telehealth: preparing advanced practice nurses to address healthcare needs in rural and underserved populations. Int J Nurs Educ Scholarsh. 2014;11(1):1–9.
169. Armstrong EG, Mackey M, Spear SJ. Medical education as a process management problem. Acad Med. 2004;79(8):721–8.
170. Ross S, Allen N. Examining the convergent validity of shared mental model measures. Behav Res. 2012;44:1052–62.

171. Langan-Fox J, Code S, Langfield-Smith K. Team mental models: techniques, methods, and analytic approaches. Hum Factors. 2000;42:242–71.
172. Hilty DM, Yellowlees PM. Collaborative mental health services using multiple technologies—the new way to practice and a new standard of practice? J Am Acad Child Adolesc Psychiatry. 2015;54(4):245–6. https://doi.org/10.1016/j.jaac.2015.01.017.
173. Fortney JC, et al. Telemedicine-based collaborative care for posttraumatic stress disorder: a randomized clinical trial. JAMA Psychiatry. 2015;72(1):58–67.
174. Akinci F, Patel PM. Quality improvement in healthcare delivery utilizing the patient-centered medical home model. Hosp Top. 2014;92(4):96–104.
175. Yellowlees PM, Nafiz N. The psychiatrist-patient relationship of the future: anytime, anywhere? Harv Rev Psychiatry. 2010;18(2):96–102.

2 Entangled in the Web: Unexpected Events with New Technologies—Safety Issues, Addiction, and Consequences on Communication

Agnes Wrobel and Janusz Wrobel

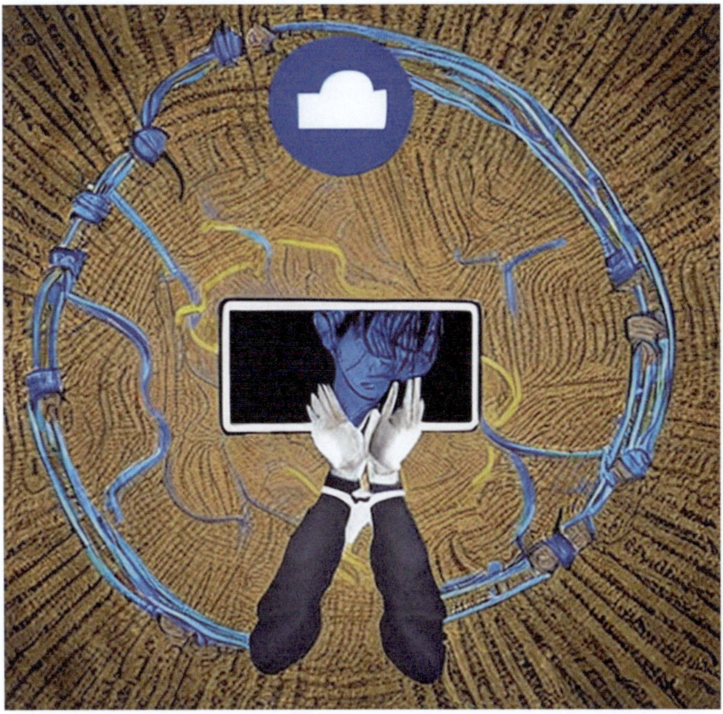

D. Mucić, D. M. Hilty (eds.), *Digital Mental Health*,
https://doi.org/10.1007/978-3-031-59936-1_2

Abstract

This chapter takes a step back to look at the landscape from which the phenomenon of telepsychiatry emerges—the Internet. Having become one of the most powerful instruments in the hands of the human race in recent decades, it is now a necessary tool in fulfilling vital elements of our daily tasks. On the one hand, the following advantages of the use of the Internet are discussed: revolutionary increase in opportunities to disseminate, share, obtain, accumulate, and store information and interpersonal contacts. On the other hand, the major disadvantages of the use of the Internet, including deception (scams and cybercrimes), hate, violence, bizarre conspiracy theories, so-called fake news, manipulation of public opinion, and the phenomenon of socially accepted and expected compromise of privacy to the point of exhibitionism, are discussed. In addition, the physiological and psychological negative side effects of abuse of the Internet, including atrophy of certain brain activities, submissiveness toward "tyranny of tiny tasks," and a gradual decrease in face-to-face interpersonal communication, which is being replaced by virtual anonymity, are debated. These deleterious effects, as well as Internet addiction, can be treated by telepsychiatry, ironically itself impossible without the Internet. The dangers of new technologies such as artificial intelligence and virtual reality are also pointed out.

About 27 years ago, the idea of instant communication on a massive scale became a reality. Today, the Internet is one the most powerful instruments in the hands of the human race that is crucial in fulfilling vital elements of our daily tasks. The Internet created unthinkable opportunities, of which the phenomenon of telepsychiatry (the topic of this book) is one of the examples. It is ironic, however, that such a web-based kind of treatment can be used in treating one of the dangerous side effects of applying this new technology, namely, Internet addiction. *Objectives*: (1) Discussion of the advantages of the Internet; (2) Exploration of the negative social consequences of malicious misuse of the Internet; and (3) Examination of physiological and psychological negative side effects of abuse of the Internet. *Results*: (1) The following are the advantages of the use of the Internet: revolutionary increase in opportunities to disseminate, share, obtain, accumulate, and store information and interpersonal contacts. (2) The major disadvantages of the use of the Internet are deception (scams, cybercrimes, and smearing), manipulation of public opinion, and

A. Wrobel
Corewell Health, Beaumont Hospital, Troy, MI, USA

Oakland University, Rochester, MI, USA
e-mail: agawrobel@yahoo.com

J. Wrobel (✉)
Department of International Studies, Oakland University, Rochester, MI, USA

Balance and Harmony Counseling, LLC, Troy, MI, USA
e-mail: obtainbalance@yahoo.com

the phenomenon of socially accepted and expected compromise of privacy to the point of exhibitionism. (3) When it comes to physiological and psychological negative side effects of abuse of the Internet, the following are mentioned: atrophy of certain brain activities, submissiveness toward "tyranny of tiny tasks," and gradual decrease in face-to-face interpersonal communication, which is being replaced by virtual anonymity.

2.1 Introduction

It was to be fast, effective, and practical; at least such hopes were triggered by the invention of the Internet—and it is. Thanks to the keyboard, writing an email takes much less time than preparing stationery, a pencil, or an envelope, addressing it after finding information on the receiver's location, and putting a stamp. Additional precious minutes are saved because we do not have to make a trip to the mailbox or post office. What is astonishing as well is the fact that later we do not have to wait for days or weeks for the person we sent it to, to receive it, and another chunk of time before we get the answer. Sure, there were telegrams available and we have checked how it works today. There is the SendTelegram.com which offers the next-day hand delivery of telegrams. In the USA the fee for the service is around $30 for a short telegram.

Now, in the free-of-charge Skyping and Zooming era, it will be difficult for our younger readers to imagine that in the 1980s, to make a call from Poland to the USA, it had to be arranged in advance with the local post office, which would contact the person in the USA to set up a time for the conversation. When the day had come, we had to arrive at the post office where we would hear the public announcement: "America, the telephone booth number 7." Later, already during the conversation, we would be interrupted from time to time by the post office clerk who was asking in your telephone receiver: "Still talking? Still talking?" In the 1990s, it was already easier because it was possible to make overseas calls from the home telephone or even from the public telephone booth, but such a pleasure cost at least 0.50¢ per minute. Then the telephone cards "epoch" followed, which could be bought in many places, and thanks to that, the cost of international telephone connections was drastically lowered. Later yet, cellular phones appeared. Finally, the Internet made existence possible that not only is free but also allows seeing the person with whom you are talking. To fully understand how revolutionary this progress is (from the necessity of visiting the post office to call somebody to watch him or her on the computer monitor or the cellular phone) let us imagine that during the future *Skype*-like conversation, we maybe will be able to touch and feel the smell of our telephone interlocutor—in other words, be physically present with such a person.

In this chapter, the reader will learn about:

1. The advantages of the Internet.
2. The negative social consequences of malicious misuse of the Internet.
3. Physiological and psychological negative side effects of abuse of the Internet.

2.2 Technology: Brings Us Together and Life to Our Fingertips?

First radio, then later the TV possessed the unimaginable power of simultaneously reaching uncountable masses of listeners or watchers at the same moment. Those who on Halloween day in October 1938 were listening to the radio drama based on the book by Orson Welles *The War of the Worlds* experienced how powerful this ability was. The use of the radio and television created an opportunity for disseminating knowledge delivering entertainment, but also issuing important messages warnings, and emergency alerts. Today's users of *Twitter* (especially more popular politicians) have the opportunity to inform an impressive number of people using cell phones about important events when they are taking place.

The existence of social networks allows ill people to blog about their fights against diseases, which has become a significant inspiration for others who experience similar conditions. This led to the creation of virtual support groups for people who have to deal with different types of challenges in their lives (i.e., parents raising children with autism). In not as serious everyday life dimension, when we need to obtain some information (how to get rid of red wine spot on the white tablecloth or effectively challenge ants in the kitchen), the most obvious thing to do, just after asking a grandmother about it, would be googling the answer.

For those who produce something, the use of the network opened the unknown potential of advertising different types of products. For those who are looking for them, it has become an excellent source of finding them and an opportunity to look for the best prices. For those who need things or services or have something to offer, it created an unlimited platform for letting others know about it. For charitable institutions, it gave a great chance for publicizing benevolent purposes and collecting resources for achieving them.

Today's lucky tourists, thanks to digital technology and the Internet, can share a link to Eiffel Tower pictures with hundreds of *Myspace* or *Instagram* contacts by sending it directly from a Parisian bistro by an iPad instead of going through the time (and money) consuming process of developing pictures, printing them, and mailing out to the friends to share happy vacation's moments. Photographic documentation of important and less essential occasions is available without time and space limits on social networks. Thanks to the common access to the Internet, the girl who was kidnapped 17 years ago (she was 15 at that time) has been recognized on *Facebook* by her sister, which finally led to the end of the suffering of the victim. Talking about criminal activities, let us mention the computer registration of the perpetrators, which makes easier the policemen's job because in their cars they have access to the registry data with information content more impressive than those of the biggest traditional archives.

The new technologies do a good job serving society with navigation issues too. From time to time, our family would get lost during car trips despite the use of quite accurate maps. It took a child to come up with the idea of presenting us with the global positioning system (GPS) to solve the problem. Today's cars are equipped with navigation tools that solve the problem. We, the former skeptics, when it came to the use of satellite-type guidance, now cannot imagine traveling without it.

2.3 Science, Education, and Technology

It is really difficult to overestimate the benefits of the Internet in the domain of science. The Internet library available for everybody with access to the net created the opportunity of entering not only very impressive data, research results, books, and articles, but also quite rare publications that in the past could be only reached in designated places in the form of microfilms.

The exchange of information and research effects does not require physical presence anymore. We can attend overseas conferences from our homes thanks to the use of many platforms, among them *Skype* and *Zoom*. Teachers can teach the students online and share links with them illustrating the most recent progress in a particular field. Students can watch the lectures, submit their assignments, interact with fellow students, and take quizzes and exams from their homes. The Internet breaks the barriers of a traditional teaching environment that requires all participants of the learning process to comply with the "HERE and NOW" requirement (synchronous type of education). The asynchronous communication allows instructors to reach learners who might be hundreds of miles away; creates a platform in which students can participate in forums devoted to particular topics by adding their own posts/or commenting on others' submissions at different, convenient times; and permits the teacher to devote individual attention to each student's needs, concerns, and questions. When one of the authors of this chapter participated in training preparing him to teach his courses in an online setting, he was not only scared but skeptical as well. It was difficult for him to imagine not facing the students in the class; he had concerns over the effectiveness of his teaching, and worried about the value of the "open book" exams. The practice of the web-teaching has changed his mind to the point in which when it comes to homework assignments for the students who are taught on-campus, it is expected to be submitted on Moodle (e-teaching the stem used at Oakland University), which is what makes evaluating them much easier and allows students to check their grades at any time. Interestingly enough, his concerns over testing students proved to be ungrounded—the average final grade for the same course taught online and on-campus is similar.

When it comes to scholars, the Internet creates an unparalleled chance for the worldwide exchange of creative thoughts and related to them, hope for the acceleration of the positive effects of attempts to deal with many plagues that haunt us, including finding cures for illnesses. On the micro-scale level, computerization of the patient data allows the emergency room (ER) doctor immediate access to the history of the disease and results of many tests and exams of the patient who comes there in the middle of the night. As Chap. 3 of this book stresses, the telemental health model creates numerous opportunities for the improvement of health care, which relates to expanding access to it, promoting prevention, and when it comes to behavioral health allowing "Cadillac treatment" at a distance. As Hilty et al. indicated [1]:

> One significant advantage of telepsychiatry has been improving access to psychiatric care in urban, suburban, and rural areas, often by providing academic specialists to areas with provider shortages.

The results of a study of 200 telepsychiatric consultations [2] showed high satisfaction among psychiatrists who performed them; the average level of positive experience was 6.6 on a scale of 1 to 8 (the highest score).

The Internet removes work barriers created by the inability to physically reach an office, a store, or the bank. The life of those who can use this opportunity is much easier—they can buy, return taxes, and do banking, including making payments by the use of the computer. Thanks to the communicative net, many people can work or look for a job from home and can use it for entertainment purposes such as watching shows and movies worldwide. They are also able to establish contact with unknown people or even, with the use of dating portals, find candidates for husbands or wives.

Recent years brought rapid changes, challenges, and opportunities related to electronic technology that are reflected in our assessment of security. The safety of the planet and its inhabitants, which was taken for granted in the first two decades of the twenty-first century, has been vehemently shaken. The "Safety Perception Index 2023" [3] found "(…) a notable rise in generalized and non-specific feelings of fear and lack of safety throughout the world, with people becoming more fearful overall but less certain about the sources of potential threats. On this note, the report finds a rise in "ambiguous risk". This refers to people's sense that risk exists in the world around them but that it cannot always be defined. The rise in ambiguous risk can be seen in the responses to a World Risk Poll question on the greatest perceived threat in people's daily lives. Between 2019 and 2021, the largest changes in response rates were for those saying that no risk existed in their lives, which fell by half, and those saying they did not know what their greatest risk was, which nearly doubled."

Let us discuss the major factors that contributed to this dramatic shift in safety perception.

2.3.1 COVID Pandemic

The expected inevitability of rising human longevity, a healthier populace, and an increased mastery over infectious diseases was utterly rebutted by the arrival of the coronavirus disease-2019 (COVID-19) pandemic for which, as it was revealed, we were completely unprepared. According to the World Health Organization (WHO): "Globally, as of 5:43 pm CEST, 17 May 2023, there have been 766,440,796 confirmed cases of COVID-19, including 6,932,591 deaths" [4]; this appalling toll is reflected in the substantial decrease in the world population's life expectancy [5]. In its aftermath, the COVID pandemic leaves behind a population more distrustful of public health officials [6] and many pessimistically wondering if the ordeal has done much to prepare society for future pandemics.

2.3.2 War in Ukraine

After the collapse of communism and the demise of "The Evil Empire," the USSR, the world expected peaceful coexistence between Europe and a democracy-aspiring Russia. Instead, the unprovoked, unjust, and inhumane Russian invasion of Ukraine in February of 2022 turned the world back to 1939, the year of Hitler's invasion of Poland, and Vladimir Putin, Russia's president, has been declared a war criminal wanted by The International Criminal Court in The Hague.

2.3.3 Gun Violence and Mass Shooting

The steadiness and predictability of gun violence, especially in the USA, do little to alleviate the growing feelings of insecurity. The data [7] indicate that between January 1, 2023, and May 17, 2023, alone there were 16,016 deaths caused by the use of guns (6908 homicides and 9108 suicides), and 226 mass shootings, many of which involved schools. Among the victims of gun violence were 100 children (aged 0–11) and 569 teens (aged 12–17).

2.3.4 The Internet Phenomenon

With its rapid expansion, the Internet was to become an instrument of effective global communication, and an extraordinary tool for disseminating useful knowledge, as well as democratic ideas [8]. In many aspects, it fulfills this role, but it simultaneously serves as an extremely efficient medium for spreading disinformation, hate, violence, bizarre conspiracy theories, defamation, and so-called fake news. This significant increase in the use of hate on the Internet, especially by so-called trolls, whose goal is to manipulate and shape the conscience and the way of thinking of entire societies (as seen in the recent presidential elections in the USA or the Russian hybrid war on Ukraine), leads to unfortunate and sometimes dangerous results in the mental well-being of the users of the web.

One of the most malicious misuse of the Internet is cyberbullying, which is unfortunately widespread. Between 2017 and 2023, internet bullying increased suicidal thinking among victims by 14.5% [9]. According to a Pew Research Center survey which was conducted in May 2022, "nearly half of U.S. teens have been bullied or harassed online, with physical appearance being seen as a relatively common reason why. Older teen girls are especially likely to report being targeted by online abuse overall and because of their appearance" [10]

2.3.5 Artificial Intelligence

The recent break-neck progress in artificial intelligence (AI) creates unimaginable opportunities for humanity in many fields. It can make our lives much easier (i.e., autonomous cars), can positively affect our decision-making, reduce human errors (i.e., in helping victims of natural disasters), and replace human labor (i.e., recently 3D-printed houses in Germany [11]). Yet, also in Germany, *Die Aktuelle* magazine published an alleged interview with Michael Schumacher, which in reality was generated by artificial intelligence. The publisher apologized later, writing: "This tasteless and misleading article should never have appeared. It does not in any way correspond to the standards of journalism that we – and our readers – expect from a publisher like Funke" [12]. The apology does little to hide the terrifying implications of the effective use of artificial intelligence in generating propaganda. Another example of manipulation with the use of AI was the news and photos of the alleged arrest of Trump and imprisonment of Putin widely spread on Twitter in March of 2023. "It does add noise during crisis events. It also increases the cynicism level," said Jevin West, a professor at the University of Washington in Seattle who focuses on the spread of misinformation. "You start to lose trust in the system and the information that you are getting" [13]. The psychological, philosophical, and moral challenges Internet users will now face when encountering artificiality generated media indiscernible from reality are unsettling, to say the least.

Currently, the most controversy surrounds ChatGPT (Generative Pre-trained Transformers), which was introduced to the public in November 2022 and used in the mentioned alleged interview with the famous racing driver. This very powerful artificial intelligence model was inspired by how natural language used by us is processed. The analysis of this phenomenon allowed ChatGPT's creators to effectively imitate human conversational dialogue. What it means in practice is that the machine can create letters, emails, essays, articles, poems, short stories, and novels in human-like language. At the current stage of development of this tool, it will be relatively easy to recognize what was generated not by a human being's mind. However, the rapid progress in technology tells us that it is probably a matter of time before intelligent robots will match or even surpass our mental capabilities, as was shown in May of 2020, when, "for the first time in history, a computer defeated a world chess champion in a match of several games. The IBM-made device dubbed 'Deep Blue' defeated the reigning champion, Garry Kasparov, in an unusually swift chess game. The sixth game lasted only 19 moves, while an average game takes around 40 to complete" [14].

It is no wonder that we now worry whether students could pass university exams or even earn an entire degree using artificial intelligence [15].

2.3.6 Virtual Reality

Another challenge that we face comes from the technological progress in virtual reality (VR). Its vast domain provides many types of entertainment, especially video games, which attract millions of users. The outstanding success of the Pokémon Go game launched in 2016 led to crowds of zombie-like people, mainly youngsters, glued to their smartphones on a mission to hunt the hidden Pokémons. Unfortunately for young minds, many video games are inviting their users to very dark, extremely violent, and aggressive spaces where the amount of murdered people is translated to success in winning the game.

The recent research on the mental health risks of using virtual reality indicates the following symptoms: nausea ("simulation sickness"), episodes of unreality after using a VR headset, fatigue, confusion, social anxiety, addiction, and symptoms of dissociation involving "breaks in the connection between the mind and body, from briefly failing to recognize oneself in the mirror all the way to thinking you're inhabiting the wrong body" [16]. Many psychologists also warn that exposure to virtual violence leads to emotional desensitization, a decrease in empathic feelings, and even triggers brutal, cruel, and inhuman behaviors (i.e., mass shootings).

There are many psychological and philosophical implications related to human exposure to this phenomenon. Ben Kenwright in his article on the ethical challenges and dangers of virtual reality offers the following findings: "The growth of VR technologies leads to an increase in new products and accelerated development of VR in industries such as education, healthcare, household management, tourism, and video games, impacting social and economic sectors. On one hand, there will be huge opportunities for new and innovative VR applications, beyond entertainment uses. On the other hand, there are numerous challenges and ethical issues that need to be addressed. More research needs to be done to investigate the psychological impact of VR, especially on young children, both in the short and long term" [17].

2.3.7 Reflections

The events and forces of these past seven years have had a serious negative effect on the state of mental health of the inhabitants of Europe and North America. All the benefits, easiness, and surges in the wealth of societies are not reflected by increased happiness. On the contrary, there are more and more mental problems reported, including depression, anxiety, and aggression.

Yet, during these years, a contemporaneous positive phenomenon also emerged. As it had with remote work and online school, the COVID pandemic catalyzed an unprecedented proliferation of e-mental health services, resulting in far greater access to psychiatric treatment and psychotherapy. The period of social isolation that exacerbated mental health problems paradoxically stimulated a greater availability of tools to combat them, making remote treatment far more prevalent in the field than could have been predicted. And as a conversation with artificial intelligence becomes ever less distinguishable from that of a fellow person, one can only imagine whether in another seven years the majority of digital mental health consultations, and mental health services in general, will be provided by humans at all.

2.4 Internet: Pitfalls and Cautions

It was to be fast, effective, and practical; at least such hopes were triggered by the invention of the Internet. We found out that despite incredible opportunities, the use of the net may lead to many serious inconveniences or even dangers. The following is a review of some of them.

2.4.1 When Technology Fails

Let us start with writing letters. In the past, writing one was a time-consuming chore; today, preparing it and sending it in electronic form takes a couple of minutes or even less. However, as Tim Wu [18] aptly noticed in his article *The Problem with Easy Technology* it does not always work for us:

> Our technologies may have made us prosthetic gods, yet they have somehow failed to deliver on the central promise of free time. The problem is that, as every individual task becomes easier, we demand much more of both ourselves and others. Instead of fewer difficult tasks (writing several long letters) we are left with a larger volume of small tasks (writing hundreds of e-mails). We have become plagued by a tyranny of tiny tasks, individually simple but collectively oppressive.

2.4.2 We Save Time (Or Not Really?)

In reality, saving time became an illusion. Instead of accumulating it, we spend more of it, when compulsively, several times per day, we first check and then respond to dozens of emails. The proud owner of an email address may expect to receive an enormous number of email letters daily of which the majority of them are advertisements (*spam*). From time to time, we can get an electronic chain letter sent to us by the horrified friend (*Tim Smith has not sent this letter immediately to fifteen persons, so on the third day his right leg was amputated, and after 14 days he died).* Sometimes a good soul would warn us about the message encouraging *see the attached birthday card sent to you by your friend*, which carries a virus that in just a moment may damage all the data on the hard disk. These are just a few among many possible scenarios.

2.4.3 Anonymity

Distant communication, without personal contact, creates a new quality of discourse in which its participants, or the sender and receiver of the message, may but not have to reveal their true identity. Anonymity, a possibility of claiming a false name, age, or gender, or using a virtual avatar is used on the net by people who want to achieve their dishonest, vile, or malicious goals. Too many times a young girl's cyber friend, who she believes is a teenage boy, is in reality an adult man with foul intentions. One of the mechanisms preventing people from acting on their repugnant impulses or temptations is the fear of being recognized, and in consequence, being punished or at least publicly stigmatized. Hiding behind the mask or even using several different individualities leads to a situation in which such a person does not feel like taking responsibility for his/her actions (because it is not him/her, etc.).

When we think about the nature of Internet communication, we conclude that when reading an email message, theoretically we cannot be fully sure who sent it to us. The same uncertainty is true when it comes to the person who is the receiver of our messages. It only takes hacking of our user profile for somebody being able on our behalf to send a request for financial assistance to all our contacts under the pretext of us being allegedly in a dramatic situation. Examples include allegedly losing our wallet and having our passport and our credit card stolen during the trip abroad. In a more innocent scenario, it would be publicizing under the auspices of our identity an advertisement of the weight loss medication (less embarrassing) or increasing sexual potency (more reprehensible). Despite everything being said, we have no choice: we are sentenced for using the net at work and in contact with our family and friends. It is really sad that instead of interacting with a real person we look at the cold light of the computer screen. Let us quote a fragment of the book by Wrobel [19]:

> Faceless and eyeless others offer unimaginable chances for the exchange of information but award no opportunity for contact. Looking at computer/telephone screens, "talking" to virtual electronic partners, texting or tweeting them, taking an ephemeral break only to listen to a voice mail and to read a routine, incoming fax, slowly but surely, we may transform ourselves into communicative robots. (p. 34)

2.4.4 Communication Without Context

Unfortunately, more troublesome questions appear as we are not only uncertain about who we communicate with, but now, more frequently, we experience the fear of being used by others. Is this request for financial support for the treatment of cancer a scam? Did we become a victim of identity theft when providing our Social Security number (and we have experienced it because somebody used one of our numbers to fill his/her tax return)? Is this demand for verification of the password an attempt to wangle it from us? Virtuality is expanding at the cost of reality and the side effect is the rise of uncertainty, suspiciousness, and lack of security. The result is that the "mechanics of trust" undergoes a dramatic change because anonymity, unfortunately, promotes deceit. On the other hand, personal communication, face-to-face type, builds trust faster and more effectively.

2.4.5 Technology "Changes" the "What" and "How"

As we have already mentioned, digital mental health creates new opportunities for providing the needed assistance to patients and clients, but certain worries related to telepsychiatry were expressed as well. McLaren et al. [20] pointed out that important verbal cues are often missed during videoconferences. Hilty et al. [1] indicated that signal delays typical of equipment that is not of state-of-the-art quality cause a turn-taking conversation problem. Overall, the psychiatrist's concerns with e-Mental Health were summarized by Hilty et al. [1] in the following way:

> Concerns surfaced about technical problems (e.g. unclear picture, video freeze); decreased ease with the process; decreased ability to express oneself; and poorer quality of the interpersonal relationship.

The following is another, quite disturbing question related to so common use of the Internet: what happened to our privacy? It happens that the writers had unfortunate personal experiences with the time when the part of Europe was under the Soviet thumb and remember well the fear of surveillance orchestrated by the secret police or the anxiety caused by the possibility that the neighbor is an informer and reports on our activities. Thirty years later, we would still sometimes speculate that there was not a Mark Zuckerberg behind the *Facebook* invention, but a "big brother" or secret agent because they do not have to spy, monitor, and eavesdrop anymore, etc. Our willingness to inform the whole world about our whereabouts, with whom, what, when, and how many times we are doing certain things, makes government spying unnecessary. We live in a world of socially accepted and widespread exhibitionism—everybody may become a celebrity under the condition of having a habit of making public announcements of whom one date, how often, and how seriously she argues/breaks up/reunite with her partner. The paradox of this phenomenon comes from the fact that matters that we would not be willing to discuss in a group of six people, are announced to hundreds of "friends" on *Facebook* in the hope of getting the widest possible approval. In this way, we became the Fausts of the twenty-first century who traded with the devil intimacy for "I like" marks. The fact of having dozens, if not hundreds, of friends, has to lead to a superficial, hackneyed communication that is focused on the spectacular effect that is to lead to wide acceptance and appreciation. We have created an informative bazaar where everything is for sale and all sale gimmicks are allowed. Authenticity is a major victim here, and the biggest winner is appearance.

2.4.6 "Orwell's 1984" Revisited

Our use of cellular phones and satellite navigation allows governmental agencies not only to track our location but also, as per the recent surveillance scandal revealed by Snowden [21], to record our telephone conversations. Because today's smartphones store an impressive amount of information about us, your privacy related to their use must be protected. Fortunately, it was recognized by the recent U.S. Supreme Court decision.

> The Wednesday [June 26, 2014 - J.W.] Supreme Court decision of Riley v. California isn't just a landmark ruling on cell phone privacy. It also represents a dramatic shift in the high court's attitude toward technology and privacy. The Supreme Court's new attitude is best summarized

by a single sentence in the opinion. The government had argued that searching a cell phone is no different from searching other items in a suspect's pocket. That, the court wrote, "is like saying a ride on horseback is materially indistinguishable from a flight to the moon." [22]

2.5 Discussion

The Internet indeed makes it possible to get many things done without leaving home, but when we are visiting the post office we have an interaction with a person, not a machine. Going to the bank creates an opportunity to exchange some words with a man who assists us, and buying a plane ticket in a tourist agency is connected with having a conversation on our vacation plans. By choosing the faster and easier way, we shut the prospect of interactions with people who were taking care of us. Of course, the computer type way will be "faster and easier," but only under the condition that we own an alphabetical notebook of all passwords where, among dozens of sophisticated codes, we can identify the one for the postal services, the one for the bank, that one we should use when buying a discount ticket, etc. A similar situation happens when it comes to pictures. In the past, we had significantly less of them, but at least we physically possessed them. Today, we are allegedly owners of thousands of pictures (we do not have to worry about the costs of the film development) but in most cases, they are somewhere in the computer's memory instead of sitting in a photo album that at least from time to time is watched.

The practically unlimited possibility of publishing everything by everybody leads sometimes to violation of privacy, to posting comments which are offensive, rude, or falsified, but accessible to all web users. In extreme situations, like posting telephone made videos that document sexual harassment of underage girls by their male colleagues, we have to deal with the suicidal deaths of the victims who were not able to carry the stigma of shame.

The Internet is indeed the well of knowledge, but is it always the objective one? Among popular news sites, information is posted that is carefully selected in a way that is to direct the opinion of the readers. They are either removed from the context or presented selectively, and even though they are true because the other news events are ignored, they say only a part of the truth and in this way manipulate the reader's way of thinking.

We have already mentioned how computerization expanded the abilities and range of the influence of science, including medicine. Are we, however, fully aware of what may happen when there will be a serious shortage of power or when terrorists will get access to the most vital centers of computer management? The cover of the American magazine *The Week* [23] issued on May 30, 2014, announces *World War 3.0. The U.S.'s new offensive against China's cyber thieves*, which suggests all of us face dangers that are difficult to imagine.

2.5.1 Hazards That Affect Mental Well-Being

The danger does not come only from outside. When we rely too much on technological shortcuts—that is, in simple arithmetic, when instead of multiplying from memory or by the means of paper and pencil, we escape to the telephone calculator—in a longer range it leads to the alarming phenomenon of biological atrophy about which the already mentioned Tim Wu writes. To our disadvantage, not only our mind becomes ponderous but our body as well; and mainly seating lifestyle promotes obesity, cardiovascular diseases, and type II diabetes.

Finally, how do we recognize that when it comes to the use of the Internet, we have already left the safe territory and entered into the domain of addiction (see Chap. 14, which discusses the pathological use of this technology)? Let us briefly formulate what creates the main criterion of addiction, based on *DSM-5* [24] criteria (pp. 282–283) for gambling disorder (there is still no Internet-related addiction officially defined). We are dealing with it when our activities negatively affect our functioning in society, at work, with family, and in contact with others. If, for example, the amount of time that is spent by a young person on social networks causes that there is a shortage of time when it comes to homework, and test preparation, or leads to sleep deprivation and taking naps during classes, then we have a problem. If a child avoids going outside, meetings with friends, or being active in sports because of the computer, then we may suspect that it is the result of compulsion. If we plan to spend just 1 h in front of the monitor, because it is the amount of time that we can afford, whereas 3 h later we are still not where we should be, it means that it is not us anymore who decides our activities. If watching pornography and masturbating in front of the computer screen translates first to the negligence of intimacy with one's wife and later lack of either strength or will to have one, it means that the time has come to see a therapist. If thinking about using a computer prevents us from drawing pleasure from what we are doing at a given moment, or if it does not allow us to focus on conversation or the task we are conducting, it means that we have lost control over the Internet domain of our life. If, when in the office, we cannot resist the temptation of looking at the web page that excites us despite knowing that somebody can notice it, and as a result we can lose our job, or if we are not able not to read and answer the text while driving and being fully aware of the danger of collision, then it means that we allowed technology that was to make our life easier to enslave us.

Inventions, including the Internet, create many opportunities for the human race but at the same time, they bring a lot of dangers. However, we should realize that the effects of the scientific progress themselves, without the prime mover of their creator, and later customer, who starts using them for his/her beneficial or destructive purposes, are mostly neutral. It is we who give meaning to our lives and their instruments. Arsenic is very useful in the production of glass, the conservation of wood, or dentistry, but it is also a deadly poison. At the beginning of the twentieth century, workers in despair were destroying machines because they believed that they were taking jobs away from them. Today, thanks to robots and automatization, a "physical laborer" description less and less frequently reflects a situation in which a worker has to indeed use the strength of his muscles. Thanks to inventions, our daily tasks are less difficult, and accomplishing them requires less time than in the past. Theoretically, we can have more, under the condition that in front of the temptation of more and more technologically sophisticated and spectacular but at the same time very possessive toys, we will have enough common sense not to allow them to enslave us.

2.6 Summary

The invention of the Internet creates enormous opportunities, and, at the same time, serious dangers. The paradox is that similar qualities, depending on who is using them and for what purpose, could be turned either to our advantage or disadvantage. This chapter discusses the opposing views on several aspects of the use of the Internet focusing on ways in which it positively and negatively affects the lives of those who depend on it.

The reasonable, balanced, and careful deployment of this technology led to a revolutionary increase in opportunities to disseminate, share, obtain, accumulate, and store information and interpersonal contacts.

The abuse and malicious misuse of the Internet—and the instruments that operate thanks to it—result in many unfortunate phenomena: "tyranny of tiny tasks" related to the use of email technology; the Internet deception, which includes scams, cyber-crimes, and smearing, that negatively affects the mechanics of trust; voluntary compromise of our privacy by the wide use of the social networking; the atrophy of certain brain activities because of choosing the technological shortcuts; manipulation of the public opinion; the phenomenon of the Internet addiction; and gradual decrease in face-to-face interpersonal communication, which is being replaced by communing with the cyber gadgets.

References

1. Hilty DM, et al. Effects of telepsychiatry on the doctor-patient relationship: communication, satisfaction, and relevant issues. Primary Psychiatry. 2002;9:29–34.
2. Hilty DM, Yellowlees PM, Nesbitt TS. Evolution of telepsychiatry to rural sites: changes over time in types of referrals and PCP knowledge, skill, and satisfaction. Gen Hosp Psychiatry. 2006;28(5):367–73.
3. Safety perceptions index 2023. Understanding the impact of risk around the world. Posted by Vision of Humanity website on 21 February 2023. https://www.visionofhumanity.org/wp-content/uploads/2023/02/SPI-2023-2.pdf.
4. WHO Coronavirus (COVID-19) Dashboard. Posted by WHO on 17 May 2023. https://covid19.who.int/.
5. Schöley J, et al. Life expectancy changes since COVID-19, Nature Journal website Posted in November 2022. https://www.nature.com/articles/s41562-022-01450-3.
6. Kirsinger A, et al. The COVID-19 pandemic: inside from three years of KFF polling, Kaiser Family Foundation website. Posted on 7 March 2023. https://www.kff.org/coronavirus-covid-19/poll-finding/the-covid-19-pandemic-insights-from-three-years-of-kff-polling/.
7. Gun Violance Archive. Posted on 18 May 2023. https://www.gunviolencearchive.org/.

8. Brown H. The role of social media in the Arab uprisings. PEW Research Center website. Posted on 28 November 2012. https://www.pewresearch.org/journalism/2012/11/28/role-social-media-arab-uprisings/.
9. Vojinovic I. Heart-breaking cyberbullying statistics for 2023. Posted on the DataProt website on 5 May 2023. https://dataprot.net/statistics/cyberbullying-statistics/.
10. Emily A. Vogels, Teens and cyberbullying 2022. PEW Research Center website. Posted on 15 December 2022. https://www.pewresearch.org/internet/2022/12/15/teens-and-cyberbullying-2022/.
11. Paving the way for future living: Germany's first 3D-printed house. Posted on GIRA website on 26 July 2022. https://www.gira.com/en/en/g-pulse-magazine/building/3d-house-germany#.
12. German publisher apologizes for fake Schumacher AI interview. AP News website Posted on 23 April 2023. https://apnews.com/article/schumacher-fake-interview-d90d3802c6e3ea49f0da6c7795e954cd.
13. LajkaA, MarceloP. Trump arrested? Putin jailed? Fake AI images spread online. Posted on AP News website 23 March 2023. https://apnews.com/article/ai-misinformation-trump-putin-new-york-42ac9c41c5504d05412b492e48bcaded.
14. Petkauskas V. Rise of the machines: when a computer beats a chess master. Posted on Cybernews website on 16 May 2022. https://cybernews.com/editorial/rise-of-the-machines-when-a-computer-beats-a-chess-master/.
15. ChatGPT: can students pass using AI tools at university? Posted on BBC News website on 9 May 2023. https://www.bbc.com/news/education-65316283.
16. None G. Is virtual reality bad for our mental health? Posted on the TECHMONITOR website on 28 April 2022. https://techmonitor.ai/technology/emerging-technology/is-virtual-reality-bad-for-mental-health.
17. Kenwright B. Virtual reality: ethical challenges and dangers, posted on technology and society website on 14 January 2019. https://technologyandsociety.org/virtual-reality-ethical-challenges-and-dangers/.
18. Wu T. The problem with easy technology. Posted on The New Yorker blog "Elements" on February 25, 2014. http://www.newyorker.com/online/blogs/elements/2014/02/the-problem-with-easy-technology.html.
19. Contact WJ. The tale of human longing for fulfilling communication. San Diego: Wisdom Moon Publishing; 2013.
20. McLaren P, et al. An evaluation of the use of interactive television in an acute psychiatric service. J Telemed Telecare. 1995;1:79–85.
21. Snowden E. Here's how we take back the internet. Posted on the TED website on March 2014. http://www.ted.com/talks/edward_snowden_here_s_how_we_take_back_the_internet.
22. Lee TB. The most important sentence in the supreme Court's cell phone privacy ruling. Posted on VOXcom website, on 26 June 2014. http://www.vox.com/2014/6/26/5843586/the-most-important-sentence-in-wednesdays-cell-phone-privacy-ruling.
23. Chinese hackers indicted for cyber theft. The editorial page (the main stories…). The Week. 2014;14(670):2.
24. American Psychiatric Association. Desk reference to the diagnostic criteria from DSM-5. Washington, DC: American Psychiatric Association; 2013.

Information Technology for Behavioral Health: Global Perspectives on Access, Services, and Stigmatization

3

Donald M. Hilty, Shalini Ahuja, John A. Naslund, Allison Crawford, and Norman Sartorius

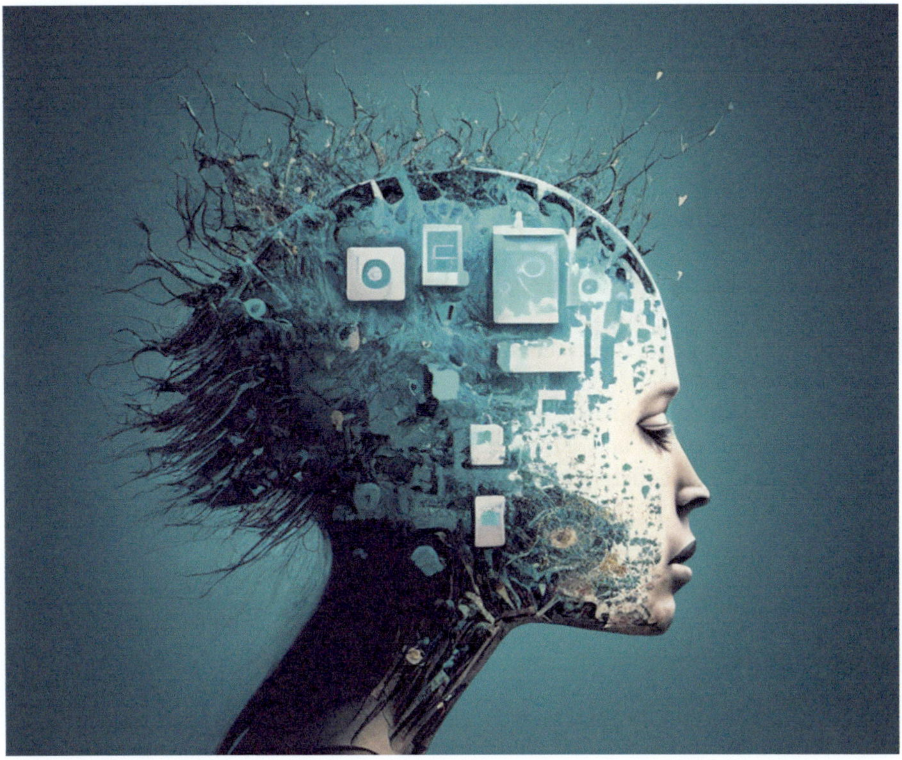

D. M. Hilty (✉)
Department of Psychiatry and Behavioral Sciences, Keck School of Medicine
University of Southern California, Los Angeles, CA, USA
e-mail: donald.hilty@uhsinc.com; hilty@med.usc.edu

D. Mucić, D. M. Hilty (eds.), *Digital Mental Health*,
https://doi.org/10.1007/978-3-031-59936-1_3

Abstract

Our exchange of information through health technologies helps to increase access to care, analyze information, and disseminate practices. Clinical informatics is a rapidly expanding area and can facilitate patient-centered care as defined by quality, affordable, and timely health care. This chapter covers developments in information systems and electronic health records for communications with patients and staff (e.g., alerts, texts), setting behavioral health indicators and developing digital advances to improve practice and research. Patient-centered care with technology facilitates quality outcomes and efficiency via sound system processes. By learning how systems are designed and tailored to collect data, clinicians can use technology to inform decisions and facilitate outcomes. Setting priorities involves input from all care participants, as well as technological competencies for the clinician and institution. Cultural safety and humility focuses on patients' experiences and values. This empowers patients' roles in clinical care and helps to avoid inadvertent perpetuation or repetition of traumatic or stigmatizing experiences. Patient, clinician, and institutional attitudes and skills in technology, equity, and diversity can align clinical care, training, and research missions and stimulate process improvement.

3.1 Introduction

Information exchange through health technologies, particularly clinical informatics, is used to access, analyze and disseminate information for facilitating high quality, affordable, and timely patient-centered care [1, 2]. Worldwide, health care systems and governmental agencies are emphasizing quality, evidence-based care with behavioral health data/indicators for individuals and populations [3]. This requires acceptable, measurable, and scalable approaches. For feasible and sustainable services, effectiveness and implementation science approaches gain input from all

S. Ahuja
Health Services and Population Research Department, King's College London, Institute of Psychiatry, Psychology and Neurosciences, Centre for Implementation Science, London, UK
e-mail: shalini.ahuja@kcl.ac.uk

J. A. Naslund
Department of Global Health and Social Medicine, Harvard Medical School, Boston, MA, USA
e-mail: John_Naslund@hms.harvard.edu

A. Crawford
Virtual Mental Health, Centre for Addiction and Mental Health, University of Toronto, Toronto, ON, Canada
e-mail: allison.crawford@utoronto.ca

N. Sartorius
Association for the Improvement of Mental Health Programmes (AMH), Geneva, Switzerland
e-mail: sartorius@normansartorius.com

stakeholders in health care settings [4, 5]. Technology is a key part of the World Health Organization (WHO) global health strategy, with the expectation of scalable behavioral health interventions, particularly for people in communities affected by adversity [6, 7]. Culturally appropriate care is important for patients and communities worldwide and informs better policy decisions [8].

The Health Information Technology for Economic and Clinical Health (HITECH) Act brought a wave of electronic health records (EHRs), and with this, meaningful use criteria standards in the U.S. The EHR or computer-based patient record (CPR) improved clinical practice through data collection, retrieval of information and decision support systems for outcome measurement. Typically, notes are more completely documented and have more appropriate clinical decisions compared to handwritten notes [9], but there are inefficiencies and EHRs are linked to burnout among health professionals [10, 11]. System management processes like health information systems (IS), telemedicine, and information technology (IT)) facilitates care delivery with clinical decision support, typically supported by advances in artificial intelligence (AI) to assist patients and clinicians with decision-making in time and across settings [12]. Advances in sensing technologies and affective computing have enabled machines to analyze data for patterns in time and longitudinally, and help users detect, assess, and respond to emotional states. Use of machine learning (ML) and pattern recognition promises to improve public and population health surveillance.

Culturally appropriate health care is a priority according to the National Academy of Science [2020] and the World Health Organization (WHO) [2017]. A common definition of cultural competence is "a set of congruent behaviours, attitudes and policies...enable...professions to work effectively in cross-cultural situations" [13]. Cultural diversity includes race, ethnicity, spirituality, religion, sexual preference, gender identity, geography (urban, rural, global), age, socioeconomic status, education, special populations (e.g., incarcerated), and language [14, 15]. More recently, some suggest a clinical, educational, and policy shift from the concept of cultural competence to cultural humility [16] and/or cultural safety [17–19], which would include Indigenous knowledge, community-centered care, understanding the role of colonialism in health and social determinants of health, as well as the ongoing impact of historical trauma and loss. This is more patient-centered and overlaps with an anthropologic definition in which people acquire knowledge and use it to interpret their world socially [20].

Many assume that good clinicians will adapt in-person care to video, telephone, mobile health, and other technologies, and intermix these options with ease in combination [2], but clinician- or learner-centered approaches that parallel patient-centered ones are needed to ensure quality care so clinicians can embrace technology as part of health care reform [6, 14]. Competencies for video [21], asynchronous technologies [2], and mobile health and culture [15, 22] help with this mission.

This chapter introduces data collection and analysis, EHRs, and information technologies, which improve services and research. Specifically, this chapter will help the reader:

1. Learn how to set goals toward quality outcomes and help clinicians and systems be efficient with patient-centered care using technology.

2. Consider how systems are designed and tailored to collect data, inform decisions, and evaluate outcomes.
3. Be aware of cultural safety, humility, and stigmatization to improve access, quality of care, and process improvement.

3.2 Setting Goals to Achieve Value and Quality in Practice and the Role of Technology

Innovation with technology is only as good as the evidence base that supports it, and the evidence-based approaches used by clinicians to provide care, as well as the process/quality improvement and evaluation of outcomes by a health care system or across a population. Technology serves to efficiently collect data to show that quality care was provided, but, to date, most of the technologies deployed to assess quality have focused on process metrics (e.g., productivity, errors, cost), and emphases on implementation, population health, and economic cost analyses are propelling a good shift to more meaningful outcome metrics across the world—one thing in common is *from* symptoms *to* social functioning and well-being.

Advances in the collection and analysis of big data hold promise to advance behavioral health practice and research. Much of this work aims toward achieving personalized behavioral health interventions, which started in high-income countries and are taking root around the globe [23, 24]. At a minimum, the treatment of mental illness relies on subjective measurement for diagnosis, treatment/intervention, and long-term monitoring. At a maximum, a variety of sensors and wearables offer new options for patient care, clinician decision-making, and population health—via mobile phones and other smart devices. This technology more precisely assesses and captures human behavior through continuous monitoring and can enable personalized digital interventions aligned with optimizing clinical outcomes. These options can reduce geographical, cost, and temporal barriers, with privacy and professionalism risks that are reasonable [3, 24].

Health care clinics and hospitals can help by identifying behavioral health domains or targets to assess [25]. Standard quality reporting metrics in the USA come from the Center for Medicare and Medicaid Services (CMS) and National Quality Forum (i.e., G-PRO), as well as the International Consortium for Health Outcomes Measurement (ICHOM), which outlines international standards of health outcome assessment in behavioral health care [26]. The Mental Health Atlas of 2017 shows discrepancies in availability of data, with almost a quarter of all countries in the African region reporting "no regular collection of data in the last two years" [27]. To improve monitoring and transparency, in 2014 the Organisation of Economic Corporation and Development recommended a list of behavioral health indicators, including those measuring: readmissions; case management and mortality with severe mental disorders; anti-cholinergic and anti-depressant drugs with elderly patients; continuity of care and timeliness of ambulatory follow-up after hospitalization; use of anti-depressant medication and visits during the acute phase of treatment; and racial and ethnic disparities and behavioral health follow-up rates [28].

In many low- and middle-income countries (LIMCs), the lack of data from primary care limits the scale-up of community mental health programs [29, 30]. This information gap is responded by formulation of contextualized behavioral health indicators, for example, a minimum set of frequently endorsed indicators were co-designed using a Delphi study across five LMICs. These indicators measure mental health coverage and performance covering domains such as needs, utilization, quality, and financial risk protection [30]. While evaluating the use of these new indicators in LMICs, interviewees perceived that new and simpler forms led to better collection of data, monitoring, and documentation [3, 30]. Iterative development with input helps with prioritization, customization, and coordination for health and governmental systems [25].

Important clinical and administrative outcomes include no-show rates, percentage of treatments completed over time, and proportion of first-time patients presenting for follow-up visits within recommended time frames. Stable, simple, and standard measures can directly shape quality evaluation and clinical decision-making—with input by patients on selection and alignment with regulatory and payor metrics—and can avoid complexity and burdening care participants. The forms and results should appear in clinician notes to inform decision-making—meaning EHR compatibility is key. The level of knowledge, competence, confidence, and motivation of health workers affects likelihood of implementation and sustainability [3]. A better look at combining technologies and in-person services (i.e., hybrid care) is needed, with care navigators helping patients understand options and providing input on design and process [2, 31].

3.3 Components and Processes of Systems for Access and Quality

3.3.1 Overview

Evaluation of clinical practice has become increasingly important in *both* the provision of a service *and* demonstration of quality care and improved patient health outcomes. A philosophical shift has occurred from efficacy-based interventions—often under ideal conditions or research protocols—to translational and effectiveness interventions, based on implementation science (i.e., acceptability, adoption, feasibility, cost, sustainability) [4, 5]. Methodologies are needed for development, implementation, and evaluation (quantitative and qualitative) of a technology. Key steps suggested for institutions to integrate video apply to other technologies: (1) assess readiness; (2) create/hardwire the culture; (3) write policies and procedures; (4) establish the curriculum and competencies; (5) train learners and faculty; and (6) evaluate/manage change [11].

3.3.2 Structural Approaches

EHRs: EHRs may be a good example for considering barriers that may interfere with the successful implementation of a technology. For users, menu-based user interfaces have been cumbersome, but are evolving into more intuitive graphical interfaces. CPR and integrated voice-recognition software is usually time-saving after the initial investment of time to learn it. For CPRs that require physician typing for data entry and analysis, patient engagement (e.g., eye contact) and rapport may be affected [9, 32]. EHR guidelines are aimed at preparing clinical practices for reporting within the new health care delivery and payment models

Dictation Dictation with voice recognition is increasingly common and reduces administrative support costs. While it is a significant adjustment for some clinicians, for systems the costs pay for themselves compared to alternatives (i.e., computer equipment, time, support staff). There are challenges of integration with legacy systems, billing systems, and practice management systems. An undeveloped area appears to be using video and audio dictations more purposely in workflow (e.g., replacing a specialist text e-consultation with a video, since it is more engaging, memorable, synthetic and user-friendly) [2].

Kiosks and Tablets Not all clinicians and patients are interested in or able to use their EHR patient portal due to inexperience with technology, or limited access to high-speed Internet (a common challenge in underserved communities, particularly in rural or low-resource areas, as well as in many regions in LMICs). A popular alternative is to have kiosks within the reception area of the practice where patients can easily complete targeted patient-reported outcomes using a touch screen. These have been used for diagnosis and treatment of depression and alcohol use disorders in primary care clinics in rural and urban settings in Colombia [33].

Patient Portals A way to assess outcomes is *a patient portal*, which is a secure electronic website that gives patients access to parts of their EHR within a clinician's EHR. One can administer questionnaires and surveys to patients through these portals, which streamlines assessment, treatment and integration of patient reported outcomes.

3.3.3 Functional Technologies

e-Consultation (i.e., e-Consult or eConsult) This generally involves a primary care provider (PCP) referral for a consultation related to questions about patient care that are outside of their expertise [34, 35]. It requires basic hardware, software, and integration within the EHR, with substantial practice, quality, and process improvement supports. e-Consultation resulted in reduced wait times for patients, lower costs, fewer in-person visits, and high satisfaction by users.

Store-and-Forward/Asynchronous Technology (ATP) Store-and-forward technologies have been used for dermatology, radiology, and many other specialties—the specialist interprets an image or a video interview for BH, while incorporating clinical history from the referring physician, and gives the PCP a plan to implement [36]. ATP has outcomes comparable to video consultation and can enable collaborative and integrated care [2, 36].

Email There appear to be several advantages to email interviewing, particularly with young populations, as it is cost-effective and offers flexibility [37]. It also provides a transcript for analysis and offers time to reflect on questions, compose answers, and respond at leisure in the comfort of familiar home surroundings. Challenges include verification of self-report, potentially compromised rapport due to lack of visual and auditory cues, privacy, and issues around quality control in studies (e.g., participants' comprehension levels).

Text Text-based chat and social media communication pose opportunities and challenges in terms of content and process issues [30]. Mobile health interventions are used in many ways (e.g., reminders, 14%; information, 17%; supportive messages, 42%; self-monitoring procedures, 42%) [38]. As keyboard characters have limitations for text, emoticons have been used since 1982 to enrich communication and comprehension [39], though they are not always used in a standard way, particularly across cultures [30].

Apps A review of apps found scant evidence-based treatment content, few comprehensive anxiety self-management apps, and few advanced features that leverage the broader functionalities of smartphone capabilities (e.g., sensors, ecological momentary assessments (EMA)) [39–41]. Furthermore, despite widespread interest in the use of apps for mental health, the quality of the evidence has been variable, with use of differing study designs and appropriate comparison conditions often driving the noticeable differences in impact on clinical outcomes rather than the use of the app [42]. Such concerns emphasize the need for rigorously designed clinical trials comparing the use of smartphone apps to established BH interventions in order to establish the clinical utility of these digital tools. The child, adolescent, and family literature show significant research on apps and text interventions related to appointment reminders, treatment adherence, well-being, suicide, and other clinically related topics [39].

Sensors and Wearables Wearable sensors are usually wireless, miniature circuits embedded in patches or bandages, wristbands, rings, or shirts (e.g., smartwatches, heart rate monitors, and smart glasses) [43]. These enable collection of behavioral data, detection, symptom monitoring, accessing and sharing of data, and providing interventions [44]. This transforms care by moving from cross-sectional, manual transfer of data to an integrated, longitudinal, minimally intrusive and interactive sharing of data that is based on the ecology of a person or patient in their natural settings, using EMA methods [12]. Wearable devices have shown promise for tracking health behaviors in BH populations, extending their utility to other lifestyle factors such as sleep or activity that are known to be associated with mental health outcomes [45].

AI and Big Data Traditional applications of clinical decision support technology have used EHRs and are being enhanced by newer technologies, such as cloud computing, AI, ML, and signal processing algorithms (i.e., neural networks, random forests, support vector machines, natural language processing [NLP]) [12]. These technologies enable context-aware, live streaming of data, and real-time feedback to enhance the assessment of clinical, lifestyle, and social activities [46]. Temporal modeling leverages dynamical information and extends methods across multiple decision time points, so clinicians iteratively reevaluate, intervene, and make new observations and sequentially make decisions [12, 44]. They can monitor, intervene, and follow trajectories longitudinally, often with quality of life and economic cost dimensions [44]. Current studies are investigating smartphone, biological, and clinical data to identify markers of risk, diagnosis, state, stage, treatment response, and prognosis in different populations (e.g., depression) [44, 47–50]. These approaches can also help with patient engagement and enrollment across a variety of international and culturally diverse populations (e.g., age, disorder, ethnicity, generation, immigrant, military, refugee). Analyzing large amounts of data will require close collaboration between partners from diverse areas of expertise, such as researchers, clinicians, statisticians, software developers, and engineers.

The Internet and Social Media Patients, families, and caregivers seek information on diseases or medical problems, support, treatments, health professionals, and other health-related topics [30]. Teenagers may have few traditional care options and feel more comfortable to share experiences and try to learn new behaviors anonymously or at a distance. At times, they may express ideas of self-harm and negative affective states, which is concerning if these things are not shared with parents and/or professionals [44]. Patients with anxiety, trauma (e.g., military personnel), and psychotic disorders use the Internet for seeking information related to their illness and medication [30], and connecting with others who share similar conditions and experiences [46]. Research using social media data is measuring self-report of key symptoms (e.g., suicidal ideation, sexting) and evaluating social media content for diagnostic and predictive analysis. Models assess affect, linguistic style, and context with supervised learning algorithms, random forests, and machine learning to discriminate between healthy, depressed, and posttraumatic stress disorder populations [51]. Postpartum depression was, as predicted from a model, related to increased social isolation and decreased social capital (i.e., less activity, interaction); this was manifested by fewer status updates, media items, and reaching out to friends compared to others and usual personal patterns [52]. Yet caution is warranted regarding safety, privacy, and viability of these platforms to characterize behavioral health conditions and provide evidence-based services [53].

3.3.4 Picking the Right Technologies and Models of Care and Integrating Them into Practice

How does one best integrate technologies into clinical practice? The application of telehealth modalities to one's practice requires reflection and purpose, discussion with patients, and staying-up on the rapidly changing literature. Overarching goals in the integration of technology include: *improving access* to care in terms of geography, time, and transportation; *triaging patients* if they need to be seen in between appointments; providing *adjunctive support* to in-person services; and *improving efficiency and continuity* of care. The specific needs and goals, preferences on what technology to use, and the requisite behaviors/skills and targeted outcomes can vary among the users: patients; primary care teams; and specialists (Table 3.1). This requires attention to: assessment and evaluation (e.g., text, e-consultation, asynchronous video or store-and-forward); management/treatment planning (e.g., secure email and text); administrative issues; and human factors. In addition, in vivo training on technology can enable the clinician to "fit" the technology with the patient's needs, develop a good digital relationship, and iteratively improve the process (Fig. 3.1). The key steps are: (1) needs assessment; (2) technology options; (3) therapeutic relationships; (4) training and support; (5) implementation; and (6) evaluation—then the cycle returns to the beginning as part of process improvement (Fig. 3.2).

The intersection of health, technology, and cultural literacy is key for participants in care—both traditional ones like the patient and clinician—and now expanding to care navigators or coordinators and others [2, 54].

1. The Patient: Depending on comfort, and familiarity with technology and/or the clinician, the individual patient may have varying degrees of receptiveness and skill (i.e., e-literacy). The patient's willingness to engage and favorable opinion may determine the success and effectiveness of the implementation. A social support system consisting of individuals who can assist them with this decision and in navigating the new technology is also helpful.
2. Health Literacy: The technology must be appropriate and effective for the course of treatment of the disease—which the patient must connect with experience [54]. For example, a condition like schizophrenia may be suited to at-home monitoring, if examinations and procedures (e.g., long-acting antipsychotic injections) can be done. Though often very ill, individuals living with schizophrenia should not be excluded from improving quality of life through exercising an online support group chat [30, 41]. Overall, interventions may be needed to integrate digital health literacy with health literacy and health information skills for self-management and participation in care.
3. Care Navigators: The concept of a new team member, the digital navigator, able to assume this role is introduced as a solution [55]. With a digital navigator, any clinic today can take advantage of mobile health and smartphone tools to augment and expand existing telehealth and in-person care. The role of a digital

Table 3.1 Goals and skills for patients, primary care teams, and specialists to use asynchronous technology for behavioral health care

Patient care	Patient	PC team member	Specialist
Assessment/ evaluation (e.g., text) • Consent • History • Engagement and communication • Administration and documentation • Medico-legal: privacy, safety, data protection/ integrity, and security	Learn from personal experience and via health care visits Reflect on purpose for use • Log/diary information • Send information to health care team for their use • Communicate with health care team: get information or make a decision Weigh relative value compared to other technology If used, what is(are) the purpose(s) for health care? Does clinic and/or health system support text use or not?	Patient care planning • Use a screening questionnaire to assess text use, OR • Have a team member ask a few screening questions Consider factors to decide if should use text before proceeding: • Time, skills, and knowhow to use text • Can text be built into information flow (e.g., EHR)? • How do we use text with patients and specialist consultants? If used, what is main purpose: log, send, or obtain information?	Include SP/device, apps, and other technologies in informed consent Elicit history/screen for personal vs. health care use Use privacy settings All: reflect and weigh impact • Positives vs. negatives • Impact on care: communication • Text vs. other technologies Clarify with patient and PC (primary care) team about effective communication Instruct on best ways to use an app • An evidence-based app with • An evidence-based approach • Simplicity with purpose
Assessment/ evaluation (e.g., e-consultation)	Learn about it and weigh versus other options (i.e., in-person or video with specialist) If used, could feel good that the PCP has access to specialists to email, telephone, e-consult, and/or refer for synchronous or in-person care	Goals: gain knowledge and skill with CDS for assessment and treatment • Gain technical assistance on safety/risk and contingency plan • Triage urgent/ emergent issues to synchronous option • Quickly diagnose and treat to improve system's capacity	Help learners and staff use decision support tools based on evidence Research/disseminate procedures to prevent problems and manage workflow Advise on specific specialty consultations with relative/absolute contraindications Train/supervise to optimize assessment (e.g., pre-consult information, tests)

(continued)

Table 3.1 (continued)

Patient care	Patient	PC team member	Specialist
Assessment/ evaluation (e.g., asynchronous video or store-and-forward)	Easy to use and glad that PCP confers with a specialist Less travel and it gets done faster Go through a guided interview and add things here and there that provide context (e.g., narrative, verbal and non-verbal behaviors)	Clinical care considerations • What skills are needed? • What technology is needed? • Training in semi-structured interviewing for reliability and validity to improve my (or PC team member's) skills, as well as our workflow • Many synchronous video consults are not needed	Train/consult PC team members to improve assessment, triage, and interventions • Diagnostic tests • Concurrent care management ATP psychiatrist needs training related to: • Clinical workflow • Primary care setting • Security, privacy, and confidentiality • Team-leading, if applicable
Management/ treatment planning (e.g., secure email and text) • Use tools within EHR for clinical decision support (CDS) • Use "best practice" with evidence-based approaches • Monitor and improve	Good ways to use email and text if privacy ensured • Follow-up details needed • Send additional documents/ information or complete questionnaires • Engage loved one to help • Capture day-to-day accurate accounts of life (e.g., mood, functioning, activity) • To "stay in contact" with a nurse, mid-level, and/or PCP	Care • Triage simple and/or sequential workflow to target goal; triage complex, urgent/emergent issues to synchronous option • Obtain clinical information for CDS for assessment/ treatment Consultation: gaining knowledge, skill development • Apply knowledge into practice • Gain technical assistance on safety/risk and back-up plans	Select "best" mode for a given task: SP/device and/or apps, email/text, telephone, and/or in-person Triage complex, urgent/emergent issues to synchronous (telephone, in-person) care Give technical assistance on safety/ risk (e.g., medication) and offer a back-up plan Prioritize SP/device and app options, email, and tools that integrate into the EHR Learn/teach pre- and intra-platform data feeds (e.g., questionnaire upload) into EHR to improve quality of care and be efficient

(continued)

Table 3.1 (continued)

Patient care	Patient	PC team member	Specialist
Administrative issues: • Workflow and documentation • Medico-legal: privacy, safety, data protection/ integrity, and security	Keep information up-to-date Review patient portal and communicate needs Learn safeguards for privacy, security, and confidentiality Use secure forms of communication (e.g., secure email within EHR not Gmail)	Develop standard consent form, treatment plan, and other procedures Adhere to clinic, health system, and professional requirements Identify and adhere to laws and regulations in the jurisdiction(s) of practice and of that of the patient Obtain clinical and legal advice	Seek input from users to plan Help administrators to: • Develop language for documentation • Adapt current practices • Develop policies/ procedures Teach/consult Adapt legal/regulatory principles Assess fit of technology for users
Human factors: • Communication • Attitude • Cultural/diversity • Social determinants • Special populations	Be flexible Be brief, clear, and spell out communications Clarify if issues are unclear Able to discuss my culture, language, and other matters related to use of technologies Do not want to be stereotyped	Be flexible Role model willingness to improve Discuss scope, timing, and agreed upon plan(s) for use Triage to other technology, if needed Consider preferences Ask about impact of culture and diversity on use and preferences Promote reflection and discussion, make adjustments, and manage language impact Generalize across generations and cultures	Teach on scope of communication with technology to clarify expectations and anticipate problems (e.g., feasibility of checking mH device at other sites, clinics) Educate/consult colleagues about asynchronous technology use Clarify expectations with questions about culture Adjust care to culture and preferences, using generalizations not stereotypes Teach/consult to PC team on cultural complexities to achieve outcomes

app application; (video), *ATP* asynchronous telepsychiatry, *BH* mental/behavioral health, *EHR* electronic health record, *mH* mobile health, *PCP* primary care provider, *SP* smartphone

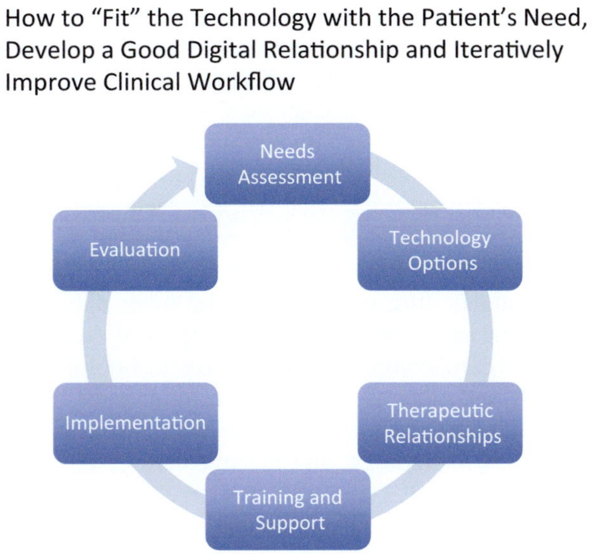

Fig. 3.1 How to "fit" the technology with the patient's need, develop a good digital relationship, and iteratively improve clinical workflow

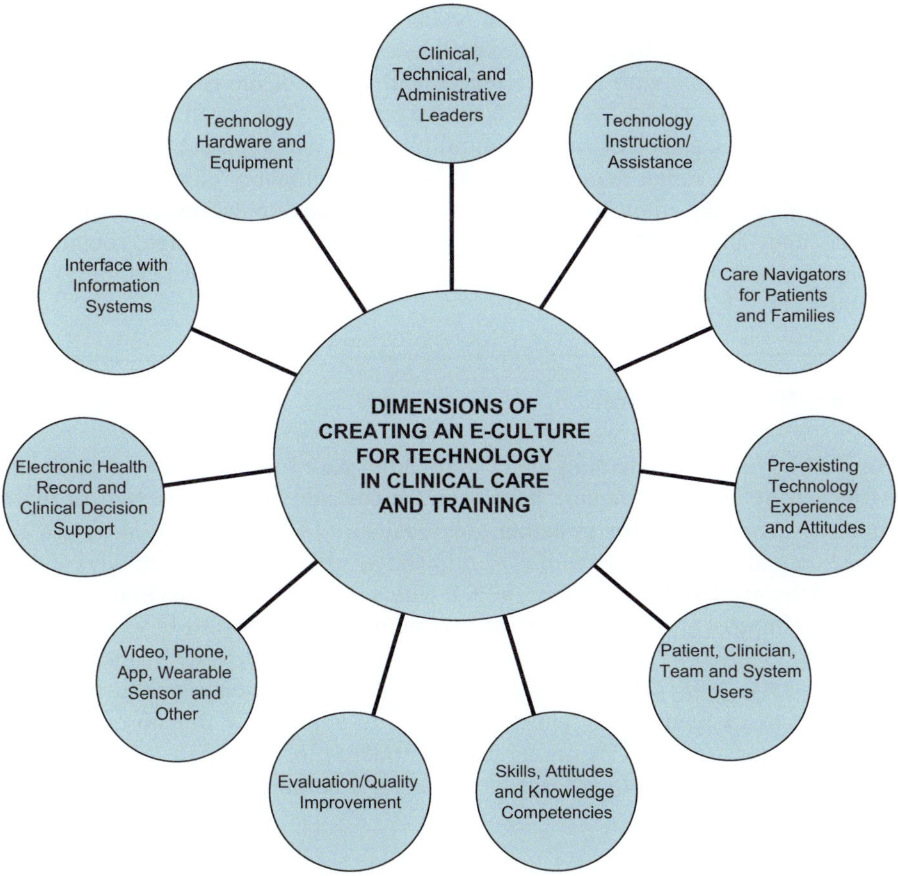

Fig. 3.2 Dimensions of creating an e-culture for technology in clinical care and training

navigator is suitable as an entry-level health care role, additional training for an experienced clinician, and well suited to peer specialists.

4. The Clinician: Before offering care to accompany in-person services with technology, the clinician must ensure that they have the expertise, time, and resources to provide quality and consistent care as is promised and expected through the new modality. Clinicians' skills need to be adapted from in-person and video care to a wide range of technologies (Table 3.1). Training for technology should include, but not be limited to: (1) use of medical libraries; (2) use of information technology for Internet-based searches and other work; (3) literature, drug information, and other databases; and (4) video, telephone, mobile health, and other technologies. With AI, ML, and other informatics topics in care, competency sets across technologies, particularly wearable sensors [44], and other asynchronous technologies [2] are needed. Specifically, mobile health competencies should include clinical decision support, prudent selection of technology, and management of flow of information across an EHR platform [44].
5. Cultural Factors: Compassionate care that is competent and safe—and provided from a place of humility—is increasingly recognized as an instrumental part of health care, including via technology like video [21], mobile health [15], and other technologies [2]. Digital care should be culturally safe—meaning that it aligns with the preferences and values of the recipient of care, as judged by that person rather than by the provider. The corollary for providers is assuming a stance of cultural humility, a reflexive approach as an other-oriented learner, rather than focusing on the development of cultural competence [56]. Racial and ethnic minorities and marginalized populations can be engaged for input about technological fluency, health literacy, language, social, economic, and other cultural issues, and support integration of technology into their care [3, 57].

3.3.5 Models of Care

Another key issue is selecting the best model of care for a patient or population. Models of telepsychiatric care have been framed into low-, moderate-, or high-intensity levels of care by updating previous work [58]. The intensity levels are based on patient acuity, technology complexity, specialist time, and who is designated the primary provider (i.e., a PCP with a secondary telepsychiatrist versus a telepsychiatrist). Low-intensity interventions involve specialists working with PCPs by: telephone, text, or email (doctor-to-doctor "curbside" consultations; case reviews) [58]. Moderate-intensity service interventions usually include a specialist assessment of the patient by video to adjust PCP diagnoses, develop treatment plans (e.g., ATP), or augment treatment [36, 58]. High-intensity interventions with video include team-based care via collaborative care and stepped care [58].

3.4 Organizational Options to Promote Culturally Safe Care and Reduce Stigmatization

3.4.1 Shift from Culturally Competent to Safe Care

Many institutions are considering shifting from cultural competence to cultural humility [13] or cultural safety (Spradley) as an organizing framework. Cultural humility emphasizes engagement, process, subjectivity, reflection, power balance, skills and attitudes, as well as individual, group, community, and institutional accountability in the commitment to an ongoing relationship with patients, communities, and colleagues [13]. When examining biases, clinicians focus on growth in terms of values, attitudes, and beliefs, and an institution shifts policy, hiring, structure, faculty, and leaders to match with the community served. Traditional clinical (i.e., diagnostic, treatment) and training approaches in medicine have etic perspectives (i.e., general, structural, objective) whereas culture, language, and public health approaches have emic perspectives (i.e., participant-based, internal/subjective, and functional) [59, 60].

The concept of cultural safety originated with the Māori of Aotearoa [New Zealand) [59, 60], with foci on: health gains and positive outcomes; relationships within healthcare; power relations between participants, with empowerment of service users; and addressing the relationship of history, political, social, and employment status, housing, education, gender and personal experience to current healthcare interactions [61, 62]. Cultural safety challenges health providers to recognize power relations and attend to social determinants of health, which are ongoing impacts of colonization and structural racism [61–63]. There is also a robust body of evidence highlighting the importance of rigorous and systematic methods to the adaptation of evidence-based interventions according to the culture, language, and context of the target population group, with growing recognition of employing these approaches to the adaptation of digital interventions [63].

3.4.2 Professional Organizations and Other Guidelines

Numerous accreditation bodies in medicine, public health, nursing education, and social work contribute to making cultural competency a standard of care [64], based on a broad international scope of position statements, policies, and guidelines for culturally competent care come from medicine, psychiatry, psychology, US social work, counseling, and marriage/family [15] (Table 3.2). The cultural competencies for First Nations, Inuit, and Metis Health Core Competencies are also an excellent prototype for a specific population, and the Canadian Psychiatric Association Guidelines for Training in Cultural Psychiatry provide a broad overview for institutions and are also consensus based [21, 22].

The Cultural and Linguistic Appropriate Services (CLAS) Standards focus on culturally competent care and organizational supports [65, 66] and include technology as a solution for barriers. The goal is to build trust [16] and improve outcomes

Table 3.2 A comparison of health organizations' cultural competency standards, practice documents, position statements, and guidelines

American Association for Marriage and Family Therapy, 2018. Competencies for Family Therapists Working in Health Care Settings
www.aamft.org/healthcare
1. Six anchoring competency domains: Systems; biological, psychological, social, and spiritual (BPSS); collaboration; leadership; ethics; and diversity
(a) Biological, psychological, social, and spiritual: Recognizing that health is comprised of all four areas of mutual influence
• 2.1b. Identifies and applies BPSS framework in relation to diseases and conditions common to the setting
• 2.1d. Understands common biological and mental/behavioral comorbidities of various health conditions (e.g., chronic pain, depression) with consideration of cultural and spiritual beliefs and practices
(b) Diversity: Recognizing various groups, communities, and cultural influences that impact the delivery, response, policies, and study of integrated behavioral health care
• 6.1a. Demonstrates understanding of different sociocultural and socioeconomic beliefs, practice, and traditions regarding health and health care (including diverse views regarding health disparities and healing across all BPSS dimensions) (e.g., identifies specific health care beliefs, practices, and/or traditions that are unique to the populations they serve)
• 6.1b. Demonstrates awareness of and sensitivity to social locations (e.g., ability, age, citizenship, geographic location, race/ethnicity, sexual/gender identity and orientation, socioeconomic status) in relation to assessment, diagnoses, and treatment options
• 6.1e. Demonstrates recognition of one's own personal biases and beliefs about diverse patient populations, health care disciplines, or settings and openness to seek support/training/supervision to improve clinical practice/clinical research
• 6.2a. Develops instructional methods that build learners' and supervisees' confidence and competence in areas of clinical services, research, and/or teaching with diverse patient/learner/participant populations and diverse inter-professional collaborators
• 6.2c. Promotes learners and supervisees' cultural humility in relational and BPSS practice, research, and teaching initiatives
• 6.3a. Recognizes and mitigates the impacts policies and laws have on diverse populations
• 6.4a. Demonstrates cultural sensitivity and humility as an integrated behavioral health care and relational researcher
• 6.4b. Addresses ethical dilemmas pertaining to implementation of research studies with vulnerable populations and minority groups
American Association of Medical Colleges, 2015. Cultural Competence Education
https://www.aamc.org/system/files/c/2/54338-culturalcomped.pdf
The Core Competencies for Entering Medical Students, 2020
https://students-residents.aamc.org/applying-medical-school/article/core-competencies/
Cultural competence: Demonstrates knowledge of sociocultural factors that affect interactions and behaviors; shows an appreciation and respect for multiple dimensions of diversity; recognizes and acts on the obligation to inform one's own judgment; engages diverse and competing perspectives as a resource for learning, citizenship, and work; recognizes and appropriately addresses bias in themselves and others; interacts effectively with people from diverse backgrounds
Tool for assessing cultural competence training (TACCT)

(continued)

Table 3.2 (continued)

https://www.aamc.org/what-we-do/mission-areas/diversity-inclusion/tool-for-assessing-cultural-competence-training
Original TACCT
• Tools for Assessing Cultural Competence Training (TACCT) (PDF)
• Tools for Assessing Cultural Competence Training (TACCT) (Excel)
• Guidelines for preparing and completing the TACCT instrument: Using TACCT
• Background: Cultural Competence Education for Medical Students: Assessing and Revising Curriculum (PDF)
• Cultural Competence Education for Medical Students: Alphabetical Bibliography (PDF)
• Cultural Competence Education for Medical Students: Categorical Bibliography (PDF)
Revised TACCT
These resources are available on MedEdPORTAL, a free repository of educational materials and resources. Please note that login information is needed for access
• A Revised Curriculum Tool for Assessing Cultural Competency Training (TACCT) in Health Professions Education (2009). (Lie REF)
• Critical Synthesis Package: Tool for Assessing Cultural Competence Training (TACCT): Boardman J. Critical synthesis package: tool for assessing cultural competence training (TACCT). (MedEdPortal REF)
Assessing Change: Evaluating Cultural Competence Education and Training
https://www.aamc.org/system/files/2019-08/document-diversityandinclusion-assessingchange-08-14-19.pdf
American Counseling Association, 2014. Code of Ethics https://www.counseling.org/resources/aca-code-of-ethics.pdf
1. Section C Professional Responsibility
(a) C.5. Nondiscrimination counselors do not condone or engage in discrimination against prospective or current clients, students, employees, supervisees, or research participants based on age, culture, disability, ethnicity, race, religion/spirituality, gender, gender identity, sexual orientation, marital/partnership status, language preference, socioeconomic status, immigration status, or any basis proscribed by law
2. Section E Evaluation, Assessment, and Interpretation
(a) E.5. Diagnosis of Mental Disorders E.5.b. Cultural Sensitivity: Counselors recognize that culture affects the manner in which clients' problems are defined and experienced. Clients' socioeconomic and cultural experiences are considered when diagnosing mental disorders
(b) E.8. Multicultural Issues/Diversity in Assessment: Counselors select and use with caution assessment techniques normed on populations other than that of the client. Counselors recognize the effects of age, color, culture, disability, ethnic group, gender, race, language preference, religion, spirituality, sexual orientation, and socioeconomic status on test administration and interpretation, and they place test results in proper perspective with other relevant factors
3. Section F Supervision, Training, and Teaching
(a) F.11. Multicultural/Diversity Competence in Counselor Education and Training ProgramsF.11.b. Student Diversity Counselor educators actively attempt to recruit and retain a diverse student body. Counselor educators demonstrate commitment to multicultural/diversity competence by recognizing and valuing the diverse cultures and types of abilities that students bring to the training experience. Counselor educators provide appropriate accommodations that enhance and support diverse student well-being and academic performance

(continued)

Table 3.2 (continued)

American Counseling Association: Other
1. Competencies for Counseling the Multiracial Population: Couples, Families, and Individuals; and Transracial Adoptees and Families, 2015 https://www.counseling.org/docs/default-source/competencies/competencies-for-counseling-the-multiracial-population-2-2-15-final.pdf?sfvrsn=c7ba412c_14
2. Competencies for Addressing Spiritual and Religious Issues in Counseling, 2009 https://www.counseling.org/docs/default-source/competencies/competencies-for-addressing-spiritual-and-religious-issues-in-counseling.pdf?sfvrsn=aad7c2c_8
3. Multicultural and Social Justice Counseling Competencies, 2015 https://www.counseling.org/docs/default-source/competencies/multicultural-and-social-justice-counseling-competencies.pdf?sfvrsn=8573422c_20
(a) Counselor Self-Awareness
(b) Client Worldview
(c) Counseling Relationship
• *Attitudes and beliefs*: Privileged and marginalized counselors are aware of how client and counselor worldviews, assumptions, attitudes, values, beliefs, biases, social identities, social group statuses, and experiences with power, privilege, and oppression influence the counseling relationship
Multicultural and social justice competent counselors:
Acknowledge that the worldviews, values, beliefs, and biases held by privileged and marginalized counselors and clients will positively or negatively influence the counseling relationship
Acknowledge that counselor and client identity development shapes the counseling relationship to varying degrees for privileged and marginalized clients
Acknowledge that the privileged and marginalized status of counselors and clients will influence the counseling relationship to varying degrees
Acknowledge that culture, stereotypes, discrimination, power, privilege, and oppression influence the counseling relationship with privileged and marginalized group clients
Acknowledge that the counseling relationship may extend beyond the traditional office setting and into the community
Acknowledge that cross-cultural communication is key to connecting with privileged and marginalized clients
• *Knowledge*: Privileged and marginalized counselors possess knowledge of how client and counselor worldviews, assumptions, attitudes, values, beliefs, biases, social identities, social group statuses, and experiences with power, privilege, and oppression influence the counseling relationship
• *Skills*: Privileged and marginalized counselors possess skills to engage in discussions with clients about how client and counselor worldviews, assumptions, attitudes, values, beliefs, biases, social identities, social group statuses, power, privilege, and oppression influence the counseling relationship
(d) Counseling and Advocacy Interventions
American Medical Association, 2020. 5 Keys to Student Diversity: Changing the Face of Medical Education. https://www.ama-assn.org/education/medical-school-diversity/5-keys-student-diversity-changing-face-medical-education and https://www.ama-assn.org/member-groups-sections/minority-affairs/about-minority-affairs-section-mas
1. Develop curricular innovations that focus on health care disparities and the social determinants of health
2. Use Liaison Committee on Medical Education (LCME) Standards to garner support

(continued)

Table 3.2 (continued)

3. Create premedical post-baccalaureate programs for underrepresented students
4. Enhance admissions processes to promote diversity
5. Develop a research agenda that measures and promotes the results of diversity-based programs
American Psychological Association. Guidelines for Providers of Psychological Services to Ethnic, Linguistic, and Culturally Diverse Populations, 2017. http://www.apa.org/pi/oema/resources/policy/provider-guidelines.aspx
American Psychiatric Association, 2020. Best Practice Highlights for Treating Diverse Patient Populations: A Guide to Help Assessment and Treatment of Patients from Diverse Populations
https://www.psychiatry.org/psychiatrists/cultural-competency/education/best-practice-highlights
American Psychiatric Association, 2020. Diversity and Health Equity Education. https://www.psychiatry.org/psychiatrists/cultural-competency/education
As part of APA's efforts to prepare culturally competent psychiatrists, the Department of Diversity and Health Equity partners with subject matter experts and psychiatrists to develop online educational resources. These resources, including fact sheets, guides, and online learning modules, help clinicians provide quality health care that addresses the needs of culturally diverse populations
• [NEW] Mental Health Facts for Bisexual Populations
• [NEW] Mental Health Facts for Refugees, Asylum-seekers, and Survivors of Forced Displacement
• [NEW CME MODULE] Gay Men's Mental Health
Topics on vulnerable populations
• Mental health disparities: Diverse populations
https://www.psychiatry.org/psychiatrists/cultural-competency/education/mental-health-facts
• A guide for working with transgender and gender nonconforming patients
https://www.psychiatry.org/psychiatrists/cultural-competency/education/transgender-and-gender-nonconforming-patients
Diverse populations
• African Americans*
• Appalachian People
• American Indian/Alaska Native/Native Hawaiian*
• Asian Americans*
• Hispanics and Latinos/as*
• International Medical Graduates*
• Lesbian, Gay, Bisexual, Transgender, and Queer/Questioning*
• Women*
• Other Vulnerable Populations
*One of APA's seven official Minority/Underrepresented Caucuses
American Psychological Association
Multicultural Guidelines: An Ecological Approach to Context, Identity, and Intersectionality, 2017 http://www.apa.org/about/policy/multicultural-guidelines.pdf
Guideline 1. Psychologists seek to recognize and understand that identity and self-definition are fluid and complex and that the interaction between the two is dynamic. To this end, psychologists appreciate that intersectionality is shaped by the multiplicity of the individual's social contexts

(continued)

Table 3.2 (continued)

Guideline 2. Psychologists aspire to recognize and understand that as cultural beings, they hold attitudes and beliefs that can influence their perceptions of and interactions with others as well as their clinical and empirical conceptualizations. As such, psychologists strive to move beyond conceptualizations rooted in categorical assumptions, biases, and/or formulations based on limited knowledge about individuals and communities
Guideline 3. Psychologists strive to recognize and understand the role of language and communication through engagement that is sensitive to the lived experience of the individual, couple, family, group, community, and/or organizations with whom they interact. Psychologists also seek to understand how they bring their own language and communication to these interactions
Guideline 4. Psychologists endeavor to be aware of the role of the social and physical environment in the lives of clients, students, research participants, and/or consultees
Guideline 5. Psychologists aspire to recognize and understand historical and contemporary experiences with power, privilege, and oppression. As such, they seek to address institutional barriers and related inequities, disproportionalities, and disparities of law enforcement, administration of criminal justice, educational, mental health, and other systems as they seek to promote justice, human rights, and access to quality and equitable mental and behavioral health services
Guideline 6. Psychologists seek to promote culturally adaptive interventions and advocacy within and across systems, including prevention, early intervention, and recovery
Guideline 7. Psychologists endeavor to examine the profession's assumptions and practices within an international context, whether domestically or internationally based, and consider how this globalization has an impact on the psychologist's self-definition, purpose, role, and function
Guideline 8. Psychologists seek awareness and understanding of how developmental stages and life transitions intersect with the larger biosociocultural context, how identity evolves as a function of such intersections, and how these different socialization and maturation experiences influence worldview and identity
Guideline 9. Psychologists strive to conduct culturally appropriate and informed research, teaching, supervision, consultation, assessment, interpretation, diagnosis, dissemination, and evaluation of efficacy as they address the first four levels of the layered ecological model of the multicultural guidelines
Guideline 10. Psychologists actively strive to take a strength-based approach when working with individuals, families, groups, communities, and organizations that seeks to build resilience and decrease trauma within the sociocultural context
Guidelines for Providers of Psychological Services to Ethnic, Linguistic, and Culturally Diverse Populations, 1990
https://www.apa.org/pi/oema/resources/policy/provider-guidelines
Preamble: The guidelines represent general principles that are intended to be aspirational in nature and are designed to provide suggestions to psychologists in working with ethnic, linguistic, and culturally diverse populations
1. Psychologists educate their clients to the processes of psychological intervention, such as goals and expectations; the scope and, where appropriate, legal limits of confidentiality; and the psychologists' orientations
2. Psychologists are cognizant of relevant research and practice issues as related to the population being served
3. Psychologists recognize ethnicity and culture as significant parameters in understanding psychological processes
4. Psychologists respect the roles of family members and community structures, hierarchies, values, and beliefs within the client's culture

(continued)

Table 3.2 (continued)

5. Psychologists respect clients' religious and/or spiritual beliefs and values, including attributions and taboos, since they affect world view, psychosocial functioning, and expressions of distress
6. Psychologists interact in the language requested by the client and, if this is not feasible, make an appropriate referral
7. Psychologists consider the impact of adverse social, environmental, and political factors in assessing problems and designing interventions
8. Psychologists attend to as well as work to eliminate biases, prejudices, and discriminatory practices
9. Psychologists working with culturally diverse populations should document culturally and sociopolitically relevant factors in the records
***Australian Indigenous Psychologists Association*, 2020**
http://www.indigenouspsychology.com.au/
1. Aboriginal and Torres Strait Islander people will have access to equitable, timely, safe, sustainable, evidence-based psychological care that respects and promotes their cultural integrity, regardless of where they live
2. Psychology in Australia will be responsive to aboriginal and Torres Strait islander cultures, values, and belief systems and will be grounded in holistic indigenous perspectives and the determinants of social and emotional well-being
3. The number of indigenous entrants into undergraduate and postgraduate psychology programs, across all specialties, will increase and parity within the profession will be improved
Australian Psychological Society, 2018. Code of Ethics
https://www.psychology.org.au/getmedia/d873e0db-7490-46de-bb57-c31bb1553025/APS-Code-of-Ethics.pdf
Explanatory statement: "...have a high regard for the diversity and uniqueness of people and their right to linguistically and culturally appropriate services. *Psychologists* acknowledge people's right to be treated fairly without discrimination or favouritism, and they Endeavour to ensure that all people have reasonable and fair access to *psychological services* and share in the benefits that the practice of psychology can offer"
British Psychological Society, 2018, Code of Ethics and 2017, Practice Guideline
Code of ethics
https://www.bps.org.uk/news-and-policy/bps-code-ethics-and-conduct
3.1. Respect: Respect for the dignity of persons and peoples is one of the most fundamental and universal ethical principles across geographical and cultural boundaries, and across professional disciplines. It provides the philosophical foundation for many of the other ethical principles. Respect for dignity recognizes the inherent worth of all human beings, regardless of perceived or real differences in social status, ethnic origin, gender, capacities, or any other such group-based characteristics. This inherent worth means that all human beings are worthy of equal moral consideration Statement of values: Psychologists value the dignity and worth of all persons, with sensitivity to the dynamics of perceived authority or influence over persons and peoples and with particular regard to people's rights
Practice guideline
https://www.bps.org.uk/news-and-policy/bps-code-ethics-and-conduct
2.0. Where psychologists work
2.1 working environment: whether the setting is culturally acceptable to clients
2.4. Working for defense and security organizations: Psychologists working with these populations should ensure they investigate and acknowledge cultural differences, particularly when working with other national cultures

(continued)

Table 3.2 (continued)

3.9. Working with detained people: Detained people may be afraid of raising a particular topic in case it is misunderstood, or too embarrassed because of cultural standards
3.11. Working with cultural difference: Psychologists need to be aware of stereotypical beliefs and assumptions that manifest in thinking about culture and ethnic groups. Psychologists should bear in mind the history of racism and the early development of Western psychology and culturally biased testing biases Psychologists need to understand the discrimination suffered by people from diverse and/or minority ethnic and religious backgrounds as a result of:
• The interchangeable use of the terms race, culture, and ethnicity leading either to the perception of black and minority culture, race, and ethnicity as unitary or an assumption that knowing about these cultures solves the problem of equality, fairness, and availability of services
• The maintenance of the color-blind approach in service where "one size fits all," resulting in a lack of formal recognition of the varied diverse needs as well as these needs being ignored, unacknowledged, or assumed to be the same
• The lack of appropriate culturally relevant psychological therapy available to certain black and minority ethnic (BME) communities
• Being discriminated against on grounds of "special" needs, effectively considered as "cultural pathology"
• Experiencing instances of indirect, subtle, or unintentional discrimination often called "micro-aggressions"
It would be expected that all practicing psychologists should develop a productive working relationship with culturally and linguistically diverse groups of people by:
• Avoiding different types of biases and finding new ways (verbally and non-verbally) to build rapport and respect
• Using and working with trained interpreters in assessment, formulation, and intervention work as well as research work
• Being aware of the impact of culture, ethnicity, and religion in assessment, formulation, and intervention processes and the use of norm-referenced tests that do not include minority ethnic groups as part of their standardization
• Pre-assessing and pre-incorporating ethnic identity (including its fine gradations, region, class, and generation), which can have impacts on processes and outcomes of psychological work
• Acknowledging their own ethnocentricity and possible underlying socially conditioned prejudice to people who are "different"; psychologists need to acknowledge that people can change, irrespective of their differences and psychological distress
• Relooking at current models of mental health, which traditionally reflect Western constructions, and incorporating other world views of psychological well-being
• Understanding and respecting the different concepts of health and illness that exist within different ethnicities, including newly arrived people from Europe and refugees from Syria, Turkey, Somalia, etc
3.12. Working with people of faith, religion, and spirituality
3.13. Working with sexual and gender minorities
3.14. Working with people who may be socially excluded

(continued)

Table 3.2 (continued)

4.0. Safeguarding. Institutional abuse is the mistreatment or neglect by a regime or individuals, in settings that people who may be at risk reside in or use. Institutional abuse may occur when routines, systems, and regimes result in poor standards of care, poor practice and behaviors, inflexible regimes, and rigid routines, which violate the dignity and human rights of the adults and place them at risk of harm. It may occur within a culture that denies, restricts, or curtails privacy, dignity, choice, and independence. It involves the collective failure of a service provider or an organization to provide safe and appropriate services and includes a failure to ensure the necessary preventative and/or protective measures are in place
Canadian Medical Association
CMA Launches New Equity and Diversity Initiative. March 6, 2020
https://www.cma.ca/news/you-cannot-be-what-you-cannot-see-cma-launches-equity-and-diversity-policy
The Health of Aboriginal Peoples, 2002
https://policybase.cma.ca/documents/policypdf/PD03-02.pdf
Recommendations
1. That the federal government adopt a comprehensive strategy for improving the health of aboriginal peoples that involves a partnership among governments, nongovernmental organizations, universities, and the aboriginal communities
2. That all stakeholders work to improve provision for the essential needs of aboriginal peoples and communities that affect their health (e.g., housing, employment, education, water supply)
3. That governments and other stakeholders work toward resolving issues of self-determination for aboriginal peoples and their communities in areas of cultural, social, political, and economic life
4. That all stakeholders actively encourage the development of integrated, holistic primary care service delivery relevant to the needs and culture of aboriginal communities and under community control
5. Promote educational initiatives in cross-cultural awareness and practice tools
6. Governments and other stakeholders simplify and clarify jurisdictional responsibilities with respect to aboriginal health at the federal, provincial, and municipal level, with a goal of simplifying access to service delivery
7. Strategies be explored to increase access to health services by remote communities; for example, through the use of technology (e.g., web sites, telemedicine) to connect them with academic medical centers
8. Medical and other health faculties increase access and support programs to encourage enrollment of aboriginal students
9. Government of Canada support the First Nations and Inuit Regional Longitudinal Health Survey Process, and the First Nations and Inuit Health Information System, and parallel interests for the Métis and Inuit
10. Government and other stakeholders support aboriginal peoples and communities in the development of aboriginal research, the means of interpreting its findings, and make public results a priority in order to facilitate its use by aboriginal communities
Canadian Psychological Association, 2018. Canadian Code of Ethics for Psychologists
https://cpa.ca/docs/File/Ethics/CPA_Code_2017_4thEd.pdf
Ethical principles
1. Respect for the Dignity of Persons and Peoples. Demonstrate appropriate respect for the knowledge, insight, experience, areas of expertise, and cultural perspectives and values of others, including those that are different from their own

(continued)

Table 3.2 (continued)

(a)	Informed consent. Accept and document non-written consent (e.g., oral, a verbal agreement, a handshake, or other culturally normative exchange)
(b)	Privacy. Respect the moral right of research participants, employees, supervisees, students, and trainees to reasonable personal privacy, and take care not to infringe, in research, teaching, supervision, or service activities, on the personally, developmentally, or culturally defined private space of individuals or groups (e.g., couples, families, organizations, communities, peoples)
2. Responsible Caring	
(a)	Cultural discrimination or oppression
(b)	Risks/benefits are appropriate to the particular cultural and social contexts of the individuals and groups involved
(c)	Maximize benefit. This information would be communicated in ways that are developmentally, linguistically, and culturally appropriate, and that are meaningful and helpful
3. Integrity in Relationships	
(a)	Fully open and straightforward disclosure might not be needed or desired by others and, in some circumstances, might be a risk to their dignity, well-being, or best interests, or considered culturally inappropriate
(b)	The risk level and acceptability of other conflicts of interest (e.g., dual or multiple relationships) might be partially dependent on cultural or geographic factors.
(c)	Conflicts of interest. Culturally contraindications
4. Responsibility to Society	
(a)	Respect for society. In their scientific and professional activities, convey respect for and abide by prevailing mores, social customs, and cultural expectations of organizations, communities, and peoples, provided that this does not contravene any of the ethical principles of this *Code*
(b)	Development of society.
•	If their work is related to societal issues, be especially careful to keep well informed of social, cultural, historical, economic, institutional, legal, and political context issues through relevant reading, peer consultation, and continuing education
•	Not promote, contribute to, nor engage in any activity that contravenes international humanitarian law (e.g., declarations, treaties, or conventions regarding: human rights; torture and other cruel, inhumane, or degrading treatment or punishment; economic, social, and cultural rights; civil and political rights; rights of indigenous peoples; children's rights; weapons of mass destruction; destruction of the environment)
Steps in Practice	
1. Consideration of how one's own biases, external pressures, personal needs, self-interest, or cultural, social, historical, economic, institutional, legal, or political context and background, might influence the development of or choice between courses of action	
2. Analysis of likely short-term, ongoing, and long-term risks and benefits of each course of action on the individuals and groups involved or likely to be affected, taking into account relevant individual and cultural, social, historical, economic, institutional, legal, and political contextual factors	
Definitions	
1. "Moral rights" means the fundamental and inalienable rights of persons and peoples… aspects may not be so contained or protected. Of particular significance to *psychologists* are moral rights to: developmentally appropriate privacy and confidentiality, self-determination, and liberty; cultural identity, cultural survival, and social participation; and distributive, social, and natural justice	

(continued)

Table 3.2 (continued)

Liaison Committee on Medical Education, 2019. Functions and Structure of a Medical School. Standards for Accreditation of Medical Education Programs Leading to the MD Degree
https://lcme.org/publications/
1. Specific competencies
(a) 3.3 (Diversity/Pipeline Programs and Partnerships) (institution rather than student)
(b) 7.5 (Social Problems) The faculty of a medical school ensure that the medical curriculum includes instruction in the diagnosis, prevention, appropriate reporting, and treatment of the medical consequences of common societal problems
(c) 7.6 (Cultural Competence/Health Care Disparities/Personal Bias)
The faculty of a medical school ensure that the medical curriculum provides opportunities for medical students to learn to recognize and appropriately address biases in themselves, in others, and in the health care delivery process. The medical curriculum includes content regarding the following:
• The diverse manner in which people perceive health and illness and respond to various symptoms, diseases, and treatments
• The basic principles of culturally competent health care
• Recognition of the impact of disparities in health care on all populations and potential methods to eliminate health care disparities The knowledge, skills, and core professional attributes needed to provide effective care in a multidimensional and diverse society
National Association of Social Workers. 2001 Standards for Cultural Competence in Social Work Practice
http://catholiccharitiesla.org/wp-content/uploads/NASW-Cultural-Competence-in-Social-Work-Practice.pdf
Standard 1. Ethics and Values. Social workers shall function in accordance with the values, ethics, and standards of the profession, recognizing how personal and professional values may conflict with or accommodate the needs of diverse clients
Standard 2. Self-Awareness. Social workers shall seek to develop an understanding of their own personal, cultural values and beliefs as one way of appreciating the importance of multicultural identities in the lives of people
Standard 3. Cross-Cultural Knowledge. Social workers shall have and continue to develop specialized knowledge and understanding about the history, traditions, values, family systems, and artistic expressions of major client groups that they serve
Standard 4. Cross-Cultural Skills. Social workers shall use appropriate methodological approaches, skills, and techniques that reflect the workers' understanding of the role of culture in the helping process
Standard 5. Service Delivery. Social workers shall be knowledgeable about and skillful in the use of services available in the community and broader society and be able to make appropriate referrals for their diverse clients
Standard 6. Empowerment and Advocacy. Social workers shall be aware of the effect of social policies and programs on diverse client populations, advocating for and with clients whenever appropriate
Standard 7. Diverse Workforce. Social workers shall support and advocate for recruitment, admissions and hiring, and retention efforts in social work programs and agencies that ensure diversity within the profession
Standard 8. Professional Education. Social workers shall advocate for and participate in educational and training programs that help advance cultural competence within the profession

(continued)

Table 3.2 (continued)

Standard 9. Language Diversity. Social workers shall seek to provide or advocate for the provision of information, referrals, and services in the language appropriate to the client, which may include use of interpreters
Standard 10. Cross-Cultural Leadership. Social workers shall be able to communicate information about diverse client groups to other professionals
Ethnicity and Race
https://www.socialworkers.org/practice/ethnicity-race
Lesbian, Gay, Bisexual, and Transgender (LGBT)
https://www.socialworkers.org/practice/LGBT
Royal College of Physicians and Surgeons Canada. CanMEDS Physician Competency Framework, 2015 http://canmeds.royalcollege.ca/uploads/en/framework/CanMEDS%202015%20Framework_EN_Reduced.pdf
1. Communicator
(a) Engage patients and their families in developing plans that reflect the patient's health care needs and goals
• Facilitate discussions with patients and their families in a way that is respectful, non-judgmental, and culturally safe
(b) Respect for diversity: 1.1, 1.6, 2.2, 4.1
2. Collaborator
(a) Respecting and valuing diversity: 1.2, 2.1, 2.2
3. Professional
(a) Respect for diversity: 1.1 "…values such as integrity, honesty, altruism, humility, respect for diversity"
4. Health Advocate.
(a) Promoting health equity, whereby individuals and populations reach their full health potential without being disadvantaged by, for example, race, ethnicity, religion, gender, sexual orientation, age, social class, economic status, or level of education
Scott K, Bourassa C, Dignan T, et al. Examining cultural safety: Indigenous health values and principles as interpreted through the CanMEDS framework. Poster, Royal College of Physicians and Surgeons of Canada Annual Meeting, 2014. https://www.hhr-rhs.ca/index.php?option=com_mtree&task=viewlink&link_id=11179&Itemid=456&lang=fr
Royal College of Physicians, UK, 2020. Doctors Can Promote Fairness and Equality in Health
https://www.rcplondon.ac.uk/news/doctors-can-promote-fairness-and-equality-health
Recommendations
• Refocus attitudes and resources in health care toward prevention rather than treatment of ill-health.
• Identify opportunities to help patients from disadvantaged backgrounds to manage their health, taking into account their social and physical environment, and to encourage patients from marginalized groups to access health information, screening, and health promotion services
• Encourage patients to undertake healthy activities such as cycling, which have co-benefits for both the patient and the environment. Persuade local authorities to supply the resources and green spaces to support more active lifestyles
• Urge doctors to join forces to advocate for health equality at all levels—from impassioned medical students to influential deans and directors. The entire profession can use its powerful voice to promote action on the social determinants of health

(continued)

Table 3.2 (continued)

• Restructure the undergraduate and postgraduate education of doctors to make the public health and social aspects of the courses more engaging. Give doctors in training the opportunities to be involved in issues around social determinants of health through innovative continuing professional development and certification
• Provide user-friendly and accessible information for socially disadvantaged groups and young people, and share information between doctors, public health teams, and researchers on best practices in reducing inequalities

for Indigenous people and those with limited English proficiency (LEP) [21]. Clinicians' increased cultural competence has been linked to increased patient satisfaction, treatment adherence, and information seeking and sharing [21]. Such leadership paradigms may transform community practices by building capacity, reducing silos, and developing partnerships. Project ECHO—a collaborative model of medical education and care management that connects rural primary care teams with specialist teams—has increased participant self-efficacy and reduced isolation of rural providers, using an Indigenous well-being curriculum with behavioral health components and a specialist team (i.e., psychiatrist, social work, and an Indigenous Elder and others) [64]. The inclusion of local, regional, and international cultural perceptions and customs may also help to scale-up behavioral health treatment for health systems regardless of resources (e.g., help refugees) [65–68].

In terms of education and training, students need to learn intellectually *and* relationally and emotionally, in a culturally rich, safe environment—an immersive educational experience that is transformative and profound (extension for Community Healthcare Outcomes, Struminger). The BPS [69] or biopsychosocial (BPS) with biopsychosocialcultural (BPSC) adaptations [70] model may help trainees and clinicians. Another practical approach would be to shorten the Cultural Formulation Interview's (CFI) 16 items to 2 items (i.e., CFI-2) for medical students and a CFI-4 for residents [71]. Terminology that combines the words technology and culture—"techture"—may also help facilitate reflection on how the patient's and clinician's background and technology's structure and programming influence communication and user adaptation [72]. Lastly, a culturally safe environment for learning can enhance skill, team, and care outcomes, with modification for Indigenous students' competing cultural obligations [73].

3.4.3 Cultural Competencies for Health Care Clinicians and Institutions

The literature revealed no operationalized skills based on cultural competence, humility, or safety—and only select cultural skills were mentioned in the accreditation council of graduate medical education (ACGME) Milestones and CanMEDS frameworks [21]. The authors built a framework using ACGME domains and subdomains with excerpts from the addiction medicine, clinical informatics, family medicine, internal medicine, psychiatry, and surgery Milestones, with Novice/Advanced Beginner, Competent/Proficient, and Expert Levels. Additional resources used to develop the depth and breadth of the competencies included: the Outline for Cultural Formulation [74]; CFI [71]; and its Supplementary Modules [75].

Likewise, telehealth, culture, and health equity affect all levels of an organization, so institutional competencies are suggested to: (1) assess readiness; (2) create/hardwire the culture; (3) write policies and procedures; (4) establish the curriculum and competencies; (5) train learners and faculty; and (6) evaluate/manage change [21, 76] (Table 3.3). For example, clinical care and technology must be adapted to age/generation, culture, and other factors. Faculty have to acknowledge Indigenous students' cultures and enable them to feel safe. Leaders have to promote culture and diversity within all missions (e.g., hiring) so the workforce and leaders match the diversity of patients and the community without unintended consequences [75–78].

Table 3.3 Competencies for institutions/academic health centers for telehealth, culture, and health equity

Competency focus	Technology competencies	Cultural competencies
Patient-centered care	Distinguish between telehealth modalities Employ inter-professional teams and care coordination Understand data warehouse, analysis, and health information exchange concepts Screen patients for use of technology Implement policies and procedures to include telehealth use Teach and educate on consumer technologies (e.g., apps, sensors/wearables) Design clinical technology workflows Import social science, health behavior, and business concepts Monitor documentation quality and timeliness Employ care and navigation coordinators to use technology	Provide effective, equitable, understandable, and respectful quality care and services that are responsive to diverse cultural health beliefs and practices, preferred languages, health literacy, and other communication needs Inform all individuals of the availability of language assistance services clearly and in their preferred language, and help those with limited English proficiency and other communication needs; use those trained in language assistance Provide easy-to-understand print and multimedia materials and signage in common languages Employ teams, care coordination, and navigation Acknowledge indigenous patients' cultures and enable them to feel safe Screen eHealth literacy and how populations seek online health information Use clinical tools, interventions, and other e-services adapted to culture

(continued)

Table 3.3 (continued)

Competency focus	Technology competencies	Cultural competencies
Evaluation and outcomes	Assess clinicians on readiness for change Link behavior to outcomes for a patient or program Use evidence-based measures and disease state measures Use accreditation principles: Goal, measure, benchmark, target, and data Build video scheduled and on-demand options Use 360 evaluation Organize care on a technology platform (e.g., electronic health record) Standardize clinician workflow, for those who work asynchronously, with training, policies, and procedures Use social science, health service, and business constructs to shift evaluation of skills and attitudes	Establish culturally and linguistically appropriate goals, policies, and procedures for accountability throughout operations Conduct ongoing assessments of the organization's cultural and linguistic appropriate services (CLAS)-related activities to assess, collect data, and monitor the impact on health equity and outcomes Assess community assets and needs to plan and implement services to fit cultural and linguistic diversity of populations Develop evaluation tools, measures, and processes that are culturally sensitive in order to assess screening, diagnosis, and intervention for individuals Assess cultural literacy in the training, clinician, and other workforce Assess patient-directed interventions, building and supporting local capacity, and the need for remote access to specialists Use evidence-based measures (e.g., Joint Commission)
Trainee/student needs/roles	Prepare as resource manager Clarify personal versus professional technology use Use technology as a lifelong learner/teacher and model healthy behaviors Integrate skill development, care, teaching, and supervision Monitor well-being and professionalism Adjust curricula (e.g., part-time rotations, supervision)	Gain experience with a variety of culturally diverse populations Use cultural paradigms (competency, humility, safety) as a lifelong learner/teacher Integrate skill and attitude development with knowledge for patient care and education Learn to use trained interpreters for in-person, video, and asynchronous care (as applicable) Acknowledge indigenous patients' and peers' cultures and enable them to feel safe

(continued)

Table 3.3 (continued)

Competency focus	Technology competencies	Cultural competencies
Faculty clinical, teaching, and leadership roles	Emphasize communication, well-being, and professionalism Emphasize resource manager technology leadership role Monitor technology impact on care, well-being/fatigue Define success based on teams, systems, and populations Use sustainable, longitudinal approaches Remember that "less is more" and evidence base is key Use technology for portfolio, curricula, dissemination, networking, and other purposes Use faculty development projects for existing/new leaders	Develop or import an indigenous-based cultural safety educational initiative Develop departmental, school, and community culture and diversity committees and interest groups Consider the role of adverse childhood experiences in patient care for health education, health promotion, and mitigation of trauma, chronic stress, and behavioral and emotional sequelae Advocate for building and supporting local capacity and access to remote specialists Acknowledge indigenous students' cultures and enable them to feel safe Support, contribute to, and build curricula Create conflict and grievance resolution processes that are culturally and linguistically appropriate to identify, prevent, and resolve conflicts or complaints
Teams, professions, and systems within institutions	Assess structure/function of social groups that govern behavior of a community Use faculty development with teams, projects, and professions to build skills and shift culture Foster alignment across systems Organize goals and outcomes for success based on teams and systems Use team-based care and virtual teams Align outcomes: patient/clinician outcomes; learner/teacher; clinic/system; and institution/community	Embrace and lead cultural safety education and application to practice to improve relationships, health outcomes, and support indigenous people entering health education programs Mentor graduates interested in working in diverse communities Explore, teach, and role model the shift of etic population health surveillance, universal screening, and diagnostic screening to emic approaches for clinical care and education Implement patient-directed interventions, build and support local capacity, and access remote specialists Identify and report potential institutional racism

(continued)

Table 3.3 (continued)

Competency focus	Technology competencies	Cultural competencies
Academic health center organizational structure, process, and finance	Evaluate/manage governance structure and change Weigh human resources, technology, and cost issues Market technology delivery of care competitively Build academic health center–community partnerships to share resources and integrate care Align clinical, educational, and research missions and values Integrate (not add or append) information technology into organizational structure Measure technology in performance evaluations and provide feedback Add research and funding infrastructure for pilot and full-scale projects Assess context, pace, scope, and drive of/for change Monitor private, federal, state, and other sectors for best practices, partner agencies, and grant funding Select incremental, sustainable solutions Adapt evidence-based approaches Develop strategies for promoting adoption/optimization of clinical information systems	Advance and sustain organizational governance and leadership that promotes CLAS and health equity through policy, practices, and allocated resources Recruit, promote, and support a culturally and linguistically diverse governance, leadership, and workforce that is responsive to the population Educate and train governance, leadership, and workforce in culturally and linguistically appropriate policies and practices on an ongoing basis Promote culture and diversity within all missions Reduce barriers to access related to culture, language, and other disparities for health care Strategically design, implement, and evaluate cultural safety curriculum policies for clinical and community sites to ensure cultural and linguistic appropriateness Reflect on current power structures and consider changes in hiring, systems, and leadership to reflect the diversity of patients and trainees Advocate toward health equity and improved health for indigenous people and communities Promote cultural safety education to increase indigenous people entering health education programs and in working in diverse communities Prioritize the shift of etic to emic care approaches Screen, assess, and intervene to promote well-being and reduce institutional racism Communicate the organization's progress in implementing and sustaining CLAS to all stakeholders, constituents, and the general public

3.5 Discussion

E-platforms in networks in communities, clinics and health care systems have empowered consumers and clinicians in day-to-day health care delivery by improving access to evidence-based information at the point of care. [79] They have also: facilitated the delivery of a wider range of health services, particularly to primary and community care; provided accurate data to policy and governance stakeholders; and ensured a sustainable, secure, reliable electronic environment [79]—in settings where there is robust technology access and infrastructure. However, across lower resource settings internationally, and in both higher and lower income countries, there remain key problem areas and limitations: (1) technology infrastructure; (2) policy, human resource and health governance challenges for behavioral health management IS (e.g., data collection, reporting, dissemination) and infrastructure (e.g., experts, technical support, supervision); (3) inadequate inclusion of behavioral health care in budgets, in general, and limited efforts to integrate behavioral health into medical settings; and (4) limited emphasis on program implementation and sustainability. [80, 81] Greater attention, though, is given to control and eradication of infectious diseases and conditions associated with reproductive, maternal and child health, as well as to disaster response.

Successful implementation of behavioral health indicators is dependent on their evidence base, and importantly is a function of acceptability, feasibility, and sustainability [4]. Unconventional and innovative approaches to collect data on indicators (e.g., using community health workers, care coordinators, mid-level providers) [82, 83] show promise for integrating behavioral health care in primary care settings. Referred to as task sharing, training non-specialist providers like community health workers is a robust approach—along with using technology—for scaling up capacity and making evidence-based services more available in both higher- and lower-income countries [84, 85]. There remain barriers to measuring new indicators related to the time consumed in recording (e.g., severity of illness, functionality), overstretched health workers, poor coordination within and across departments, and poor service delivery [3]. At the organizational level, utilization-focused evaluation may reduce uncertainties, improve effectiveness, and inform decisions on the goals, concerns, and perspectives of stakeholders [2, 21].

Improvement in culturally safe practices with technology for health care includes better assessment, evaluation of technological fluency and health literacy, and training on cultural/language factors for patients, families, clinicians, and trainees. The good news is that professional organizations are moving forward with efforts to improve care by outlining best practices and goals (e.g., Tables 3.1 and 3.2)—including model programs, delivery systems, and administration. But awareness of these issues does not translate into tangible and sustainable practices for most health systems, which can be facilitated by evidence- and consensus-based approaches to cultural safety and humility (e.g., competencies to ensure quality for trainees *and* clinicians in practice as well as institutional competencies for organizational change) [2], particularly for creating a diverse workforce [84–87].

3.6 Conclusions

Various technologies are employed for many types of patient-centered care, with information systems, electronic health records, electronic communication, behavioral health indicators, and related digital advances playing instrumental roles in advancing practice and research. Needs assessments help to develop appropriate outcomes for patients, clinicians, and systems, which then need to be aligned with technological, quality improvement, and other workflows used by health systems. By grasping how systems are designed and tailored to collect data, patients are empowered to make decisions and clinicians benefit from decision support. Setting priorities involves input from all care participants, and patient, clinician, and institutional competencies for skills, attitudes, and behaviors can align missions and stimulate quality improvement. Cultural safety and humility focuses on patients' experiences and values, and this empowers patients' roles in clinical care. A culturally safe approach would also ensure that digital health services are designed with communities, and do not create a system of health care that ignores local context, strengths, and knowledge. A culturally safe approach would help prevent the perpetuation of mistrust in health care and to mitigate the inequities that are the result of racism within health care.

Acknowledgments American Telemedicine Association and the Telemental Health Interest Group.

- Department of Psychiatry and Behavioral Sciences, University of California, Davis School of Medicine.
- European Psychiatric Association and World Psychiatric Association.
- Veteran Affairs Northern California Health Care System and Mental Health Service.
- World Health Organization and Psychiatric Association.

Conflicts of Interest None.

References

1. Institute of Medicine. Crossing the quality chasm; 2001. http://www.iom.edu/~/media/Files/Report%20Files/2001/Crossing-the-Quality-Chasm/Quality%20Chasm%202001%20%20report%20brief.pdf. Accessed 1 Aug 2020.
2. Hilty DM, Torous J, Parish M, et al. A literature review comparing clinicians' approaches and skills to in-person, synchronous and asynchronous care: moving toward asynchronous competencies to ensure quality care. Telemed J E-Health. 2020;27:356. https://doi.org/10.1089/tmj.2020.0054.
3. Ahuja S, Hanlon C, Chisholm D, et al. Experience of implementing new mental health indicators within information systems in six low- and middle-income countries. BJPsych Open. 2019;5(5):e71. Published 2019 Aug 6. https://doi.org/10.1192/bjo.2019.29.
4. Proctor E, Silmere H, Raghavan R, et al. Outcomes for implementation research: conceptual distinctions, measurement challenges, and research agenda. Adm Policy Ment Health. 2010;38(2):65–76.

5. Gargon E, Gorst SL, Williamson PR. Choosing important health outcomes for comparative effectiveness research: 5th annual update to a systematic review of core outcome sets for research. PLoS One. 2019;14(12):e0225980. https://doi.org/10.1371/journal.pone.0225980.
6. World Health Organization. Technology report on scalable psychological interventions for people in communities affected by adversity; 2017. https://www.who.int/mental_health/management/scalable_psychological_interventions/en/.
7. World Health Organization. Draft global strategy on digital health, 2020–2024; 2020. https://www.who.int/docs/default-source/documents/gs4dhdaa2a9f352b0445bafbc79ca799dce4d.pdf. Published 26 Jun 2020.
8. World Health Association. Culture matters: using a cultural context of health approach to enhance policy-making; 2017. http://www.euro.who.int/__data/assets/pdf_file/0009/334269/14780_World-Health-Organisation_Context-of-Health_TEXT-AW-WEB.pdf?ua=1.
9. Luo JL, Hilty DM, Worley LLM, et al. Considerations in change management related to technology. Acad Psychiatry. 2006;30(6):465–9.
10. Shanafelt TD, Dyrbye LN, West CP, et al. Potential impact of burnout on the US physician workforce. Mayo Clin Proc. 2016;91(11):1667–8. https://doi.org/10.1016/j.mayocp.2016.08.016.
11. Hilty DM, Armstrong CM, Smout SA, Crawford A, Maheu MM, Drude K, et al. Findings and guidelines on provider technology, fatigue, and well-being: scoping review. J Med Internet Res. 2022;24(5):e34451. Published 2022 May 25.
12. Luxton DD. Artificial intelligence in behavioral health care. Boston, MA: Elsevier; 2016.
13. Cross TL, Bazron B, Dennis K, et al. Towards a culturally competent system of care: a monograph on effective services for minority children who are severely emotionally disturbed. Washington, DC: Georgetown University Child Development Center; 1989. https://www.ncjrs.gov/App/Publications/abstract.aspx?ID=124939.
14. The National Academy of Sciences, engineering, and medicine. Health and Medicine Division; 2020. http://www.nationalacademies.org/hmd/Global/Meetings.aspx.
15. Hilty DM, Crawford A, Teshima J, Nasatir-Hilty SE, Luo J, Chisler LSM, et al. Mobile health and cultural competencies as a foundation for telehealth care: scoping review. J Tech Behav Sci. 2021;6:197–230.
16. Fisher-Borne M, Cain JM, Martin SL. From mastery to accountability: cultural humility as an alternative to cultural competence. Soc Work Educ. 2015;34(2):165–81.
17. Fleming T, Creedy DK, West R. Cultural safety continuing professional development for midwifery academics: an integrative literature review. Women Birth. 2019;32:318–26.
18. Crawford A, Waddell C, Lund C. Unsettling healthcare with Inuit in Canada: cultural safety education for healthcare providers. In: Schiff R, Molle H, editors. Health and healthcare in northern Canada. Toronto, ON: University of Toronto Press; 2021.
19. Kemp J, Zhang T, Inglis F, et al. Delivery of compassionate mental health care in a digital technology–driven age: scoping review. J Med Internet Res. 2020;22(3):e16263. https://doi.org/10.2196/16263.
20. Spradley JP, McCurdy DW. Conformity and conflict: readings in cultural anthropology. New York: Jill Potash; 2012.
21. Hilty DM, Crawford A, Teshima J, et al. A framework for telepsychiatric training and e-health: competency-based education, evaluation and implications. Int Rev Psychiatry. 2015;27(6):569–92.
22. Crawford A, Sunderji N, López J, et al. Defining competencies for the practice of telepsychiatry through an assessment of resident learning needs. BMC Med Educ. 2016;16:28. Published 2016 Jan 26. https://doi.org/10.1186/s12909-016-0529-0.
23. Naslund JA, Aschbrenner KA, Araya R, et al. Digital technology for treating and preventing mental disorders in low-income and middle-income countries: a narrative review of the literature. Lancet Psychiatry. 2017;4(6):486–500.
24. Torous J, Roberts LW. The ethical use of mobile health technology in clinical psychiatry. J Nerv Ment Dis. 2017;205(1):4–8. https://doi.org/10.1097/nmd.0000000000000596.

25. Obbarius A, van Maasakkers L, Baer L, et al. Standardization of health outcomes assessment for depression and anxiety: recommendations from the ICHOM depression and anxiety working group. Qual Life Res. 2017;26(12):3211–5.
26. World Health Organization. Mental Health ATLAS 2017 Report; 2017. https://www.who.int/mental_health/evidence/atlas/mental_health_atlas_2017/en/. Organisation of Economic Corporation and Development. Perspectives on Global Development 2014: Boosting Productivity to Meet the Middle-Income Challenge; 2014. https://www.oecd.org/dev/pgd/EN_Pocket%20Edition_PGD2014_web.pdf.
27. Cohen A, Eaton J, Radtke B, et al. Three models of community mental health services in low-income countries. Int J Ment Health Syst. 2011;5(1):3. Published 2011 Jan 25. https://doi.org/10.1186/1752-4458-5-3.
28. Ajuha S, Shidhaye R, Semrau M, et al. Mental health information systems in resource-challenged countries: experiences from India. BJPsych Int. 2018;15(2):43–6. https://doi.org/10.1192/bji.2017.6.
29. Jordans M, Chisholm D, Semrau M, et al. Evaluation of performance and perceived utility of mental healthcare indicators in routine health information systems in five low- and middle-income countries. BJPsych Open. 2019;5(5):e70. https://doi.org/10.1192/bjo.2019.22.
30. Hilty DM, Chan S, Torous J, et al. New frontiers in healthcare and technology: internet- and web-based mental options emerge to complement in-person and telepsychiatric care options. J Health Med Inform. 2015;6(4):1–14.
31. Hendrickson MA, Melton GB, Pitt MB. The review of systems, the electronic health record, and billing. JAMA. 2019;322(2):115–6. https://doi.org/10.1001/jama.2019.5667.
32. Hilty DM, Randhawa K, Maheu MM, et al. A review of telepresence, virtual reality and augmented reality applied to clinical care. J Tech Behav Sci. 2020;5:178. https://doi.org/10.1007/s41347-020-00126-x.
33. Torrey WC, Cepeda M, Castro S, et al. Implementing technology-supported care for depression and alcohol use disorder in primary care in Colombia: preliminary findings. Psychiatr Serv. 2020;71(7):678–83. https://doi.org/10.1176/appi.ps.201900457.
34. Liddy C, Drosinis P, Keely E. Electronic consultation systems: worldwide prevalence and their impact on patient care—a systematic review. Fam Pract. 2016;33(3):274–85.
35. Archibald D, Stratton J, Liddy C, et al. Evaluation of an electronic consultation service in psychiatry for primary care providers. BMC Psychiatry. 2018;18(1):119. https://doi.org/10.1186/s12888-018-1701-3.
36. Yellowlees P, Burke Parish M, González Á, et al. Asynchronous telepsychiatry: a component of stepped integrated care. Telemed J E Health. 2018;24(5):375–8.
37. Cleary M, Walter G. Is e-mail communication a feasible method to interview young people with mental health problems? J Child Adolesc Psychiatr Nurs. 2011;24(3):150–2. https://doi.org/10.1111/j.1744-6171.2010.00257.x.
38. Berrouiguet S, Baca-García E, Brandt S, et al. Fundamentals for future mobile-health (mHealth): a systematic review of mobile phone and web-based text messaging in mental health. JMIR. 2016;18(6):e135. https://doi.org/10.2196/jmir.5066.
39. Bry LJ, Chou T, Miguel E, et al. Consumer smartphone apps marketed for child and adolescent anxiety: a systematic review and content analysis. Behav Ther. 2018;49(2):249–61. https://doi.org/10.1016/j.beth.2017.07.008.
40. Goldberg SB, Lam SU, Simonsson O, et al. Mobile phone-based interventions for mental health: a systematic meta-review of 14 meta-analyses of randomized controlled trials. PLoS Digit Health. 2022;1(1):e0000002.
41. Chan S, Li L, Torous J, Gratzer D, et al. Review of use of asynchronous technologies incorporated in mental health care. Curr Psychiatry Rep. 2018;20(10):85. Published 2018 Aug 28. https://doi.org/10.1007/s11920-018-0954-3.
42. Pisani AR, Wyman PA, Gurditta K, et al. Mobile phone intervention to reduce youth suicide in rural communities: field test. JMIR Ment Health. 2018;5(2):e10425. Published 2018 May 31. https://doi.org/10.2196/10425.

43. L'Hommedieu M, L'Hommedieu J, Begay C, et al. Lessons learned: recommendations for implementing a longitudinal study using wearable and environmental sensors in a health care organization. JMIR Mhealth Uhealth. 2019;7(12):e13305. https://doi.org/10.2196/13305.
44. Hilty DM, Armstrong CM, Luxton DD, et al. A scoping review of sensors, wearables and remote monitoring for behavioral health: uses, outcomes, clinical competencies and research directions. J Tech Behav Sci. 2020;6:278.
45. Aledavood T, Torous J, Triana Hoyos AM, et al. Smartphone-based tracking of sleep in depression, anxiety, and psychotic disorders. Curr Psychiatry Rep. 2019;21:1–9.
46. Naslund JA, Aschbrenner KA, McHugo GJ, et al. Exploring opportunities to support mental health care using social media: a survey of social media users with mental illness. Early Interv Psychiatry. 2019;13(3):405–13.
47. Greenes RA, Bates DW, Kawamoto K, et al. Clinical decision support models and frameworks: seeking to address research issues underlying implementation successes and failures. J Biomed Inform. 2018;78:134–43.
48. Rus-Calafell M, Garety P, Sason E, et al. Virtual reality in the assessment and treatment of psychosis: a systematic review of its utility, acceptability and effectiveness. Psychol Med. 2018;48(3):362–91. https://doi.org/10.1017/S0033291717001945.
49. Torous J, Baker JT. Why psychiatry needs data science and data science needs psychiatry: connecting with technology. JAMA Psychiatry. 2016;73(1):3–4.
50. Faurholt-Jepsen M, Munkholm K, Frost M, et al. Electronic self-monitoring of mood using IT platforms in adult patients with bipolar disorder: a systematic review of the validity and evidence. BMC Psychiatry. 2016;16(1):7. https://doi.org/10.1186/s12888-016-0713-0.
51. Reece AG, Reagan AJ, Lix KLM, et al. Forecasting the onset and course of mental illness with Twitter data. Sci Rep. 2017;7(1):13006. Published 2017 Oct 11. https://doi.org/10.1038/s41598-017-12961-9.
52. De Choudhury M, Counts S, Horvitz E, et al. Characterizing and predicting postpartum depression from shared Facebook data. In: 2014 Presented at: 17th ACM conference on Computer supported cooperative work & social computing—CSCW '14; Feb 15–19, Baltimore, MD, USA; 2014. p. 626–38. https://doi.org/10.1145/2531602.2531675.
53. Naslund JA, Bondre A, Torous J, et al. Social media and mental health: benefits, risks, and opportunities for research and practice. J Tech Behav Sci. 2020;5:1–13.
54. Verweel L, Newman A, Michaelchuk W, Packham T, Goldstein R, Brooks D. The effect of digital interventions on related health literacy and skills for individuals living with chronic diseases: a systematic review and meta-analysis [published online ahead of print, 2023 Jun 8]. Int J Med Inform. 2023;177:105114.
55. Wisniewski H, Gorrindo T, Rauseo-Ricupero N, Hilty D, Torous J. The role of digital navigators in promoting clinical care and technology integration into practice. Digit Biomark. 2020;4(Suppl 1):119–35. Published 2020 Nov 26. https://doi.org/10.1159/000510144.
56. Indigenous Physicians Association of Canada. First Nations, Inuit, Metis Health Core Competencies; 2019. https://www.ipac-amac.ca/downloads/core-competencies.pdf. Accessed 1 Aug 2020.
57. Doshi R, Aseltine RH, Sabina AB, et al. Interventions to improve management of chronic conditions among racial and ethnic minorities. J Racial Ethn Health Disparities. 2017;4(6):1033–41.
58. Hilty DM, Rabinowitz TR, McCarron RM, et al. Telepsychiatry and e-mental health models leverage stepped, collaborative, and integrated services to primary care. Psychosomatics. 2018;59(3):227–50.
59. Leininger MM. Culture care diversity & universality: a theory of nursing. New York, NY: National League for Nursing Press; 1991.
60. Yan MC, Wong YR. Rethinking self-awareness in cultural competence: toward a dialogic self in cross-cultural social work. Fam Soc J Contemp Soc Serv. 2005;86:181–8.
61. Tervalon M, Murray-García J. Cultural humility versus cultural competence: a critical distinction in defining physician training outcomes in multicultural education. J Health Care Poor Underserv. 1998;9(2):117–25.

62. Dube SR. Continuing conversations about adverse childhood experiences (ACEs) screening: a public health perspective. Child Abuse Negl. 2018;85:180–4.
63. Naslund JA, Spagnolo J. Cultural adaptation of digital therapeutics. In: Jacobson N, Kowatsch T, Marsch L, editors. Digital therapeutics for mental health and addiction: state of the science and vision for the future. Amsterdam: Elsevier; 2023. p. 151–64.
64. Indigenous Physicians Association of Canada. IPAC. http://www.cpa-apc.org/wp-content/uploads/Training_in_Cultural_Psychiatry-2012-53-web-EN.pdf.
65. Danso R. Cultural competence and cultural humility: a critical reflection on key cultural diversity concepts. J Soc Work. 2016;18:410. https://doi.org/10.1177/1468017316654341.
66. U.S. Department of Health and Human Services. Office of Minority Health. National Standards for Culturally and Linguistically Appropriate Services (CLAS) in Health and Health Care. https://www.thinkculturalhealth.hhs.gov/clas; 2018.
67. Kim H, Xie B. Health literacy in the eHealth era: a systematic review of the literature. Patient Educ Couns. 2017;100(6):1073–82.
68. Shapiro ML, Miller J, White K. Community transformation through culturally competent nursing leadership: application of theory of culture care diversity and universality and tri-dimensional leader effectiveness model. J Transcult Nurs. 2006;17(2):113–8.
69. Engel GL. The clinical application of the biopsychosocial model. Am J Psychiatry. 1980;137(5):535–44.
70. Hilty DM. Advancing science, clinical care and education: shall we update Engel's biopsychosocial model to a bio-psycho-socio-cultural model? Psychol Cogn Sci. 2015;1(1):e1. https://doi.org/10.17140/pcsoj-1-e001.
71. American Psychiatric Association. Cultural Formulation Interview. Patient Version. http://www.dsm5.org/Pages/Feedback-Form.aspx, and Informant Version 2013; 2013. http://www.multiculturalmentalhealth.ca/wp-content/uploads/2013/10/2013_DSM5_CFI_InformantVersion.pdf.
72. Shore JH. Intended and unintended consequence in the digital age of psychiatry: the interface of culture and technology in psychiatric treatments. Psychiatr Clin North Am. 2019;42(4):659–68.
73. Oliver R, Rochecouste J, Anderson R, et al. Understanding Australian aboriginal tertiary student needs. Int J High Educ. 2013;2(4):52–64.
74. American Psychiatric Association. Diagnostic and statistical manual of mental disorders, text revision. 5th ed. Washington, DC: American Psychiatric Publishing, Outline for Cultural Formulation; 2013.
75. American Psychiatric Association. Cultural Formulation Interview Supplementary Modules. http://www.multiculturalmentalhealth.ca/wp-content/uploads/2013/10/2013_CFI_supplementarymodules.pdf.
76. Hilty DM, Unutzer J, Ko DK, et al. Approaches for departments, schools and health systems to better implement technologies used for clinical care and education. Acad Psychiatry. 2019;43(6):611–6.
77. Kurtz DLM, Janke R, Vinek J, Wells T, et al. Health sciences cultural safety education in Australia, Canada, New Zealand, and the United States: a literature review. Int J Med Educ. 2018;9:271–85.
78. Curtis E, Jones R, Tipene-Leach D, et al. Why cultural safety rather than cultural competency is required to achieve health equity: a literature review and recommended definition. Int J Equity Health. 2019;18:174. https://doi.org/10.1186/s12939-019-1082-3.
79. Yellowlees PM, Hogarth MA, Hilty DM. The development of distributed academic networks in America. Acad Psychiatry. 2006;30(6):451–5.
80. Upadhaya N, Jordans MJD, Abdulmalik J, et al. Information systems for mental health in six low and middle income countries: cross country situation analysis. Int J Ment Health Syst. 2016;10:60. Published 2016 Sep 26. https://doi.org/10.1186/s13033-016-0094-2.
81. Mugisha J, Abdulmalik J, Hanlon C, et al. Health systems context(s) for integrating mental health into primary health care in six emerald countries: a situation analysis. Int J Ment Health Syst. 2017;11:7. Published 2017 Jan 5. https://doi.org/10.1186/s13033-016-0114-2.

82. Singla DR, Kohrt BA, Murray LK, et al. Psychological treatments for the world: lessons from low- and middle-income countries. Annu Rev Clin Psychol. 2017;13:149–81. https://doi.org/10.1146/annurev-clinpsy-032816-045217.
83. Hoeft TJ, Fortney JC, Patel V, et al. Task-sharing approaches to improve mental health care in rural and other low-resource settings: a systematic review. J Rural Health. 2018;34(1):48–62. https://doi.org/10.1111/jrh.12229.
84. Raviola G, Naslund JA, Smith SL, et al. Innovative models in mental health delivery systems: task sharing care with non-specialist providers to close the mental health treatment gap. Curr Psychiatry Rep. 2019;21(6):44. Published 2019 Apr 30. https://doi.org/10.1007/s11920-019-1028-x.
85. Naslund JA, Gonsalves PP, Gruebner O, et al. Digital innovations for global mental health: opportunities for data science, task sharing, and early intervention. Curr Treat Options Psychiatry. 2019;6(4):337–51. https://doi.org/10.1007/s40501-019-00186-8.
86. Institute for Healthcare Improvement. Quality Improvement Essentials Toolkit. 2018. http://www.ihi.org/resources/Pages/Tools/Quality-Improvement-Essentials-Toolkit.aspx.
87. National Academy of Science. Integrating Health Literacy, Cultural Competence, and Language Access Services. 2016. https://www.nap.edu/catalog/23498/integrating-health-literacy-cultural-competence-and-language-access-services-workshop.

4 Detection, Evaluation, and Best Practices for Technology-Based Fatigue to Promote Well-Being

Donald M. Hilty, Christina M. Armstrong, Shawna D. Wright, Shelby A. Smout, Kenneth P. Drude, Marlene M. Maheu, and Elizabeth A. Krupinski

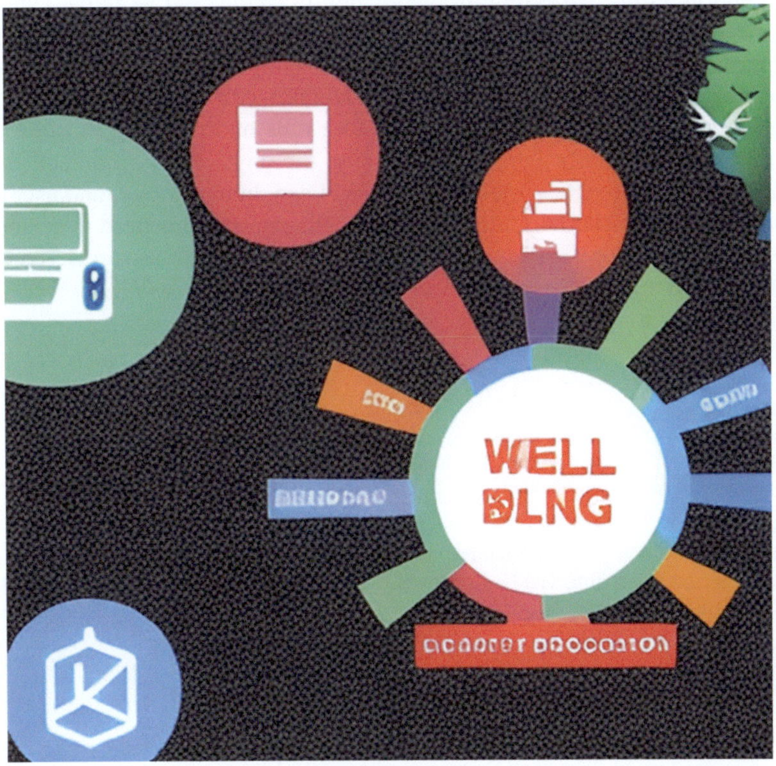

D. M. Hilty (✉)
Department of Psychiatry and Behavioral Sciences, Keck School of Medicine
University of Southern California, Los Angeles, CA, USA
e-mail: donald.hilty@uhsinc.com; hilty@med.usc.edu

D. Mucić, D. M. Hilty (eds.), *Digital Mental Health*,
https://doi.org/10.1007/978-3-031-59936-1_4

Abstract

As telehealth, mobile health, and other technologies reshape the delivery of health care, a thorough evaluation is needed for barriers related to workflow that contribute to provider fatigue and may affect quality of care. The relationship between technology, fatigue, and health care needs to be explored in order to improve conditions for providers. The literature about synchronous video, telephone, informatics systems, asynchronous wearable sensors, and mobile health technologies used in health care suggests substantial behavioral, cognitive, emotional, and physical impact on users. This may vary based on individual, clinic, hospital, and system/organizational workplaces. Video and electronic health record use are associated with fatigue with: physical eye fatigue, neck pain, stress, and tiredness; behavioral impact related to additional effort due to barriers, trouble with engagement, emotional wear and tear, and exhaustion; cognitive inattention, effort, expecting problems, multi-tasking, and workload; and emotional experiences like anger, irritability, stress, and concern about well-being. Other studies not focusing on fatigue also found high user ratings on data quality, accuracy, and processing, but low satisfaction with clerical tasks, the effort required in work, and interruptions costing time and resulting in more errors, stress, and frustration. Few studies discuss the physical environment, occupational health approaches, mobile, telework, Lean, human factor, and user design approaches to workflow. Clinicians and health care systems need to evaluate the impact of technology and consider implementation approaches, process improvement, and human factors to promote well-being and reduce fatigue.

C. M. Armstrong
Connected Health Implementation Strategies, Office of Connected Care, U.S. Department of Veterans Affairs, Washington, DC, USA
e-mail: Christina.Armstrong@va.gov

S. D. Wright
Department of Psychiatry and Behavioral Sciences, University of Kansas Center for Telemedicine and Telehealth, The University of Kansas Medical Center, Fairway, KS, USA
e-mail: swright6@kumc.edu

S. A. Smout
Virginia Commonwealth University, Richmond, VA, USA
e-mail: smoutsa@vcu.edu

K. P. Drude
Coalition Technology in Behavioral Science, Fairborn, OH, USA

M. M. Maheu
Coalition for Technology in Behavioral Sciences, Telebehavioral Health Institute, Inc, San Diego, CA, USA
e-mail: mmaheu@telehealth.org

E. A. Krupinski
Department of Radiology and Imaging Sciences, Emory University, Atlanta, GA, USA
e-mail: ekrupin@emory.edu

4.1 Introduction

Technology is reshaping the delivery of health care worldwide as a facilitator, practice extender, and virtual team member for person- and patient-centered care [1, 2]. Health care systems and governmental agencies across the world are promoting quality and evidence-based care by implementing the Quadruple Aim, which emphasizes reducing costs and improving population health, patient experience, and team well-being [1–3]. Fatigue is a very complex and multidimensional construct and a review of research across cognitive science, exercise physiology, and clinical practice suggests that its most promising common feature is the notion of "perceived effort"—this accounts for inter-individual differences and situational variations, includes both mental and physical constructs, and integrates motivational and emotional dimensions [4]. Providers and other employees have increasingly noted problems related to fatigue and excessive workflow steps, particularly electronic health records (EHRs), which may affect well-being and contribute to burnout [5].

Technology challenges include learning to use it personally/professionally, integrating it into workflow and screen time [6–8]. Subjective phrases like "technology fatigue" or in the Coronavirus Disease-2019 (COVID-19) era, "Zoom fatigue," suggest technology *causes* fatigue. Past research on employees' subjective and physical issues (e.g., eye strain) related to computer displays [9–14] suggests there are many additional occupational health factors related to fatigue, burnout, and accidents [15–17]. Competitive industries in business have had to contend with technological challenges and systematically changed workflows for users to transform and avoid extinction—in health care, there appears to be a gap between the system's perception of processes and users' or participants' experiences [18].

It appears there is a gap in how the EHR and other technologies affect clinician workflow, particularly the amount of effort and the development of fatigue or burnout [2]. Health care is evaluating work engagement, burnout, job demands versus resources, and the role of working conditions [19, 20]. Assessment of well-being [2, 21, 22], burnout [23–28], burnout with EHRs [29, 30], and related risk factors [31] is underway, including in psychiatry and behavioral health providers [2, 32–34]. Interventions can help to prevent and ameliorate burnout [35, 36] and changes to organizational structure (e.g., shared leadership), process improvement (e.g., Lean), employee support (e.g., leisure, fitness, diet), and professional development are in order [2, 37–39]. Another gap is that systems have approached burnout as an individual's problem (e.g., depression) rather than an organizational problem (i.e., a shared problem). Less focus has been spent on resilience. Key stressors that put people at risk of burnout need to be identified, so that changes can be made to reduce their impact and create healthier workplaces. For example, models for reducing stress are needed for health care (e.g., social workers) [40], information and communication technology (ICT) [41], and information technology (IT) [42] professionals, as well as systems in general [43].

The relationship between technology, fatigue, and health care is reviewed by looking at health, business, and technology literature to:

1. Reflect on the intersection of technology, fatigue, and health care.

2. Consider business, occupational health, and well-being literature that might apply to health care technology-based fatigue.
3. Suggest guidelines for health care related to technology, well-being, and fatigue for providers and systems in order to promote a culture of well-being.

4.2 The Landscape of Technology and Fatigue

The notion of "perceived effort" leading to fatigue accounts for inter-individual differences and situational variations and includes both mental and physical constructs [4]. It also integrates motivational and emotional dimensions. Searches on the topic have considered categories and keywords like these:

- Physical impact (ache, back, distress, exhaustion, eye, fatigue, headache, neck, pain, problems, strain, stress, tiredness, visual).
- Behavioral impact (anxious, barriers, boredom, complain(t;ing), concerns, depressed-, detach(ed;ment), distance, effort(ful), engage(d;ment), emotional-, enjoy(able), exhaustion, experience, factor, fatigue, insomnia, intimacy, isolation, mental, onerous, positive, readiness, reward(s;ing), social, substance, suicide, team, worry).
- Cognitive impact (attention, alertness, critical, cynicism, distraction, (self)-efficacy, effort, expectation, incompetence, indecision, motivation, multi-tasking, negative, steps, task(s), workflow, workload).
- Emotional impact (alone, anger, anxiety, compassion(ate), complex, confidence, empower, esteem, irritability, lonely, positive, quality of life, resilience, sadness, satisfaction, share(ing), trauma, satisfaction, stress, support, susceptible, therapeutic, wellness, well-being).

It also is important to consider the workplace environment: technology accessories and video display; workload burden; clerical support; sense of control; competing demands; distractions or interruptions; home, work, telework, or mobile settings; breaks or naps; recognition and accolades; productivity measures like the relative value unit (RVU); and organization of workflow. For well-being, burnout, and stress, it may be important to consider how adaptable workers are, if they can make adjustments or have coping strategies. Overall, their sense of confidence and control may help with esteem, fitness, happy, mindfulness, purpose, relaxation, and overall resilience and wellness. Providers bring perceptions regarding technology to work, including attitudes, willingness to change, motivation, readiness to use technology, biases, and a range of experiences with technology.

4.3 Results

4.3.1 Technology, Health Care, and Fatigue

A recent review [2] found 12 papers focused on technology, fatigue, and well-being [8, 13, 14, 45–53], mostly from the USA. These studies assessed behavioral (8;

66.7%), emotional (4; 33.3%), cognitive (7; 58.7%), and physical (4; 33.3%) impact of workflow at the individual (11; 91.7%), clinic (8; 66.7%), hospital (6; 50.0%), and system/organizational (6; 50.0%) levels; only 3 included all levels. Video and electronic health record use are associated with physical issues, usually reported as eye fatigue, neck pain, stress, and tiredness. Behavioral impact involved additional effort regarding barriers, trouble with engagement with patients, emotional wear and tear, exhaustion, and fatigue. Cognitive impact has focused on inattention, effort, expecting problems, multi-tasking, and workload. Emotional impact was related to anger, irritability, stress, and concerns about well-being.

Only two of these studies looked at the workplace broadly, discussing the physical environment, occupational health issues, Lean, human factor, and user design approaches to workflow. System on-boarding and training typically gets users oriented and informally sets expectations, but often there are no processes for ongoing self-, peer-, and system-assessment of experience or skill development. Workplace, workspace, ergonomic, and technology implementation are gaining more attention in health care [54, 55] and other industries for those who function at work and home [56]; mobile and telework are being researched outside of health care, primarily. Most studies are unidirectional in association, mediation, and causation—technology causing fatigue—and like other studies in the literature [11, 12, 57, 58], they lack standard assessment, monitoring, and interventions.

Studies have focused on the technology use [8, 45, 53], survey of providers [46, 51], visual strain or fatigue [13, 14], implementation/usability [47, 52], and consensus reports [61, 62] (Table 4.1). Table 4.1 is organized by study, sample size (*N*), length of time, population, country, design, type of technology, area of focus of the assessment (i.e., behavioral, cognitive, emotional, and physical impact), and level of the assessment (i.e., individual, clinic, hospital, and system/organizational). Physician participants experienced physiological fatigue at least once during simulation exercises involving 4 patient cases, with 80% experiencing physiological fatigue within the first 22 min of use [8]. Those who experienced EHR-related fatigue in one patient case were less efficient in the subsequent patient case, as demonstrated by longer task completion times ($r = -0.521$; $P = 0.007$), higher numbers of mouse clicks ($r = -0.562$; $P = 0.003$), and more EHR screen visits ($r = -0.486$; $P = 0.01$). Visual strain and fatigue studies have focused on individual-level adjustments for accommodation at near distances, with lack of energy, physical discomfort, and sleepiness being statistically significantly higher as a function of the length of session [13, 14].

Studies have determined that physicians spend 4–6 h on EHR and desk work during the day and another 1–2 h after work, often for clerical and administrative tasks (e.g., documentation, order entry, billing, coding, and system security) [52]. US providers—compared to non-US counterparts—spent substantially more time actively using the EHR (mean time, 90.2 min vs. 59.1 min; $P < 0.001$), composed more automated note texts (77.5% vs. 60.8% of note text; $P < 0.001$), and received statistically significantly more messages per day (33.8 vs. 12.8; $P < 0.001$). Furthermore, US clinicians used the EHR for a longer time after hours, logging in 26.5 min per day versus 19.5 min per day for non-US clinicians ($P = 0.01$). These findings did not vary according to daily patient volume or organizational structure, type, and size. Scientific evidence, workflow, ordering efficiency, and user satisfaction may reduce mouse clicks and unproductive thinking time [53].

An additional 14 studies that explored provider experiences or perceptions about technology that may apply to fatigue—but did not directly investigate it—focused on combination or solitary use of EHR, video, video display terminals (VDTs), computers, smartphones, and personal digital assistants (PDAs) (Table 4.1) [6, 56, 63–74]. Methods were heterogeneous with surveys, semi-structured interviews, qualitative methods, and comparison groups. Studies of physicians who spent 11 h a day in the hospital found that clerical and administrative tasks (e.g., documentation, order entry, billing, coding) accounted for 44.2% of their time, inbox management 23.7%, and additional time was consumed communicating with patients, refilling prescriptions, or reviewing test results each day [63, 73]. User ratings were high on data quality, accuracy, and processing [64], but low for satisfaction with clerical tasks [6]. Interrupted tasks required more time and resulted in more errors, stress, and frustration [74]. There were differences between generations regarding adaptability, perceived benefits and drawbacks, and perceptions of other generations' ability to adapt.

There appears to be room for organizational responses to improve provider experiences by attending to human factors related to technology [47, 52] (Table 4.2). Table 4.2 summarizes human factors and technology in health care: organizational responses for prevention and adjustment of workflow, as organized in terms of evidence/findings, manifestations and analysis of technology problems, and individual user versus organizational adjustments being made. A change management plan with process management [59] requires training, supervision, and evaluation to adjust competencies/skills, improve quality/performance, and re-allocate resources in health care [2, 60].

4.3.2 Business, Occupational Health, and Well-Being Literature to Contextualize Technology-Based Fatigue

Over the past 40 years, a shift has occurred regarding the origin of technology-related problems in business, occupational health, and other walks of life [46, 75]. The earlier perception attributed problems of production, efficiency, and outputs as being related to ergonomic, mechanical, workplace, and other factors for individuals, cohorts (e.g., VDT employees), and systems. Findings from VDT studies related to occupational hygiene (e.g., climate, lighting, electrostatic conditions) and ophthalmologic dimensions appear to be quite pertinent to video, EHR, and psychosocial work commonly associated with "technology fatigue" [9, 10, 76]. Job stress is higher, quality of life is lower, and visual strain, discomfort, and fatigue are higher in VDT workers than non-VDT users [77]. Combined/interactive communication causes more discomfort than data entry or acquisition. Postural risk factors and job strain in the environment seemed to increase musculoskeletal symptoms for those with 7+ hours of VDT use/day.

Table 4.1 Studies at the intersection of technology, health care, and fatigue for clinicians

Article #	Study	*N*	Length (of study)	Population	Country	Design	Methods	Key findings	Technology (i.e. hardware, software)	Area of focus[a] (1 = yes, 0 = no) B	E	C	P	Level of focus[b] (1 = yes, 0 = no) I	C	H	S
Technology, health care, and fatigue																	
1	Galt et al. (2019) [46]	2195	Not specified	Pharmacists	USA	Cross-sectional descriptive analytic study	Survey	Integration of health technology into pharmacy practice introduced new error types and alert fatigue	Video monitor, computer	0	0	1	0	1	1	0	1
2	Holmgren et al. (2020) [45]	N/A	10 months	Providers	USA, Canada, northern Europe, Western Europe, Middle East, and Oceania	Cross-sectional descriptive analytic study of full-time use	Cross-sectional; controlling for organizational characteristics, including structure, type, size, and daily patient volume	EHR (mean time, 90.2 min vs. 59.1 min; $P < 0.001$), including doing notes, orders, in-basket messages, and clinical review [43]. They also composed more automated note text than their non-US counterparts (77.5% vs. 60.8% of note text; $P < 0.001$) and received statistically significantly more messages per day (33.8 vs. 12.8; $P < 0.001$). Furthermore, US clinicians used the EHR for a longer time after hours, logging in 26.5 min per day versus 19.5 min per day for non-US clinicians ($P = 0.01$)	EHR, video monitor, computer	1	0	0	0	1	0	0	1
3	Khairat et al. (2020) [8]	25	Not specified	Physicians	USA	Cross-sectional descriptive analytic study	EHR simulation exercise involving 4 patient cases (mean [SD] completion time, 34:43 [11:41] min) recorded a total of 14 h and 27 min of EHR activity	Physicians: 20 of 25 participants (80%) experienced physiological fatigue within the first 22 min of EHR use. Physicians who experienced EHR-related fatigue in 1 patient case were less efficient in the subsequent patient case, as demonstrated by longer task completion times ($r = -0.521$; $P = 0.007$), higher numbers of mouse clicks ($r = -0.562$; $P = 0.003$), and more EHR screen visits ($r = -0.486$; $P = 0.01$)	EHR, video monitor, computer	1	0	0	1	1	0	0	0

(continued)

Table 4.1 (continued)

Article #	Study	N	Length (of study)	Population	Country	Design	Methods	Key findings	Technology (i.e. hardware, software)	Area of focus[a] (1 = yes, 0 = no)				Level of focus[b] (1 = yes, 0 = no)			
										B	E	C	P	I	C	H	S
4	Krupinski et al. (2009) [13]	6	Not specified	Radiologists	USA	Observational study of full-time use	Use of an autorefractor to measure eye strain at various reading distances; on average, participants had been reading CT or X-rays 5.73 h (SD = 1.24) in late afternoon	Nearer user distance to video displays increased eye strain. There was a statistically significant difference ($F = 1188.36$; $p < 0.0001$) in the data as a function of target distance, as a function of time of day ($F = 316.10$; $p < 0.0001$), and radiologists more than residents ($F = 271.47$; $p < 0.0001$)	Video monitor, computer, autorefractor	0	0	0	1	1	0	0	0
5	Krupinski et al. (2010) [14]	40	Not specified	Radiologists	USA	Observational study of full-time use	Reading time, visual accommodations, and symptoms of fatigue were measured after varied reading schedules (prior to workday and after workday)	After a day of clinical reading, radiologists have reduced ability to focus, increased symptoms of fatigue and oculomotor strain, and reduced ability to detect fractures. Lack of energy, physical discomfort, and sleepiness were statistically significantly higher as a function of the length of session	Video monitor, computer	0	0	1	1	1	0	0	0
6	Lopez et al. (2018) [47]	N/A	Not specified	Nurses	USA	Usability study	Assessment of technology usability in health care can be categorized into 4 major types: Inspection methods, formal usability testing, summative testing, and field studies	Technologies are, and will be for the foreseeable future, central to the work of intensive care nurses. These technologies must be highly usable to ensure high-quality and safe care delivery without unnecessary increases in workload	Technology (general)	1	0	1	0	1	1	1	0

Article #	Study	*N*	Length (of study)	Population	Country	Design	Methods	Key findings	Technology (i.e. hardware, software)	Area of focus[a] (1 = yes, 0 = no)				Level of focus[b] (1 = yes, 0 = no)			
										B	E	C	P	I	C	H	S
7	Mylod et al. (2017) [48]	N/A	Not specified	Physicians	USA	Intervention related to full-time use	Framework	A two-pronged approach to clinician burnout is proposed whereby inherent stress is addressed separately from external stress so as to best manage the various stressors present in clinical settings that contribute to clinician burnout	EHR, video monitor, computer	0	1	1	0	1	1	1	1
8	Nakagawa et al. (2020) [49]	N/A	Not specified	Physicians	USA	Model intervention for full-time use	Consensus	Technological advancements improve efficiency, allow more flexible working arrangements, and increase convenience for patients and physicians	EHR, video monitor, computer + (phone, email, tablet, social media, virtual assistants)	1	1	1	0	1	1	1	1
9	National Academies of Science (2019) [50]	N/A	Not specified	Providers	USA	Consensus	Consensus methodology	Health care technology is always evolving and that these developments are likely to be disruptive to the care delivery system as we know it today	EHR, video monitor, computer	1	1	1	0	0	1	1	1
10	Shanafelt et al. (2017) [51]	N/A	Not specified	Physicians, health care admin-istrators	USA	Assessment related to full-time use	Survey	Deliberate, sustained, and comprehensive efforts by the organization to reduce burnout and promote engagement can make a difference. Many effective interventions are relatively inexpensive, and small investments can have a large impact Approximately 45% of physicians work more than 60 h per week compared with less than 10% of US workers in other fields	Technology (general)	1	1	0	0	1	1	1	1

(continued)

Table 4.1 (continued)

Article #	Study	*N*	Length (of study)	Population	Country	Design	Methods	Key findings	Technology (i.e. hardware, software)	Area of focus[a] (1 = yes, 0 = no) B	E	C	P	Level of focus[b] (1 = yes, 0 = no) I	C	H	S
11	Tutty et al. (2019) [52]	N/A	Not specified	Physicians	USA	Identification of intervention options for full-time use	Implementation	Multiple opportunities for regulators, policymakers, EHR developers, payers, health system leadership, and users to make changes collectively to improve the use of efficacy of EHRs. Studies have determined that physicians spend 4–6 h on EHR and desk work during the day and another 1–2 h after work, often for clerical and administrative tasks (e.g., documentation, order entry, billing, coding, and system security)	EHR, video monitor, computer	1	0	0	1	1	1	1	1
12	Zhang et al. (2013) [53]	388	Not specified	Physicians	USA	Quasi-experimental for full-time use	Measure cognitive workload via number of clicks for different order set combinations	Excessive cognitive workload on physicians imposed by technology impacts the cognitive behavior of users. The most important three factors that separate ideal order sets from the rest are patient safety, efficiency, and user satisfaction. Scientific evidence, workflow, ordering efficiency, and user satisfaction reduce mouse clicks and unproductive thinking time	EHR, video monitor, computer	1	0	1	0	1	1	0	0
# of 12										8	4	7	4	11	8	6	6
Average										66.7%	33.3%	58.3%	33.3%	91.7%	66.7%	50.0%	50.0%
Studies of other technology-related experiences in health care for clinician																	
1	Arndt et al. (2017) [61]	142	3 years	Physicians	USA	Retrospective cohort study	EHR time log data	Clinicians spent 355 min (5.9 h) of an 11.4-h workday in the EHR per weekday per 1.0 clinical full-time equivalent: 269 min (4.5 h) during clinic hours and 86 min (1.4 h) after clinic hours	EHR, video monitor, computer, tablet	1	0	1	0	1	0	0	0

Article #	Study	N	Length (of study)	Population	Country	Design	Methods	Key findings	Technology (i.e. hardware, software)	Area of focus[a] (1 = yes, 0 = no)				Level of focus[b] (1 = yes, 0 = no)			
										B	E	C	P	I	C	H	S
2	Campbell et al. (2007) [62]	95	3–4 days per site	Physicians	USA	Qualitative	Qualitative surveys and interviews with physicians	Technology can create chaos when there are insufficient backup systems in place, users have false expectations regarding data accuracy and processing, and some clinicians cannot work efficiently without computerized systems	EHR	1	0	1	0	1	1	1	0
3	Hilty et al. (2007) [63]	94	3 years	Physicians, rural patients with depression	USA	Mixed methods	Qualitative and quantitative	Intensive modules using telepsychiatric educational interventions toward PCPs may be superior, but the most critical ingredient may be administrative tracking of patients	Video monitor, computer, phone	0	1	0	0	1	1	0	0
4	McAlearney et al. (2005) [64]	161	6 months	Physicians	USA	Qualitative	Qualitative interviews and focus groups using standard, semi-structured guide with open-ended questions to promote discussion	Organizational strategies should include active support for broad-based and niche use, active support for niche use, and basic support for individual physicians	Smartphones, personal data assistants (PDAs)	1	1	1	0	1	0	0	1
5	McAlearney et al. (2015) [65]	82	Not specified	Physicians	USA	Qualitative	Qualitative interviews and focus groups to explore physician and administrative barriers to EHR: Financial, technical, time, psychological, social, legal, organizational, and change process	Recommendations provided regarding how to facilitate physician adoption and use and address organizational concerns	EHR, video monitor, computer	1	1	1	0	1	1	1	1

(continued)

Table 4.1 (continued)

Article #	Study	*N*	Length (of study)	Population	Country	Design	Methods	Key findings	Technology (i.e. hardware, software)	Area of focus[a] (1 = yes, 0 = no)				Level of focus[b] (1 = yes, 0 = no)			
										B	E	C	P	I	C	H	S
6	Middleton et al. (2013) [56]	=	Not specified	Health care profes-sionals	USA	Consensus	2011 Health care technology foundation clinical alarms survey	Provided recommendations regarding human factors, health information technology research, health IT policy, industry recommendations, and recommendations for the clinician end-user of EHR software	EHR, video monitor, computer	1	1	1	0	0	1	1	1
7	Mirhafez et al. (2019) [66]	197	5 months	Nurses	Iran	Cross-sectional descriptive analytical study	Surveys from nurses across three hospitals	Hospitals need to manage alarms to decrease alarm fatigue, improve alarm system safety, and further develop clinical policies and procedures	EHR, video monitor, computer	0	1	1	0	1	0	0	0
8	Nakagawa et al. (2019) [67]	–	Not specified	Physicians	USA	Mixed methods	Semi-structured interviews with focus groups or individual physicians	Despite the increasing adoption of technology into medical practice, the benefits that technology can offer to physician health remain largely untapped. It is time to start evaluating the impact of health technologies on physician well-being using tools	EHR, video monitor, computer, phone, email	1	1	1	0	1	0	0	1
9	Nimjee et al. (2020) [68]	11	1 month	Physicians	Canada	Qualitative	Semi-structured interviews	Common problems encountered included usability issues, downtimes, alarm fatigue, and administrative tasks. There were differences between generations regarding adaptability, perceived benefits and drawbacks, and perceptions of other generations' ability to adapt	EHR, video monitor, computer	1	0	0	0	0	1	1	1
10	Paterick et al. (2018) [69]	–	Not specified	Physicians	USA	Qualitative	Qualitative methods were used to gather and analyze data describing unintended adverse consequences of computerized provider order entry	–	EHR, video monitor, computer	1	0	1	0	1	1	1	0

Article #	Study	*N*	Length (of study)	Population	Country	Design	Methods	Key findings	Technology (i.e. hardware, software)	Area of focus[a] (1 = yes, 0 = no)				Level of focus[b] (1 = yes, 0 = no)			
										B	E	C	P	I	C	H	S
11	Shanafelt et al. (2016) [6]	6375	3 months	Physicians	USA	Non-experimental quantitative survey	US physicians across all specialties were surveyed from August to October 2014 and provided information regarding their use to EHR, electronic patient portals, and computerized physician order entry	Physicians who used EHRs were less satisfied with the amount of time spent on clerical tasks and were at higher risk for professional burnout	EHR, video monitor, computer, electronic patient portal	0	1	0	0	1	0	0	0
12	Sockalingam et al. (2020) [70]	426	Not specified	Health care profes-sionals	Canada	Implementation study	Rapid implementation and survey	Using an iterative curriculum design approach and existing implementation frameworks, the tele-education model can be rapidly mobilized to address health needs during the COVID-19 pandemic	Video monitor, computer, real-time polling	0	1	0	0	1	0	0	0
13	Tai-Seale et al. (2017) [71]	471	3 years	Physicians, health care admin-istrators	USA	Retrospective cohorts	Measure amount of time physician spent in EHR versus face-to-face care provided to patients	Physicians had an increase in computer-related tasks and decrease in face-to-face time with patients over time	EHR, video monitor, computer, phone, email	1	1	1	0	1	0	1	1
14	Westbrook et al. (2010) [72]	40	Not specified	Physicians	Australia	System redesign	Observational time and motion study conducted in the 400-bed emergency department of a teaching hospital	Task completion times are shorter for interrupted tasks; tasks with high frequency of interruptions have lower accuracy; stress and frustration are higher during interrupted tasks	Personal digital assistant (PDA)	1	0	1	0	1	0	0	0
# out of 14										9	9	10	1	12	6	6	6
Concept area 1a average										64.3%	64.3%	71.4%	7.1%	85.7%	42.9%	42.9%	46.2%

COVID-19 Coronavirus Disease-2019, *EHR* electronic health record, *UK* United Kingdom, *USA* United States of America, *VDT* video monitor

[a]Area of focus: B = Behavioral, E = Emotional, C = Cognitive, P = Physical

[b]Level of focus: I = Individual, C = Clinic, H = Hospital, S = System

Table 4.2 How to identify, minimize, and prevent fatigue related to technology

Evidence and findings.	Manifestations	Analysis	User adjustments
Clinical care			
Engagement and communication problems	Different quality eye contact Missed non-verbals Feels less responsive	Video ≠ in-person Requires more concentration, fewer distractions	Use an "ice breaker" Adjust communication (e.g., verbal not tissue for tears) Fit equipment to task
Requires effort: –Cognitive –Emotional –Physical	Fatigue with workflow –Less focus/attention –Irritability, criticism –Aches, strain	Individual (e.g., trait or state) versus work environment issues	Prepare and assist others Avoid multi-tasking Take breaks to refresh Attend to ergonomics
Excessive screen time	Eye, wrist, and other complaints Tired and finishing late	Retrieving, analyzing, and entry Extra time needed	Adjust eyewear, furniture, and length of day; take breaks
Interruptions	Texts, calls, and other alarms	Required, purposeful interruptions	Silence alarms and limit email/text; notify patients
Care and workflow metrics needed	Adjustments for video, EHR, and other	Detect if experience is good and effective	Identify data needed to assess issues and give input
Technology and office adjustments			
Selection of primary technology	Solo desktop or laptop screen is challenging	Funding is needed for equipment (e.g., two screens, accessories)	Pre-plan basic needs and customize to individual needs
Planning for other technology needed	Using personal phone for work Mobile devices may not feed into EHR	Assess resources versus needs, particularly for mobile health Use telework checklist	Administrative, clerical, and technical support upfront and ongoing
Work space, screen time, and ease of work	Eye, wrist, neck, head, and other complaints Substantial effort and late days	Ergonomic furniture, screen, and issues—Use occupational health and design studio principles	Adjust eyewear, furniture, and length of day Pilot workflow and any changes
Workflow alignment across settings	Home office is not adequate Going mobile results in problems	New settings raise challenges Standardize as much as possible	Align settings in design (e.g., arrangement of furniture)
Space and efficiency issues	Delays, problems, and fatigue Lack of back-up systems	Technology and task fit for workflow	Re-invest space $ to home setting Sound, décor, and environment positive for patient and clinician

Table 4.2 (continued)

Evidence and findings.	Manifestations	Analysis	User adjustments
Technology failure(s)	Battery, hardware/ software, other Wi-Fi availability, and cost	Technology and task fit Help in time may be needed	Pilot, log, and feed problem to IT staff and administration
Training and professional development			
Task-specific training and monitoring	Video okay but other technologies not	Skills, optimizing experience, and flow	Attend training and have forum to share tips
Skills/competencies	Asynchronous less routine and more challenges	Identify need (skill, knowledge) and triage	Schedule regular time (rather than free time)
Learning online may not be less effective	Limited discourse and less PD acculturation	Distractions, multi-tasking interruptions	Identify in-person: Skills, attitudes, and networking
Teaching effectiveness and flow	Virtual: Need time to shift material/ method	Virtual plan reduces errors and disruptions	Set learner expectation and create virtual culture
Social factors and relationships	Less networking and venting	Evaluate teamwork and connection to others	Do little things before and after meeting; use rewards
Human factors			
Amplification (shift from seldom to frequent use)	Physical ailments Fatigue complaints	Minor issues become problems; fatigue turns into burnout	Identify tedious or problematic workflow context(s) and modify
Cumulative load of technology in work and life	Emotional, cognitive, physical fatigue Put off/delayed events	Recreation, social (media), training, and care add up	Identify what needs to be/in-person and triage/shift Diversify activity modes
Fitness (emotional, physical, spiritual) versus fatigue	Concerns, worries, appearance, and personal disclosures	Personal/professional, individual/team/group evaluation	Localize problem and check-in with supervisor Add good habits
Isolation versus social/interpersonal connection	Missing discussions, meetings, and shifts Poor teamwork	Temporary or prolonged State versus trait/chronic	Evaluate culture of care, training, and faculty development
Errors and missed details	Poor outcomes and EHR alerts/alarms	Individual, group, team, and IS factor(s)	Identify common errors via performance data
Myth of multi-tasking	Poor patient engagement and errors	Facilitate reflection, use peer observation	Engage/focus on task and rare purposeful multi-tasking

Abbreviations/Definitions/Key: *$* financial, *EHR* electronic health record, *IS* information systems, *IT* information technology, *PD* professional development

Display and workflow interventions have been successful in many regards, including ergonomic interventions, which improved functioning [57, 78]. A 15-min work period with micro breaks [79] and physically large displays help employee performance. A 15-degree rather than 40-degree video display curvature (display curvature impacts effort to visualize displayed text) [80] and a case manuscript and luminance ratio of 3 (used for the useful contrast of a display) also help users' performance [9–14]. Co-working spaces are an alternative to the home office since professional isolation negatively impacts job performance, and employees with inhibitory deficits (e.g., prone to distraction) and poorer boundaries experience more stress [58, 81].

Content, discourse, and framework qualitative analysis techniques appear to indicate a continuum from health/resilience to risk of fatigue to manifestations of burnout [2]. Burnout manifests as exhaustion (physical, emotional), cynicism, and detachment from the job and others, and a sense of ineffectiveness and lack of accomplishment [24, 25]. Low job dissatisfaction is associated with low organizational commitment, with more frequent absenteeism, intention to leave the job, and turnover, as well as lower productivity and impaired quality of work. Those who suffer from burnout also disrupt others' job tasks and are more interpersonally aggressive. The Areas of Worklife (AW) Model considers workload, sense of control, reward, community, fairness, and values as important to burnout [75]. Reward and recognition provide opportunities for intrinsic satisfaction and self-efficacy. A good community provides social support, trust, effective means of working out disagreements, and better job engagement. The job demands-resources (JD-R) model posits that burnout is related to experience of incessant job demands and inadequate resources, whereas the conservation of resources (COR) model follows basic motivational theory in assuming that burnout arises as a result of persistent threats to available resources.

Conceptualization of fatigue and burnout may also be organized by engagement and job stress [24, 25, 82]. Engagement is considered a state of high energy, strong involvement, and a sense of efficacy. It is a persistent, positive affective-motivational state of fulfillment that is characterized by the three components of vigor, dedication, and absorption. Engagement is considered an independent and distinct concept, which is not the opposite of burnout, although is negatively related to it. Interventions at the *individual level* may involve: (1) changing work patterns; (2) developing coping skills; (3) obtaining social support; (4) utilizing relaxation strategies; (5) promoting good health and fitness; and (6) developing a better self-understanding. At the *workplace level*, it may mean: (1) redesigning job tasks; (2) improving recognition of notable work by both teams and individuals; and (3) developing more fair and equitable policies.

4.3.3 Guidelines for Providers and Organizations in Health Care for Use of Technology and Well-Being

A shift to a culture of well-being with technology use requires implementation, evaluation, and monitoring of individual, workplace, workflow, and institutional strategies [2]. If the link between technology and fatigue is poorly recognized, changes in workflow processes and policies may not be carried out until professional well-being is already at risk due to burnout [49]. Guidelines for health care, well-being, and use of technology (e.g., EHRs) are somewhat focused on burnout, but not fatigue. A shift to a culture of well-being that incorporates technology will require adaptations and quality improvement in the areas of technology, physical environment, and other occupational health factors. Objective measures to promote, evaluate, and enhance well-being are suggested to improve workflow at all levels: the individual; clinic; hospital; and system/organizational (Table 4.3). This could include adjustments in information systems and technology (IS, IT), use of

Table 4.3 Best practices in technology use for the workplace to promote well-being and prevent stress and fatigue

General
• Create reasonable workflow at work office, mobile/virtual, and home contexts [40]
– Consider alignment of values to standardize structure, process, and workflow
– Identify benefits (e.g., facility, convenience) and challenges (e.g., boundaries)
– Assess, monitor, and plan for change via lean or other processes [74]
– Emphasize "top of the license" and create new coordination care positions [48]
• Create a culture to reflect on impact of technology
– Provide initial and longitudinal training and promote adaptation for challenges
– Discuss impact of technology in educational and professional development forums
– Discuss what is working and what things need to change in workflow, particularly workload related to intensification via technology
– Employ employee experiential (i.e., user participation and training effectiveness) and psychological (i.e., user involvement and management support) engagement strategies [24, 25]
• Promote self-care, resilience, and well-being related to technology
– Seek organizational assistance for self-care [66, 67]
– Monitor stress, unexpected events, and challenges in workflow
– Use cognitive, mindfulness, fitness, and emotional strategies for coping and managing demands [25, 42]
– Consider the person, workplace, and person–workplace interaction [41]
Human factors
• Use an approach for technology use that is simple, customized to key constituents, and sustainable over time to promote stable interrelationships between the technology, production, organization, and the culture [2]
• Promote spirituality, social activities, help-seeking, and quality interpersonal relationships, and affirm strengths, perseverance, elasticity, and flexibility [39]
• Work toward and promote technological competencies; in health care, video [44], mobile health, and asynchronous technologies [18]
• Adjust work schedule and routines to observed/experienced rather than theoretical plans [24, 25]
– Avoid interruption and multi-tasking, as interruption self-efficacy can help offset interruption-based stress
– Take regular work breaks and technology breaks throughout the workday [79, 80, 87]
– Utilize expectation setting and help from team members to support boundaries on time [87]
– Manage time and life–work balance [17, 39]
– Resolve work–home conflicts [90]

(continued)

Table 4.3 (continued)

• Assess physical (e.g., eyewear, musculoskeletal, light) and professional environment needs [13]
• Ergonomic interventions improved eye (e.g., fatigue, burning, red eyes, and double/hazy vision) and physical pain (e.g., neck, shoulder, forearm, and back) symptoms, and wrist/hand discomfort [11, 78–80]
Ease of workflow
• Consider usability attributes: Simplicity; natural-ness; efficient interactions; effective information presentation; preserved context; and minimized cognitive load [47, 63]
• Get help with the selection and implementation of the technology for clinical workflow
– Identify approach and responsible party for initial and ongoing help
– Log accurate and meaningful data on successful and problematic events for analysis
• Align structure, process, and workflow across settings and contexts (e.g., work, home, mobile/virtual) [90]
• Assess impact of video and mobile health, stress, and workflow challenges, which are more common for those working across work and home settings compared to separators [2]
Site and workplace factors and interventions
• Balance outcome- and process-driven workflow and evaluation [39]
• Promote self-care and evaluate/monitor Well-being, health, and resilience versus fatigue and burnout [6, 18, 29, 50, 69, 83]
• Facilitate individual/team coordination and collaboration [58]
• Create presence with others while using technology by managing and considering time and environmental factors [87]
• Suggest leader behaviors that encourage and support employees' autonomy, participative decision-making, and meaning of work by reinforcing proactive employee behaviors
• Employ technology design and physical environment adjustments (e.g., ergonomics) based on business and occupational health principles [7, 78]
• Apply technology competency domains used for organizations to individuals and teams to increase digital literacy [18, 60]
• Provide technical support to reduce technostress/overload [43]
• Consider digital native (i.e., persons born or brought up during the age of the internet and digital technology) and digital immigrant perspectives on a continuum rather than by generation and age, regarding the concept of digital fluency [70]
• The 40-degree video display terminal position showed significantly greater head tilt angles and higher muscle activity levels than the preferred 15-degree position [2]
Evaluation and process improvement [18, 89] to promote: Good device visuals; in time help options; ease of use and learning; and quality of support [6, 7, 30, 52, 80]
• Use a 360-degree perspective to evaluate well-being related to technological integration [17, 52]
• Consider quantitative and qualitative analysis of each technology to see associated factors, types of fatigue, and resilience patterns to guide prevention and amelioration efforts
• Employ user design approaches/studios with focus groups, studies, and surveys [47, 53, 56]
• Apply joy in practice framework principles to identify and address human needs/factors, and develop leaders' participative management competency [28]
• Incorporate evaluations of technology, Well-being, and fatigue with regular, traditional outcomes like quality of care (e.g., engagement, improvement) and quality of life (e.g., enjoyment, facility/natural) [2]
• Use a business model to determine such an implementation strategy by involving all important stakeholders in a value-driven dialogue on what the technology should accomplish [2]
• Employ trust-based work time arrangements for information and communications technology use that allow for discretion over when, where, and how to perform work-related tasks

Lean methods, and emphasis on interprofessional education efforts with technology team-based care from the Institute of Healthcare Improvement and Agency for Healthcare Research and Quality [18].

Methods based on institutional competencies are also needed to promote provider competencies with technology and self-care. Deliberate, sustained, and comprehensive efforts by the organization, often inexpensive, reduce burnout and promote engagement [24, 25, 49–51]. It appears that provider well-being and health is related to technological integration—or lack of integration—of video, EHR, and mobile health over time. While the release of new technologies is common in the marketplace, introduction (or in some cases integration) of technologies into workflow for health care systems often occurs later—with initial training and the assumption that users will adapt, as needed [2]. Organizations vary widely in their efforts and resultant outcomes: (1) high—substantial institutional support to seek user input, optimize clinical skill/workflow, and monitor resilience and well-being; (2) mid—good, but limited institutional support to include user input, improve some workflow processes, but not systematically; and (3) low—minimal institutional support with expectations that users learn, adapt workflow, and maintain well-being individually [2].

4.4 Discussion

Studies are increasingly sophisticated related to implementation and evaluation of provider behavioral, emotional, cognitive, and physical adjustments to technology [8, 13, 14, 45–53]. Video and electronic health record use are associated with fatigue with: physical eye fatigue, neck pain, stress, and tiredness; behavioral impact related to additional effort due to barriers, trouble with engagement, emotional wear and tear, and exhaustion; cognitive inattention, effort, expecting problems, multitasking, and workload; and emotional experiences like anger, irritability, stress, and concern about well-being. While user ratings may be high on data quality, accuracy, and processing, cumbersome clerical tasks, the effort required in work, and interruptions cost time and result in more errors, stress, and frustration [6, 56, 63–74]. Other problems contributing to fatigue may include the addition of workflow steps before and after clinical care is provided, often requiring sustained periods of technology use. Few organizations consider the physical environment, occupational health approaches, Lean or process improvement, human factor, and user design approaches to workflow. Qualitative analysis of the literature suggests a continuum from health/resilience to risk of fatigue to manifestations of digital burnout [2]. Few data were found to contextually evaluate differences according to health professions and practice contexts.

Movements in workplace culture, well-being, and prevention of burnout from other fields are beginning to be used in health care [29, 49, 83], but an accurate evaluation of the problems is just beginning. Areas of specific focus include clinical care, human, training, professional development, workflow, and administration factors. The conceptualization of "burnout" is also undergoing change, with a shift toward the recognition of burnout as an occupational phenomenon rather than solely as an individual medical disease (e.g., depression) per the World Health Organization

[84]. Thus, deployment of health care and administrative resources should move beyond the individual (e.g., Family and Medical Leave Act) and look at structural, educational, cultural, and social factors. To begin to address challenges in health care related to fatigue and burnout—including those associated with technology—a substantial, collaborative effort is needed from health system leadership, organizational researchers, IT/IS specialists, and potentially the government [2, 3, 28, 29], as changes in financing, reimbursement, and regulatory processes may need adjustment. To transform organizational culture, "wrap-around" support for providers—not just patients—may be needed, as done in the culture of business organizations [38, 85]. An IT-business-medicine understanding or conceptual framework has been likewise suggested with individual and institutional competencies [38, 60] based on IT architecture [86], as well as a 360-degree perspective with qualitative approaches to collect input from providers (e.g., what makes care "therapeutic," enjoyable and easy to provide) [87]. Human factors engineering and usability assessment has a rich set of scientific methods, a strong evidence base, and is widely applied effectively in other industries [88–90].

Health care delivery and systems are increasingly incorporating technology, but need to evaluate its impact for all users, including providers.

- Acknowledgments American Telemedicine Association and the Telemental Health Interest Group.
- The Coalition for Technology in Behavioral Science.
- Department of Psychiatry and Behavioral Sciences, University of California, Davis School of Medicine.
- Veteran Affairs Northern California Health Care System and Mental Health Service Office of Connected Care, Department of Veterans Affairs.

References

1. Pew Research Center: Experts Say the 'New Normal' in 2025 Will Be Far More Tech-Driven, Presenting More Big Challenges. https://www.pewresearch.org/internet/2021/02/18/experts-say-the-new-normal-in-2025-will-be-far-more-tech-driven-presenting-more-big-challenges/. Accessed 1 Jul 2023.
2. Hilty DM, Armstrong CM, Smout SA, Crawford A, Maheu MM, Drude K, et al. Findings and guidelines on provider technology, fatigue, and well-being: scoping review. J Med Internet Res. 2022;24(5):e34451. Published 2022 May 25. https://doi.org/10.2196/34451.
3. Bodenheimer T, Sinsky C. From triple to quadruple aim: care of the patient requires care of the provider. Ann Fam Med. 2014;12(6):573–6.
4. Pattyn N, Van Cutsem J, Dessy E, Mairesse O. Bridging exercise science, cognitive psychology, and medical practice: is "cognitive fatigue" a remake of "the emperor's new clothes"? Front Psychol. 2018;9:1246. Published 2018 Sep 10. https://doi.org/10.3389/fpsyg.2018.01246.
5. Montgomery A, Panagopoulou E, Esmail A, Richards T, Maslach C. Burnout in healthcare: the case for organisational change. BMJ. 2019;366:l4774. https://doi.org/10.1136/bmj.l4774.
6. Shanafelt TD, Dyrbye LN, Sinsky C, Hasan O, Satele D, Sloan J, et al. Relationship between clerical burden and characteristics of the electronic environment with physician burnout and professional satisfaction. Mayo Clin Proc. 2016;91(7):836–48. https://doi.org/10.1016/j.mayocp.2016.05.007.

7. Nguyen OT, Jenkins NJ, Khanna N, Shah S, Gartland AJ, Turner K, et al. A systematic review of contributing factors of and solutions to electronic health record-related impacts on physician well-being [published online ahead of print, 2021 Feb 1]. J Am Med Inform Assoc. 2021;28:ocaa339. https://doi.org/10.1093/jamia/ocaa339.
8. Khairat S, Coleman C, Ottmar P, Jayachander DI, Bice T, Carson SS. Association of electronic health record use with physician fatigue and efficiency. JAMA Netw Open. 2020;3(6):e207385. Published 2020 Jun 1. https://doi.org/10.1001/jamanetworkopen.2020.7385.
9. Knave BG, Wibom RI, Bergqvist UO, Carlsson LL, Levin MI, Nylén PR. Work with video display terminals among office employees. II. Physical exposure factors. Scand J Work Environ Health. 1985;11(6):467–74. https://doi.org/10.5271/sjweh.2199.
10. Böös SR, Calissendorff BM, Knave BG, Nyman KG, Voss M. Work with video display terminals among office employees. III. Ophthalmologic factors. Scand J Work Environ Health. 1985;11(6):475–81. https://doi.org/10.5271/sjweh.2207.
11. Travers PH, Stanton BA. Office workers and video display terminals: physical, psychological and ergonomic factors. AAOHN J. 2002;50(11):489–93.
12. Mocci F, Serra A, Corrias GA. Psychological factors and visual fatigue in working with video display terminals. Occup Environ Med. 2001;58(4):267–71.
13. Krupinski EA, Berbaum KS. Measurement of visual strain in radiologists. Acad Radiol. 2009;16(8):947–50.
14. Krupinski EA, Berbaum KS, Caldwell MFA, et al. Long radiology workdays reduce detection and accommodation accuracy. J Am Coll Radiol. 2010;7(9):698–704. https://doi.org/10.1016/j.jacr.2010.03.004.
15. Dawson D, Ian Noy Y, Härmä M, Akerstedt T, Belenky G. Modelling fatigue and the use of fatigue models in work settings. Accid Anal Prev. 2011;43(2):549–64. https://doi.org/10.1016/j.aap.2009.12.030.
16. Caldwell JA, Caldwell JL, Thompson LA, Lieberman HR. Fatigue and its management in the workplace. Neurosci Biobehav Rev. 2019;96:272–89. https://doi.org/10.1016/j.neubiorev.2018.10.024.
17. Verret CI, Nguyen J, Verret C, Albert TJ, Fufa DT. How do areas of work life drive burnout in orthopaedic attending surgeons, fellows, and residents? Clin Orthop Relat Res. 2020;479:251. https://doi.org/10.1097/CORR.0000000000001457.
18. Hilty DM, Torous J, Parish M, Chan SR, Xiong G, Scher L, et al. A literature review comparing clinicians' approaches and skills to in-person, synchronous and asynchronous care: moving toward asynchronous competencies to ensure quality care. Telemed J E-Health. 2020;27:356. https://doi.org/10.1089/tmj.2020.0054.
19. Maricuțoiu LP, Sulea C, Iancu A. Work engagement or burnout: which comes first? A meta-analysis of longitudinal evidence. Burn Res. 2017;5:35–43. Accessed 1 July 1 2023. https://doi.org/10.1016/j.burn.2017.05.001.
20. Mäkikangas A, Leiter MP, Kinnunen U, Feldt T. Profiling development of burnout over eight years: relation with job demands and resources. European J Work Org Psychology Published online. 2020;30:720. Accessed 1 July 1 2023. https://doi.org/10.1080/1359432X.2020.1790651.
21. Schneider A, Weigl M. Associations between psychosocial work factors and provider mental well-being in emergency departments: a systematic review. PLoS One. 2018;13(6):e0197375. Published 2018 Jun 4. https://doi.org/10.1371/journal.pone.0197375.
22. Sakuraya A, Imamura K, Watanabe K, Asai Y, Ando E, Eguchi H, et al. What kind of intervention is effective for improving subjective well-being among workers? A systematic review and meta-analysis of randomized controlled trials. Front Psychol. 2020;11:528656. Published 2020 Nov 13. https://doi.org/10.3389/fpsyg.2020.528656.
23. American Medical Association: 7 steps to prevent burnout in your practice [internet]. AMA Wired, Aug 11, 2015. https://wire.ama-assn.org/practice-management/7-steps-prevent-burnout-your-practice. Accessed 1 Jul 2023.
24. Maslach C, Leiter MP. Understanding the burnout experience: recent research and its implications for psychiatry. World Psychiatry. 2016;15(2):103–11.

25. Maslach C, Leiter MP. New insights into burnout and health care: strategies for improving civility and alleviating burnout. Med Teach. 2017;39(2):160–3. Epub 2016 Nov 13. https://doi.org/10.1080/0142159X.2016.1248918.
26. West CP, Dyrbye LN, Erwin PJ, Shanafelt TD. Interventions to prevent and reduce physician burnout: a systematic review and meta-analysis. Lancet. 2016;388(10057):2272–81. https://doi.org/10.1016/S0140-6736(16)31279-X.
27. Stehman CR, Testo Z, Gershaw RS, Kellogg AR. Burnout, drop out, suicide: physician loss in emergency medicine, part I [published correction appears in West J Emerg med. 2019 Aug 21;20(5):840-841]. West J Emerg Med. 2019;20(3):485–94. https://doi.org/10.5811/westjem.2019.4.40970.
28. Swensen SJ, Shanafelt T. An organizational framework to reduce professional burnout and bring back joy in practice. J Comm J Qual Patient Saf. 2017;43(6):308–13. https://doi.org/10.1016/j.jcjq.2017.01.007.
29. Shanafelt TD, Noseworthy JH. Executive leadership and physician well-being: nine organizational strategies to promote engagement and reduce burnout. Mayo Clin Proc. 2017;92(1):129–46. https://doi.org/10.1016/j.mayocp.2016.10.004.
30. Downing NL, Bates DW, Longhurst CA. Physician burnout in the electronic health record era: are we ignoring the real cause? Ann Intern Med. 2018;169(1):50–1. https://doi.org/10.7326/M18-0139.
31. Gleichgerrcht E, Decety J. Empathy in clinical practice: how individual dispositions, gender, and experience moderate empathic concern, burnout, and emotional distress in physicians. PLoS One. 2013;8(4):e61526. https://doi.org/10.1371/journal.pone.0061526.
32. Fothergill A, Edwards D, Burnard P. Stress, burnout, coping and stress management in psychiatrists: findings from a systematic review. Int J Soc Psychiatry. 2004;50(1):54–65. https://doi.org/10.1177/0020764004040953.
33. Rössler W. Stress, burnout, and job dissatisfaction in mental health workers. Eur Arch Psychiatry Clin Neurosci. 2012;262(Suppl 2):65–9. Epub 2012 Aug 28. Erratum in: Eur Arch Psychiatry Clin Neurosci. 2016 Jun;266(4):381. 10.1007/s00406-016-0688-3. https://doi.org/10.1007/s00406-012-0353-4.
34. O'Connor K, Muller Neff D, Pitman S. Burnout in mental health professionals: a systematic review and meta-analysis of prevalence and determinants. Eur Psychiatry. 2018;53:74–99. https://doi.org/10.1016/j.eurpsy.2018.06.003.
35. Panagioti M, Panagopoulou E, Bower P, Lewith G, Kontopantelis E, Chew-Graham C, et al. Controlled interventions to reduce burnout in physicians: a systematic review and meta-analysis. JAMA Intern Med. 2017;177(2):195–205. https://doi.org/10.1001/jamainternmed.2016.7674.
36. Van Steenbergen EF, van der Ven C, Peeters MCW, Taris TW. Transitioning towards new ways of working: do job demands, job resources, burnout, and engagement change? Psychol Rep. 2018;121(4):736–66. https://doi.org/10.1177/0033294117740134.
37. Hilty DM, Crawford A, Teshima J, Chan S, Sunderji N, Yellowlees PM, et al. A framework for telepsychiatric training and e-health: competency-based education, evaluation and implications. Int Rev Psychiatry. 2015;27(6):569–92.
38. Hilty DM, Luo J, Giron E, Ko D-K. A shared information technology-business-health model: lessons for health care leaders on integrating technology from investment banking. Psychol Cogn Sci Open J. 2021;7(1):1–18. https://doi.org/10.17140/PCSOJ-7-159.
39. Adamson C, Beddoe L, Davys A. Building resilient practitioners: definitions and practitioner understandings. Br J Soc Work. 2014;44(3):522–41. http://www.jstor.org/stable/43687656.
40. Hilty DM, Groshong LW, Coleman M, Maheu MM, Armstrong CM, Smout SS, et al. Best practices for technology in clinical social work to promote Well-being and prevent fatigue. Clin Soc Work J. 2023;51:211. https://doi.org/10.1007/s10615-023-00865-3.
41. Wulansari NA, Ranihusna D, Witiastuti RS. Reduction effect of technostress with role of perceived organizational support. Indian J Appl Bus Econ Res. 2015;13(7):5159–71.
42. Upadhyay P, Chang TFH, Hariri S, et al. The effect of inner engineering online (IEO) program on reducing stress for information technology professionals: a randomized control study.

Evid Based Complement Alternat Med. 2022;2022:9001828. Published 2022 Jan 4. https://doi.org/10.1155/2022/9001828.
43. Vogt F, Seidl F, Santarpino G, et al. Healthcare information management and systems society technology utilization and penetration among physicians: novel IT solutions in healthcare - use and acceptance in hospitals. Eur Surg Res. 2018;59(1–2):100–13. https://doi.org/10.1159/000490241.
44. Maheu M, Drude K, Hertlein K, Hilty DM. An interdisciplinary framework for telebehavioral health competencies. J Tech Behav Sci. 2018;3(2):108–40; correction 3(2):107.
45. Holmgren AJ, Downing NL, Bates DW, Shanafelt TD, Milstein A, Sharp CD, et al. Assessment of electronic health record use between us and non-us health systems [published correction appears in JAMA intern med. 2021 Feb 1;181(2):296]. JAMA Intern Med. 2021;181(2):251–9. https://doi.org/10.1001/jamainternmed.2020.707.
46. Galt KA, Fuji KT, Kaufman TK, Shah SR. Health information technology use and patient safety: study of pharmacists in Nebraska. Pharmacy (Basel). 2019;7(1):7. Published 2019 Jan 10. https://doi.org/10.3390/pharmacy7010007.
47. Lopez KD, Fahey L. Advocating for greater usability in clinical technologies: the role of the practicing nurse. Crit Care Nurs Clin North Am. 2018;30(2):247–57. https://doi.org/10.1016/j.cnc.2018.02.007.
48. Mylod DE. One way to prevent clinician burnout. Harvard Bus Rev. https://hbr.org/2017/10/one-way-to-prevent-clinician-burnout. Published October 12, 2017. Accessed 1 Jul 2023.
49. Nakagawa K, Yellowlees P. Inter-generational effects of technology: why millennial physicians may be less at risk for burnout than baby boomers. Curr Psychiatry Rep. 2020;22(9):45. Published 2020 Jul 13. https://doi.org/10.1007/s11920-020-01171-2.
50. National Academies of Sciences, Engineering & Medicine. Taking action against clinician burnout: a systems approach to professional well-being. National Academies Press; 2019. https://nam.edu/systems-approaches-to-improve-patient-care-by-supporting-clinician-well-being/?gclid=CjwKCAjw2P-KBhByEiwADBYWChB818zZC1PzDVuR9MKjU8Thn-ChfUeuctyVtenux0W84tBeCBY4WQBoCPpcQAvD_BwE. Accessed 1 Jul 2023.
51. Shanafelt TD, Lightner DJ, Conley CR, Petrou SP, Richardson JW, Schroeder PJ, et al. An organization model to assist individual physicians, scientists, and senior health care administrators with personal and professional needs. Mayo Clin Proc. 2017;92(11):1688–96. https://doi.org/10.1016/j.mayocp.2017.08.020.
52. Tutty MA, Carlasare LE, Lloyd S, Sinsky CA. The complex case of EHRs: examining the factors impacting the EHR user experience [published correction appears in J Am Med Inform Assoc. 2019 Nov 1;26(11):1424]. J Am Med Inform Assoc. 2019;26(7):673–7. https://doi.org/10.1093/jamia/ocz021.
53. Zhang Y, Padman R, Levin JE. Reducing provider cognitive workload in CPOE use: optimizing order sets. Stud Health Technol Inform. 2013;192:734–8.
54. Braithwaite J, Churruca K, Long JC, Ellis LA, Herkes J. When complexity science meets implementation science: a theoretical and empirical analysis of systems change. BMC Med. 2018;16(1):63. https://doi.org/10.1186/s12916-018-1057-z.
55. Keyworth C, Hart J, Armitage CJ, Tully MP. What maximizes the effectiveness and implementation of technology-based interventions to support healthcare professional practice? A systematic literature review. BMC Med Inform Decis Mak. 2018;18(1):93. . Published 2018 Nov 7. https://doi.org/10.1186/s12911-018-0661-3.
56. Middleton B, Bloomrosen M, Dente MA, Hashmat B, Koppel R, Overhage JM, et al. Enhancing patient safety and quality of care by improving the usability of electronic health record systems: recommendations from AMIA. J Am Med Inform Assoc. 2013;20(e1):e2–8. https://doi.org/10.1136/amiajnl-2012-001458.
57. Karwowski W, Eberts R, Salvendy G, Noland S. The effects of computer interface design on human postural dynamics. Ergonomics. 1994;37(4):703–24. https://doi.org/10.1080/00140139408963684.

58. Robelski S, Keller H, Harth V, Mache S. Coworking spaces: the better home office? A psychosocial and health-related perspective on an emerging work environment. Int J Environ Res Public Health. 2019;16(13):2379. Published 2019 Jul 4. https://doi.org/10.3390/ijerph16132379.
59. Christensen CM. Disruptive innovation: can health care learn from other industries? A conversation with Clayton M. Christensen. Interview by Smith MD. Health Aff (Millwood). 2007;26(3):w288–95.
60. Hilty DM, Unutzer J, Ko DK, Luo J, Worley LLM, Yager J. Approaches for departments, schools and health systems to better implement technologies used for clinical care and education. Acad Psychiatry. 2019;43(6):611–6.
61. Aij KH, Rapsaniotis S. Leadership requirements for lean versus servant leadership in health care: a systematic review of the literature. J Healthc Leadersh. 2017;9:1–14. Published 2017 Jan 18. https://doi.org/10.2147/JHL.S120166.
62. Maijala R, Eloranta S, Reunanen T, Ikonen TS. Successful implementation of lean as a managerial principle in health care: a conceptual analysis from systematic literature review. Int J Technol Assess Health Care. 2018;34(2):134–46. https://doi.org/10.1017/S0266462318000193.
63. Arndt BG, Beasley JW, Watkinson MD, Temte JL, Tuan WJ, Sinsky CA, et al. Tethered to the EHR: primary care physician workload assessment using EHR event log data and time-motion observations. Ann Fam Med. 2017;15(5):419–26. https://doi.org/10.1370/afm.2121.
64. Campbell EM, Sittig DF, Guappone KP, Dykstra RH, Ash JS. Overdependence on technology: an unintended adverse consequence of computerized provider order entry. AMIA Annu Symp Proc. 2007;2007:94–8. Published 2007 Oct 11.
65. Hilty DM, Marks S, Wegelin J, Callahan EJ, Nesbitt TS. A randomized, controlled trial of disease management modules, including telepsychiatric care, for depression in rural primary care. Psychiatry (Edgmont). 2007;4(2):58–65.
66. McAlearney AS, Schweikhart SB, Medow MA. Organizational and physician perspectives about facilitating handheld computer use in clinical practice: results of a cross-site qualitative study. J Am Med Inform Assoc. 2005;12(5):568–75. https://doi.org/10.1197/jamia.M1816.
67. McAlearney AS, Hefner JL, Sieck CJ, Huerta TR. The journey through grief: insights from a qualitative study of electronic health record implementation. Health Serv Res. 2015;50(2):462–88. https://doi.org/10.1111/1475-6773.12227.
68. Mirhafez SR, Movahedi A, Moghadam-Pasha A, Mohammadi G, Moeini V, Moradi Z, et al. Perceptions and practices related to clinical alarms. Nurs Forum. 2019;54(3):369–75. https://doi.org/10.1111/nuf.12338.
69. Nakagawa K, Yellowlees PM. University of California Technology Wellness Index: a physician-centered framework to assess technologies' impact on physician well-being. Psychiatr Clin North Am. 2019;42(4):669–81. https://doi.org/10.1016/j.psc.2019.08.005.
70. Nimjee T, Miller E, Solomon S. Exploring generational differences in physicians' perspectives on the proliferation of technology within the medical field: a narrative study. Healthc Q. 2020;23:53–9. https://doi.org/10.12927/hcq.2020.26172.
71. Paterick ZR, Patel NJ, Paterick TE. Unintended consequences of the electronic medical record on physicians in training and their mentors. Postgrad Med J. 2018;94(1117):659–61. https://doi.org/10.1136/postgradmedj-2018-135849.
72. Sockalingam S, Clarkin C, Serhal E, Pereira C, Crawford A. Responding to health care professionals' mental health needs during COVID-19 through the rapid implementation of project echo. J Contin Educ Health Prof. 2020;40:211–4. https://doi.org/10.1097/CEH.0000000000000311.
73. Tai-Seale M, Olson CW, Li J, Chan AS, Morikawa C, Durban M, et al. Electronic health record logs indicate that physicians split time evenly between seeing patients and desktop medicine. Health Aff (Millwood). 2017;36:655–62.
74. Westbrook JI, Coiera E, Dunsmuir WT, Brown BM, Kelk N, Paoloni R, Tran C. The impact of interruptions on clinical task completion. Qual Saf Health Care. 2010;19(4):284–9. Epub 2010 May 12. https://doi.org/10.1136/qshc.2009.039255.
75. Leiter MP, Maslach C. Areas of worklife survey manual and sampler set. 5th ed. Menlo Park, CA: Mind Garden; 2011.

76. Steffy BD, Jones JW. The psychological impact of video display terminals on employees' well-being. Am J Health Promot. 1989;4(2):101–7. https://doi.org/10.4278/0890-1171-4.2.101.
77. Turville KL, Psihogios JP, Ulmer TR, Mirka GA. The effects of video display terminal height on the operator: a comparison of the 15 degree and 40 degree recommendations. Appl Ergon. 1998;29(4):239–46. https://doi.org/10.1016/s0003-6870(97)00048-3.
78. Aarås A, Horgen G, Ro O, Konarska M, Larsen S, Thoresen M, et al. The effect of an ergonomic intervention on musculoskeletal, psychosocial and visual strain of VDT data entry work: the Norwegian part of the international study. Int J Occup Saf Ergon. 2005;11(1):25–47. https://doi.org/10.1080/10803548.2005.11076627.
79. Balci R, Aghazadeh F. The effect of work-rest schedules and type of task on the discomfort and performance of VDT users. Ergonomics. 2003;46(5):455–65. https://doi.org/10.1080/0014013021000047557.
80. Park S, Kyung G, Choi D, Lee S, Lee JE, Choi B, et al. Effects of display curvature and task duration on proofreading performance, visual discomfort, visual fatigue, mental workload, and user satisfaction. Appl Ergon. 2019;78:26–36. https://doi.org/10.1016/j.apergo.2019.01.014.
81. Golden TD, Veiga JF, Dino RN. The impact of professional isolation on teleworker job performance and turnover intentions: does time spent teleworking, interacting face-to-face, or having access to communication-enhancing technology matter? J Appl Psychol. 2008;93(6):1412–21. https://doi.org/10.1037/a0012722.
82. Molino M, Cortese CG, Ghislieri C. The promotion of technology acceptance and work engagement in industry 4.0: from personal resources to information and training. Int J Environ Res Public Health. 2020;17(7):2438. Published 2020 Apr 3. https://doi.org/10.3390/ijerph17072438.
83. Perlo J, Balik B, Swensen S, Landsman J, Feeley D. IHI framework for improving joy in work. IHI White Paper. Cambridge, MA: Institute for Healthcare Improvement; 2017. http://www.ihi.org/resources/Pages/IHIWhitePapers/Framework-Improving-Joy-in-Work.aspx. Accessed 1 Jul 2023.
84. World Health Organization. Burn-out an "occupational phenomenon:" International Classification of Diseases, 2019. https://www.who.int/mental_health/evidence/burn-out/en/. Accessed 1 Jul 2023.
85. Ray G, Muhanna WA, Barney JB. Competing with IT: the role of shared IT-business understanding. Commun ACM. 2007;50(12):87–91.
86. Ross JW. Creating a strategic IT architecture competency: learning in stages. In: MIT Sloan School of Management Working Paper, 4314–03, Center for Information Systems Research Working Paper, No. 335; 2003. http://dspace.mit.edu/handle/1721.1/3526. Accessed 1 Jul 2023.
87. Brown-Johnson C, Schwartz R, Maitra A, Haverfield MC, Tierney A, Shaw JG, et al. What is clinician presence? A qualitative interview study comparing physician and non-physician insights about practices of human connection. BMJ Open. 2019;9(11):e030831. Published 2019 Nov 3. https://doi.org/10.1136/bmjopen-2019-030831.
88. Szalma JL. On the application of motivation theory to human factors/ergonomics: motivational design principles for human-technology interaction. Hum Factors. 2014;56(8):1453–71. https://doi.org/10.1177/0018720814553471.
89. Pelayo S, Kaipio J. Section editors for the IMIA yearbook section on human factors and organizational issues. Findings from the 2018 yearbook section on human factors and organizational issues. Yearb Med Inform. 2018;27(1):79–82. https://doi.org/10.1055/s-0038-1667074.
90. Camacho S, Barrios A. Teleworking and technostress: early consequences of a COVID-19 lockdown. Cogn Technol Work. 2022;24(3):441–57. https://doi.org/10.1007/s10111-022-00693-4.

Part II

Access, Evaluation, User Design

Designing New Technology for Neurodevelopmental Disorders and the Importance of Involving Users (Not Only Robots)

5

Thomas Gargot, Arzu Guneysu, Carlos Cifuentes, and Silvia Orlandi

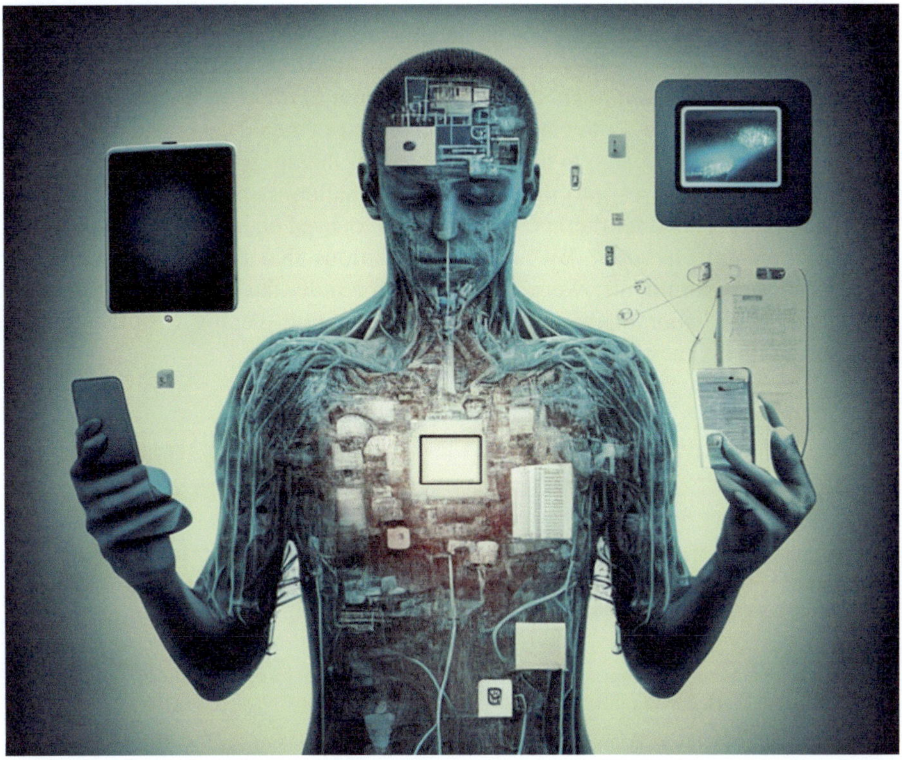

D. Mucić, D. M. Hilty (eds.), *Digital Mental Health*,
https://doi.org/10.1007/978-3-031-59936-1_5

Abstract

Mental disorders including neurodevelopmental difficulties are frequent, creating a substantial disparity between the demand for mental health care and the available resources. The potential of therapeutic technologies to address this treatment gap is immense, offering scalable solutions to enhance access. Yet, the intricate nature of mental disorders, woven with diverse risk factors, poses challenges to a comprehensive understanding of their mechanisms and assessment of this potential.

Current assessments of mental disorders heavily rely on the expertise of trained clinicians, making it imperative to explore innovative avenues such as "digital phenotyping" to capture nuanced behaviors. However, integrating technology into healthcare encounters obstacles exacerbated by the divergent cultures of medical professionals and engineers. While technical feasibility is a priority for engineers, it often needs to match the acceptability standards set by healthcare professionals.

Navigating the complexity of the healthcare ecosystem compounds the challenge of identifying precise needs. Furthermore, the time-intensive nature of clinical research methods hinders the swift evaluation of efficacy. To surmount these hurdles, we advocate for the incorporation of user-centered design methodologies and participatory research in the development of therapeutic technologies.

This chapter delves into the multifaceted challenges of designing technologies, such as robots, for therapeutic programs focused on individuals with neurodevelopmental disorders. By proposing solutions that prioritize participatory co-design environments, we aim to empower individuals from diverse backgrounds to collaboratively support those undergoing therapy with technology, ensuring its efficacy and benefits.

T. Gargot (✉)
Child and Adolescent Psychiatry Department, University Hospital of Tours, Tours, France

EXcellence Center in Autism and Neurodevelopmental Disorders—Tours ExAC-T, iBrain U1253, University of Tours, Tours, France

Université de Tours, INSERM, Imaging Brain and Neuropsychiatry, iBraiN U1253, Tours, France
e-mail: thomas.gargot@univ-tours.fr

A. Guneysu
Department of Biomedical Engineering and Health Systems, KTH Royal Institute of Technology, CBH, Stockholm, Sweden

Department of Computing Science, Umeå University, Umeå, Sweden
e-mail: arzu.guneysu@umu.se

C. Cifuentes
Bristol Robotics Laboratory, University of the West of England, Bristol, UK
e-mail: carlos.cifuentes@uwe.ac.uk

S. Orlandi
Department of Electrical, Electronic, and Information Engineering—Guglielmo Marconi (DEI), University of Bologna, Bologna, Italy

IRCCS Istituto delle Scienze Neurologiche di Bologna, Bologna, Italy
e-mail: silvia.orlandi9@unibo.it

5.1 Unmet Needs of Access to Care

5.1.1 Treatment Gaps in Mental Care

Mental disorders are very frequent and impairing [1]. World Health Organization reports that, independently of all mental disorders, depression is the first cause of disability in the world [2]. However, access to care is very limited. The bulletin of the World Health Organization reports that between 32.2% of schizophrenia, 56% of depression, and 78.1% of alcohol abuse and dependence patients did not have access to care [3]. Even when the difficulties are emerging and easier to resolve in child and adolescent psychiatry, the situation is poor. In France, access to care is around 50% in child and adolescent psychiatry (*Cour des comptes* 2023) and can be much lower in other countries. Neurodevelopment disorders are frequent in 10–15% of the population. They have the highest cost per patient [4]. Autism spectrum disorder prevalence is 0.70–3%. Developmental coordination disorder prevalence is 0.76–17%. Learning disorders prevalence is 3–10%. Attention deficit hyperactivity disorder prevalence is 5–11%. Language disorders and communication prevalence is 1–3.42%. Intellectual deficiency prevalence is 0.63% [5]. Many emerging technologies aim to tackle the mental health treatment gap, particularly mobile applications [6].

5.1.2 Potential of New Technologies

New technologies were already used to facilitate communication in psychiatry (telepsychiatry). In this chapter, we will discuss emerging technologies using either special sensors and machine learning techniques (automatic assessment and rehabilitation) or technologies giving (semi-) autonomous care (applications -apps-, interaction scenarios, robots).

New technologies could help to tackle access to care thanks to several properties: (1) better measure and monitoring of the behavior of the user ("digital phenotyping") [7] with proper measures, (2) the ability to integrate these measures to regroup the users in categories and predict the evolution (prognostic) (precision psychiatry), and (3) the possibility to scale up and adapt the measures and therapeutic strategies more easily.

In more detail:

1. New technologies are prone to precisely record the interaction with the user (use of an app, interaction with a robot, a remote control, an interface). For instance, digital phenotyping is a field of research that aims to characterize it. It could be helpful to support either screening of the disorder or to guide the reeducation based on appropriate features. We can measure movements using machine vision (posture, movement characteristics, head pose, gaze), e.g. in autism [8, 9], measures of emotions affective computing (sadness, fear, frustration, stress)

with cameras or wearables [10], analyzing language with natural language processing [11].
2. From these features, it is possible to use models to make categories or predict evolution that could be useful for a final aim to adapt clinician or technological system accordingly, for instance, from writing features, a model based on electronic tablet features [12] could extract different clusters/subtypes of handwriting [13] that could have different prognosis for rehabilitation needs (precision psychiatry). These new technologies allow us to go beyond the classical categorical and symptoms-based Diagnostic and Statistical Manual of Mental Disorders (DSM) criteria [14]. For instance, they could help better define psychiatric disorders with network symptoms analysis [15].
3. Like any software, they can be quite easily scalable. Software is easy to copy and then scale up without any loss from the sharer. The field of open data aims to share databases and models that enable the transfer of knowledge and tools more easily between users and researchers with a minimal cost, thanks to the internet to facilitate reusability, transparency, and development. Meditation apps like "Headspace" were downloaded by 70 million users, and "Petit Bambou" was used by eight million.

Beyond communication, new technologies offer tremendous perspectives in care like recording thoughts and emotions (ecological momentary assessment [16]), training sensory or motor difficulties that are early impaired in children with neurodevelopmental disorders and offering possibilities of compensation to alleviate memory, planning and time management, emotion regulation strategies, reading difficulties.

Broadly speaking, emerging technologies can potentially enhance the characterization of behaviors associated with mental disorders, a concept known as "digital phenotyping" [17]. Currently, such behaviors are primarily evaluated by trained clinicians. The integration of new technologies can contribute to a more comprehensive understanding of mechanisms underlying mental disorders, particularly in the context of normal and pathological human development, shedding light on the dynamics of behavioral changes.

Unfortunately, very often, technologies are not developed, either with end-users, or experts in the mental health field like psychiatrists or psychologists (that can limit their customization to the needs of the field). Also, they are not based on an evidence framework (e.g. , learning principles and cognitive and behavioral therapy), and their efficacy (is it working at the end on the field?) needs to be assessed properly.

Beyond their efficacy, several concerns can be raised. Are they acceptable [18]? Can some technologies be palliative of a poor organization of society or healthcare? Technology development informs what is possible, but some technologies should not be used. Are they usable for the user? Are they respecting their practice? In the end, are they cost-efficient? A good design involving users early in the process can help to understand the challenges better and answer the relevant needs of the end-users.

5.1.3 Usage Scenarios Should Be Defined from the Field

5.1.3.1 Acceptability, Expectancy, and Organizational Challenges

Technologies should enhance the psychiatrist/therapist–patient relationship and improve access to care, rather than replace it. We propose a model to describe the development process of new technologies spanning from addressing the treatment gap to their integration into the healthcare system. This model highlights several challenges involved in designing and evaluating new technologies in psychiatry and healthcare in general (Fig. 5.1). This process takes several years to implement.

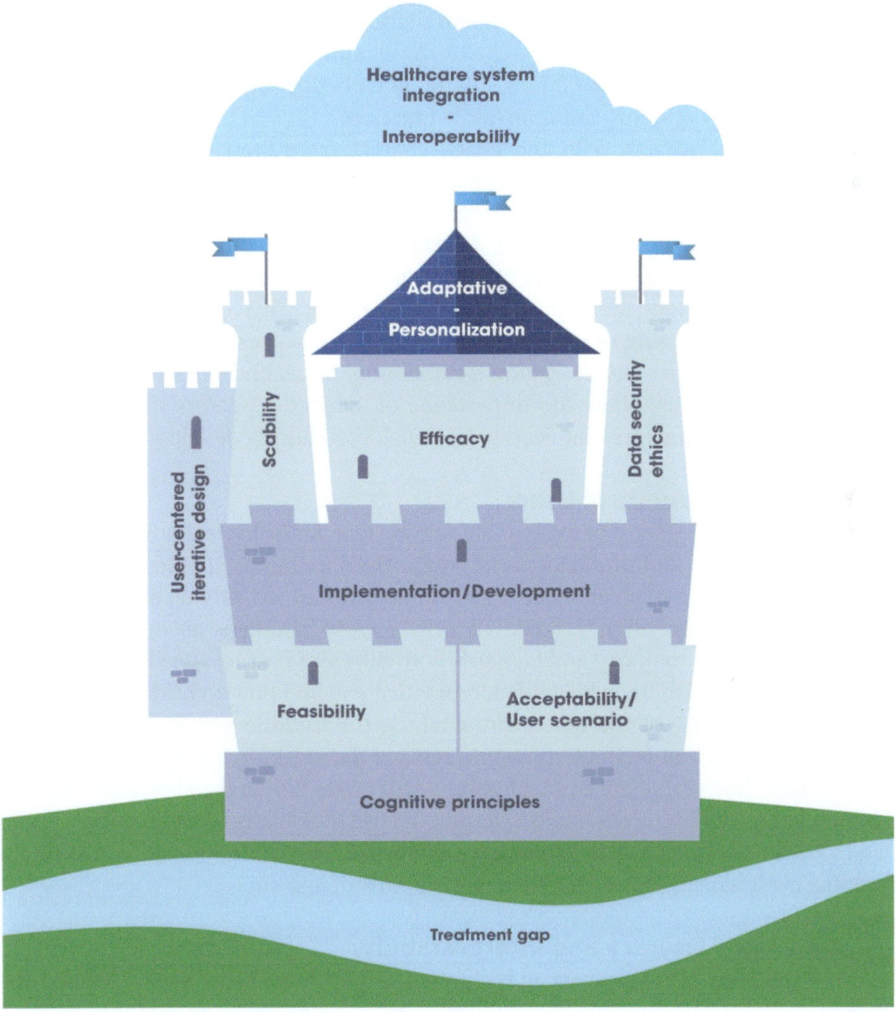

Fig. 5.1 Different steps involved in the design process

Defining the usage scenario can be difficult, and some practices can induce some reluctance in professionals (are they replacing the professional that feels threatened?, what is the system's performance, and how to deal with the accountability of the professional?) As a result, it is important to define well the user scenario (when it should or should not be used) and the usability needs to be assessed early before any dissemination [19, 20].

Venkatesh et al. [21] described the Unified Theory of Acceptance and Use of Technology model (UTAUT). It is a technology acceptance model defined in four constructs: (1) performance expectancy, (2) effort expectancy, (3) social influence, and (4) enabling conditions. In a survey, Alaiad and Zhou assessed the determinants of home healthcare robot adoption. The most important determinants were performance expectancy, social influence, trust, privacy concerns, ethical concerns, and facilitating conditions with social influence (the extent to which a stakeholder perceives that significant others believe he or she should use the device) [22]. Stahl and Coeckelbergh [23] argue that ethics should be embedded in practical settings from the design of new systems and innovative practices.

In a literature review, Alla and Pazos characterized the (1) technological, (2) human, and (3) organizational contexts as key factors that affect robot adoption in healthcare. (1) Design and technical issues, system reliability, and system compatibility represent technological factors. (2) Human factors are trust, perceived usefulness, ease of use, privacy concern, attitude, and confidence towards technology. (3) Organizational factors are represented by legal, security, cost, interoperability, recruitment, and training of manpower relevant to the process [24].

These studies show that designing a technology in healthcare is a complex engineering process. They show the importance of subjective factors like expectancy and organizational factors that need to be considered during development.

5.1.3.2 Heterogeneity of Users

There are two extremes. Some people could be fascinated by technology, or others could be reluctant and afraid of technology. Both extremes should raise caution. There can be a large mismatch between routine practice and proven evidence-based strategies. Implementation science describes early adopters as opposed to the extreme of the late majority and laggards with different profiles, needs, and motivations [25] and why there is an evidence-practice gap and how to bridge it.

At the beginning of the nineteenth century, the Luddite movement was raised because of a fear that technology would replace the workforce among English textile workers. Such reluctance of technology still exists [26] and can be legitimate. In healthy aging studies, older adults fear that the use of socially assistive robots could lead to dehumanized care, in general, in which social isolation of older adults might become even worse, or they may become victims of ageism.

5.1.3.3 Digital Literacy and Interpretability

The transparency of the device can be limited, which could be driven by technology literacy and poor design. When technology helps in the decision-making during a diagnosis (screening of some disorders like writing difficulties, behavior, or malformation), the professionals need to understand the features used by the system to categorize the disorder. Are the features (semiology to describe the difficulties) interpretable? Is the model (how the features are used to classify the children) easy to understand? Some advanced machine learning techniques can have very good performance but poor interpretability. Using feature extraction and simpler/older techniques like Random Forest instead of deep learning could be better to keep this interpretability [12] since the model's accuracy can be less important than interpretability. Another strategy is trying to bypass this problem by keeping the advantages of deep learning, especially for image analysis, with a second step to make it more interpretable for the user (e.g., if the model suggests that an image/behavior is suspicious, it shows and describes the region that is considered problematic). This field of research is called Explainable artificial intelligence [27–30].

Thinking of synergies between scalable technological needs and specific, face-to-face, and tailored strategies that a human would better handle is more relevant. Technologies can be more complementary to the therapist, especially when they empower him/her (with special sensors, repetitive tasks, and integration of a large amount of data).

5.1.3.4 Specificities in Children and Their Family

It seems relevant to target the development of new technologies specifically for children and adolescents. Most disorders appear in childhood/adolescence, in particular neurodevelopmental disorders. In a large-scale meta-analysis of 192 epidemiological studies, Solmi et al. showed that mental disorders were already frequent in children and adolescents with a pick age of onset at 14.5 years [31]. The former director of the National Institute of Mental Health in the United States of America goes further by stating that “Mental disorders are chronic diseases of the young” [32]. There was a strong debate in the literature about the impact of screens on the development of children, with some concerns that were more ideological than evidence-based [33].

Children and younger patients, in general, could be less reluctant to change and use new technologies [34]. They grew up with new technologies and can seem more at ease even if they are not technology-literate. Since the brain is more plastic, an early intervention could be more useful. It seems important to focus these efforts, especially in the young population [35]. They can have the support of their parents who want to help their children and can, for instance, do it by using jointly an app (e.g., relaxation exercises) or a robot in cooperative mode. They could be more creative and more prone to use their imagination. However, since this population is more sensitive, ethics could be more stringent because this brain plasticity diagnosis can change more often than in adults [36].

5.1.3.5 Medico Economic Studies

We have demonstrated that the demand for technology in psychiatry, especially child and adolescent psychiatry, is substantial. Nevertheless, one significant barrier could be the considerable costs involved, which warrants careful consideration [4]. There could be a potential for acceptable and scalable approaches. Since the cost of new technology can be important, it is important to consider the medico-economic approach of a new technological strategy.[1] In the E-goliath-eco study, two tablets are given to the child with autism spectrum disorder and the parent to do imitation and turn-taking activities based on early start Denver model (ESDM) therapy. The ESDM is a well-established therapy. We can expect that the intervention with a tablet will be less engaging and tailored to the needs of the child and his/her parents than face-to-face ESDM therapy. Still, scalability would be much better and could improve the treatment provided by the services as usual.

Hence, design processes and strategies when developing new technologies are complex and require good communication between engineers and clinicians.

5.2 Communication Between Different Worlds: Engineers Vs. Clinicians

5.2.1 Building an Effective Communication Between Engineers and Clinicians

Effective communication between engineers and clinicians is essential for developing new medical technologies and devices that meet the needs of therapists and patients. Engineers bring technical expertise, while clinicians bring medical knowledge (how to diagnose, treat, and the rationale) and an understanding of patient needs. When they work together, they can develop innovative solutions that are both effective and user-friendly. However, each group's language and processes can differ, making communication challenging. To overcome these obstacles, it is important to establish clear and open lines of communication, foster a culture of collaboration, and encourage the exchange of information between both groups to ensure the development of effective and innovative medical technologies.

Clear and productive communication and team efforts are crucial in every multidisciplinary work, especially for the success of healthcare projects. To foster this communication, it is important for both parties, engineers and clinicians, to take the time to understand each other's perspectives and constraints.

A few articles focused on effective communication between clinical and engineering staff to develop medical devices [37, 38]. This good communication facilitates the understanding of each stakeholder. While engineers could be interested in solving very defined problems, the problems are only sometimes replicable or well-defined in clinical practice. A doctor's goal is to personalize medicine to the specific needs of his/her patient, which is much closer to craft work than industrial practice. The ultimate model in medical research to assess the efficacy of an approach is the randomized control trial. However, different steps are required before assessing the goal of the device, in which case (user scenario). Based on this best case, is the device feasible?

[1] https://clinicaltrials.gov/study/NCT05271955.

5.2.2 How to Speak to an Engineer?

When engaging with engineers, it is important to understand their mindset and communication preferences. Engineers often desire to classify and categorize information, drawing upon their technical expertise and experience to create systematic frameworks [39]. Providing clear priorities and assertively expressing needs is crucial to effectively communicate with engineers. Engineers appreciate synchronization between different components and systems and the opportunity to reuse and integrate existing solutions, although this may vary depending on the context [39]. Acknowledging what may be useful and important from a clinical perspective can pose technical challenges. Conversely, concepts that seem trivial to clinicians may require considerable technical implementation [39]. Furthermore, it is crucial to respect the constraints of clinician and hospital schedules, as time management can greatly impact collaborative efforts. For example, clinicians should consider that a software tool or a piece of hardware requires development time and a lot of testing before it is ready for deployment or applied in a clinical research study. In particular, if engineers are also researchers or professors, technical parts are often conducted in collaboration with students and trainees due to a lack of personnel resources and time constraints. These considerations can lead to additional testing even with participants and patients. Sometimes, this can present challenges as clinicians must explain to participants recruited in a clinical study that they need to return to the hospital for additional sessions because something was not ready or properly tested. This may require ethics amendments and can result in delays. Therefore, involving end-users in a research study's developmental and design phases can benefit everyone, for instance, via focus group meetings, pilot testing, and feasibility studies before running the clinical study. It is crucial to consider the technical deployment in the project timeline of a clinical study, even if it is optional by the Research Ethics Board (REB) offices.

Engaging with engineers involves intellectual property considerations, open access strategy, and patents. Engineers appreciate early discussions about valorization and protecting intellectual property rights [39]. Additionally, engineers value clean code and efficiency in implementation, as their focus lies primarily on technical aspects rather than clinical methodology [39]. However, it is important to note that engineers have diverse technical backgrounds. Furthermore, while some engineers may be more technology-centered, others may possess broader perspectives, especially in robotics [39, 40], or have direct experience with participants and individuals with disabilities, such as rehabilitation engineers.

5.2.3 How to Speak to a Clinician?

When engaging with clinicians in a research context, it is important to approach communication with an understanding of their mindset and specific needs. Like engineers, clinicians also use specialized jargon, although it may not be the same terminology [41, 42]. To effectively communicate with clinicians, it is essential to start the conversation by addressing the problem first rather than focusing on the technology [41]. However, the problem is sometimes tailor-made, even if an industrial or a researcher should provide a replicable solution. Taking the time to develop a strong understanding of the needs of clinicians can facilitate better communication and collaboration.

Central reasons behind failures can be listed as follows: "the technology versus human approach" which is adopted by several technical experts and researchers (creating a fear of technology), "technology-oriented design rather than problem-oriented design," and "lack of communication of engineers or designers with clinicians, caregivers, and patients." Multiple domain experts and stakeholders of healthcare systems, including occupational therapists, psychometricians, nurses, medical doctors, patient groups, and patients' ecosystem of caregivers, must be involved in every design step as lasting partners in developing and implementing effective technologies.

For instance, technology-oriented approaches are common in the robotics field, where the design process of robotic systems targets multiple user groups without considering the expectations or possible adoption problems [24]. Within the initial engineering principle, the collaboration between humans and technology should be the leading response. A study for identifying metastatic breast cancer shows that when the intelligent system's predictions are combined with the human pathologist's diagnoses, they get the best prediction results [43]. We believe new embedded technologies should be designed as tools that will collaboratively support humans. This is particularly important, considering the medical responsibility/accountability an algorithm cannot hold.

Due to a lack of communication, the technological solution envisioned by engineers might not serve a real problem. Even if various technologies offered brilliant solutions, they might not be accepted in real environments or natural settings. For instance, in healthy aging studies, older adults fear that the use of socially assistive robots could lead to dehumanized care, in general, in which social isolation of older adults might become even worse [44]. This example shows how research might be disconnected from the expectations and perceptions of the targeted group. This kind of technology-oriented approach tends to focus on the functionality of the technology instead of considering its impact on the user's healthcare behavior and potential user resistance [45].

Acceptance refers to the extent to which potential users are willing to use a specific system [46], while acceptability is the judgment made before the system is actually introduced. Acceptance is based on the attitudes and behavioral responses of respondents after the introduction of the system. In contrast, acceptability is closely linked with usage and depends on how user needs are incorporated into the system's development. Previous studies [47–51] have shown that clinicians generally have a positive view of the potential of robotic devices, but lack of knowledge about the systems currently being developed. They also expressed concerns about patient confidentiality, cost, and usability. A survey revealed that clinicians consider safety, positioning, movement control, patient feedback, and access to information important features of robotic devices [52]. It is important to note that there are different parameters for technology when considering their practicality and acceptability.

Clinicians often need more time due to their demanding schedules and the need for efficient integration of technology into their routines [41, 42]. Special methods to assess usability can be very useful for clinicians, such as using usability questionnaires, as measured by tools like the system usability scale (SUS) and user experience (UX), which becomes a critical factor in the successful adoption of technology [53–55]. There are several reasons clinicians might reject a device, such as difficulty with donning/doffing, handling complications, or triggering fear in patients. Therefore, it is crucial to ensure the technology is acceptable and practical. Therefore, it is important to consider the ease of implementation when discussing potential solutions with clinicians. Design guidelines can be very useful to share the best practices in the field [56, 57] (Figs. 5.2 and 5.3).

Clinicians bear the ultimate responsibility for the well-being of their patients and are accountable to both the patients and their families [41]. They must prioritize patient safety and ethical considerations, including data privacy and compliance with regulations such as the General Data Protection Regulation (GDPR) [58]. Technology design should consider how, why, where, and by whom a technology is used. Understanding the importance of these ethical considerations and ensuring data privacy and security measures are in place is crucial when speaking to clinicians.

While clinicians may possess a different technical background than engineers, they rely on fundamental sciences like neuroscience and experimental biology, clinical methodology, and evidence-based approaches that are not pragmatic or mechanistic driven [41, 42]. Integration of new technologies in healthcare emphasize role of sociology of organizations [59]. They require coherent integration of new technologies with established care practices and clinical trials, like randomized control trials. Providing interpretable numbers and a basic understanding of the underlying

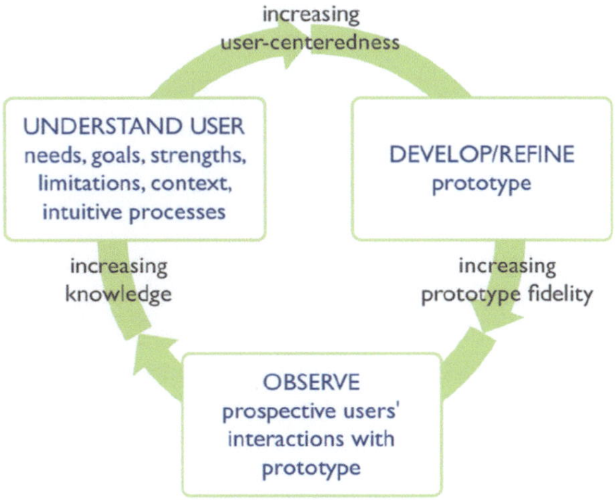

Fig. 5.2 User-centered design framework in Witteman 2021, licensed under CC-BY 4.0 International License

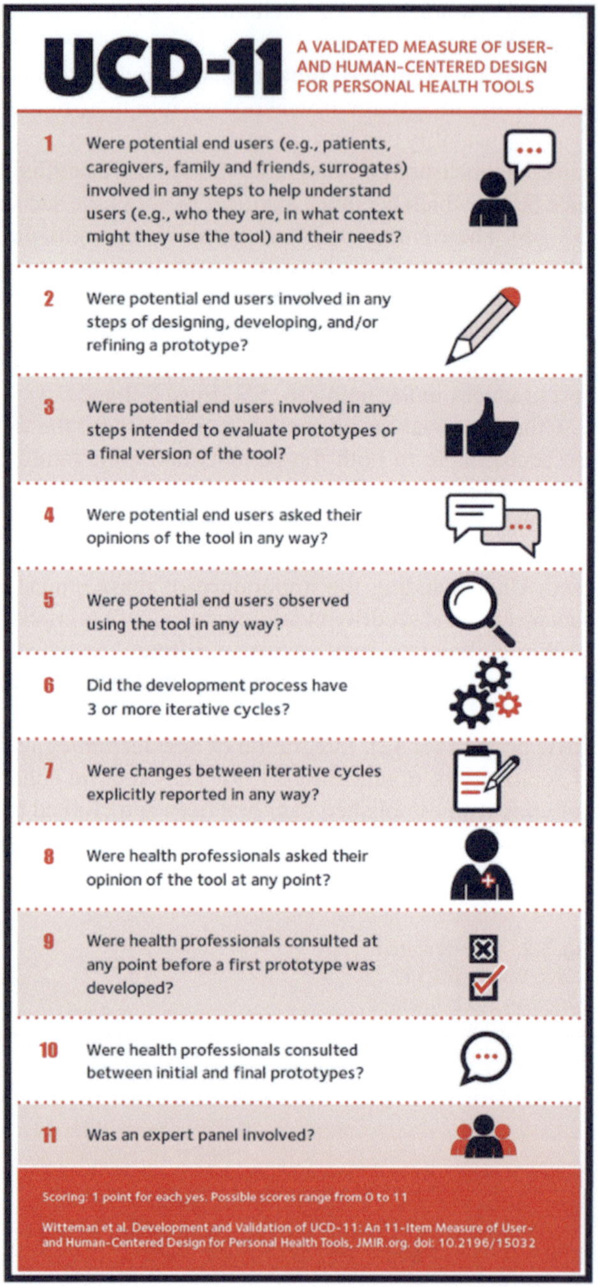

Fig. 5.3 Items and scoring of the User-Centered Design 11-item measure (UCD-11) in [57], licensed under CC-BY 4.0 International License

system's cognitive principles (intermediate markers that the clinician can track) and physiopathological models can facilitate their decision-making process [41, 42].

It is important to acknowledge that clinicians have diverse specializations and areas of expertise. They may have different perspectives and priorities. Collaborating with clinicians from the early stages of research and valuing their input can lead to more successful outcomes. Discussions regarding intellectual property, contracts, and potential valorization opportunities should be initiated early in collaboration [41].

In summary, effective communication with clinicians in research requires understanding their time constraints, incorporating usability considerations, addressing ethical concerns, respecting clinical methodology, and valuing their specialized expertise. Researchers can establish fruitful partnerships with clinicians in developing and implementing technology solutions by considering these factors and fostering a collaborative approach.

Regarding using robots in healthcare, there are four important factors to consider for acceptance. First, the robot should not cause harm—this is a crucial design principle clinicians understand well. A training and familiarization phase can be necessary for the professional and the patient using the device. Clinicians understand how long a patient can become accustomed to a new device. They can clarify its goals [60] and limits to prevent deception, noncompliance, and disappointment. Second, the robot should not induce fear and provide patients safety and comfort. Clinicians can ensure this by understanding the device well and using it accurately during therapy sessions [61–63]. They can also provide empathy due to their experience with patients and their conditions.

5.3 Potential Solutions: Design Methodologies

5.3.1 Different Levels of Users Involvement

In the last decades, researchers have developed several technology-enhanced applications in multiple healthcare domains, such as monitoring or assisting the elderly, assisting physical therapy of stroke survivors, and training the cognitive skills of neurodivergent children to contribute to healthcare.

To better understand the needs in the clinical field, it is important to involve end-users in participatory design (sometimes called co-design or cooperative design) [64]. Anderberg stated that technology and design are "too important to be left only to technicians and designers" [65].

The importance of co-participatory design of end-users in developing new tech approaches and technologies to support people with disabilities, children, and adults cannot be overstated. Understanding clinicians' and users' needs, expectations, and limits is crucial in the assessment phase.

The most appropriate participation form may vary depending on the project, the children, and resources [64] (Fig. 5.4). In some studies, the children can undertake several roles [64].

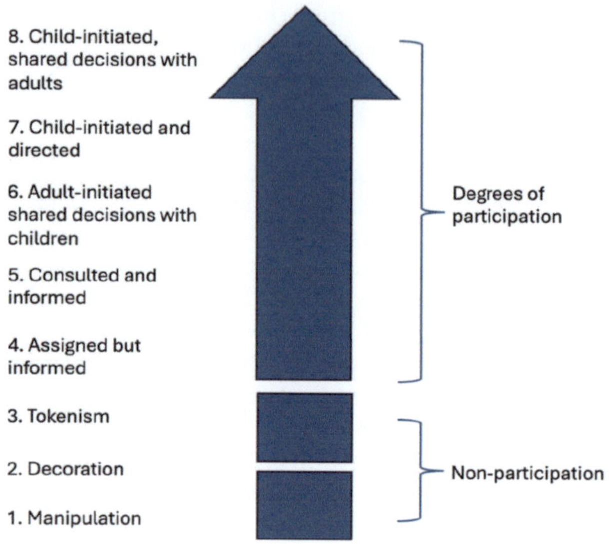

Fig. 5.4 Hart [66] suggests the different levels of child participation. (Adapted from [64])

In a review about how to involve children with educational needs and difficulties to improve participation in technology design, Benton and Johnson report that Druin [67] identified several levels of child participation: user, tester, informant (that gives input at several points of developments), design partner (they can elaborate on ideas of other children and adults, act as equal stakeholders), and co-designer [64]. The child's involvement can be measured through external observer metrics (by being observed using the technology, offering direct verbal or written feedback, for example, on a prototype), or more active in the design process while engaging in a dialogue with the adults.

Sometimes, a predesign phase is necessary, during which the designer assumes the role of an anthropologist. In this step, they immerse themselves in the environment where the technology might be used—such as hospitals, other healthcare settings, homes, or schools—to observe and gain a deeper understanding of the needs and constraints present in the field [68].

Children and adults seek inspiration from each other's ideas during idea elaboration. "This inspiration is then used to create new ideas or design direction as well as build directly upon another participant's idea, where "ultimately it may be difficult to remember whose ideas they were originally" ([64], citing [69]). This engagement can benefit the participant who can enjoy himself, feel empowered, take more responsibility, feel competent, develop teamwork, and learn social or creative skills [64].

However, there are debates on how technologies fail to adopt or fulfil the demanded actions envisioned by engineers [22–24].

Sierra Marín et al. [70] investigated the expectations and perceptions of healthcare professionals regarding robot deployment in hospital environments during the coronavirus disease 2019 (COVID-19) pandemic, highlighting the significance of involving clinicians in the design process. Similarly, Raigoso et al. [71] surveyed socially assistive robotics. They found that clinicians' and patients' perceptions play a vital role in successfully integrating a social robot within gait rehabilitation therapies.

Moving into the deployment/implementation phase, Casas et al. [72] emphasized the importance of aligning expectations with reality regarding attitudes towards a socially assistive robot in cardiac rehabilitation. Additionally, Múnera et al. [73] explored clinicians' experiences using rehabilitation robotics, emphasizing the value of incorporating their insights in refining and improving the technology. By involving end- users and clinicians throughout the design and deployment phases, we can create technologies that effectively meet the needs and expectations of those they aim to support, ultimately leading to enhanced outcomes and improved quality of life.

5.3.1.1 How to Reach the Design of a Technology with a Participatory Approach

To incorporate a participatory approach, the end- users should be seen as experts, rather than as subjects or participants in studies. Technology itself is not the solution itself since there are multidimensional complexities in each healthcare environment. Therefore, fast prototyping (minimum viable product) and in-the-wild testing are necessary to observe and understand these dynamics. Moreover, the design should facilitate high adaptability, personalization, and customization, tailored to the specific dynamics of each environment and the relationships between various stakeholders involved.

Creating engagement and fostering involvement are crucial goals in designing any activity. Several environmental dimensions affecting the engagement and involvement of users are identified in literature as follows [45, 74]:

- *Availability*: Objective provision of activities and services, including time of use and frequency of attending the activity.
- *Accessibility*: Stakeholders' ability, or perceived ability, to access the activity or situation. The actual or perceived ability of stakeholders to access an activity or situation, including both subjective perceptions of accessibility and objective opportunities to do so.
- *Affordability*: Resource constraints to the activity, including financial cost, time costs, and energy costs. An activity having less resource cost will potentially have a higher reach, impact, and adoption.
- *Accommodability*: The ability of the situation to be adapted or modified. Modifiability of an activity to be adjusted, changed, or customized to suit different needs, situations, or preferences.
- *Acceptability*: The affected person's and other people's acceptance of the activity and its situational context, including the person's acceptance of the situation and other people's acceptance of the individual in the activity setting. It could be important to conduct simulation phases with users and focus groups to assess these questions during the design phase or at least before an efficacy trial. Specific guidelines to report qualitative research exist like the COREQ [75] or SRQR [76] guidelines.

Due to this multidimensionality, designing technology-enhanced solutions for multiple ecosystems becomes more complicated. Although the provided solutions should be adaptable to multiple factors, what should be adapted and what to adapt for need to be clarified within these complex environments. Therefore, observational experiences within multiple healthcare environment with patients with ranging profiles are crucial for the design and successful integration of new technology in such environments in a more sustainable way.

Designing technology-enhanced activities within therapy sessions presents numerous challenges and uncertainties. These include managing the arrangement of activities, utilizing space effectively, and determining the composition of groups comprising children or patients with diverse learning goals and varying physical and cognitive capabilities, particularly those with special needs. Considering these complexities, envisioning a traditional study setup or a singular ideal solution for developing and testing a functional design to demonstrate positive learning outcomes becomes impractical [77]. Multiple setbacks and learning experiences arise, necessitating active engagement with stakeholders to refine the current design and enhance its functionality and flexibility to cater to patients facing different challenges.

Due to these factors, apart from following an iterative design methodology where the system is tested and improved repeatedly at different stages of maturity and practicality, the studies should be implemented in the wild in their natural settings to consider the different contexts and complexities of these specific ecosystems. Throughout each cycle of refinement, the improved design must undergo thorough verification to identify weaknesses and collect insights and feedback that can assist in further enhancements and adjustments for integration into various settings.

Several lessons learned can be drawn from the wild therapy ecosystems [78]. Some of the observational insights are as follows:

- Allowing the therapists to intervene the interaction between technology and the patient is crucial. The technological solution for therapy should not exclude the therapist and might need to allow therapists to intervene in the therapeutic activity (Accessibility).
- The design targeting young children, particularly those aged 3 to 5 years old, should prioritize the incorporation of simple rules or possibly provide unstructured free play (Accessibility).
- Computer–human interaction studies should go beyond using engagement scales with robots or technologies in activities that target functional training, especially for younger children who might refuse to use the technology (Acceptability).
- Children's perception of technologies (especially robots) influences their behavior, interaction, and expectations on the role and capabilities of the system [79, 80]. This might affect the learning goals or therapeutic output. For instance, the design of verbal, visual, and motion-based feedback should account for the perception of children below 5 years old [81]. This includes understanding how much attention they typically allocate to each type of feedback mechanism or to the overall system [82]. Additionally, considering their limited comprehension of

virtual or visual elements is essential in creating effective feedback systems (Accommodability).

- Robots or new technologies might not serve multiple purposes and learning goals of a complex therapy or learning environment. They are just tools that might be integrated as "one alternative" into the natural activity flow and structure of the current ecosystem. Therefore, such technologies.
  - require to allow integration of traditional practices into the activity flow,
  - need adaptation of activity content according to the schedule, current methodology, and objectives of the therapists/psychologists (accommodability),
  - need ease of setup for the unique room settings and change of rooms within a limited time (5–10 min setup time) (affordability),
  - Also, the duration of the technological activity has to be adapted to the attention levels of the children and the therapy duration (Affordability). This limited duration of practice sessions (30 or 40 min) and the limited space available in therapy centers and schools (Availability) are important factors to be considered in the design [83].
- Studying the potential impact of technology on group dynamics is crucial for group therapy, along with examining how different roles assigned to robots might influence children's behavior. Additionally, it's essential to explore how group dynamics can influence the overall interaction between children and technology (especially robots). During the design phase, it's important to account for elements like peer pressure, the need for peer approval, and the tendency to imitate peers. These factors can significantly impact how children interact with and respond to the designed elements, particularly in social settings or group environments [83, 84]. In group therapy, systems targeting multi-child systems should account for the fluctuating or dynamic changes in the number of children involved. To accommodate the varying number of children from one session to another, the design approach could involve creating adaptable setups with a flexible number of robots working simultaneously. Alternatively, it could focus on crafting activities that allow multiple children to interact synchronously with a single robot or participate together in a game (accommodability).

These insights play a significant role in shaping the design of new technology for therapy, taking into account various facets of diverse care environments. Adapting the design and elements of a technology-enhanced activity to suit different user groups and settings, enhances the potential for integrating such systems into various care environments in a sustainable manner.

5.3.2 User-Centered Design

User-centered design is a fundamental approach that emphasizes the active involvement of end- users in the design and development process of new technologies. This chapter section explores the importance of customization for specific populations and contexts, recognizing that users' needs and preferences can vary greatly. It also highlights the significance of user participation and the use of various participatory design methods to create inclusive and effective solutions [64]. The concept of informant design was introduced to actively involve users in the design process. Experience centered design goes even further, aiming to maximize user engagement throughout the process [64].

Designing for different populations and contexts requires a deep understanding of their unique requirements and challenges. For instance, the needs of children with disabilities may differ significantly from those of adults. Moreover, the environment inside a hospital setting may present distinct considerations compared to the outside world. Recognizing these differences is crucial in tailoring technologies that truly address the specific needs of the target population.

To achieve customization and user-centeredness, a range of participatory design methods can be employed. Visual templates, drawing materials, games, sculptures, and narrative-based participatory methods can facilitate user engagement and the expression of their preferences and ideas [85]. Additionally, simulation and roleplay techniques can help users envision the potential impact of the technology in their daily lives.

Participation goes beyond individual users and extends to the involvement of the community and relevant associations. Engaging stakeholders who represent the target population helps to ensure that the design process reflects a broader range of perspectives and experiences. By including community members and associations, the design team can gain valuable insights and create contextually appropriate and meaningful solutions to the end-users.

Measuring the success of user-centered design efforts is also important. The development and validation of measures such as the user- and human-centered design for personal health tools (UCD-11) provide a framework for evaluating the effectiveness of user-centered design practices [57] (Figs. 5.2 and 5.3). These measures help assess the extent to which the design process prioritizes user needs, preferences, and usability. For instance, during the development of the "oto chair"[2] that allows to perform deep pressure on children with autism, several versions of a prototype were designed. The use with psychometricians and end-users like children with autism and intellectual deficiency allowed researchers to design an easy and simple interface. A small light on the remote control that could be sensory stimulating was suppressed after these tests, and the noise accompanying the inflation and deflation was decreased.

A good animation of such design sessions is important, especially in children groups, particularly when they may have special educational needs and disabilities. According to Benton, the role of adults is (1) to ensure the children's well-being, (2) to encourage every opportunity to engage in activities they want to, (3) to provide the support and environment so the children can feel empowered whenever possible, (4) to provide an environment to foster mutual learning, and (5) to create an experience that is positive enough to encourage them to repeat the experience.

[2] https://www.oto-chair.com/ [67].

In conclusion, user-centered design with customization for specific populations and contexts is a time-intensive yet essential approach. Incorporating participatory design methods, involving the community, and utilizing validated measurement tools can enhance the effectiveness and inclusivity of technology solutions. By prioritizing the active engagement of end- users and considering their unique needs, we can create technologies that positively impact their lives.

5.4 Conclusion

There is a great treatment gap between the needs and what the healthcare system can provide. New technologies offer interesting opportunities in mental health and in the healthcare system in general. It is important to develop and apply good practice and good evidence to have clear cognitive principles on which to build upon new technology, for instance, the cognitive behavior therapy principle, feedback loops, flow theory, and proximal zone of development and gamification in serious games (see Fig. 5.1 for the different development phases). It is important to know precisely when the technology intervenes and how (what is the user scenario? Is it acceptable?). For instance, in an iterative design process of a writing serious game, we measured handwriting improvement before and after the robot activity within an occupational therapy context [86] while adapting the system into multiple occupational therapy environments which demanded variants of adaptations throughout the iterations. Parallelly, it is important to assess technological feasibility based on needed resources. After these steps, the next stage involves initiating a user-centered design process directly in the field [57]. With these elements in place, the implementation and development of the technology can proceed effectively. Once the technology is mature (see for instance, the Technology readiness levels [87], it is time to assess the efficacy. The design can continue with new usage. These technologies can offer new possibilities in terms of scalability to reduce the treatment gap but also raise new challenges about data security and ethics. The adaptation and personalization of the system to the specific needs of the patient and the context will need to be considered. In a complex system like a healthcare organization, the last steps would be integrating the new device with pre-existing technologies and allowing proper communication between these systems.

References

1. Vigo D, Thornicroft G, Atun R. Estimating the true global burden of mental illness. Lancet Psychiatry. 2016;3(2):171–8. https://doi.org/10.1016/S2215-0366(15)00505-2.
2. WHO. Depression and other common mental disorders: global health estimates. Geneva: World Health Organization; 2017.
3. Kohn R, Saxena S, Levav I, Saraceno B. The treatment gap in mental health care. Bulletin of the world health organization. 2004;82(11):858–66.

4. Christensen MK, Lim CCW, Saha S, Plana-Ripoll O, Cannon D, Presley F, Weye N, Momen NC, Whiteford HA, Iburg KM. The cost of mental disorders: a systematic review. Epidemiol Psychiatr Sci. 2020;29:e161.
5. Francés L, Quintero J, Fernández A, Ruiz A, Caules J, Fillon G, Soler CV. Current state of knowledge on the prevalence of neurodevelopmental disorders in childhood according to the DSM-5: a systematic review in accordance with the PRISMA criteria. Child and adolescent psychiatry and mental health. 2022;16(1):27.
6. Torous J, Bucci S, Bell IH, Kessing LV, Faurholt-Jepsen M, Whelan P, Firth J. The growing field of digital psychiatry: current evidence and the future of apps, social media, chatbots, and virtual reality. World Psychiatry. 2021;20(3):318–35.
7. Oudin A, Maatoug R, Bourla A, Ferreri F, Bonnot O, Millet B, Schoeller F, Mouchabac S, Adrien V. Digital phenotyping: data-driven psychiatry to redefine mental health. J Med Internet Res. 2023;25:e44502.
8. Gargot T, Archambault D, Chetouani M, Cohen D, Johal W, Anzalone SM. Automatic assessment of motor impairments in Autism Spectrum Disorders: a systematic review. Cognitive Computation. 2022:1–36.
9. de Belen RAJ, Bednarz T, Sowmya A, Del Favero D. Computer vision in autism spectrum disorder research: a systematic review of published studies from 2009 to 2019. Translational psychiatry. 2020;10(1):1–20.
10. Kaliouby RE, Picard R, Baron-Cohen S. Affective computing and autism. Annals of the New York Academy of Sciences. 2006;1093(1):228–248.
11. Le Glaz A, Haralambous Y, Kim-Dufor DH, Lenca P, Billot R, Ryan TC, Lemey C. Machine learning and natural language processing in mental health: systematic review. Journal of Medical Internet Research. 2021;23(5):e15708.
12. Asselborn T, Gargot T, Kidziński Ł, Johal W, Cohen D, Jolly C, Dillenbourg P. Automated human-level diagnosis of dysgraphia using a consumer tablet. NPJ Digit Med. 2018;1(1):42. https://doi.org/10.1038/s41746-018-0049-x.
13. Gargot T, Asselborn T, Pellerin H, Zammouri I, Anzalone SM, Casteran L, Johal W, Dillenbourg P, Cohen D, Jolly C. Acquisition of handwriting in children with and without dysgraphia: a computational approach. PLoS One. 2020;15(9):e0237575.
14. American Psychiatric Association. Diagnostic and statistical manual of mental disorders (DSM-5®). Washington, DC: American Psychiatric Association; 2013.
15. Borsboom D. A network theory of mental disorders. World Psychiatry. 2017;16(1):5–13.
16. Shiffman S, Stone AA, Hufford MR. Ecological momentary assessment. Annu Rev Clin Psychol. 2008;4:1–32. https://doi.org/10.1146/annurev.clinpsy.3.022806.091415.
17. Insel TR. Digital phenotyping: technology for a new science of behavior. Jama. 2017;318(13):1215–16.
18. Bourla A, Ferreri F, Ogorzelec L, Peretti CS, Guinchard C, Mouchabac S. Psychiatrists' attitudes toward disruptive new technologies: mixed-methods study. JMIR mental health. 2018;5(4):e10240.
19. Blankenhagel KJ. Identifying usability challenges of ehealth applications for people with mental disorders: errors and design recommendations. In proceedings of the 13th EAI international conference on pervasive computing technologies for healthcare. 2019;(pp. 91–100).
20. Inal Y, Wake JD, Guribye F, Nordgreen T. Usability evaluations of mobile mental health technologies: systematic review. Journal of Medical Internet Research. 2020;22(1):e15337.
21. Venkatesh V, Morris MG, Davis GB, Davis FD. User acceptance of information technology: toward a unified view. MIS Q. 2003;27:425–78.
22. Alaiad A, Zhou L. The determinants of home healthcare robots adoption: an empirical investigation. Int J Med Inform. 2014;83(11):825–40.
23. Stahl BC, Coeckelbergh M. Ethics of healthcare robotics: towards responsible research and innovation. Robot Auton Syst. 2016;86:152–61.
24. Alla S, Pazos P. Healthcare robotics: key factors that impact robot adoption in healthcare. Orlando, FL: Institute of Industrial and Systems Engineers; 2019. p. 1121–6.

25. Feijt MA, de Kort YA, Bongers IM, IJsselsteijn, W. A. Perceived drivers and barriers to the adoption of eMental health by psychologists: the construction of the levels of adoption of eMental health model. J Med Internet Res. 2018;20(4):e9485. https://doi.org/10.2196/jmir.9485.
26. Jones SE. Against technology: from the luddites to neo-luddism. London: Routledge; 2013.
27. Baur T, Heimerl A, Lingenfelser F, Wagner J, Valstar MF, Schuller B, André E. eXplainable cooperative machine learning with NOVA. KI-Künstliche Intelligenz. 2020;34:143–64.
28. Gunning D, Stefik M, Choi J, Miller T, Stumpf S, Yang G-Z. XAI—explainable artificial intelligence. Sci Robot. 2019;4(37):eaay7120.
29. Quellec G, Al Hajj H, Lamard M, Conze P-H, Massin P, Cochener B. ExplAIn: explanatory artificial intelligence for diabetic retinopathy diagnosis. Med Image Anal. 2021;72:102118.
30. Xu F, Uszkoreit H, Du Y, Fan W, Zhao D, Zhu J. Explainable AI: a brief survey on history, research areas, approaches and challenges. In: Natural language processing and Chinese computing: 8th CCF International Conference, NLPCC 2019, Dunhuang, China, October 9–14, 2019, Proceedings, Part II 8; 2019. p. 563–74.
31. Solmi M, Radua J, Olivola M, Croce E, Soardo L, Salazar de Pablo G, Fusar-Poli P. Age at onset of mental disorders worldwide: large-scale meta-analysis of 192 epidemiological studies. Molecular psychiatry. 2022;27(1):281–95.
32. Insel TR, Fenton WS. Psychiatric epidemiology: it's not just about counting anymore. Arch Gen Psychiatry. 2005;62(6):590–2.
33. Sanders T, Noetel M, Parker P, Del Pozo Cruz B, Biddle S, Ronto R, Hulteen R, Parker R, Thomas G, De Cocker K, Salmon J, Hesketh K, Weeks N, Arnott H, Devine E, Vasconcellos R, Pagano R, Sherson J, Conigrave J, Lonsdale C. An umbrella review of the benefits and risks associated with youths' interactions with electronic screens. Nat Hum Behav. 2023;8:82–99. https://doi.org/10.1038/s41562-023-01712-8.
34. Lopez-Morinigo J-D, Barrigón ML, Porras-Segovia A, Ruiz-Ruano VG, Martínez ASE, Escobedo-Aedo PJ, Alonso SS, Iturralde LM, Lorenzo LM, Artés-Rodríguez A, David AS, Baca-García E. Use of ecological momentary assessment through a passive smartphone-based app (eB2) by patients with schizophrenia: acceptability study. J Med Internet Res. 2021;23(7):e26548. https://doi.org/10.2196/26548.
35. Doyle O, Harmon CP, Heckman JJ, Tremblay RE. Investing in early human development: timing and economic efficiency. Economics & Human Biology. 2009;7(1):1–6.
36. Caspi A, Houts RM, Ambler A, Danese A, Elliott ML, Hariri A, Harrington H, Hogan S, Poulton R, Ramrakha S. Longitudinal assessment of mental health disorders and comorbidities across 4 decades among participants in the Dunedin birth cohort study. JAMA Netw Open. 2020;3(4):e203221.
37. Morschauser M. Improving patient safety through collaboration between clinical staff and engineering staff in hospitals. J Clin Eng. 2014;39(3):129–31.
38. Yoda T. The effect of collaborative relationship between medical doctors and engineers on the productivity of developing medical devices. R&D Manag. 2016;46(S1):193–206.
39. Norman D. The design of everyday things: revised and expanded edition. New York: Basic Books; 2013.
40. Lemley MA, Merges RP, Balganesh S. Intellectual property in the new technological age: 2016. Clause 8 Publishing; 2016.
41. Liss DT, Peprah YA, Brown T, Ciolino JD, Jackson K, Kho AN, Murakami L, Walunas TL, Persell SD. Using electronic health records to measure quality improvement efforts: findings from a large practice facilitation initiative. Jt Comm J Qual Patient Saf. 2020;46(1):11–7.
42. Ryan KA, Smith SN, Yocum AK, Carley I, Liebrecht C, Navis B, Vest E, Bertram H, McInnis MG, Kilbourne AM. The life goals self-management mobile app for bipolar disorder: Consumer feasibility, usability, and acceptability study. JMIR Formative Research. 2021;5(12):e32450.
43. Wang D, Khosla A, Gargeya R, Irshad H, Beck AH. Deep learning for identifying metastatic breast cancer. arXiv preprint arXiv:1606.05718. 2016.

44. Vandemeulebroucke T, de Casterlé BD, Gastmans C. How do older adults experience and perceive socially assistive robots in aged care: a systematic review of qualitative evidence. Aging Ment Health. 2018;22(2):149–67.
45. Imms C, Adair B, Keen D, Ullenhag A, Rosenbaum P, Granlund M. 'Participation': a systematic review of language, definitions, and constructs used in intervention research with children with disabilities. Dev Med Child Neurol. 2016;58(1):29–38.
46. Vlassenroot S, Brookhuis K, Marchau V, Witlox F. Towards defining a unified concept for the acceptability of Intelligent Transport Systems (ITS): a conceptual analysis based on the case of Intelligent Speed Adaptation (ISA). Transport Res F Traffic Psychol Behav. 2010;13(3):164–78. https://doi.org/10.1016/j.trf.2010.02.001.
47. Casas-Bocanegra D, Gomez-Vargas D, Pinto-Bernal MJ, Maldonado J, Munera M, Villa-Moreno A, Stoelen MF, Belpaeme T, Cifuentes CA. An open-source social robot based on compliant soft robotics for therapy with children with ASD. Actuators. 2020;9(3):Article 3. https://doi.org/10.3390/act9030091.
48. Céspedes N, Irfan B, Senft E, Cifuentes CA, Gutierrez LF, Rincon-Roncancio M, Belpaeme T, Múnera M. A socially assistive robot for long-term cardiac rehabilitation in the real world. Front Neurorobot. 2021a;15:633248. https://doi.org/10.3389/fnbot.2021.633248.
49. Céspedes N, Múnera M, Gómez C, Cifuentes CA. Social human-robot interaction for gait rehabilitation. IEEE Trans Neural Syst Rehabil Eng. 2020;28(6):1299–307. https://doi.org/10.1109/TNSRE.2020.2987428.
50. Céspedes N, Raigoso D, Múnera M, Cifuentes CA. Long-term social human-robot interaction for neurorehabilitation: robots as a tool to support gait therapy in the pandemic. Front Neurorobot. 2021b;15:10. https://doi.org/10.3389/fnbot.2021.612034.
51. Cifuentes CA, Pinto MJ, Céspedes N, Múnera M. Social robots in therapy and care. Curr Robot Rep. 2020;1(3):59–74. https://doi.org/10.1007/s43154-020-00009-2.
52. Lee M, Rittenhouse M, Abdullah HA. Design issues for therapeutic robot systems: results from a survey of physiotherapists. J Intell Robot Syst. 2005;42(3):239–52. https://doi.org/10.1007/s10846-004-7194-y.
53. Brooke J. SUS—a quick and dirty usability scale. In: Usability evaluation in industry, vol. 189; 1996. p. 4–7.
54. Davis FD, Bagozzi RP, Warshaw PR. User acceptance of computer technology: a comparison of two theoretical models. Manag Sci. 1989;35(8):982–1003.
55. Nielsen J. Usability engineering. Burlington, MA: Morgan Kaufmann; 1994.
56. Grossard C, Bettencourt C, Kellems R, Chetouani M, Cohen D. Building the design ICT inventory (DICTI): a Delphi study. Comput Hum Behav Rep. 2023;9:100261.
57. Witteman HO, Vaisson G, Provencher T, Chipenda Dansokho S, Colquhoun H, Dugas M, Fagerlin A, Giguere AM, Haslett L, Hoffman A. An 11-item measure of user-and human-centered design for personal health tools (UCD-11): development and validation. J Med Internet Res. 2021;23(3):e15032.
58. Ienca M, Ferretti A, Hurst S, Puhan M, Lovis C, Vayena E. Considerations for ethics review of big data health research: a scoping review. PLoS One. 2018;13(10):e0204937.
59. Birken SA, Bunger AC, Powell BJ et al. Organizational theory for dissemination and implementation research. Implementation Sci. 2017;12:62. https://doi.org/10.1186/s13012-017-0592-x
60. Chen CC, Bode RK. Factors influencing therapists' decision-making in the acceptance of new technology devices in stroke rehabilitation. Am J Phys Med Rehabil. 2011;90(5):415. https://doi.org/10.1097/PHM.0b013e318214f5d8.
61. Chen N, Liu X, Sun Y. Study on acceptance of social robots by aging adults living alone. In: Stephanidis IC, Antona M, Gao Q, Zhou J, editors. HCI international 2020—late breaking papers: universal access and inclusive design. Berlin: Springer International; 2020. p. 482–94. https://doi.org/10.1007/978-3-030-60149-2_37.
62. Conti D, Commodari E, Buono S. Personality factors and acceptability of socially assistive robotics in teachers with and without specialized training for children with disability. Life Span Disabil. 2017;20(2):Article 2.

63. Liu X, He X, Wang M, Shen H. What influences patients' continuance intention to use AI-powered service robots at hospitals? The role of individual characteristics. Technol Soc. 2022;70:101996. https://doi.org/10.1016/j.techsoc.2022.101996.
64. Benton L, Johnson H. Widening participation in technology design: a review of the involvement of children with special educational needs and disabilities. Int J Child Comput Interact. 2015;3-4:23–40. https://doi.org/10.1016/j.ijcci.2015.07.001.
65. Anderberg P. Making both ends meet. Disabil Stud Q. 2005;25(3):Article 3. https://doi.org/10.18061/dsq.v25i3.585.
66. Hart RA. Children's participation: from tokenism to citizenship. Papers, Article inness 92/6. 1992. https://ideas.repec.org//p/ucf/inness/inness92-6.html.
67. Druin A. The role of children in the design of new technology. Behav Inform Technol. 2002;21(1):1–25.
68. Gargot T, Vachaud A, Gilard C, Audrain A, Gomot M, Guidotti M. et al. A Compressive Armchair (OTO) to Perform Deep Pressure Therapy in Children With Autism Spectrum Disorder: User-Centered Design and Feasibility Study. JMIR Human Factors. 2024. 11, e55754.
69. Guha ML, Druin A, Fails JA. Cooperative inquiry revisited: reflections of the past and guidelines for the future of intergenerational co-design. Int J Child Comput Interact. 2013;1(1):14–23.
70. Sierra Marín SD, Gomez-Vargas D, Céspedes N, Múnera M, Roberti F, Barria P, Ramamoorthy S, Becker M, Carelli R, Cifuentes CA. Expectations and perceptions of healthcare professionals for robot deployment in hospital environments during the COVID-19 pandemic. Front Robot AI. 2021;8:612746. https://doi.org/10.3389/frobt.2021.612746.
71. Raigoso D, Céspedes N, Cifuentes CA, del Ama AJ, Múnera M. A survey on socially assistive robotics: clinicians' and patients' perception of a social robot within gait rehabilitation therapies. Brain Sci. 2021;11(6):Article 6. https://doi.org/10.3390/brainsci11060738.
72. Casas JA, Céspedes N, Cifuentes CA, Gutierrez LF, Rincón-Roncancio M, Múnera M. Expectation vs. reality: attitudes towards a socially assistive robot in cardiac rehabilitation. Appl Sci. 2019;9(21):4651.
73. Múnera M, Pinto-Bernal MJ, Zwickl N, Gil-Agudo A, Barria P, Cifuentes CA. Experiences of clinicians using rehabilitation robotics. In: Cifuentes CA, Múnera M, editors. Interfacing humans and robots for gait assistance and rehabilitation. Berlin: Springer International; 2022. p. 349–75. https://doi.org/10.1007/978-3-030-79630-3_14.
74. Maxwell G, Alves I, Granlund M. Participation and environmental aspects in education and the ICF and the ICF-CY: findings from a systematic literature review. Dev Neurorehabil. 2012;15(1):63–78.
75. Tong A, Sainsbury P, Craig J. Consolidated criteria for reporting qualitative research (COREQ): a 32-item checklist for interviews and focus groups. International J Qual Health Care. 2007;19(6):349–57. https://doi.org/10.1093/intqhc/mzm042.
76. O'Brien BC, Harris IB, Beckman TJ, Reed DA, Cook DA. Standards for reporting qualitative research: a synthesis of recommendations. Acad Med. 2014;89(9):1245–51. https://doi.org/10.1097/ACM.0000000000000388.
77. Rosner DK. Critical fabulations: reworking the methods and margins of design. Cambridge, MA: MIT Press; 2018.
78. Guneysu A, Yadollahi E, Indurkhya B. Lessons learned from in the wild child robot interaction in multiple ecosystems of care and education. In: The 11th International Conference on human-agent interaction. New York, NY: ACM; 2023.
79. Gargot T, Hermier C, Wobrock D, Anzalone S. What are children's beliefs on robots during a "learning by teaching" writing scenario? 2023. https://www.psycharchives.org/en/item/4c89cf8a-c037-4be3-a48a-14c865a33b9e.
80. Rubegni E, Malinverni L, Yip J. "Don't let the robots walk our dogs, but it's ok for them to do our homework": children's perceptions, fears, and hopes in social robots. In: Interaction design and children; 2022. p. 352–61.
81. Guneysu A, Arnrich B. Socially assistive child-robot interaction in physical exercise coaching. In: In 2017 26th IEEE international symposium on robot and human interactive communication (RO-MAN). Piscataway, NJ: IEEE; 2017. p. 670–5.

82. Olsen JK, Ozgur AG, Sharma K, Johal W. Leveraging eye tracking to understand children's attention during game-based, tangible robotics activities. Int J Child Comput Interact. 2022;31:100447.
83. Guneysu Ozgur A, Özgür A, Asselborn T, Johal W, Yadollahi E, Bruno B, Skweres M, Dillenbourg P. Iterative design and evaluation of a tangible robot-assisted handwriting activity for special education. Front Robot AI. 2020;7:29.
84. Guneysu A, Karatas I, Asık O, Indurkhya B. Attitudes of children towards dancing robot NAO: a kindergarden observation. In: Proceedings of the international conference on social robotics (ICSR 2013): workshop on taking care of each other: synchronisation and reciprocity for social companion robots, Bristol, UK; 2013. p. 27–9.
85. https://studiolab.ide.tudelft.nl/studiolab/codesignwithkids/ accessed January 10th, 2024.
86. Gargot T, Asselborn T, Zammouri I, Brunelle J, Johal W, Dillenbourg P, Archambault D, Chetouani M, Cohen D, Anzalone SM. "It Is Not the Robot Who Learns, It Is Me." Treating severe dysgraphia using child–robot interaction. Front Psychiatry. 2021;12:596055. https://doi.org/10.3389/fpsyt.2021.596055.
87. Mankins JC. Technology readiness levels. White paper, April 6, 1995.

6 Digital Mental Health Improves Access to Care, Facilitates Early Intervention, and Provides Evidence-Based Treatments at a Distance

Donald M. Hilty, Alice Zhang, Annaleis K. Giovanetti, Dorothy Stubbe, and Eve-Lynn Nelson

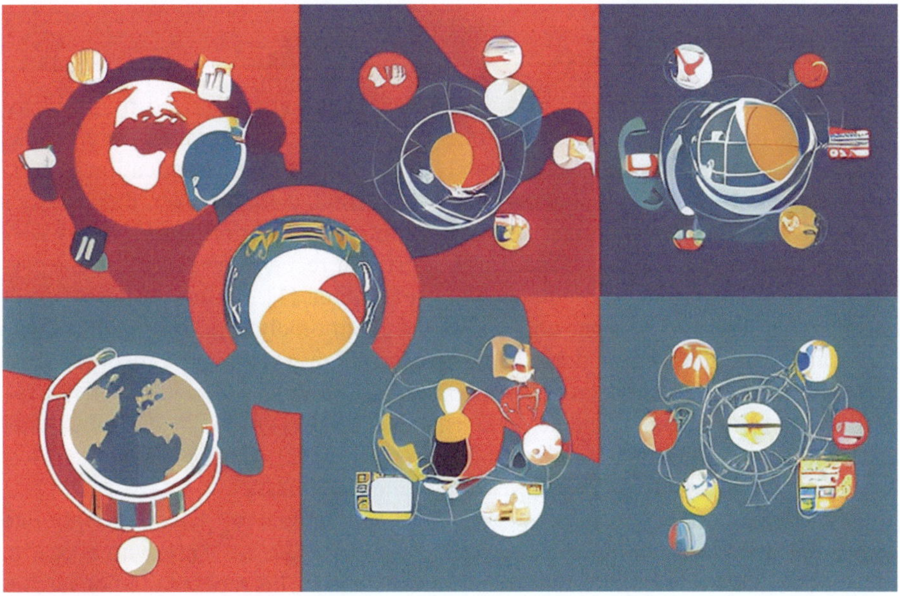

D. M. Hilty (✉)
Department of Psychiatry and Behavioral Sciences, Keck School of Medicine University of Southern California, Los Angeles, CA, USA
e-mail: donald.hilty@uhsinc.com; hilty@med.usc.edu

A. Zhang
Department of Occupational Therapy Education, University of Kansas Medical Center, Kansas City, KS, USA
e-mail: ezhang@kumc.edu

D. Mucić, D. M. Hilty (eds.), *Digital Mental Health*,
https://doi.org/10.1007/978-3-031-59936-1_6

Abstract

Most healthcare systems are striving to improve access to timely, evidence-based, and cost-friendly healthcare, particularly for mental disorders. Telemental health video improves access to care regardless of the point-of-service or barriers involved, and it is effective across age, diagnosis, and populations. Asynchronous technologies like mobile health are also effective modes of service delivery to a variety of settings and populations. Early evidence-based intervention is easier to distribute via telehealth and is particularly helpful for very young children and their families, diverse populations, and others with medical disadvantages. Research is needed on how to implement and evaluate synchronous and asynchronous technologies for clinical care and training, as well as across cultures and across users' health, lifestyle, and clinical care experiences.

6.1 Introduction

Our current healthcare system in the United States is characterized by problems with access to timely care, especially timely care for mental disorders. For example, an examination of data from the National Comorbidity Survey Replication in 2005 found that only 41% of Americans with a mental disorder over the previous 12 months received any treatment for their condition in the prior year [1]. Only 28% of Americans with a mental disorder in the past year received treatment from a psychiatrist or nonpsychiatrist mental health professional [1]. Further examination of this same survey showed very worrisome data about timely care: among those who do receive care, the median delay in treatment initiation after initial disorder onset ranges from 6 to 23 years across disorders [2]. Of those with common disorders—mood, generalized anxiety, panic, or substance disorders—only 25–40% make initial treatment contact in the first year of disorder onset [2]. Thus, critical time is lost in the identification and early intervention of mental illness.

A 2012 Institute of Medicine report, Crossing the Quality Chasm, brought into focus that the American healthcare system has challenges not only with access to *any* care but access to quality, evidence-based care [3]. This report called on healthcare providers and organizations in the United States to close the gap between care

A. K. Giovanetti
Clinical Psychology, University of Kansas, Lawrence, KS, USA
e-mail: annaleis@ku.edu

D. Stubbe
Child Study Center and Child and Adolescent Psychiatry and Program Director of Residency Training, Yale School of Medicine, New Haven, CT, USA
e-mail: dorothy.stubbe@yale.edu

E.-L. Nelson
Pediatrics, Telemedicine & Telehealth, Kansas City Medical Center, University of Kansas School of Medicine, Kansas City, KS, USA
e-mail: enelson2@kumc.edu

that we know is effective (i.e., evidence-based care) and care that we actually deliver (often fragmented care with interventions that are convenient but not necessarily evidence-based). Nowhere is this chasm wider than in our healthcare system's treatment of mental disorders in patients. This is despite the remarkable proliferation of somatic and psychosocial treatments that are well-tolerated and research supported in recent decades [4].

Clinicians and health systems emphasize improvement in science and patient safety to advance and sustain better outcomes in health. The quadruple aim consists of: (1) better population health, (2) better patient experience of care and better quality and safety of care, (3) reduced cost, and (4) team well-being. In order to achieve better population health—the population here being a medical center's patients or an insurance company's subscriber—a healthcare system can improve the mental health of its patient population by investing in interventions to promptly treat minor and major mental illness. Telemental health's (TMH) effectiveness has gone through three phases [5]. First, it was judged effective in terms of increasing access to care, being well-accepted, and having good educational outcomes [5]. Second, the validity and reliability of TMH compared to in-person care showed no differences [6, 7]. This assessment moved forward into formal "as good as" or noninferiority studies [8], which have also had positive results.

Access is only as good as sustainability—and perhaps the most important factor in that is cost feasibility. TMH cost analyses are limited in quality, with few using cost-comparison, -effectiveness or -benefit methodology, which is more common with telehealth studies; the few studies show favorable clinical, quality of life, and economic impact though. A standard framework for economic cost analysis should include: implementation and evaluation; a toolkit or guideline; comprehensive analysis with an incremental cost-effectiveness ratio; measures for health, quality of life, and utility outcomes for populations; methods to convert outcomes into economic benefits (e.g., monetary, quality of adjusted life year); broad perspective (e.g., societal perspective); sensitivity analysis for uncertainty in modeling; and adjustments for differential timing (e.g., discounting and future costs) [9]. Fortunately, many new excellent approaches and frameworks involve synchronous video or a wide range of asynchronous technologies like mobile health [10] and models of care [11] that extend worldwide [12].

This chapter will help the reader to:

1. Highlight TMH's role in improving access to care for people with access, medical, cultural, geographic, and other barriers.
2. Highlight TMH's role in bringing evidence-based child and adolescent care to children and families, especially intensive psychosocial care.

6.2 Access and Service Delivery

The service points at which TMH can be used to enhance care are theoretically limitless: clinics, emergency rooms, patients' homes, nursing homes, homeless shelters, hospices, schools, forensic facilities, and at the battlefront. A full range of evaluation, consultation, and treatment services have been carried out by telemedicine. Especially surprising is the breadth of psychotherapeutic interventions that have been provided using TMH, with satisfaction, working alliance, and communication quite good, including with therapy [7, 13]. Technology is a key part of the World Health Organization's (WHO) global health strategy, with the expectation of scalable behavioral health (BH) interventions, particularly for people in communities affected by adversity [14, 15]. In our immediate context, care is needed during the COVID pandemic, so that the innovation curve does not reinforce the social gradient of health and worsen healthcare inequities [16].

6.2.1 Child and Adolescent Populations

The evidence base telebehavioral health (TBH) for children and adolescents is growing—following the work in adults with effectiveness and efficacy reviews, summarized in the American Telemedicine Association child and adolescent guideline [17, 18]. Initial concerns about therapeutic engagement and the ability to simulate in-person care have subsided, and outcomes are comparable. One review of assessment/treatment between 1976 and 2016 in narrative style for pharmacotherapy, psychotherapy, pediatric psychology intervention, and/or developmental medicine found limited, but overall positive results [19]. Another review indicated good impact via video, computerized cognitive behavioral therapy (CBT), online therapy, and other technologies from 2005 to 2015 [20]. Four small trials have demonstrated the effectiveness of providing family interventions and parent-management training through videoconferencing (VC) (attention deficit; epilepsy; general) [21–24]. Multiple studies/reviews have demonstrated the feasibility of implementing VC with young people across diverse settings (e.g., rural, pediatrics) [25]. The most described settings are primary care clinics, community mental health centers, and schools, but others include correctional settings, residential treatment facilities, critical access hospitals, group homes, area health education centers, colleges, sites serving foster care, military bases, and daycares care [19, 25]. Unsupervised settings, including patient homes, bring both new benefits and risks [25]. Recent studies have also focused on inpatient psychiatry and emergency departments [26].

Particularly, youth may feel less self-conscious, less worried about confidentiality as the provider is outside of the local community, and freer with the personal space it affords. For video care, adjustments appear to be necessary based on developmental status, family involvement, and patient-site modifications for space and sound. Additional clinical issues include the need to specify who, exactly, is the "patient" (i.e., the patient, family, and/or other stakeholders), modalities of care (i.e., age-related psychotherapies such as play therapy or behavior management), and psychopharmacology. Treatment modalities like parent management, play therapy, or behavior training require site- and technology-based modifications that may not be considered in work with adults (e.g., remote site room design, camera options like zoom/control/tracking, audio/sound detection). Some patient populations and treatment settings—corrections/juvenile hall, home health, and school settings—require additional skill sets, particularly with nonclinical professionals. Clinicians must extrapolate knowledge and skills from usual settings.

6.2.2 Adult and Geriatric Populations

Reports in adult patients show TMH results in an improvement in depression [27–29], reductions in length of hospitalization [30, 31], more appropriate medication use [28, 31], symptom reduction in disorders [28, 30, 31], and improvements in a portion of psychotherapy judged to be evidence-based for posttraumatic stress disorder (PTSD) [31, 32]. With the number of people aging and older adults at-risk for other health problems, more outreach will be needed to the rural elderly to help families/caregivers who are profoundly affected and require in-home TMH options [33].

Geriatric data are emerging, but more studies are needed in medicine and TMH [34]. Obstacles include access to service, functional challenges, primary care provider attitudes, and lack of psychiatrists [35], and perhaps what could be called a lack of nursing home "ownership" by any one provider to formalize a clinical approach. Nursing home TMH studies have been effective in terms of informal measures [36], mainly focusing on depression or dementia, with evaluation of more facile and more efficient use of consultant time. Assessment, cognitive intervention, and outcomes have been similar to in-person [34], and a new development is telemonitoring of depression in the home, which facilitates connectedness [35]. Extra attention to helping older adults access the technology, especially if they have difficulties with their hearing or vision, is required, but acceptance of TMH appears fine.

6.3 Case Examples of Evidence-Based Care

6.3.1 Example 1: Providing Linguistically and Culturally Expert Care

Many suggest a clinical, educational, and policy shift from the concept of cultural competence to cultural humility [37] and/or cultural safety [38, 39], which would include Indigenous community, colonialism, and historical trauma perspectives. This is more patient-centered and consistent with an anthropologic definition is "the acquired knowledge that people use to interpret their world and generate social behavior" [40]. The concept of cultural safety originated with the Māori of Aotearoa [New Zealand] [38, 39], with foci on health gains and positive outcomes; relationships within healthcare; power relations between participants, the empowerment of service users; and addressing the relationship of history, political, social, and employment status, housing, education, gender and personal experience to current healthcare interactions [41, 42]. Cultural safety challenges health providers to recognize power relations and attend to social determinants of health.

The utility of tele-translation services is obvious. While most healthcare providers aim to use in-person providers, these interpreters are often staff members who serve a double function and have received little formal training. The use of family members for interpreting is fraught with pitfalls, both practical and ethical. Staff members—even nurses—and family members are prone to miscommunicate patient complaints or de-emphasize critical pieces of the patient report [43, 44]. Use of interpreters via videoconferencing therapy technology may be especially useful for languages that are relatively rare, such as sign language [45].

Beyond language expertise, TMH has been shown to be useful in bringing culturally expert services to populations who have specialized cultural needs [6, 7, 10]. Culture is known to influence a number of aspects of an individual's healthcare, including attitudes toward different treatments, the provider–patient relationship, and an individual's willingness to engage in the use of technology. While culture may affect outcomes, poverty, and education for all populations, these may have a greater impact for African Americans [46]. Just like with in-person psychiatry, when cultural issues seem especially relevant, a clinician can use the Outline for Cultural Formulation and Cultural Formulation Interview from the Diagnostic and Statistical Manual of Mental Disorders, Fifth Edition [47] to clarify their formulation of a patient.

The University of Colorado School of Medicine's Center for Native American TeleHealth and TeleEducation (CNATT) has done several studies looking at acceptability of mental health services delivered by interactive videoconferencing with patients from Native American populations. They have conducted studies with children and adolescent patients in Rapid City, South Dakota [48], and with adult male veterans from a Northern Plains tribe [49]. In both studies, the authors were concerned that videoconferencing technology itself might be off-putting to this population and result in low patient satisfaction. They likewise theorized, however, that both the patient-side and teleprovider side clinicians were experts and experienced in the treatment of people from local Native American populations, and this expertise might offset patient discomfort about the videoconference technology.

6.3.2 Example 2:Providing Expert Care for Disorders Requiring Combination Inpatient Hospitalization and Family Psychotherapy

Anorexia nervosa is a severe and life-threatening mental illness. Treatment for this disorder may require inpatient stabilization, nutritional rehabilitation, and multidimensional psychotherapeutic care [50]. In adolescents, the addition of family therapy has been found to help patients gain weight, reduce depression, and reduce family conflict. Modern e-health psychological approaches in the treatment of eating disorders provide potential bases of continuous assistance that are decidedly less burdensome in the costs of territorial services in the case that they are not identified as necessary [51]. In case eight sessions of family therapy were delivered via TMH to a girl with anorexia in an inpatient psychiatric unit in Ottawa while her family was at home in a small town in Northern Ontario [52]. This girl's eating disorder was severe enough that she required specialized inpatient hospitalization, but it was not feasible for the family to travel from rural Ontario to Ottawa to participate in family therapy. TMH allowed them to add family therapy—an evidence-based intervention—to their usual inpatient care. They reported that by the end of her hospitalization, the patient felt emotionally closer to her father, had accepted that she had an eating disorder, and was taking responsibility for her recovery. She was discharged with a body mass index (BMI) of 19.5. The staff of the inpatient unit felt that provision of this family therapy was integral to this girl's recovery in their unit [52].

6.3.3 Example 3: TMH May Be More Acceptable for Veterans with PTSD Patients Than In-Person Care

Patients with anxiety disorders and PTSD often experience worry, fear, phobic avoidance, panic attacks, and other anxiety experiences that prohibit seeking help. Ironically, symptoms of their mental illness prevent them from seeking treatment for their mental illness. Military veterans may be burdened with attitudes that make them feel even more stigmatized by mental illness than their civilian peers, and this feeling of stigmatization raises the psychological obstacles to local treatment even higher. Many studies are in progress to reach veterans by phone, e-mail, chat rooms, and other technologies—for individual and group contact—to overcome some of these obstacles and to reduce isolation [26, 53]. In order to address the needs of veterans, investigators have studied TMH for the treatment of veterans with PTSD, panic, and depression. Telephone and TMH studies employing CBT for PTSD have been found effective [54]. In the Bouchard study, patients and providers reported a strong therapeutic alliance was noted in all three dimensions of the treatment alliance. Both provider and patients reported that the technology did not interfere with feeling immersed in the treatment, and patients made comments like, "I'm glad you are here, it helps me so much".

6.3.4 Example 4: Pharmacotherapy Through Videoconferencing

The delivery of pharmacotherapy through VC has been described with youth in schools, mental health centers and daycare, outpatient settings, and juvenile justice facilities [18], but one short-term randomized controlled trial (RCT) for attention-deficit hyperactivity disorder (ADHD) by child and adolescent telepsychiatrists was positive compared to treatment in primary care complemented by a single telepsychiatry consultation [55], with good adherence to guideline-based pharmacotherapy [56]. While telepsychiatrists are the most frequent providers of pharmacotherapy via VC, the guidance is applicable across providers serving youth, including developmental pediatricians, general pediatricians, family practice physicians, nurse practitioners, and physician assistants. Telehealth behavioral treatment has also helped for medication nonadherence [57].

6.3.5 Example 5: Teenagers' Affinity for Technology Leads to High Acceptability of TMH and Mobile Health with Ecological Validity

Another population that may prefer TMH and mobile health options to in-person services is teenagers. Teenagers are notorious for two characteristics that can be leveraged to one's advantage: (1) their affinity for technology and (2) their preoccupation with privacy and confidentiality. A review of the use of TMH in juvenile justice settings noted, "youths seem to be more open in disclosing personal information, and the interactions are more relaxed than in a traditional face-to-face encounter with this population," and that, in general, "the kids really like it" [58]. Focus groups, studies, and surveys for improvement also suggest involvement and supervision of caregiver(s); better visuals; and chat options [59]. Children and youth using technology for health/medicine have more commonly reported problems related to ease of use, ease of learning, quality of support information, and event errors. Teenagers appear much more offput by automatic responses at the end of sequences like "thank you for your message," and kids want to still participate in water or contact sports despite wearables. Human-centered co-design studios work well to engage children and youth by interactive methods and observations of nonverbal behavior are used to better develop and pre-test technology [60, 61].

6.4 Discussion

We began this chapter by discussing the directive for healthcare systems to provide services mental health services that are not limited by geographical proximity to urban areas with large numbers of mental health professionals. We have shown that TMH can provide access to mental healthcare for diverse populations in a variety of settings. This would include care within the patient-centered medical home (primary care clinic), as well as care delivered in the home or school setting.

However, for the large number of patients who require specialized care delivered by a highly-trained and expert clinician, TMH also provides a way to provide so-called "Cadillac care." This Cadillac care may be highly acceptable to patients, as the patient can stay in a comfortable environment of their home or school. TMH has tremendous potential advantages for providers as well. Comer and Barlow posit that future specialty mental health clinics may be located, not in a brick-and-mortar setting, but online. This arrangement would liberate providers to specialize in a narrow band of populations, disorders, and treatments in which they could become truly experts. It would also liberate patients with specialty conditions from having to receive their expert treatment in large metropolitan areas or at large teaching hospitals [4] (Tables 6.1 and 6.2).

Table 6.1 Summary of advantages of TMH

Geographic access	Bring care to where the patients are	• Rural areas
		• Underserved urban areas
		• Primary care clinics
		• School
		• Juvenile justice settings
		• Nursing homes
		• Homes
Access to evidence-based practices, administered by highly-trained providers	Cadillac care	• Linguistically or culturally-specialized care
		• Children's ADHD TMH treatment study
		• CBT for obsessive compulsive disorder (OCD)
		• Parent–child interaction therapy for disruptive behavior disorders
		• Family therapy for anorexia nervosa
May be superior to in-person care	Patients may prefer it	• Anxious and autistic patients may be relieved by the added distance and less confrontation
	Providers may prefer it	• Patients who feel stigmatized by having to seek treatment may be more likely to participate (military veterans)
	Ecological validity	• Teenagers may be attracted to the technology
		• When done in-home, very private
		• Better continuity:
		– Allows providers' safety in situations perceived as dangerous (correctional)
		– Provider can continue to treat patient even if the provider moves
		• Allows specialization
		– Providers can specialize in certain EBP and provide enough volume of services to be financially viable
		– Providers can provide specialized linguistic and cultural services
		• Child and adult behavior can be observed in the home
		• Child behavior observed in the classroom
		• Family-based treatments can be provided in the home

Table 6.2 Common factors in situations in which TMH may be superior to in-person care: common denominators of this success

Anxiety/ avoidance	Anxious patients may prefer TMH as feeling less confrontational, less intimate (and therefore more tolerable)
Novelty	Teenagers may find TMH fun or "more like a videogame"
Direction or cueing	Patients with autism or ADHD may be better able to attend technological interface better than an in-person interview
Distance and privacy	Patients who live in small communities (tribal reservations) or who feel a high degree of stigma (military veterans, patients with substance abuse problems) may especially appreciate more physical and psychological distance
Authenticity of the interaction	Patients may "let their guard down" and demonstrate more ecologically-valid behavior over TMH than in-person

As we better learn how to integrate synchronous TMH and asynchronous technologies throughout our system, we will likely evolve to using hybrid care, providing a spectrum of generalist in-person care to TMH used for expert consultation to expert treatment via videoconferencing therapy [62, 63]. This hybrid care has the potential to provide care that is superior for many patients and many mental health conditions. For asynchronous technologies, this means: (1) patient- and learner-centered technology approaches; (2) effectiveness research; and (3) implementation science rather than randomized controlled trials research to focus outcomes based on acceptability, adoption, feasibility, cost, and sustainability.

6.5 Conclusions

The potential for TMH to broaden access to care and access to high-quality specialized care is starting to be recognized widely. This development is exciting not only because it has the potential to relieve the suffering caused by mental disorders in the population currently but also because the early intervention (especially with young children) that is feasible through TMH has the potential to prevent suffering and disability in future populations. Even the World Health Organization is surveying telemedicine opportunities and developments in member states [14].

References

1. Wang PS, Lane M, Olfson M, et al. Twelve-month use of mental health services in the United States results from the National Comorbidity Survey Replication. Arch Gen Psychiatry. 2005;62:629–40.
2. Wang PS, Berglund P, Olfson M, et al. Failure and delay in initial treatment contact after first onset of mental disorders in the National Comorbidity Survey Replication. Arch Gen Psychiatry. 2005;62:603–13.
3. Institute of Medicine (US) Committee on Quality of Health Care in America. Crossing the quality chasm: a new health system for the 21st century. Washington, DC: National Academies

Press (US); 2001. https://www.iom.edu/Reports/2001/Crossing-the-Quality-Chasm-A-New-Health-System-for-the-21st-Century.aspx.
4. Comer JS, Barlow DH. The occasional case against broad dissemination and implementation: retaining a role for specialty care in the delivery of psychological treatments. Am Psychol. 2014;69:1–18.
5. Hilty DM, Liu W, Marks SL, et al. Effectiveness of telepsychiatry: a brief review. Can Psychiat Assoc Bull. 2003;35(5):10–7.
6. Yellowlees PM, Shore JH, Roberts L, et al. Practice guidelines for videoconferencing-based telemental health. Telemed J E Health. 2010;16:1074–89.
7. Hilty DM, Ferrer D, Callahan EJ, et al. The effectiveness of telemental health: a 2013 review. Telemed J E Health. 2013;19(6):444–54.
8. Richardson LK, Frueh BC, Grubaugh AL, et al. Current directions in videoconferencing telemental health research. Clin Psychol. 2009;16(3):323–8.
9. Hilty DM, Serhal E, Crawford A. A telehealth and telepsychiatry economic cost analysis framework: scoping review. Telemed J E Health. 2023;29:23–37. https://doi.org/10.1089/tmj.2022.0016.
10. Hilty DM, Torous J, Parish M, et al. A literature review comparing clinicians' approaches and skills to in-person, synchronous and asynchronous care: moving toward asynchronous competencies to ensure quality care. Telemed J E Health. 2021;27:356. https://doi.org/10.1089/tmj.2020.0054.
11. Hilty DM, Marks SL, Wegeland JE, et al. A randomized controlled trial of disease management modules, including telepsychiatric care, for depression in rural primary care. Psychiatry. 2007;4(2):58–65.
12. Ahuja S, Hanlon C, Chisholm D, et al. Experience of implementing new mental health indicators within information systems in six low- and middle-income countries. BJPsych Open. 2019;5(5):e71. Published 2019 Aug 6. https://doi.org/10.1192/bjo.2019.29.
13. Nelson EL, Duncan AB, Lillis T. Special considerations for conducting psychotherapy via videoconferencing. In: Myers K, Turvey CL, editors. Telemental health: clinical, technical and administrative foundations for evidenced-based practice. San Francisco: Elsevier; 2013. p. 295–314.
14. World Health Organization. Technology report on scalable psychological interventions for people in communities affected by adversity. 2017. https://www.who.int/mental_health/management/scalable_psychological_interventions/en/. Accessed 8 Jan 2023.
15. World Health Organization. Draft global strategy on digital health, 2020–2024. 2020. https://www.who.int/docs/default-source/documents/gs4dhdaa2a9f352b0445bafbc79ca799dce4d.pdf. Published 26-06-20. Accessed 8 Jan 2023.
16. Crawford A, Serhal E. Digital health equity and COVID-19: the innovation curve cannot reinforce the social gradient of health. J Med Internet Res. 2020;22(6):e19361. Published 2020 Jun 2. https://doi.org/10.2196/19361.
17. Pesamaa L, Ebeling H, Kuusimaki ML, et al. Videoconferencing in child and adolescent telepsychiatry: a systematic review of the literature. J Telemed Telecare. 2004;10:187–92.
18. Myers K, Nelson EL, Rabinowitz T, Hilty D, Baker D, Barnwell SS, et al. American telemedicine association practice guidelines for telemental health with children and adolescents. Telemed J E Health. 2017;23(10):779–804.
19. Nelson E-L, Patton S. Using videoconferencing to deliver individual therapy and pediatric psychology interventions with children and adolescents. J Child Adolesc Psychopharmacol. 2016;26:212–20.
20. Aboujaoude E, Salame W. Technology at the service of pediatric mental health: review and assessment. J Pediatr. 2016;171:20–4. https://doi.org/10.1016/j.jpeds.2015.12.009.
21. Xie Y, Dixon JF, Yee OM, Zhang J, Chen YA, Deangelo S, et al. A study on the effectiveness of videoconferencing on teaching parent training skills to parents of children with ADHD. Telemed J E Health. 2013;19:192–9.

22. Tse YJ, McCarty CA, Stoep AV, Myers KM. Teletherapy delivery of caregiver behavior training for children with attention-deficit hyperactivity disorder. Telemed J E Health. 2015;21:451–8.
23. Glueckauf RL, Fritz SP, Ecklund-Johnson EP, Liss HJ, Dages P, Carney P. Videoconferencing-based family counseling for rural teenagers with epilepsy: phase 1 findings. Rehabil Psychol. 2002;47:49–72.
24. Reese RM, Jamison R, Wendland M, Fleming K, Braun MJ, Schuttler JO, et al. Evaluating interactive videoconferencing for assessing symptoms of autism. Telemed J E Health. 2013;19:671–7.
25. Nelson EL, Cain S, Sharp S. Considerations for conducting telemental health with children and adolescents. Child Adolesc Psychiatr Clin N Am. 2017;26(1):77–91. https://doi.org/10.1016/j.chc.2016.07.008.
26. Reliford A, Adebanjo B. Use of telepsychiatry in pediatric emergency room to decrease length of stay for psychiatric patients, improve resident on-call burden, and reduce factors related to physician burnout. Telemed J E Health. 2019;25(9):828–32. https://doi.org/10.1089/tmj.2018.0124.
27. Fortney JC, Pyne JM, Kembrell TA, et al. Telemedicine-based collaborative care for posttraumatic stress disorder: a randomized clinical trial. JAMA Psychiatry. 2015;72:58–67.
28. Moreno FA, Chong J, Dumbauld J, et al. Use of standard webcam and internet equipment for telepsychiatry treatment of depression among underserved Hispanics. Psychiatr Serv. 2012;63:1213–7.
29. O'Reilly R, Bishop J, Maddox K, et al. Is telepsychiatry equivalent to face to face psychiatry: results from a randomized controlled equivalence trial. Psychiatr Serv. 2007;258:836–43.
30. De Las Cuevas C, Arrendondo MT, Cabrera MF, et al. Randomized controlled trial of telepsychiatry through videoconference versus face-to-face conventional psychiatric treatment. Telemed J E Health. 2006;12:341–50.
31. Morland LA, Greene CJ, Rosen CS, et al. Telemedicine for anger management therapy in a rural population of combat veterans with posttraumatic stress disorder: a randomized noninferiority trial. J Clin Psychiatry. 2010;71:855–63.
32. Frueh BC, Monnier J, Yim E. Randomized trial for post-traumatic stress disorder. J Telemed Telecare. 2007;13:142–7.
33. Schulz R, Martire LM. Family caregiving of persons with dementia: prevalence, health effects, and support strategies. Am J Geriatr Psychiatry. 2004;12(3):240–9.
34. Botsis T, Demiris G, Peterson S, et al. Home telecare technologies for the elderly. J Telemed Telecare. 2008;14:333–7.
35. Sheeran T, Dealy J, Rabinowitz T. Geriatric telemental health. In: Myers K, Turvey CL, editors. Telemental health. New York, NY: Elsevier; 2013. p. 171–95.
36. Rabinowitz T, Murphy K, Amour JL, et al. Benefits of a telepsychiatry consultation service for rural nursing home residents. Telemed J E Health. 2010;16:34–40.
37. Sheeran T, Rabinowitz T, Lotterman J, et al. Feasibility and impact of telemonitor-based depression care management for geriatric homecare patients. Telemed J E Health. 2011;17:620–6.
38. Spradley JP, McCurdy DW. Conformity and conflict: readings in cultural anthropology. Jill Potash; 2012.
39. Leininger MM. Culture care diversity & universality: a theory of nursing. New York, NY: National League for Nursing Press; 1991.
40. Kemp J, Zhang T, Inglis F, et al. Delivery of compassionate mental health care in a digital technology-driven age: scoping review. J Med Internet Res. 2020;22(3):e16263. https://doi.org/10.2196/16263.
41. Yan MC, Wong YR. Rethinking self-awareness in cultural competence: toward a dialogic self in cross-cultural social work. Fam Soc J Contemp Soc Serv. 2005;86:181–8.
42. Brooks TR. Pitfalls in communication with Hispanic and African-American patients: do translators help or harm? J Nat Med Assoc. 1992;84:941.
43. Brua C. Role-blurring and ethical grey zones associated with lay interpreters: three case studies. Commun Med. 2008;5:73.

44. Elderkin-Thompson V, Silver RC, Waitzkin H. When nurses double as interpreters: a study of Spanish-speaking patients in a US primary care setting. Soc Sci Med. 2001;52:1343–58.
45. Lopez AM, Cruz M, Lazarus S, et al. Use of American sign language in telepsychiatry consultation. Telemed J E Health. 2004;10:389–91.
46. Mossberger K, Tolbert CJ, Gilbert M. Race, place, and information technology. Urban Aff Rev. 2006;41:583–620.
47. American Psychiatric Association. Diagnostic criteria from DSM-5. Washington, DC: American Psychiatric Publishing; 2013.
48. Savin DM, Legha RK, Cordaro AR, et al. Spanning distance and culture in psychiatric education: a teleconferencing collaboration between Cambodia and the United States. Acad Psychiatry. 2013;37(5):355–9.
49. Shore JH, Brooks E, Savin D, et al. Acceptability of telepsychiatry in American Indians. Telemed J E Health. 2008;14(5):461–6.
50. American Psychiatric Association Practice Guidelines. Eating disorders (anorexia nervosa). 2015. http://www.psychiatry.org/practice/clinical-practice-guidelines.
51. Goldfield GS, Boachie A. Delivery of family therapy in the treatment of anorexia nervosa using telehealth. Telemed J E Health. 2003;9(1):111–4.
52. Maglia M, Corello G, Caponnetto P. Evaluation of the effects of telepsychotherapy in the treatment and prevention of eating disorders in adolescents. Int J Environ Res Public Health. 2021;18(23):12573. Published 2021 Nov 29. https://doi.org/10.3390/ijerph182312573.
53. Price M, Gros DF. Examination of prior experience with telehealth and comfort with telehealth technology as a moderator of treatment response for PTSD and depression in veterans. Int J Psychiatry Med. 2014;48(1):57–67.
54. Bouchard S, Paquin B, Payeur R, et al. Delivering cognitive-behavior therapy for panic disorder with agoraphobia in videoconference. Telemed J E Health. 2004;10(1):13–25.
55. Myers K, Vander Stoep A, Zhou C, McCarty CA, Katon W. Effectiveness of a telehealth service delivery model for treating attention-deficit/hyperactivity disorder: a community-based randomized controlled trial. J Am Acad Child Adolesc Psychiatry. 2015;54:263–74.
56. Rockhill CM, Tse YJ, Fesinmeyer MD, Garcia J, Myers K. Telepsychiatrists' medication treatment strategies in the children's attention-deficit/hyperactivity disorder telemental health treatment study. J Child Adolesc Psychopharmacol. 2016;26(8):662–71.
57. Hommel KA, Hente E, Herzer M, Ingerski LM, Denson LA. Telehealth behavioral treatment for medication nonadherence: a pilot and feasibility study. Eur J Gastroenterol Hepatol. 2013;25:469–73.
58. Kaliebe K, Heneghan J, Kim TJ. Telepsychiatry in juvenile justice settings. Child Adolesc Psychiatr Clin N Am. 2011;20(1):113–23.
59. Hilty DM, Zalpuri I, Torous J, Nelson EL. Child and adolescent asynchronous technology competencies for clinical care and training: scoping review. Fam Syst Health. 2021;39(1):121–52. https://doi.org/10.1037/fsh0000536.
60. Whittaker R, Maddison R, McRobbie H, et al. A multimedia mobile phone-based youth smoking cessation intervention: findings from content development and piloting studies. J Med Internet Res. 2008;10(5):e49. Published 2008 Nov 25. https://doi.org/10.2196/jmir.1007.
61. Hetrick SE, Robinson J, Burge E, et al. Youth codesign of a mobile phone app to facilitate self-monitoring and management of mood symptoms in young people with major depression, suicidal ideation, and self-harm. JMIR Ment Health. 2018;5(1):e9. Published 2018 Jan 23. https://doi.org/10.2196/mental.9041.
62. Yellowlees PM, Nafiz N. The psychiatrist-patient relationship of the future: anytime, anywhere? Harv Rev Psychiatry. 2010;18(2):96–102.
63. Hilty DM, Yellowlees PM. Collaborative mental health services using multiple technologies—the new way to practice and a new standard of practice? J Am Acad Child Adolesc Psychiatry. 2015;54(4):245–6. https://doi.org/10.1016/j.jaac.2015.01.017.

How to Build, Evaluate, and Improve Your Telemental Health Program

7

Donald M. Hilty and Jay Shore

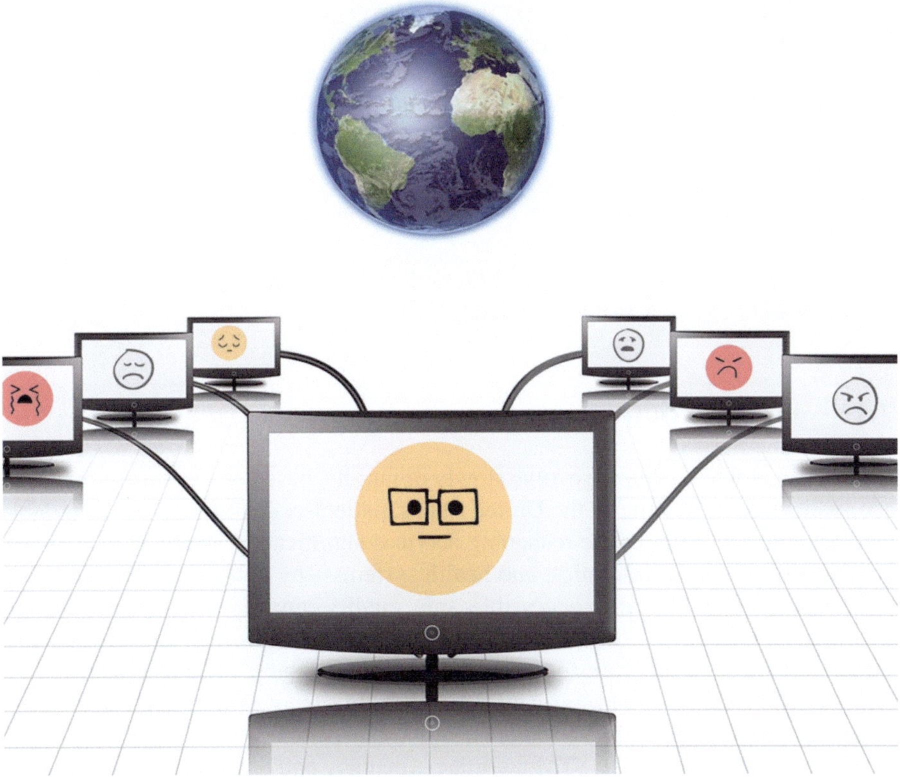

D. M. Hilty (✉)
Department of Psychiatry and Behavioral Sciences, Keck School of Medicine
University of Southern California, Los Angeles, CA, USA
e-mail: donald.hilty@uhsinc.com

D. Mucić, D. M. Hilty (eds.), *Digital Mental Health*,
https://doi.org/10.1007/978-3-031-59936-1_7

Abstract

Objective

This chapter discusses the prioritization of outcomes and evaluation in the provision of synchronous telemedicine (STM or videoconferencing; STM) services.

Methods

This organizational approach may be a shift from seeing what happens with planned services to planning the outcomes and then designing the services in advance.

Results

Basic and advanced areas of evaluation (e.g., satisfaction, technology, cost, clinical and other outcomes) are suggested and involve the many participants in STM in a systematic framework. It also offers suggestions on how to do a needs assessment and how to adjust priorities based on specific needs and available resources in a program. Examples of project improvement apply ideas from theory to clinical and other associated outcomes. References and resources of information are provided for further review.

Conclusions

The readers acquire knowledge, skill, and a framework to improve existing programs and help their many participants.

7.1 Introduction

Changes in global healthcare evolve slowly or rapidly, based on existing clinical and economic models of care. In the United States, patient-centered care, the affordable care act, and other forces are reshaping services significantly. More accountability is expected of clinicians, clinics, and health systems—by both consumers and payers. Focus is being placed on accessible, safe, quality care. New models move quality improvement from a "good" peripheral idea to a central role in the care process. Integrative methods for care (e.g., medicine and psychiatry), health systems (e.g., stepped care), and an emphasis on team work shift us from solitary interest in medicine to a combined interest in medicine, economics, and evaluation.

Versatile approaches like STM facilitate efficiency and flexibility in approach for thoughtful program evaluation. Telemental health (TMH) or synchronous telepsychiatry (STP) have shifted the focus from efficacy of interventions to effectiveness,

J. Shore
Psychiatry and Public Health, University of Colorado, Anschutz, Aurora, CO, USA
e-mail: jay.shore@cuanschutz.edu

with an emphasis on comparing it to in-person care [1]. TMH's almost immediate adaptation into primary care services led to new implementation of collaborative care models [1–3] in addition to standard phone/email "curbside" consultations between physicians and regular consultation models. Additionally, web-based data management, electronic health records (EHR), stepped models of care, and other innovations are facilitating increased reliance on STP methods [4–6], but asynchronous TP (ATP) [7] and other technologies are fast moving due to regular life (e.g., smartphones for reflection, self-assessment, and communication to providers) [8].

Program evaluation has become increasingly important to meet program, patient, provider, and externally driven (Joint Commission, reimbursement) needs—and more accountability is expected by both consumers and payers. A contemporary view is that we want to do "good" care, make a difference, and self-improve rather than being attached to the slow evolution of changes in care (i.e., "doing things the same old way")—a partially true criticism of medicine's attempts to preserve healing through the doctor-patient relationship, standards of care, and best practices. Contemporary program evaluation and outcome work is *a substantial shift* in philosophical approach for some, from seeing what happens with planned services to planning the outcomes and then designing the services—in advance. Now, it is patient, learner, and outcome-centered, whereby the end-product determines what is built or put in place—hence assessment includes satisfaction, technology, cost, clinical, process of care, and other outcomes. Accordingly, the contemporary program evaluation incorporates programmatic changes based on iterative evaluations and trials.

This chapter will help the reader to: (1) grasp the philosophical approach and methods of clinical, program, and system evaluation; (2) assess the program from clinical care coordinators to specialists, team/interdisciplinary roles, administration and leadership through use of a needs assessments and accountability; and (3) focus on clinical evaluation to set "appropriate" goals and make meaningful changes using regular standards of care, built-in "required" payer/accreditation measures, and advanced (i.e., screening, self-report questionnaires, clinician-administered) options for quality improvement. Examples of project improvement apply ideas from theory to clinical and other associated outcomes. References and resources of information are provided for further review.

7.2 Program Evaluation: The Basics, Formal Steps, and Input from Business

7.2.1 Effectiveness Defined: New and Old Ideas

Evaluation of TMH and now other modalities has gone through three phases. First, a review of TMH's effectiveness considered it effective in terms of providing access to care, being well accepted, having good educational outcomes [9]. Second, a transition moved into satisfaction beyond patients, costs/economics, and validity and reliability of clinical care compared to in-person services [10]. Third, a recent publication focused on clinical effectiveness as a bottom line way to evaluate TMH [1] and the current evidence base generally supports the assumption that a broad array of in-person services can be replicated effectively via TMH. Yet we must remain cognizant of this assumption and therefore not gear program evaluation to consider if TMH services are effective, in general, but are the services effective for specific users or participants and at what financial, administrative and clinical costs.

7.2.2 Overview of "Good" Program Evaluation

The depth and breadth of TMH program evaluation depend on a program's goals, resources, and limitations. Informal, semi-formal, and formal assessment procedures can be chosen or mixed and matched to meet a specific program's needs. Well-planned informal procedures (such as conversations with staff, group-based identification of weekly struggles and successes) can be powerful tools to help guide ongoing implementation. Semi-formal assessment could be limited to well-timed four-question survey at the start of care and on follow-up. Formal inclusion of clinician-administered instruments is highly valid and reliable, but time consuming, and sometimes the data are unused or unanalyzed.

Feasibility is a good starting (and ending) place for program evaluation. It is usually defined in terms of operational, economic, technical, market, resource, and cultural or financial feasibility. Demonstrating the feasibility of a program would come before demonstrating the clinical effectiveness of a program—this is simply tested in research (pilot study), business (test market) and in politics (straw poll). Quantitative aspects of feasibility are often based on needs identified in historical data, financial or service utilization projections, or measures of how desirable the planned services are to patients, providers, managers, and stakeholders. Qualitative aspects may include a description of the product or service, descriptions of how well a proposed system solves current problems and takes advantage of opportunities, or fits in with existing business environments, policies, and overarching goals. Lastly, the concept of feasibility remains important at every new phase of program development and evaluation—it informs the next step(s) by iterative process.

Finally, program evaluation helps to plan most, but not all, outcomes, so there are some basic rules. First, an early as possible is key. If we are committed to the principals of ongoing program evaluation for the improvement of services, it makes little sense to do the hard part (i.e., building those services) without the benefit of thoughtful step-wise evaluation. The challenge is to operationalize and merge the evaluative process with external, defined, and measurable set of hypotheses and goals. Second, incremental planning is suggested as time is limited and ultimately it is safer to be responsible and conservative in implementation. A basic plan with an option or two for expansion can work well. Third, there will be problems and conflicts—how you handle them is key, particularly for the working culture and moving ahead. For TMH, there are at least two or more sites of care, scheduling, technology, shared clinical space, and other issues.

7.2.3 Organizational, Leadership, and Team Fitness

Good evaluation of outcomes related to TMH begins with a program and its fitness: organization, function, leadership, team members, experience, and many other parameters. When designing a program, thought should be given to team members, affiliations, personnel competencies, level of on-site and remote-site buy-in, and resources all in relation to specific and measurable program goals. A brief analysis of setting up a team well suited for ongoing program evaluation will be helpful. Each component of a high-functioning TMH team should have a plan for evaluation, and plans can be as simple, involved, formal, or informal as you think necessary. A "good" or responsive team adapts to and creates change. An under-identified area of program evaluation is in attending to team characteristics and mores that promote responsiveness and effectiveness. Assessing shared team processes promotes efficiency in leadership and course correction. Team-based resources and the qualities of a high functioning of a team are shown in Table 7.1.

Table 7.1 Team-based resources and the qualities of a high-functioning of a team

Team resources:
• Leadership staff
• Clinical staff
• Patient-side clinical support staff: walk patients to TMH rooms, administer measures
• Patient- and provider-side referral sources: clinical staff to provide referrals for TMH
• Patient- and provider-side technical support: hands-on responsive personnel
• Administrative support: business manager, scheduling staff, clerks
• Data entry support: for program evaluation
• Statistician/analyst: to investigate data
• Protected team time: meetings to celebrate success, review, and problem solve
• Protected clinician time: adequate time for clinicians to manage TMH encounters
• Time for resource protection: to effectively convey evaluation results to stakeholders
• Evaluation resources: assessment plans, clinical measures, process-oriented measures
Qualities of a high-functioning TMH program:
• Unified goals
• Vitality, purpose and sense of professional well-being
• Interdisciplinary collaboration: ability share knowledge and respect varied experiences and skill-sets
• Role definition with overlapping/interchangeable responsibilities
• Clear non-defensive communication
• Personal support
• Stability
• Productive conflict resolution

7.2.4 Questions to Reflect on for Setting Appropriate Goals

Question 1 How formal does a team member's training or a program plan have to be, in order to do "good" evaluation of outcomes and improve our program?

Ultimately, there is a range of how ambitious a program's goals are, its funding, skills of team members (e.g., rural groups may not have all parts) and the level of support from administration. Deciding on the depth and breadth of TMH evaluation and outcomes is comparable to someone considering additional degrees or training. Let's assume a person has a role in a TMH program and who has an undergraduate degree, 5 years of experience, and some professional training, wants to learn more about business to learn an approach to grants, managing a team, financial stability and outcomes/evaluation. What are his/her options?

- *Informal approach*: This might be a clinician who wants to better evaluate his/her impact, or whose medical/hospital director wants to demonstrate quality improvement related to the clinical care. He/she might learn from another colleague with a model or project, take a course on quality improvement, or become familiar with some scale (completed by the patient, spouse or him/herself) to add to the services. He/she spends limited time, has a tangible outcome and improve to improve it.
- *Semi-formal approach*: This team member, a clinic manager, may be doing well and be promoted to a managerial position in a program, but lacks the "next" skill or knowledge set (or the approach to re-frame his/her new role within the organization). Mentoring will help but takes time. An executive M.B.A. full-time for about 1 year or spread half-time over 2 years might provide knowledge, some skills of business administration, and teach him/her how to hire or supervise additional team members with skill sets needed. (Another example of this level of approach may be a clinician who takes a course on research design and outcomes for clinical trials.)
- *Formal approach*: This team member, a skilled clinician and novice researcher, wants to take a leadership role and improve evaluation. He/she may be unsure of the way to move forward or there may be more than one viable option, but the requisite goal is more expertise, independent function and leadership. An M.P.H. with a focus in health services or a 2-year M.B.A. (both business and team evaluation skills) or a master's in clinical research (design, outcomes, quantitative/qualitative skills, logic models/approach, clinical measures, statistical analyses) may be good.

Question 2 Is the program aligned with the overall organization's goals?

Alignment of missions involves multiple levels. First, consider the missions of the program and its organization. Second, consider the missions of collaborating programs/sites/organizations. Lastly, consider the overall mission.

Key demonstrations of alignment are in contract agreements, negotiated time of consultants (if applicable) and of is setting up the program team; these are related to alignment of clinical, administrative, technical and financial aspects?

Funding and payment usually set up the framework for the infrastructure and all of this affects the ease and scope of evaluation. Health system design and ability to adapt varies widely. Private practice, academic health center, public sector and other settings adapt their practices, staffing, and organization of information (e.g. EHR) to meet many goals. Caution is warranted before automatically assuming that in-place EHR, quality improvement (QI) and other processes can easily be used to save time/money or avoid duplication. Key issues are who controls access, the primary mission of a committee versus the evaluation mission, and flexibility of all the parties.

Question 3 What are the do's and don'ts of program evaluation?

There are some very effective do's and don'ts of program evaluation (Table 7.2). Consensus of breadth and depth is a starting place. Re-evaluation occurs a time or two as things move forward and questions arise about priorities, options, scope, and practical issues (e.g., how much data to collect).

Question 4 Evaluating costs outcomes: what scope to choose and how much to spend?

Cost and value assessment overlap [11] and a standard semi-systematic plan would aid programs significantly. Typically, there is a cost for clinicians' time, travel (provider or patient, direct and/or indirect), technology (bandwidth, hard- and soft-ware), staff (direct and indirect), administration, and others. This topic is parsed out in the section below.

7.3 Measuring Outcomes: An Overview on the Approach and Setting Targets

7.3.1 Overview

The drive to provide quality care is the primary stimulus for evaluation and research into outcomes. These are probably best summarized by three resources:

1. The TMH group of the American Telemedicine Association (ATA) has thoroughly evaluated specific dimensions [11]: an expert consensus process which resulted in a lexicon for outcomes in the areas of patient satisfaction (i.e., access, distance to service, use of), provider satisfaction, process of care (e.g., no-shows, coordination, completion of treatment), communication (e.g., rapport), reliability/validity (e.g., assessment, treatment vs. in-person), specific disorder measures (e.g., symptoms), cost (i.e., length of service, travel, hard and software),

Table 7.2 Do's and don'ts of evaluation

The "*Do's*" of evaluation almost always include:
• Adopt standardized measures already used, in this case in in-person care or in TMH published projects. They typically have undergone multiple iterations, levels of review and sometimes psychometric testing
• Use specific measures unless generalized measures with different parts are efficient. This arises and is demonstrated in the project section (below) for the study on the treatment of depression (and anxiety) in primary care. The Beck Depression Inventory (BDI) [41, 42] could be used to grade severity of depression or a broader net of information could be obtained by using the Symptom Checklist (SCL)-90 (or a shorter version; has anxiety, somatoform and other screening) [43]. The compromise was using the BDI because the primary interest of the study was depression
• Check for disorders that confound measures. Checklist screened for anxiety and somatic symptoms that were confounding variables of outcomes (a 20-item version that had been researched to be consistent with findings of the SCL-90-R); no separate anxiety scale was therefore needed. For substance abuse, the Alcohol Use Disorders Identification Test was recommended (AUDIT) [44]
• Have self-report/patient completion if it is accurate. This comes down to time and money. The clinician administered alcohol 4-item CAGE [45] alternative was better than the AUDIT, but patients could fill out the latter one. The BDI is patient-completed. So was the SCL-20. How much can a patient do, particularly one is depressed? The BDI-30 original is the best, but the BDI-13 was chosen due to little drop off statistically; the drop off was judged as too much for the BDI-7 [46]. Many now use the BDI-II [47]. If this is a mania study, using a screening scale that is patient self-report is notoriously poor, though, and is best avoided altogether
• Collect data and do the evaluation prospectively rather than retrospectively. Why? If you look back and analyze data, it will double or triple your administration/staff time and there will be "holes" in what was collected compared to what you really "want" or need
• Make sure you know (or someone knows) what you are doing. If you don't, does a team member know about these things? Do you need an academic type, a statistician or a person who does evaluation for a living to help? Get them involved earlier, not later. The time is worth the money every time
• For a grant or contract, on the "good" end shoot for 30% of the budget for evaluation; at a minimum 20%; less then that will probably haunt you unless the research/evaluation is so engrained in a clinical EHR that things are truly automatically collected AND can be extracted and analyzed with ease…in other words…one you literally set it up and control it
• Evolve from nascent to specific targets
– *From…*Aim 1: To determine the efficacy of telemedicine for the provision of mental health services in rural primary care settings. *Hypothesis 1*: the intervention group, when compared to the control group, will demonstrate significantly decreased depressive symptoms per structured psychiatric interview and better outcomes
– *To…Aim 2*: To determine the effectiveness of collaborative care facilitated by telemedicine for the provision of mental health services in rural primary care settings. *Hypothesis 2*: The intervention group, when compared to the control group, will demonstrate significantly decreased depressive symptoms as determined by BDI self-report questionnaires and a structured psychiatric interview at 3, 6, and 12 months after study entry
• General "Don'ts" are many and these may be considered in two groups. First, one set of don'ts is inferred from reading the do's. Another set of don'ts includes, but is not limited to
• Collect "extra" data. If it is not immediately relevant, do not spend time on it. Folks put too much in front of patients to self-report, have clinicians fill out too many needless surveys, and have more data—so much—they will never get to it

(continued)

Table 7.2 (continued)

• Measure obvious things unless you have to. Satisfaction studies never got off the ground as telemedicine was so well-received (i.e., 95+% of patients and providers had high satisfaction). If a grant agency wants it measured, then you have no choice
• Ignore even minor expectations the grant agency
• Ignore the changes or upgrades in the literature; don't try to update everything with the latest and the best—not always necessary
• Automatically assume that in-place EHR, quality improvement (QI) and other processes can easily be used to save time/money

and other administrative factors (e.g., facility management, team staffing). Limitations were that the group had a difficult time prioritizing which factors were the "most" important and thus could not prioritize recommendations. The suggested approach above is shaped significantly by a customized plan for each program.

2. A review on effectiveness specific to models, populations, settings and other topics [1]: highly organized and comparative tables of clinical, cost, ethnic populations, and other outcomes for adult populations, along with prose descriptions of the rest. It was limited in scope such that tables for child and adolescent patients and many settings were not included.
3. An extensive chapter on program evaluation that has sections on clinical, cost, and other areas of TMH care [12]: even great depth than this chapter, but not including examples of project improvement nor (now) the latest outcomes, including the child and adolescent studies in depth.

7.3.2 Evaluation Parameters

7.3.2.1 Feasibility

Feasibility may be described in terms of operational, economic, technical, market, resource, or financial feasibility. Feasibility parameters include a description of the product or service, accounting statements, details of the operations and management, and policies, financial data, and legal requirements. Generally, feasibility studies precede technical development and project implementation.

7.3.2.2 Validity

For TMH and medicine, the most important issue is whether TMH works similar to the way we know in-person care works for a variety of disorders and treatments. Good satisfaction, ability to establish a therapeutic relationship to "experience" the provider, and a user-friendly perception are all good indicators of validity. TMH does most if not all things done in-person (e.g., smell alcohol on a patient, check for extrapyramidal side effects or tremor, see all movements); proxies at the remote site may be trained and used.

7.3.2.3 Reliability

In the psychometrics, reliability is used to describe the overall consistency of a measure. Measurements of people's height and weight are often extremely reliable. A recent study of attention deficit hyperactivity disorder (ADHD) at a distance used STP and ATP (i.e., web-based) approaches for further training, data collection, and monitoring with positive clinical outcomes [13]. Other TMH evidence-bases show high reliability and validity via video [14, 15].

7.3.2.4 Satisfaction

Satisfaction is colloquially used in relationship to life, purchases, work, relationships, and other common experiences. It is affected by culture, personality, state (e.g., depression), trait (i.e., personality), values, past experiences, expectations, and other factors. The TMH evidence-base for satisfaction is soundly superior (STP more so than Skype-level technologies) with patients and providers willing to use it in order to connect despite state (e.g., depression), trait (i.e., personality), culture, and language dimensions. Patient satisfaction is a proxy for quality, access, affordability, and ability to connect, while provider satisfaction has additional dimensions of the ease of technology integration into clinical workflow, perceived value of better the service, or access to specialists.

TMH appears better in overcoming obstacles related to geography, time zones, and delays of time for treatment. Cultural issues highlight how technology might better connect folks (e.g., providing access to the patient's primary language, same culture providers, communication with a provider outside of one's in-group). Ironically, the medical home's focus of care on the primary care clinic may work or not, as some prefer other settings (e.g., religion or spiritual centers) or other practitioners (e.g., shaman, priest, other). TMH has cued patients to think about things they should have (or had) already in their doctor's visit or in using technology. There are subtle differences like not hand-shaking or using empathic comments rather than passing a tissue.

7.3.2.5 Cost/Economics

With regard to cost, there is benefit to delineate between differing types of cost analyses [12, 16]. The cost-offset model, which implies treating mental conditions may reduce other health costs, is widely used. Cost-minimization analysis implies the same effectiveness model, but different (lower) costs. Cost-effectiveness assesses intervention costs versus alternative expenditures; a subtype is cost-utility analysis, which includes data on health-related quality-of-life measures (i.e., quality-adjusted life years). Cost-benefit analysis values all outcomes by translating them into economic terms to the degree possible and is particularly important when an intervention appears far too expensive at face value (or cross section), but not longitudinally (e.g., a transplant helps someone live and work an additional 50 years; this calculation gets into quality of life years analysis).

The TMH group of the ATA has thoroughly evaluated specific dimensions [11]. Generally, programs vary in calculations in terms of cost, but these may be potentially, arbitrarily, stratified into tiers of quality of assessment, though technically these should be formally stratified by research and data:

7.3.2.6 Regular Tier Quality

- Patient only.
- Technology direct, but limited (e.g., rent of lines).
- One-time (i.e., one service) cost, the cost if a certain number of consultations are done, or the cost per additional service (that is, using TMH sometimes we provide services not previously available).

7.3.2.7 Above Average Quality

- Patient, provider, and clinic, limited direct and indirect (e.g., cost of travel, missed work, avoiding higher care option, cost offset by reduced visits to PCP by treatment of depression).
- Technology, direct and indirect, but limited (e.g., above, hardware, software).
- A "break-even" model cost based on number of consultations or use over time, some cost-benefit calculation.

7.3.2.8 Very High Quality

- Patient, provider, staff, clinic, community (e.g., cost of flow of services and associated spending on gas, shopping, and hotels for travel to urban center), and administrative.
- Technology, direct and indirect, comprehensive (above, depreciation, upgrades) and including "live" technical participation (e.g., remote control or live Q&A to problem-solve one or both ends of video).
- Sophisticated analyses including impact on utilization of services, calculation of quality of life years, cost-effectiveness; need for economist or other expert.

Cost-effectiveness, cost-benefit, and other analytic models are more common with telehealth than telepsychiatry studies, and these studies show favorable clinical, quality of life and economic impact [16]. A standard framework for economic cost analysis should include: implementation and evaluation; a toolkit or guideline; comprehensive analysis (e.g., cost-effectiveness or cost-benefit) with an incremental cost-effectiveness ratio; measures for health, quality of life and utility outcomes for populations; methods to convert outcomes into economic benefits (e.g., monetary, quality of adjusted life year); broad perspective (e.g., societal perspective); sensitivity analysis for uncertainty in modeling; and adjustments for differential timing (e.g., discounting and future costs). Technology assessment and economic cost analysis contribute to clinical, training, research and other organizational missions.

7.3.3 Models of Care: How to Select Them and Impact on Evaluation

A summary of TMH models of care reviewed the pros and cons of each model [1, 17] and other models have been thoroughly studied and well articulated [18].

7.3.3.1 Low Intensity

- Case review of diagnosis and discussion may change the diagnosis and treatment plan significantly [19, 20]. Provider knowledge, skills, and complexity of questions improve over time [21], particularly in rural PCPs [22].
- In-person, telephone or email doctor-to-doctor "curbside" consultations are a central feature of clinical practice [17, 23], meeting 33% of PCPs' informational needs [24–27]. Overall, these consultations do not include patient evaluations, but they are inexpensive, rapid, brief, and often readily available [28]. A more in-depth system was a 24-h warm-line, multi-specialty phone and email physician-to-provider consultation system for adults and children with developmental disabilities [29].
- Cultural consultation to rural primary care using telemedicine [30, 31].
- Disaster response to a bioterrorism attack was evaluated as feasible in terms of training and consultations [32].

7.3.3.2 Moderate Intensity

- An integrated program of mental health screening, therapy on site, and telepsychiatric consultation (phone, email or video), with continuing medical education (CME) and training on screening questionnaires [33, 34] has improved outcomes and site-based staff skills.
- A randomized controlled trial (RCT) for depression in adults, using disease management and telepsychiatric consultation versus usual care over 12 months, improved the care of both groups, as the "usual care" group benefitted from the Hawthorne effect and skill development of the providers, in addition to curbside consultations [35].
- Asynchronous telepsychiatry (ATP) to primary care is feasible, valid, and reliable in English and Spanish-speaking patients in primary care [31, 36]. (Similar methods are used in radiology, dermatology, ophthalmology, cardiology and pathology.) One ATP model uses a basic questionnaire for screening by the provider of the patient, video capture of that interview, and uploading of patient histories for a remote psychiatrist for review in a Health Insurance Portability and Accountability Act (HIPAA)-adherent manner [37]. Diagnosis and treatment recommendations are made and PCPs implement care successfully about 80% of the time and the model is cost-effective [38].

7.3.3.3 High Intensity

- Collaborative care, which has now been more formally applied to telemedicine [2, 39, 40], has encouraging results. The virtual collaborative care team was able to produce better outcomes than the traditional "gold standard" methodology of primary care psychiatry [2].
- Child collaborative care for children with ADHD at a distance used STP and ATP (i.e., web-based) approaches for further training, data collection and monitoring showed positive clinical outcomes [14].

7.4 Evaluation Tips and Case Example

7.4.1 Program Evaluation Philosophy

Program evaluation and outcome work is *a substantial shift* in philosophical approach for some. Usually in medicine, we have assessed and treated patients, then looked at outcomes—we assumed doing it at the end would suffice. This is akin to the old style of education, in which we taught "good" ideas via elaborate curricula, with the assumption that that mastery enabled the learner to succeed. Evaluation was often cursory and added on at the end. The contemporary view of education is different—it is learner- and outcome-centered, whereby the end-product determines what is built or put in place. A useful idiom for revising one's philosophical stance like this is that the "*tail wags the dog.*" That is, the outcome or "tail" pre-determines our methods or "dog."

Program change requires in-depth analysis of real-world examples or scenarios. The Harvard-Macy Program has imported leaders and examples of what works and doesn't work—and why—from all areas of life. Detailed analysis leads to questions, approaches to solutions and literal things to change. Part of the reason this case example analysis works is that projects vary in complexity of the approach (e.g., "good" idea vs. formal hypothesis), amount of preparation/depth of work (e.g., adding a little something to pre-existing clinical programs vs. marked improvement of one), how user-friendly and proactive the approach is, and how systematic the evaluation is. Rarely, can the "big answer" or "easy" answer be gained with a quick discussion. Expert learners, by nature, instinctively question what they don't know. Another formative program is the case study used by the Harvard Business Review. These ask a fundamental question for executives like, "Do managers matter?" Then, a multi-year research project demonstrates a comprehensive program development and analysis, built key management attributes, designed to help employees become better managers. Over several years, an outcome dataset might show statistically significant improvements in managerial effectiveness and performance.

7.4.2 Project Example: Program Improvement, Development, and Augmentation Through Consultation on Grant Writing, Evaluation, and Integrated MH/Primary Care Services

7.4.2.1 Overview

The rural health network is a consortium of rural health clinics that pulled together to combine ideas, resources, and grant applications. The network director sought help from an academic medical center for the primary need of telepsychiatry service. The specific objectives were to:

1. Increase access to psychiatric and behavioral health services for consumers of primary care
2. Improve regional primary care providers' capacity to respond to consumers' behavioral health needs by providing clinical training, and technical assistance, and
3. Improve collaboration between county and primary care behavioral health providers, consumers, and community-based services to support a continuum of behavioral healthcare services through shared resources, mutual referrals and policy development

The discussion and consultation led to a substantially revised grant proposal to the California Endowment, whose mission includes facilitating care of the underserved and provision of services of high quality akin to the research philosophy of the Robert Wood Johnson Foundation.

7.4.2.2 Logistics

- Assessment of initial proposal. The proposal was a good start and well-researched in terms of rural health, underserved populations, mental health services and a plan of services to be covered. The project for 10 sites had projections of obtaining 600 h of telepsychiatry consultation and the hope was that that would improve prescribing by PCPs. In addition, they would add 7000 of on-site mental health services by an interdisciplinary team of MH providers, to increase assessment for mental illness by 50% at each site and decrease depression via treatment in 65% of diagnosed consumers accepting care. That was the entirety of the intervention and assessment plan. There was no budget for evaluation.

Project component	Objective	Outcome
Direct Service Delivery	Provides 7000 h of mental health services at seven primary care sites in NSRHN region. (28 h a month clinical, 4 h on data) per site. Mid-level provider 1 day a week	Increases assessment for mental illness by 50% at each site. Decreases depression via treatment in 65% of diagnosed consumers accepting care
Telepsychiatry Consultation	Provides 600 h of psychiatrist services via on-site care and telemedicine	Assures high-quality assessment and knowledgeable prescription of psychotropic medication for diagnosed consumers in need of medication

- Grant writing and evaluation plan. The consultant took over the proposal and it went through four iterations before arriving at the following assessment.

Project components	Objectives	Outcomes
1. Direct Service Delivery	50% more consumers at six primary care clinics will be screened for behavioral illness	Increased identification and treatment of behavioral health problems

Project components	Objectives	Outcomes
	Consumers treated for depression will show a 25% reduction in depression	Increased consumer health and well-being
	90–100% of the consumers who are receiving inadequate psychotropic medication doses, will be identified so that interventions can take place	Improved consumer behavioral health outcomes
	25% improvement in consumer satisfaction with primary behavioral healthcare services	Increased consumer health and well-being
2. Training and Technical Assistance	Increases by 25% primary care providers' knowledge and skills in assessment, diagnosis, and treatment of mental illness	Improved service delivery and increased consumer access to behavioral healthcare services delivered at their primary care clinic
	Increases by 25% the knowledge and understanding of all clinic staff about how to integrate behavioral health into primary care practices	Full integration of behavioral healthcare services into six primary care clinic sites
	Development of integrated care protocols, policies, and procedures, and use of outcomes data to inform quality improvement activities at each site	Full integration of behavioral healthcare services into six primary care clinic sites
3. Collaborate along the Continuum of BH/MH Services	Identifies and documents the entire continuum of care in each county	Improved knowledge of available care for consumers
	Holds a minimum of 10 interdisciplinary team meetings for didactics, case-based discussions, and collaboration on difficult cases. Teams will solicit consumer and front-line provider recommendations to alleviate barriers to care	Improved referral relationships, case management, and better informed service providers along the behavioral healthcare continuum
4. Policy Development	Makes recommendations to decision makers based on outcome data and clinical provider and consumer identified barriers	Increased awareness of service delivery barriers and identification of policies to improve access to care
	Develops options to address service delivery concerns	Improved systems of care. Increased access to consumer-focused, collaborative services

The final budget and evaluation plan was substantial. There was no initial evaluation plan and the final plan was formatted into three groups:

1. Patients: objectives, methods, and outcomes for diagnosis, treatment of depression, and satisfaction.
2. PCPs: skills and knowledge objectives, methods, and outcomes.

3. Administrative/clinic function: (a) integrated care protocols, policies and procedures, and use of outcomes data to inform quality improvement activities at each site; (b) and documentation of the continuum of care in each county; (c) interdisciplinary team meetings for didactics, case-based discussions and collaboration on difficult cases; and (d) policy development.

7.4.2.3 Results/Discussion

- The majority of services were provided and the initial academic TMH consultant stayed in place for the duration, but the project was divided with two colleagues (one experienced with TMH and another groomed by this project).
- The rural health network used the consultation to:
  - Improve health services,
  - Recruit MH providers and help support and recruit PCPs,
  - Integrate screening questionnaires for depressive, substance and anxiety disorders,
  - Employ screening, diagnostic and outcome questionnaires/clinician-administered short scales (e.g., child behavioral checklist),
  - Learning integrated care principles, and
  - Maintain telepsychiatry consultation.
- Four academic publications occurred and other reports were disseminated, including the case mix population of patients served by telepsychiatry and another specific to child.

7.5 Discussion and Conclusions

This chapter addressed prioritization of outcomes and evaluation in the provision of TMH services. Basic and advanced areas of evaluation (e.g., satisfaction, technology, cost, clinical and other outcomes) are suggested for the many participants in TMH in a systematic framework. Process, procedures, levels of depth, and do's and don'ts were offered to give the reader options to learn basic or advanced approaches to TMH, program change, and evaluation/outcomes. It also offers suggestions on how to do a needs assessment and how to adjust priorities based on specific needs and available resources in a program. Examples of project improvement apply ideas from theory to clinical and other associated outcomes.

The overall administrative approach should attend to process, procedures, policy and evaluation—there are many do's and don'ts related to planning, implementing, and managing a program. In particular, the fundamentals about evaluation are necessary for clinical managers, clinicians, and TBH experts because the approach and processes that guide "good" evaluation and outcome targets may require a fundamental shift in philosophy—from seeing what happens with planned services—to advanced planning of outcome targets and then subsequent design of the services. The foundation of good program administration includes support from all levels of the organization and an interdisciplinary team who shares responsibilities and overlaps roles. The administrative plan/approach considers a change in the context of the amount of preparation/depth of work, ease of implementation and scope).

At the organizational level, utilization-focused evaluation—the systematic collection of information about the activities, characteristics, and outcomes of programs—will reduce uncertainties, improve effectiveness, and make decisions focuses on the goals, concerns, and perspectives of program stakeholders. This facilitates effectiveness and accountability of organizations and helps infuse evaluative logic, values, and thinking into the planning and management processes. Furthermore, stakeholders can identify program priorities, what constitutes "success," and the data sources that could serve to answer questions about the acceptability, possible participation levels, and short- and long-term impact of proposed programs.

Acknowledgements American Telemedicine Association, and in particular, the Mental Health Interest Group.

UC Davis Department of Psychiatry and Behavioral Sciences.

References

1. Hilty DM, Ferrer D, Callahan EJ, et al. The effectiveness of telemental health: a 2013 review. Telemed J E Health. 2013;19(6):444–54.
2. Fortney JC, Pyne JM, Mouden SP, et al. Practice-based versus telemedicine-based collaborative care for depression in rural federally qualified health centers: a pragmatic randomized comparative effectiveness trial. Am J Psychiatry. 2013;170(4):414–25.
3. Katon W, Von Korff M, Lin E, et al. Collaborative management to achieve depression treatment guidelines. J Clin Psychiatry. 1997;58(Suppl 1):20–4.
4. Moreno FA, Chong J, Dumbauld J, et al. Use of standard webcam and Internet equipment for telepsychiatry treatment of depression among underserved Hispanics. Psychiatr Serv. 2012;63(12):1213–7.
5. Unutzer J, Choi Y, Cook IA, et al. A web-based data management system to improve care for depression in a multicenter clinical trial. Psychiatr Serv. 2002;53:671–8.
6. Geyer J, Myers K, Vander Stoep A, et al. Implementing a low-cost web-based clinical trial management system for community studies: a case study. Clin Trials. 2011;8:634–44.
7. Yellowlees PM, Odor A, Burke MM, et al. A feasibility study of asynchronous telepsychiatry for psychiatric consultations. Psychiatr Serv. 2010;61(8):838–40.
8. Ottawa ON. Personal wireless device use for wound care consultation: a review of safety, clinical benefits and guidelines. Canadian Agency for Drugs and Technologies in Health, May, 2014. 2023. http://www.cadth.ca/en/products/rapid-response.
9. Hilty DM, Liu W, Marks SL, et al. Effectiveness of telepsychiatry: a brief review. Can Psychiatry Assoc Bull. 2003:10–7.
10. Yellowlees PM, Shore JH, Roberts L, et al. Practice guidelines for videoconferencing-based telemental health. Telemed J E Health. 2010;16(10):1074–89.
11. Shore JH, Mishkind MC, Bernard J, et al. A lexicon of assessment and outcome measures for telemental health. Telemed J E Health. 2014;20(3):282–92. http://www.americantelemed.org/practice/standards/ata-standards-guidelines/a-lexicon-of-assessment-and-outcome-measurements-for-telemental-health#.UwF5Dv0_3-Y or http://www.americantelemed.org/resources/standards/ata-standards-guidelines/a-lexicon-of-assessment-and-outcome-measurements-for-telemental-health#.U2bG2xYrfdk.
12. Hilty DM, Yellowlees PM, Nasatir SEH, et al. Program evaluation and practical, step-by-step program modification in telemental health. In: Behavioral telehealth series volume 1—clinical video conferencing: program development and practice. Berlin: Springer; 2014. p. 75–104.

13. Myers K, Vander Stoep A, Zhou C, McCarty CA, Katon W. Effectiveness of a telehealth service delivery model for treating attention-deficit/hyperactivity disorder: a community-based randomized controlled trial. J Am Acad Child Adolesc Psychiatry. 2015;54:263–74.
14. Koenig HG, Cohen HJ, Goli V, et al. Major depression and the NIMH Diagnostic Interview Schedule: validation in medically ill hospitalized patients. Int J Psychiatry Med. 1989;19:123–32.
15. Wells KB, Burnam MA, Leake B, et al. Agreement between face-to-face and telephone administered versions of the depression section of the NIMH Diagnostic Interview Schedule. J Psychiatr Res. 1988;22:207–20.
16. Hilty DM, Serhal E, Crawford A. A telehealth and telepsychiatry economic cost analysis framework: scoping review. Telemed J E Health. 2023;29(1):23–37. https://doi.org/10.1089/tmj.2022.0016.
17. Hilty DM, Rabinowitz TR, McCarron RM, et al. Telepsychiatry and e-mental health models leverage stepped, collaborative, and integrated services to primary care. Psychosomatics. 2018;59(3):227–50.
18. World Health Organization. Telemedicine opportunities and developments in Member States. Results of the second global survey on eHealth. Geneva: WHO Press; 2011.
19. Hilty DM, Marks SL, Urness D, et al. Clinical and educational applications of telepsychiatry: a review. Can J Psychiatry. 2004;49(1):12–23.
20. Dobbins ML, Roberts N, Vicari SK, et al. The consulting conference: a new model of collaboration for child psychiatry and primary care. Acad Psychiatry. 2011;35:260–2.
21. Hilty DM, Yellowlees PM, Nesbitt TS. Evolution of telepsychiatry to rural sites: change over time in types of referral and PCP knowledge, skill, and satisfaction. Gen Hosp Psychiatry. 2006;28(5):367–73.
22. Hilty DM, Nesbitt TS, Kuenneth TA, et al. Telepsychiatric consultation to primary care: rural vs. suburban needs, utilization and provider satisfaction. J Rural Health. 2007;23(2):163–5.
23. Manian FA, Janssen DA. Curbside consultations. JAMA. 1996;275:145–6.
24. Gruppen LD, Wolf FM, Van Voorhees CV, et al. Information-seeking strategies and differences among primary care physicians. Mobius. 1987;7:18–26.
25. Ely JW, Burch RJ, Vinson DC. The information needs of family physicians: case specific clinical questions. J Fam Pract. 1992;25:265–9.
26. Gorman PN, Ash J, Wykoff L. Can primary care physicians' questions be answered using the medical journal literature? Bull Med Libr Assoc. 1994;82:140–6.
27. Dee C, Blazek R. Information needs of the rural physician. A descriptive study. Bull Med Libr Assoc. 1993;81:259–64.
28. Bergus GR, Sinift D, Randall CS, et al. Use of an e-mail curbside consultation service by family physicians. J Fam Pract. 1998;47(5):357–60.
29. Hilty DM, Ingraham RL, Yang RP, et al. Multispecialty phone and email consultation to primary care providers for patients with developmental disabilities in rural California. Telemed J E Health. 2004;10:413–21.
30. Cerda GC, Hilty DM, Hales RE, et al. Use of telemedicine with ethnic groups (letter). Psychiatr Serv. 1999;50:1364.
31. Yellowlees PM, Marks SL, Hilty DM, et al. Using e-health to enable culturally appropriate mental health care in rural areas. Telemed J E Health. 2008;14(5):486–92.
32. Ayers K, Yellowlees PM. Mental health considerations during a pandemic influenza outbreak. Int J Rescue Disaster Med. 2009;9(1). https://doi.org/10.5580/1481.
33. Neufeld JD, Bourgeois JA, Hilty DM, et al. The e-Mental Health Consult Service: providing enhanced primary care mental health services through telemedicine. Psychosomatics. 2007;48:135–41.
34. Yellowlees PM, Hilty DM, Marks SL, et al. A retrospective analysis of child and adolescent e-mental health. J Am Acad Child Adolesc Psychiatry. 2008;47(1):1–5.
35. Hilty DM, Marks SL, Wegeland JE, et al. A randomized controlled trial of disease management modules, including telepsychiatric care, for depression in rural primary care. Psychiatry. 2007;4(2):58–65.

36. Yellowlees PM, Odor A, Patrice K, et al. Transcultural psychiatry made simple: asynchronous telepsychiatry as an approach to providing culturally relevant care. Telemed J E Health. 2013;19(4):259–64.
37. Yellowlees PM, Odor A, Patrice K, et al. PsychVACS: a system for asynchronous telepsychiatry. Telemed J E Health. 2011;17(4):299–303.
38. Butler TN, Yellowlees P. Cost analysis of store-and-forward telepsychiatry as a consultation model for primary care. Telemed J E Health. 2012;18(1):74–7.
39. Fortney JC, Pyne JM, Edlund MJ, et al. A randomized trial of telemedicine-based collaborative care for depression. J Gen Intern Med. 2007;22(8):1086–93.
40. Richardson L, McCauley E, Katon W. Collaborative care for adolescent depression: a pilot study. Gen Hosp Psychiatry. 2009;31:36–45.
41. Beck AT, Ward CH, Mendelson M. An inventory for measuring depression. Arch Gen Psychiatry 1961;18:561–67.
42. Beck AT, Steer RA, Garbin MG. Psychometric properties of the Beck Depression Inventory: twenty-five years of evaluation. Clin Psychol Rev 1988;8:77–100.
43. Derogatis LR, Rickels K, Rock AF. The SCL-90 and the MMPI: a step in the validation of a new self-report scale. Br J Psychiatry 1976;128:280–9.
44. Saunders JB, Aasland OG, Babor TF, et al. Development of the Alcohol Use Disorders Identification Test (AUDIT): WHO Collaborative Project on Identification and Treatment of Persons with Harmful Alcohol Consumption, Phase II. Addiction 1993;88:791–804.
45. Ewing JA. Detecting Alcoholism: The CAGE Questionnaire. J Amer Med Asso 1984;252:1905–07.
46. Steer RA, Ball R, Ranieri RF, et al. Dimensions of the Beck depression inventory-II in clinically depressed outpatients. J Clin Psychol 1999;55(1):117–28.
47. Steer RA, Rissmiller DJ, Beck AT. Use of the Beck Depression Inventory with depressed geriatric patients. Behav Res Therapy 2000;38(3):311–8.

Digital Mental Health Toward Cross-cultural Populations Worldwide

8

Davor Mucić, Donald M. Hilty, and Peter M. Yellowlees

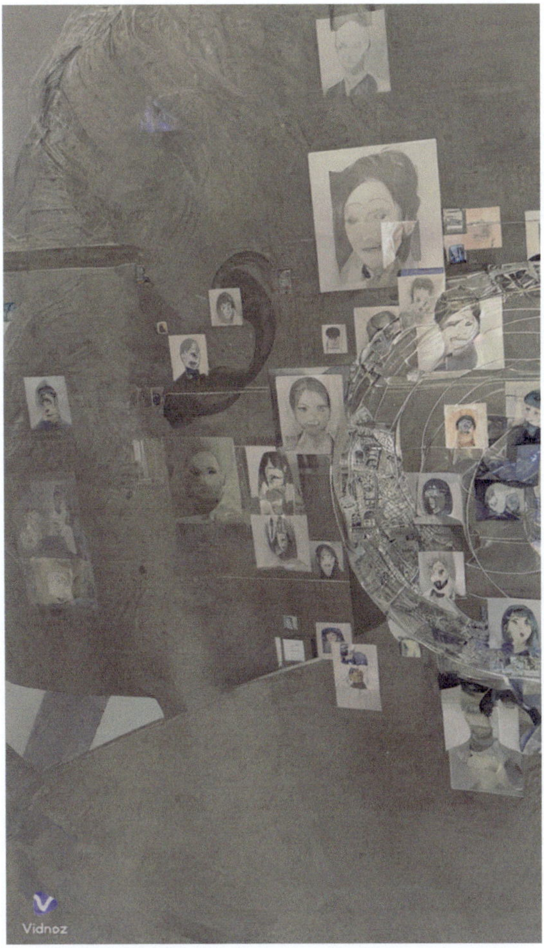

D. Mucić, D. M. Hilty (eds.), *Digital Mental Health*,
https://doi.org/10.1007/978-3-031-59936-1_8

Abstract

Refugees and immigrants in the European Union (EU) have mental health needs and present difficulties for mental health systems due to increasing numbers. These challenges call for language services, culturally skilled clinicians, staff training and adaptation, and tailored-care interventions. Effective communication between patients and providers is crucial for cross-cultural mental health care, as linguistic and other differences can impact care quality and satisfaction. The landscape of cultural competence has expanded with cultural humility and safety constructs. Factors such as geographical distances, culture, religion, and language can make it challenging for some patient populations to access mental health professionals as needed. Clinicians who embrace diversity and advocate for patients may explore digital mental health innovations to overcome obstacles, improve mental health care quality for ethnic minorities, and expand their own knowledge. Digital mental health applications provide new opportunities to lessen disparities in access to vital mental health care for vulnerable patient groups, such as refugees, migrants, and asylum seekers globally. National and international cross-cultural telepsychiatry services can help reduce stigma and enhance the quality of health care for these groups in their host countries. Equal access to culturally safe mental health services is a human right for all individuals, both domestic and immigrant, in contemporary communities worldwide.

8.1 Introduction

The coronavirus disease 2019 (COVID-19) pandemic has brought about health and social care disruptions for people with complex health needs such as refugees and migrants. From mistrust of authorities to language and cultural barriers, the COVID-19 pandemic has added an extra burden on the shoulders of some of the most vulnerable populations. However, the pandemic opened the doors for more remote healthcare and care coordination, with both services and care receivers being increasingly more receptive to virtual and digital solutions, so long as they are fit for purpose and do improve care.

D. Mucić (✉)
The Little Prince Psychiatric Centre, Copenhagen, Denmark
e-mail: davor@denlilleprins.org

D. M. Hilty
Department of Psychiatry and Behavioral Sciences, Keck School of Medicine University of Southern California, Los Angeles, CA, USA
e-mail: donald.hilty@uhsinc.com

P. M. Yellowlees
Department of Psychiatry and Behavioral Sciences, UC Davis, Sacramento, CA, USA
e-mail: pmyellowlees@ucdavis.edu

Many government and professional organizations [1] have identified the challenge of providing culturally appropriate rural health care as a health care priority. As demographic shifts continue to rapidly alter the healthcare landscape, healthcare professionals such as physicians and other healthcare workers are increasingly encountering the challenge of navigating cultural differences between themselves and their patients. This task is becoming more pressing as the composition of the healthcare workforce itself grows more diverse. In order to effectively communicate with both patients and colleagues, healthcare providers must be equipped with the skills and knowledge necessary to navigate cultural differences and promote effective and culturally responsive care.

The culture of the patient, clinician, and the setting significantly affects health and illness research [2]. Culture encompasses the shared beliefs, norms, and values of a particular group, be it a religious community, a group of athletes, or professionals in the same field. It also encompasses the unique cultural factors that influence a patient's symptoms, presentation, and perception of their health, such as family dynamics, coping mechanisms, and treatment-seeking behaviors. Additionally, a clinician's cultural background plays a role in communication with patients, primary care practices, and any biases they may hold. Culture, society, and mental health service setting issues include financing, evidence-based treatment, culturally competent service, medication, and other factors [3]. Recently, a clinical, educational, and policy shift has occurred from the concept of cultural competence to cultural humility and/or cultural safety, which would include Indigenous community, colonialism, and historical trauma perspectives [4]. There are barriers to accessing mental healthcare: limited availability of healthcare services; a lack of culturally competent healthcare providers; and the stigma surrounding mental illness. Another obstacle is the need for interpreters, which can complicate communication between mental health professionals and ethnic minority patients [5]. Having a third person involved in the conversation adds another layer of complexity to an already challenging situation.

Fortunately, the use of DMH applications enables opportunities to build the bridges over cultural and linguistic barriers, by connecting patients with professionals that "match" culturally and linguistically [3]. There are two potential solutions that healthcare providers may use to address language barriers when communicating with patients who have limited proficiency in the dominant language. The first solution involves videoconferencing with an interpreter who speaks the same language as the patient. However, if the interpreter comes from a different ethnic or cultural background than the patient, this could potentially create additional complications or misunderstandings that stem from differences in cultural norms or experiences. The second solution involves using interpreters who work at an academic center to facilitate a three-party conference call between the patient, the healthcare provider, and the interpreter. This can help ensure that the interpretation is accurate and reliable, while also allowing the interpreter to provide additional context or cultural insights that could aid in the communication process. Unfortunately, neither of these is the same as in-person service with patient-interpreter cultural, ethnic, and language matching.

This chapter is a comprehensive review of the use of digital technologies in mental health interventions for diverse populations around the world. It will review the literature, program descriptions, and case examples (e.g., innovative programs; the first international cross-cultural service), the reader will learn:

1. How DMH can facilitate clinical services to culturally diverse population, which promotes adaptation, values differences, and reduces stigma/discrimination.
2. How cross-cultural DMH can facilitate clinical services, which promotes adaptation, values differences, reduces stigma/discrimination, and results in good patient satisfaction.
3. How to achieve culturally competent care and deliver it remote.
4. International perspectives about culturally sensitive collaborative treatment of ethnic minorities worldwide, when interpreters may not be accessed, and innovative programs to overcome this issue.

8.2 Cross-cultural Psychiatry and the Approach to Clinical Care

Culturally appropriate care has been defined as "the delivery of mental health services that are responsive to the cultural and linguistic concerns of all racial or ethnic minority groups and non-minority groups, including their psychosocial issues, characteristic styles of problem presentation, family and immigration histories, traditions, beliefs and values" [2]. Approaches to clinical care [4] and educational interventions [5, 6] have been described.

More fundamental are concepts that have been defined in the literature that underlie the potential achievement of cultural competence, often referred to as culturally appropriate/sensitive care or individualized personal care [7]. These have been defined as:

- *Stereotyping* versus *generalization*: Interactions with individuals from a different cultural or ethnic background than one's own have long been characterized by stereotyping. A more appropriate approach would be to make a generalization as to which specific details about the individual can be made, which avoids the derogatory nature of many cultural and ethnic stereotypes.
- *Values of cultural and individual importance*: Different cultural and ethnic groups value the role and perspective of the individual differently. Certain cultural groups are highly individualistic, such as many individuals in the United States and in many Western European countries. Other cultural groups, such as many Asian societies, value instead the goals and needs of the group/society as a whole. With regard to mental health care, they may see the problems as individual, family, community, or societal challenges.
- *Worldview*: Individuals, particularly from different cultures, may have great differences in their view of mental health, well-being, treatments, and approaches to care.

- *Ethnocentrism and cultural relativism*: *This* involves comparing one's own culture's way of doing things with other cultures' approaches. Ethnocentrism refers to the attitude that one's own culture is the "correct" one, while the relativist approach compares other cultures to one's own in a less punitive way.
- *Time orientation*: Adherence to time varies with some cultures predominately present oriented (i.e., attentive almost exclusively to their immediate needs), while other cultures are traditionally past or future oriented.
- *Inequity* versus *egalitarianism*: Cultures are set up in different ways. In theory, America has a fairly egalitarian structure where everyone is intended to be equal, with success and power dependent on an individual's personal qualities and accomplishments. Other cultures, such as India, have a very precise social caste system where it is hard to move between different levels.

8.3 Mental Health Care Issues and Needs of Ethnic Minorities

At the end of 2020, the UNHCR documented a total of 82.4 million individuals who were forcibly displaced, with 34.4 million of those individuals being displaced outside of their home country [8]. The large number of forcibly displaced people, particularly those who have been displaced abroad, presents significant challenges for healthcare systems in the host countries [9–12].

Refugees are often exposed to numerous stressors both before, during, and after their flight, which can have a significant impact on their physical and mental health [13, 14]. These stressors can include conflict and violence in their home country, hazardous conditions during their journey, and the challenges of adapting to a new environment and culture upon arrival. As a result, refugees often require specialized healthcare services that can address their unique needs and experiences.

Forcibly displaced individuals, including refugees, have a higher prevalence of trauma-associated disorders such as posttraumatic stress disorder (PTSD) or depression [15–18]. The experiences of violence, persecution, and displacement that many refugees have endured can lead to long-lasting psychological effects that require ongoing treatment and support. Thus, access to mental healthcare services is crucial for promoting the well-being and resilience of forcibly displaced individuals [15–18].

Although there is a critical need for mental healthcare services among forcibly displaced individuals, there is often a significant treatment gap [19], meaning that many individuals do not receive the care that they need. This can be due to a variety of factors, including limited resources and funding for mental health services, stigma and cultural barriers to seeking help, and a lack of trained mental health professionals in some areas. As a result, addressing the mental health needs of forcibly displaced individuals remains a significant challenge, and efforts are needed to improve access to care and promote mental health awareness and support in affected communities [19].

Individual barriers (e.g., language barriers, somatic concept of mental health, stigmatization) [20, 21] and structural barriers (e.g., lack of treatment resources or financing opportunities) [22] hinder refugees from seeking help for mental disorders [23].

To overcome mental healthcare barriers, various approaches have been proposed [24, 25]. Barriers could be reduced by culturally adapting treatments. This involves taking into account the refugees' contexts and strains in their treatment [26, 27].

Additional solution could be to offer low-threshold treatments that are specifically adapted to the needs and experiences of this population [28].

Low-threshold treatments are designed to be easily accessible and scalable, with the goal of reaching a large number of people who may not otherwise have access to mental health services. This can involve culturally adapting treatments to be more relevant and acceptable to refugees, providing them in a format that is easy to use and understand, and addressing transdiagnostic symptoms that are common across different mental health disorders.

For example, digital mental health interventions, such as online therapy or mobile apps, could be culturally adapted to meet the needs of refugees, providing them with flexible and convenient access to care. Peer support groups, which involve individuals with similar experiences coming together to provide mutual support and encouragement, could also be an effective low-threshold treatment option for refugees.

However, the effectiveness of digital interventions among refugees appears to be inconsistent [29–31]. While a randomized controlled trial of a digital intervention to reduce posttraumatic stress disorder did not yield significant results [32], two randomized controlled pilot trials demonstrated significant reductions in depressive symptoms through the use of digital interventions [33, 34].

Addressing somatically perceived and transdiagnostic symptoms could be another viable option for overcoming barriers to mental healthcare among refugees [35–37]. Somatic symptoms, such as headaches or stomach pain, are common among individuals who have experienced trauma or stress and may be a more acceptable way for refugees to express their psychological distress.

Refugees often experience mental distress, which is frequently expressed as somatic symptoms in their countries of origin [38]. In these countries, somatic concepts of mental health are prevalent, meaning that mental health issues are often understood and communicated in terms of physical symptoms or illness [39, 40].

Physical symptoms such as sleep disturbances [41–43], headaches, stomach pain, and others can be valuable targets for mental healthcare interventions that aim to address the shared symptoms of refugees, rather than specific diagnoses. By targeting these physical symptoms, mental healthcare providers can address the broader mental health needs of refugees and help alleviate the distress caused by their displacement and experiences [44, 45].

Research has shown that treating sleep disturbances, including through the use of digital interventions, can effectively reduce associated mental health disorders such as depression and posttraumatic stress disorder among refugee populations [46–49].

By targeting sleep disturbances, interventions can address a transdiagnostic symptom that is commonly experienced by refugees and may serve as a more acceptable way to address mental health issues.

Studies have demonstrated the effectiveness of culturally adapted digital interventions in reducing mental health disorders among refugees and other forcibly displaced individuals [50–53]. By tailoring interventions to the cultural and linguistic backgrounds of the target population, digital interventions can be more accessible and acceptable to refugees and may be more effective in promoting their overall well-being and resilience.

Despite the potential benefits of culturally adapted digital interventions, only a limited number of interventions have been specifically designed and adapted for refugee populations [54–57]. However, the efficacy of some of these interventions has been demonstrated in randomized controlled pilot trials, highlighting the potential of this approach to improve mental health outcomes for refugees [33, 34].

Culturally adapted digital interventions can play an important role in addressing the mental health needs of refugees and promoting their overall well-being and resilience [28].

8.4 Barriers to Mental Health Treatment for Ethnic Minorities

There are several barriers that can hinder the assessment and/or treatment of ethnic minorities (immigrants, refugees, indigenous populations) for mental health issues. Some of these barriers include:

1. Language barriers: Limited proficiency in the dominant language can make it difficult for ethnic minorities to communicate their symptoms and needs effectively to healthcare providers.
2. Stigma: Ethnic minorities may experience greater stigma and discrimination surrounding mental health issues, which can prevent them from seeking help or being open about their symptoms.
3. Cultural differences: Differences in cultural norms, beliefs, and values can impact how mental health is perceived and treated, which can create challenges for healthcare providers trying to understand and address the needs of ethnic minority patients.
4. Access to care: Ethnic minorities may face economic, geographic, and other barriers to accessing mental health services, such as lack of transportation, financial resources, or health insurance.
5. Lack of diversity in the healthcare workforce: A lack of diversity in the healthcare workforce can make it difficult for ethnic minority patients to find providers who understand their cultural and linguistic needs and can provide appropriate care.

8.4.1 Language Barriers

Language problem is the major obstacle in the provision of a satisfactory treatment. Mental illness is such a complicated condition that the patient's choice of words is crucial to understand and thus give proper treatment. Doctor cannot settle for "sign language," which he/she may use when the problem is, e.g., a broken leg. When evaluating a patient in a language that is not their primary language, there is a risk of incomplete or distorted mental status assessment [58].

Studies have indicated that psychiatric assessments conducted in a non-native language may have reduced reliability, although the impact on overall impressions of psychopathology may differ depending on the type of symptoms being assessed [59–61]. Individuals with limited language proficiency may have worse access to psychiatric care [62]. They are less likely than others to have a usual source of medical care; frequently receive preventive services at reduced rates; have an increased risk of non-adherence to medications; are less likely than others to return for follow-up appointments after visits to the emergency room; and have higher rates of hospitalization and drug complications [63, 64]. They are less likely to receive empathy, establish rapport, receive information and encouragement to participate in decision making [65–70]. Language barriers are associated with lower rates of patient satisfaction and poor care delivery in comparison with care received by patients who speak the language of the care provider.

Ethnic minorities may have fewer psychiatric disorders, and mental health disparities are often linked to the receipt of lower-quality care. On the other hand, adequate language concordance is significantly associated with higher reporting of past experiences of traumatic events and of severe psychological symptoms, contrasting with much fewer referrals to psychological care when language concordance is inadequate. Clearly, language and even racial concordance are associated with better patient compliance, better adherence to treatment, and higher patient satisfaction within mental health as well as in other healthcare settings [67, 71]. Finally, adequate language concordance between patient and provider (compared to no concordance) was associated with higher rates of referral for psychiatric but not medical care [58].

Common strategies for overcoming language discordance and conducting reliable cross-cultural interviews are to use:

- Professionally trained medical interpreters;
- Ad hoc interpreters, i.e., family members, friends, and bilingual clinicians;
- Culturally competent bilingual clinicians who have the same ethnic and cultural background as their respective patients (sometimes known as the "ethnic matching" model).

When a patient and doctor do not share the same language, whether it be the mother tongue or a third common language like English, the use of translators or interpreters is necessary to ensure a satisfactory understanding of the patient's needs and to provide the patient and their family members with an idea of diagnosis and treatment suggestions. This approach can give rise to various disruptions, such as the following:

The presence of a third person, i.e., an interpreter, in a confidential relationship, affects patient satisfaction, as it influences both transference and countertransference between individuals involved, with unavoidable consequences on a doctor–patient relationship [72]. Interpreter-mediated communication is linked to an increase risk of loss of confidentiality which is why the most asylum seekers, refugees, and migrants exposed to such kind of communication tend to be suspicious wondering: "How soon will everyone in this little city speak about my illness?" [73]. Errors in interpretation can result from a variety of factors, such as inadequate language proficiency by the interpreter, a lack of psychiatric knowledge leading to normalization of the patient's disordered thought process, the interpreter's interjection of their own attitudes or editorializing comments, or the interpreter providing answers for the patient without first consulting with the patient.

The use of professional interpreters may improve patient-provider communication, referral to specialty care, and patient satisfaction. Studies have shown that more asylum-seekers were referred for psychiatric care when professional interpreters were used or when language concordance was deemed adequate by healthcare providers [74]. Use of ad hoc interpreters may impede the disclosure of sensitive material and contribute to distortions [75, 76]. On the other hand, the presence of an ad hoc interpreter, who is usually a family member or friend, has been found to be associated with reports of many physical symptoms but few psychological symptoms [75]. Both ad hoc interpreters, such as bilingual nurses, and professional interpreters have been found to fail in accurately translating the actual statements of psychotic patients [77]. While both trained and untrained interpreters may make errors, the errors of untrained interpreters can have a greater clinical impact, compromising diagnostic accuracy and a clinician's ability to detect disordered thoughts or delusional content.

Thus clinicians have been found to prefer working with ad hoc interpreters like bilingual nurses over professional interpreters who may withhold judgments or editorialize, even though ad hoc interpreters may not always accurately translate the patient's statements [77]. Compromised disclosure with ad hoc interpreters may yield fewer referrals for follow-up care [74, 75], potentially impacting treatment and health outcomes. Professional interpreters, however, may facilitate improved disclosure [74, 75]. In the absence of standards for interpreters, both ad hoc and professional interpreters may lack sufficient language skills to facilitate the communication needed for quality psychiatric care [78, 79].

Summarizing, errors in interpretation are common, with a higher incidence among acutely ill patients [78], and can lead to over- or underestimation of psychopathology [76].

Nevertheless, some clinicians are confident in assessments conducted with interpreters [80].

Language barriers are also likely to affect patients' trust in their providers. Patients who do not speak the language of their respective care providers have reported feelings of being discriminated against in clinical settings, whereas communicating with health professionals in a common language is associated with increased trust and confidence [81]. Nevertheless, the most ethnic minorities brought their stigma already from their respective home countries.

By a review of available scientific surveys one learns that: the presence of a third person (i.e., an interpreter) in a confidential relationship affects patient satisfaction, as it influences both transference and countertransference between individuals involved, with unavoidable consequences on a doctor–patient relationship [46]. Mistakes in interpretation (omissions, distorted questions, additions) occur frequently due to common practice where family members and non-trained interpreters involve as mediators in doctor–patient communication [79, 82]. The use of a shared language (whether that of the patient or a third language shared by both patient and clinician) seems to be the most effective approach to ensure patient satisfaction and mutual comprehension [67]. There is no doubt that language-concordance plays a significant role in building sustainable doctor–patient relationship. However, not only linguistic but also cultural and even racial concordance affect patient satisfaction as well as the satisfaction of the providers and are associated with better patient compliance, better adherence to treatment, and higher patient and provider satisfaction [83–87].

The use of professional interpreters is associated with improved clinical care and patient satisfaction more than the use of ad hoc interpreters [88]. Nevertheless, "ethnic matching" appears to be the most desirable model used in addressing language barriers and cultural disparities in mental health-care provision. Ethnic matching, supplemented by culture-competency training, has been proved as a common strategy to address a number of barriers in cross-cultural-related health-care provision [89, 90]. However, "ethnic matching" model is not that easy to implement. When the patient and the "matching" clinician are located in different places, a consultation is likely to require travel, either for the patient or the clinician. This is where a videoconference becomes an obvious solution.

8.4.2 Stigma

Stigma of mental illness has been identified as a significant barrier to help-seeking and care. The nature and extent of stigma and discrimination associated with mental health vary across and within communities and are influenced by beliefs and conceptualizations of mental health. Many Chinese, Japanese, Malayan, Tahitian, and other cultural groups frequently somatize the symptoms of psychological distress to various bodily parts, such as the abdomen, liver, intestines, or heart. This is due to the fact that somatic symptoms are less stigmatizing than psychiatric symptoms because they are explained by a perceived imbalance in bodily processes [91]. However, population-based approaches to addressing stigma often fail to account for the diverse cultural understandings of mental health [92–94]. Among ethnic and racial minorities, in comparison to the majority group, mental illness may be even more stigmatized [95].

Language barriers can impede the identification of important factors that influence the process of care, such as stigma, shame, patients' explanatory models of illness, their acceptance of the diagnosis and treatment, and the development of a therapeutic patient-provider alliance [58].

For instance, in many Middle Eastern countries, psychological treatment is not widely available or well-accepted, and there may be cultural barriers to seeking help for mental health issues. The ongoing conflicts in countries like Syria have also disrupted mental health services and led to a high prevalence of PTSD and other mental health conditions among the population while psychological treatment is not common or well accepted [96].

It is important to study mental illness and stigma within its sociocultural context, as findings from Western cultures may not be applicable to Eastern cultures or minority groups from Eastern cultures living in a Western dominant host culture, such as South Asians in the UK. Cultural factors, including beliefs about mental illness, help-seeking behaviors, and perceptions of stigma, can differ across cultures and may impact the effectiveness of interventions [97]. Therefore, culturally sensitive and contextually appropriate approaches are necessary to address mental health disparities and reduce stigma in diverse populations.

8.4.3 Culture and Religion

As mental illness is closely related to one person/personality (as opposed to a broken leg), it can cause significant problems in the treatment. In cases where refugees and migrants have a different religion and culture than the domestic population, certain difficulties may arise. These difficulties can include:

- Misunderstandings or miscommunications due to differences in cultural norms or customs.
- Stigmatization or discrimination based on cultural or religious differences.
- Challenges in accessing appropriate mental health care due to a lack of culturally sensitive or linguistically appropriate services.
- Difficulties in building trust or rapport with healthcare providers who may not share the same cultural or religious background.
- Increased risk of social isolation or marginalization within the larger community.

Possible conflicts or tensions between different cultural or religious groups can impact the overall social and political climate. Communication difficulties based on cultural differences are unfortunately particularly relevant to ethnic minority patients (EMPs). For instance, during consultations with EMPs, physicians behave less affectively, more misunderstandings occur, patients report lower satisfaction with care and communication, and studies document poorer adherence to treatment [98, 99]. Cultural differences between patient and provider are often highlighted in telepsychiatry by the patient and provider location (e.g., rural versus urban differences). Familiarity with the rural community and regular contact and feedback are important [100]. Among many cultural differences regarding the use of mental health system, involuntarily admissions are relatively frequent among mentally ill ethnic minorities compared to domicile population. This might be due to poorer contact with general practitioners and outpatient psychiatric services, thereby causing a greater risk of serious deterioration in mental health and mental illness before treatment is started [5, 101–103].

8.4.4 Access to Care

A conceptual framework by Levesque and colleagues composites five dimensions of accessibility: approachability (the ability to perceive), availability (the ability to reach), affordability (the ability to pay), acceptability (the ability to seek), and appropriateness (the ability to engage) [104]. The most prevalent barriers to healthcare access link to issues with affordability [105]. Ethnic minorities such as refugees and migrants may face difficulties in accessing relevant care in a host country due to socioeconomic, geographical, and other obstacles mentioned so far and further.

8.4.5 Lack of Diversity in the Healthcare Workforce

Despite progress made in the field of healthcare, health disparities still persist among people of color, particularly in relation to race and ethnicity, income and education, disability status, and other social characteristics. These disparities have significant consequences on the health and well-being of affected individuals [106]. The need to increase the diversity of the healthcare workforce in all fields of allied health is a continuing need [107].

One common theme in the literature on culture and language is the benefit of using the primary language for expression and more "comfort" in-person than by video [108]. Communication between providers (mental health professionals) and patients (ethnic minorities) is therefore more complicated with a third person involved as an interpreter. Cultural differences and language disabilities result in communication gaps where important nuances are either obscured or missed. In such a situation, both patients and professionals are often exposed to the "lost-in-translation syndrome." The most desirable model for addressing language barriers and cultural disparities in mental health care for cross-cultural patient populations is "ethnic matching," which involves the use of culturally competent bilingual clinicians who share the same ethnic and cultural background as their patients. Ethnic matching, supplemented by culture-competency training, has been proved as a common strategy to address a number of barriers in cross-cultural related health-care provision [86, 87]. But, ethnic matching is not that easy to implement. When the patient and the "matching" clinician are located in different places, a consultation may require travel for either the patient or the clinician. However, technology can facilitate "closeness despite the distance," making it possible for remote consultations to take place.

Furthermore, there are other strategies that have been used to overcome language discordance and conduct reliable cross-cultural interviews. Some of these strategies include:

- Using teleinterpreting or videoconferencing services to connect with interpreters remotely.
- Using language assistance technology, such as automated translation apps or phone-based translation services.
- Providing translated materials, such as brochures or patient education materials, in the patient's preferred language.
- Offering language classes or cultural competency training to healthcare providers to improve communication and understanding.
- Using community health workers or patient navigators who share the same cultural or linguistic background as the patient to facilitate communication and provide support.

These strategies may also be used in combination with the ones mentioned earlier to create a comprehensive and individualized approach to language discordance and cross-cultural communication. However, technology-related strategies belong under the common umbrella of DMH.

8.5 The Role of DMH in Providing Clinical Services to Culturally Diverse Populations

The mental health needs of refugees and migrants are primarily related to PTSD. International studies indicate that refugees experience higher rates of both short-term and long-term mental health issues, with approximately one in three refugees suffering from PTSD or other trauma-related mental disorders [11–52, 54–63, 65–69, 71–98, 100–114].

Effective responses to the issues mentioned above require innovation, the capacity to "think outside the box," culturally competence, and institutional support. One solution is to bring (cultural) expertise to the patient by use of the DMH. Culturally appropriate DMH care refers to the use of digital technologies, including videoconference, i.e., telepsychiatry, smartphone apps, and web-based interventions that are tailored to the cultural, linguistic, and social needs of diverse populations. It involves the adaptation of digital mental health interventions to the specific cultural beliefs, practices, and norms of different communities, with the aim of providing equitable and accessible mental health care that respects and acknowledges the diversity of patients' backgrounds and experiences.

DMH is certainly useful in reducing barriers to mental healthcare access for traditionally marginalized communities, such as those living in remote locations, migrants, refugees, and asylum seekers. Because of the near-ubiquity of smartphones and other Internet-enabled devices, DMH can cater to the needs of such populations [115].

Digital health technologies have expanded beyond just providing treatment to include support for individuals before and after experiencing (psycho)trauma. These technologies are used for various purposes, such as training, assessment, prevention, and treatment. Various technological advancements have been utilized to support individuals before and after traumatic experiences [116].

DMH interventions as a means of addressing the mental health needs of refugees include web-based interventions, mobile applications, and telemedicine services providing self-help tools, psychoeducation, and evidence-based treatment options.

Websites offering psychoeducation [117–119], and self-guided interventions for both youth and adults have emerged, providing services through a website [120, 121] or web-based games [122, 123].

Over the past two decades, there has been a growing body of research on Internet-based interventions for individuals with a history of trauma, and in the last decade, the number of studies has increased exponentially [124].

Studies have reported on the effectiveness of web-based learning on peer support after work-related trauma [125], and virtual reality (VR) technology for predeployment training to prevent posttrauma problems in the military [126] with the ability to control the level of exposure to potentially traumatic stimuli. Additionally, smartphone technology [127], teleconferencing [128], and VR [126] have been used for the assessment of trauma-related symptoms. Smartphone applications have been proposed to deliver self-help tools [127–130] with potential for prevention. Videoconferencing [131] and VR as PTSD treatment modalities have also been suggested [132, 133]. Despite the potential of DMH, there is still a limited number of studies assessing the clinical and cost-effectiveness of digital interventions for traumatic stress [134, 135]. However, positive experiences were reported with the similarities of teletherapy to face-to-face therapy, the flexibility, having control over their own environment and improvements in PTSD symptoms. Difficulties faced included teletherapy feeling impersonal, less support between sessions, technical difficulties, and having to manage their own therapy time [136].

The Swedish version of the PTSD Coach smartphone app was evaluated in a pilot study among 11 individuals, most of whom met the criteria for (partial) PTSD. While the app's self-reported helpfulness was only modest, which contradicts the founders' previous findings, the study found that the app's specific psychoeducation components and relaxation exercises were rated as the most helpful [137]. Digital methods have the potential to improve the assessment, monitoring, and prediction of PTSD. A simple check-up email question after completing an online grief questionnaire may lead to a positive participant experience in vulnerable populations, according to the analysis of qualitative responses [138]. Mobile mental health assessments were well accepted in the acute period after an emergency department admission. Easily accessible tools like mobile assessments may improve response rates to mental health monitoring devices [139].

Support from a therapist through email or instant messaging may improve intervention utilization and adherence [137]. Studies have shown that DMH interventions, such as Internet-based cognitive-behavioral therapy (CBT) with remote guidance from a therapist, can be effective in reducing PTSD symptoms among refugees [140–142].

The use of videoconferencing as a means of providing mental healthcare to ethnic minorities is commonly known as cross-cultural telepsychiatry and is considered one of the earliest forms of digital mental health applications. It is in "real-time" synchronous telepsychiatry (STP; or videoconferencing) and/or asynchronous (formerly store-and-forward) telepsychiatry (ATP). The clinical service provided via telepsychiatry may include the interview, other assessments, psychiatric consultation between referring physicians and specialists, and other components. Detailed telepsychiatry elaboration is available in Chap. 9. Telepsychiatry applications have been tested and developed over the last five to six decades, but most published reports of care to cultural populations are descriptive over the last 15 years.

The first description—in the form of a case or letter—discussed *videoconferencing and culture*, that being a telepsychiatric consultation to primary care of a Hispanic patient [143]. It involved a 90 min diagnostic interview of a 56-year-old Mexican American woman conducted via videoconference by a Spanish-speaking psychiatrist located at an academic medical center 60 miles away. The local PCP spoke some Spanish, but there were no mental health (MH) providers in the vicinity, much less ones speaking Spanish, and the patient was concerned about seeing an MH provider anyway in her community for fear of being stigmatized.

A few years later, in 2004, on the other side of the globe, a cross-cultural telepsychiatry service was launched due to a pilot project in order to overcome the burden of poor service access for ethnic minorities in Denmark and promote a new way of delivering mental health care by use of videoconference [144]. Thereafter, different approaches have been described [3, 145, 146]. More specifically, the current sites face many challenges in terms of specific needs of Hispanics/Latinos [147–150], Native American [151, 152], Eastern European [153], and other populations (e.g., sign language) [154].

Barriers related to the use of cross-cultural telepsychiatry services were related to various technical difficulties, such as logging into the videoconferencing software and equipment issues [155], poor Internet connection, and difficulty using the equipment [156]. Additionally, concerns regarding patient literacy and managing the intervention alone at home were also reported [156].

Telehealth has the potential to benefit racial/ethnic minorities in managing various health conditions and achieving better outcomes, especially when delivered in their preferred language. Nevertheless, its usefulness can be limited due to factors such as cost and low digital and health literacy [157]. However, patients, caregivers, and healthcare professionals have reported high levels of satisfaction with telehealth, as per various studies [150, 151, 153, 155, 158–162]. Telehealth consultations were preferred due to their increased efficiency, convenience, enhanced privacy, and reduced need for travel when compared to face-to-face consultations. Despite the potential benefits of telehealth consultations for patients from racial/

ethnic minority backgrounds, some barriers and challenges were identified. These include the cost of equipment, limited understanding of the use of technology, limited health literacy, and their challenges in navigating mainstream healthcare systems [157, 163, 164], which may hinder access to telehealth services.

Asynchronous telepsychiatry (ATP), which involves recording a video of local providers and patients, is a less commonly used but still noteworthy form of telepsychiatry. It uses a basic questionnaire and uploads videos and patient histories for a remote psychiatrist to review. The psychiatrist then evaluates the information, diagnoses the patient, and makes 2–3 treatment recommendations in a report. It was demonstrated to be feasible, valid, and reliable in English- and Spanish-speaking patients in primary care [165, 166]. In addition, it may obviate the need for real-time interpreters and be cost-effective [167]. If an interpreter's voice translates interview though, caution must be exercised to ensure that the affective tone is not lost; in this study, the historical information and video compensated for any of these impacts.

A model project is *The Little Prince Treatment Centre* in Copenhagen (Denmark), which has telepsychiatry cross-cultural expertise more than other places in Europe [168].

When the center launched the pioneer telepsychiatry pilot project in Denmark in 2004, ethnic minorities amounted to 8.6% of the country's population, and MH care was burdened by long waiting times (3–6 months at private practitioners and even 12–36 months at specialized centers for treatment of refugees and torture victims); there was also a lack of bilingual resources and most services were provided via interpreters. Four stations (i.e., two hospitals, one asylum seekers center, and one social institution for rehabilitation of refugees and migrants) used bilingual clinicians at a distance that via video conference made it possible to assess and/or treat patients via their own language, to enhance reliable assessment, and provide valid treatment for a wide variety of psychiatric disorders.

A patient satisfaction questionnaire was specially designed (Table 8.1) for completion at the end of the visit. High acceptance and satisfaction, regardless of their ethnicity or educational level, were noted [153]. Furthermore, all participants preferred "remote" contact with a bilingual clinician, that is, via mother tongue, compared to in-person care with a translator, partly due to perceived higher anonymity, confidence/trust in providers, and self-efficacy to express intimate thoughts and feelings without a third person involved [153]. It was also believed that distance bilingual clinicians had additional experience with other frameworks of care, which was perceived as helpful, rather than a disadvantage of not knowing local or regional services. As expected, there was a clear correlation between the number of sessions, reported satisfaction level, and quality of care [153]. The patients' judgment of enhanced safety and comfort by telepsychiatry might also be due to less likelihood of meeting the doctor on the street and the risks of spreading rumors in the patients' neighborhood; this is similar to Native American populations in small tribes in the United States [169]. The telepsychiatry-based service continued after the pilot project ended in 2007 and is still functioning between the psychiatric department on the island Bornholm and The Little Prince Treatment Centre in Copenhagen. It is so far the only such service in the EU where assessment and treatment of ethnic minorities

Table 8.1 Telepsychiatry user satisfaction questionnaire

Questions		Yes, in high degree (%)	Yes, in some degree (%)	No, only in less degree (%)	No, not at all (%)
1.	Did you get enough information about telepsychiatry?				
2.	Do you perceive "contact via TV" as uncomfortable?				
3.	Did you feel safe under telepsychiatry contact?				
4.	Have you been satisfied with sound quality?				
5.	Have you been satisfied with picture quality?				
6.	Did you achieve your goal via telepsychiatry/could you express everything you wanted to?				
7.	Would you recommend telepsychiatry to others?				
8	Would you prefer contact via translator in future?				
9.	What advantages did you perceive by telepsychiatry contact?				
10.	What disadvantages did you perceive by telepsychiatry contact?				

are provided via bilingual specialists through videoconference mostly and not using interpreters [168].

8.6 Cultural Competencies

Patients gain trust in clinicians and clinics if culturally sensitive treatment is available [170]. Meaning of interactions, family factors, coping styles, treatment seeking, immigration, and overall health status influence diagnosis. Providing culturally appropriate healthcare is important for racial/ethnic minorities [171, 172].

The cultural appropriateness and acceptability of telehealth consultations and the development of cultural frameworks to guide telehealth use should be considered more broadly, particularly if services are being delivered transnationally [172–174]. Although the use of bilingual staff or interpreters to deliver a telehealth consultation may mitigate some of the challenges experienced by racial/ethnic minorities when using telehealth, patients may still face significant barriers due to poor digital literacy skills. Digital literacy refers to a person's ability to use digital tools (e.g., health applications, patient portals, appointment booking) to access, understand and analyze information and communicate with others [172] . Previous studies suggest low digital literacy and cultural safety to be contributing factors to racial/ethnic disparities among telehealth users [4, 157, 175, 176].

Technology enables easier communication between cross-cultural patient populations and clinicians. However, the technology does not apply cultural competencies by itself. 68% of participants in the recent study reported that the DMH resources they used were not culturally tailored, despite 65% indicating that the resources were available in their preferred language [177]. Focus group discussions revealed issues around limited language diversity, cultural representation, competency, and stigma. Participants recommended including culturally tailored content, graphics, phrases, and lived experiences of culturally diverse populations. These findings emphasize the importance of culturally sensitive eMH interventions that go beyond language translation and the need for healthcare providers to gain a more comprehensive awareness of treatment requirements in different cultural groups.

Culture includes race, ethnicity, spirituality, religion, sexual orientation, gender identity, geography (urban, rural, global), age, socioeconomic status, education, special populations (e.g., prisoners), and language [178]; others add socioeconomic, educational and other parameters to this list [179, 180]. Core characteristics or components of culturally competent telebehavioral health care include, but are not limited to: leaders, clinicians, administrators, cultural consultant(s), technology (i.e., EHR computers, telemedicine), program evaluators (e.g., design, outcomes, approach, methods, analyses), scholarship/dissemination (e.g., grant/funding proposal, reports), and/or economist/business experts (e.g., business plans, costs). Interdisciplinary teamwork to share knowledge, skills, attitudes, and experience is usually the best approach since most systems cannot build such "dream" teams. Management of communication, change, and conflict is essential. Cultural competence training can therefore include: understanding the central role of culture in all lives and how it shapes behavior; respecting and accepting cultural differences; learning to effectively use culturally adapted and culturally specific practices; and the continuous development of one's own awareness of personal cultural influences, prejudices or biases [181]. The literature emphasizes the need for clinicians to translate knowledge and awareness into concrete behaviors that can be assessed in vivo [182]. The greater the cultural competence of the clinician, the greater the satisfaction of patients [183], compliance with treatment, and the search for and sharing of information [184]. The culture of the clinician affects the interaction, as some speak the patient's language but have a different cultural background. These factors affect the development of trust versus fear of stigmatization [1, 185].

Significant steps toward culturally competent care over the past three decades include: (1) a focus on skills in addition to knowledge for clinician training; (2) linkage of skills to patient outcomes; (3) equipping clinicians with skills to flexibly help many diverse populations rather than specialize in one population; and (4) emphasis of team- and interdisciplinary-based [186].

8.7 Telepsychiatric and Telebehavioral Health Competencies for Clinical Care and Training

A series of telepsychiatric (i.e., video) [186–188] social media [189, 190], mobile health competencies have some emphasis on culture [191–193].

They were developed to improve clinical care and they serve as a prototype for institutions to adjust teaching methods (e.g., curricula), faculty development, and administrative policies. They were organized into novice/advanced beginner, competent/proficient, and expert levels; andragogical methods to teach and evaluate skills were also suggested [194].

The social media and networking competencies [189, 190] pose substantial challenges compared to in-person and telepsychiatric care, in that the process of care: (1) is asynchronous, not synchronous, so it cannot be "organized" or structured like traditional care; (2) creates additional boundary issues; (3) is conducted over public, private and health system sites, making the data integration and security difficult, if not impossible; and (4) provides anonymity, with verification needed since false identities are not uncommon [191]. The clinical work should be documented since a clinician represents her/himself, the institution, and the profession. Mobile health poses similar challenges and skills/competencies are needed for additional dimensions like clinical decision support, technology selection, information flow management across an e-platform, and additional features (e.g., context-aware interventions).

Successful teaching of telehealth competencies requires a combination of methods that can be adapted to the different needs of different students, teachers, and environments [194]. For patient care, regardless of technology (e.g., email, text messaging, phone, videoconferencing, apps, instructional videos, machine learning, affective computing, wearables), professionals are expected to use technology and engage patients therapeutically, clearly communicate and attend without compromising the patient's personal boundaries and safety. Supervision with observation, modeling, and feedback are key to determining whether competencies have been achieved and to provide formative feedback [189, 194]. A conceptual framework has been suggested for video cultural competencies to improve patient-centered care, inclusion of the family and community, and training [186, 191, 195]. Fortunately, mobile health [191, 193, 196], and broader asynchronous [197] competencies have been developed in addition to those for video and social media.

An overarching goal is better assessment, training, and evaluation of technological fluency, health literacy, and cultural/language factors for patients, families, clinicians, and trainees. Approaches to increasing the impact of culturally safe practices and technology on health outcomes include implementation [198], effectiveness [199], effectiveness-implementation hybrid [200], and the model of assessment of technology [201] paradigms.

8.8 International Perspectives: Culturally Sensitive Collaborative Treatment of Ethnic Minorities Worldwide

The use of technology enables users and providers to be located in different parts of the world while still being connected via various applications of telecommunications technologies. DMH services/applications described in this book have a potential to provide an efficient and cost-effective opportunity to reach individuals and groups with poor service access despite geographical distances and/or national borders.

8.8.1 International, Cross-border Studies

When it comes to remote real-time DMH consultations via videoconferencing, there are only few studies describing international, cross-border studies, and none involve developing countries [88]:

- A consulting psychiatrist, who was licensed in Australia but living in New Zealand, provided care for two patients in a facility in Australia; one of the cases was a new consultation and the other was a follow-up [89].
- A 6-month trial of telepsychiatric tertiary care from South London to the island of Jersey reported five teleconsultations of a single second opinion and four case reviews [90].
- International DMH and teleeducation for Swedish medical students about cross-cultural issues in refugees with MH problems was conducted between Sweden, the United States, and Australia. There was one real patient at the American site and one simulated patient at the Australian site, with patient interviews by experts, while medical students exercised observation on videoconference and participated in the discussion [88].
- Videoconferencing provided psychoanalytic clinical care and training to psychoanalytic candidates in China by US psychoanalysts, and this involved 40 psychoanalytic and 30 psychodynamic psychotherapies [202].
- The most comprehensive international DMH service in the world was established via *The Little Prince Treatment Centre* in Denmark in mid-2006 as a part of the above-mentioned cross-cultural telepsychiatry project [203]. It became apparent that the lack of certain bilingual clinicians posed a greater problem than previously estimated. Bilingual clinicians from Sweden were employed to provide care due to their cross-cultural skills, including clinicians who spoke Arabic, Polish, Kurdish, and ex-Yugoslavian languages. Over a period of 18 months, 31 cross-cultural patients (i.e., refugees, migrants, and asylum seekers) were assessed and treated by videoconferencing from providers who spoke the patients' own language. Videoconferencing equipment connected the Swedish Department of the Little Prince Psychiatric Centre with two hospitals: one asy-

lum seekers' center and one social institution in Denmark. The distances from the Swedish station located in Malmö to the Danish telepsychiatry stations were from 140 to 300 km. Overall, high patient satisfaction was reported and minor disadvantages of DMH were offset by doctor–patient language and cultural matching.

8.9 Development of International DMH Networks

Experiences from the above-mentioned projects might pave the way for the development of an International DMH Network within the European Union (EU). Most European countries have established rehabilitation and research centers for torture victims. DMH-mediated collaboration between the centers will enable international exchange of expertise and enhance research in the field. Such a network could, by the use of various DMH applications, improve the assessment and/or treatment of primarily asylum seekers, refugees, and migrants within the EU. At the same time, mental health care of all other patient population groups could be improved as a result of increased access to specialized expertise, especially in outlying underserved areas and in urban communities with considerable limitations in access to specialized mental health care (see also Chap. 17).

National implementation of cross-cultural telepsychiatry service predicts patients' acceptance as well. Religious patients are less likely to accept DMH when compared to those who are secular [204]. However, increasing public awareness of the use and effectiveness of technology may help facilitate patients' acceptance [205]. Several studies have found that improving public awareness and understanding of telemedicine can help to overcome barriers to its adoption and promote its use in healthcare [205–208]. These studies highlight the importance of considering factors such as ease of use, compatibility with existing systems, and cost-effectiveness when evaluating the effectiveness of telemedicine interventions. Overall, these references support the idea that improving public awareness and understanding of telemedicine can help to promote its adoption and use in healthcare.

It is certainly true, but ... if the only alternative to videoconference via respective mother tongue is mental health-care provision via interpreters or no care at all, then the patient's acceptance of remote consultation is just a very logical choice, of course, predicted by the service that includes cultural competent bilingual mental health providers. Clear and transparent communication about privacy and confidentiality is of utmost importance in promoting the use of telemental health. The brief and easily understandable information received prior to the session, which is followed by reassurance that no one is listening, watching, or recording the sessions, and that the setting is absolutely private and confidential may contribute to increase acceptance of the model [153] (Table 8.2).

Table 8.2 Questions and policy implications for the intersection of TMH programs and culturally competent clinical care

Questions:
1. What kind of assessment methods and measures are needed to assess the clinical care and the roles of patients, providers, interpreters, and technology related to the provision of culturally appropriate or competent mental health (MH) care?
2. What are the intersections of culture, language, class, geography, and technology in our current MH system, and how do these intersections vary across racial/ethnic and class subgroups?
3. To what extent can technology be used to increase access to high quality MH services—along a continuum of options (e.g., web-based information, interactive sites, self-help assessment, and treatment strategies, evidence-based treatment with asynchronous interaction, asynchronous TMH, and fully synchronous treatments similar to in-person care)?
4. Can culturally and linguistically appropriate MH outcomes (acceptability, accessibility, utilization, continuity of care, improved MH status) be achieved electronically and if so, what types of electronic platforms work best for patients and providers?
5. Will patients' disorder, racial/ethnic identity, socioeconomic status, and geographic characteristics determine whether e-mental health or in-person care is more effective?
6. Should a hybrid model of in-person and electronic services provide more accurate diagnosis and a higher quality outcome?
7. Will patients' disorder, racial, or ethnic identity, or other factors determine whether e-mental health or in-person care is more effective?
Policy implications:
8. Should policy makers downplay the influence of culture on the use of technology and is it economically realistic to target e-mental healthcare toward existing monocultural clinics where it is common to have a clinic primarily focused on, for instance Asian Americans, north American Indians, or similar ethnic groupings?
9. What is the most cost-effective and logistically feasible way to provide language and interpreting support for e-mental health programs? How should policy makers maximize automated written translation services, now available on many websites, which clearly could be used in the health industry to rapidly translate the written word for e-mail or instant messaging follow-up and treatment? What is the most effective way to link cultural interpreters to the language interpretation process?
10. What new approaches to care should be the core options and which others to be used, if needed?
11. How does one educate patients, providers, systems, and others on how to effectively participate in, and contribute to, culturally competent care?

Adapted from Yellowlees et al. [3]

8.10 Discussion and Conclusions: Change from Within and Without

8.10.1 Changes from "Within" Patients and Providers?

Research suggests that many patients prefer DMH compared to in-person care with a translator due to perceived higher anonymity, trust in providers, and increased self-efficacy [153]. Patients report feeling more comfortable expressing intimate thoughts and feelings without a third person involved and appreciate the convenience and privacy that DMH provides [153]. Understanding patient preferences is essential for promoting the acceptance and use of DMH in diverse populations [209]. Overall, these references highlight the potential benefits of DMH in improving access to mental health care for underserved populations, including those with language barriers or limited access to in-person care [210].

The patients' judgment of enhanced safety and comfort by DMH might also be due to less likelihood of meeting the doctor on the street and the risks of spreading rumors in the patients' neighborhood; this is similar to Native American populations in small tribes in the United States [169].

Clinicians' attitudes and perceptions of DMH influence their intention to use the technology with their patients. The key predictor of the intention to use DMH is not clinicians' attitude toward it, but essentially how useful they expect it to be for their cross-cultural patients. Perceived usefulness has a positive impact on attitudes toward technology, and that perceived ease of use positively influences perceived usefulness [211–214]. These findings highlight the importance of considering factors such as ease of use and perceived usefulness when developing and implementing new technologies. Understanding how these factors influence attitudes toward technology can help to promote its acceptance and use in various contexts.

Furthermore, mental health providers working with, e.g., Aboriginal and Torres Strait Islander clients show initially a high level of acceptability of DMH application in the provision of mental health [215]. Finally, clinicians do not share thoughts or feelings of incompetence about adapting too many cultures and languages, but they herald DMH as a tool capable of finding "other therapists" who match culturally, racially, linguistically, and even nationally and/or religiously. They may be aware of local limitations compared to remote consultation benefits.

As long as cross-cultural-related DMH applications are not seen as a substitute but as a supplement to existing systems, the providers' acceptability level is likely to be high. Nevertheless, (un)expected resistance from the non-bilingual clinicians employed in centers for the treatment of refugees, asylum seekers, and migrants occurs the moment they feel threatened by being replaced and/or losing the control. Indeed, the introduction of an alternative means of treatment for ethnic minorities' based via telepsychiatry with professionals from other countries poses a number of threats and concerns. These threats included: accountability for care, consistency in the provision of care in accordance with the countries' medical policies and guidelines as well as the costs associated with treatment [216, 217].

8.10.2 From "Without"...Societal Perspectives?

A delicate issue in dealing with the culture and language of patients is the tension between a goal generalizing an approach or the search for "standard" nuances of specific tribes, with the difficulty of stereotyping groups, and making clinical errors [3]. Meeting with members of the community, including the health clinic, in advance, is recommended to understand cultural issues. In addition, some nuances are best learned "in vivo" (e.g., during a consultation with "real" patients).

Ethnocentrism refers to the attitude that one's own culture is the "correct" one, while the relativist approach compares other cultures to one's own in a less punitive way. Adopting a relativist approach to providing e-mental healthcare to individuals from diverse backgrounds is a minimal, essential step toward culturally appropriate care.

Different cultural and ethnic groups value the role and perspective of the individual differently [3]. Certain cultural groups are highly individualistic, such as many individuals in the United States and in many Western European countries. Other cultural groups, such as many Asian societies, value instead the goals and needs of the group/society as a whole. With regard to their mental healthcare, they may not see mental health problems as individual challenges that can be successfully treated, but as shameful or burdensome to themselves or to their families. The value of the individual should be a consideration when planning e-mental health interventions.

Refugees and asylum seekers are very often traumatized and are quite vulnerable when they seek therapy. Trust, confidentiality, and safety in a therapeutic context decrease due to the presence of a third person, i.e., an interpreter. However, the majority of refugees and asylum seekers worldwide are still exposed to assessments and/or treatments provided via interpreters that very often belong to "wrong" nationality and even speak with "wrong" dialect. Decreased level of confidentiality leads consequently to a patient's unwillingness to divulge intimate personal information, thoughts, and feelings to the interpreter. Professionals have a part of responsibility for such situations, as we must aim to match culture, language, and other differences between patients and providers, allied MH staff, and interpreters—all in our advocacy of those with mental illness, prone to stigma, and likely to have difficulty accessing services [21, 218]. Healthcare providers, hospitals, clinics, and other healthcare systems must strive to ensure accessibility, availability, acceptability, and good quality care while making every effort to facilitate effective communication, preferably in the patient's primary language. Alternatively, it may be possible to use computer-based systems to overcome national, regional, and local legislative, legal, or bureaucratic barriers by entering diversity parameters such as culture, ethnicity, language, and other relevant criteria. This approach could help patients find appropriate care and resources, much like the way companies provide language support through phone or online systems. However, this approach may not be accessible to individuals without access to financial resources, the Internet, or in situations of war, discrimination, or intolerance [219]. Formal DMH guidelines and policies, while scarce internationally, are a start but do not overcome such barriers (Table 8.2).

8.11 Conclusion

Mental health systems are faced with the global challenge of providing timely, evidence-based care for culturally diverse patients, i.e., refugees and migrants. Healthcare professionals should be aware of how to engage with cross-cultural populations, including how to navigate not just language barriers, but cultural ones as well, both in person as well as remote. The COVID-19 pandemic has brought about health and social care disruptions for people with complex health needs such as refugees and migrants [220]. COVID19 pandemic has catalyzed innovation and the widespread use of "virtual mental health care," which is seeing a significant increase in demand for all ages. The impact of the pandemic on mental health has been described, while the potential solutions are still neither widely promoted nor adopted in the daily practice of clinicians. The global COVID-19 pandemic has led to a rapid increase in the use of telehealth as an alternative to face-to-face consultations. As a result, telehealth has become a widely adopted method of delivering healthcare services. However, the implementation of this rapid transition has been largely ad hoc and lacks sufficient evidence to guide its widespread adoption. As a result, there is a risk that the quality of care could be compromised, and new access barriers may emerge for underserved groups such as racial and ethnic minorities who already experience health disparities. Therefore, providing refugees in need with free and easily accessible DMH applications is highly necessary [221].

The implementation of telehealth guidelines, policies, and practices for racial and ethnic minorities should take into account the barriers and facilitators identified to prevent exacerbating existing health disparities [157].

Telepsychiatry improves access to care. However, sets of telecompetencies integrating cultural and telehealth skills are not widely distributed. Program and system administrators can support culturally competent telehealth care through clinical, educational, and quality improvement training and evaluation. It is especially important to build, train, and maintain the capacity of the workforce. Interprofessional, interdisciplinary, and interorganizational team approaches in local, regional, and (inter)national communities are proposed [195].

Culturally sensitive care, with attention to differences, facilitates quality care, trust, safety, respect, and privacy—all essential when working with cross-cultural patient populations worldwide. Satisfaction is clearly tied to culture, ethnicity, and(when possible) language matching. The literature, model programs, and others' descriptions give us good insight into successful programs and the ingredients involved. DMH certainly facilitates care and will continue to, as international collaboration and global networks of cross-cultural experts, address the MH and other healthcare needs of ethnic minorities. Clinicians' attitudes, advocacy, and enhanced performance through supervision, teleeducation, and "second opinion" service are essential, too. DMH has the potential to significantly impact—reduce—the burden of disease associated with mental illness worldwide. Telehealth, by reducing distance as a barrier to treatment, has the potential to improve care if clinicians have cultural and telehealth skills. Training is one way to bring both clinicians and trainees together to focus on technology and cultural competency sets; many programs have neither cultural nor telepsychiatric training. Faculty/clinicians, though, need to have attitudes and skills to assess both sets, though theoretically two sets of faculty could be used. Training curricula need to set goals and align teaching and evaluation toward both sets of clinical skills. Public/rural healthcare systems are challenged to provide timely, evidence-based care, particularly for culturally diverse patients with behavioral disorders. Telepsychiatry improves access to care and tele-competency sets are beginning to integrate cultural and telehealth skills. Program and system administrators can support culturally competent care through telehealth via clinical, educational, and quality improvement training and evaluation. It is particularly important to build, train, and sustain the capacity of workforce. Interprofessional, interdisciplinary and interorganizational team approaches are suggested across local, regional, and (inter)national communities. While several training programs have incorporated formal competency-based training that emphasizes cultural competency and telepsychiatry, it is still not a routine part of daily clinical practice. This suggests that there is a need to further promote and integrate training in cultural competency and DMH for healthcare professionals. Such training could improve healthcare professionals' ability to effectively address the unique needs and preferences of diverse patient populations and increase their willingness to adopt DMH as a viable treatment option.

References

1. Office of the Surgeon General Center for Mental Health Services and National Institute of Mental Health. Mental health: culture, race, and ethnicity: a supplement to mental health: a report of the surgeon general. 2009. http://www.ncbi.nlm.nih.gov/books/NBK44242/.
2. Office of the Surgeon General (US), Center for Mental Health Services (US), National Institute of Mental Health (US). Chapter 4: Mental health care for American Indians and Alaska Natives. In: Mental health: culture, race, and ethnicity: a supplement to mental health: a report of the surgeon general. Rockville: Substance Abuse and Mental Health Services Administration (US); 2001.
3. Yellowlees PM, Marks SL, Hilty DM, et al. Using e-health to enable culturally appropriate mental health care in rural areas. Telemed J E Health. 2008;14(5):486–92.
4. Hilty DM, Crawford A, Teshima J, et al. Mobile health and cultural competencies as a foundation for telehealth care: scoping review. J Technol Behav Sci. 2021;6(2):197–230. https://doi.org/10.1007/s41347-020-00180-5.
5. Beach MC, Price EG, Gary TL, et al. Cultural competency: a systematic review of health care provider educational interventions. Med Care. 2005;43(4):356.
6. Sherrill WW, Crew L, Mayo RM, et al. Educational and health services innovation to improve care for rural Hispanic communities in the US. Educ Health (Abingdon). 2005;18:356–67.
7. Galanti GA. Caring for patients from different cultures. 3rd ed. Philadelphia: University of Pennsylvania Press; 2004.
8. Global trends: forced displacement in 2020. UNHCR The UN Refugee Agency. 2021. https://www.unhcr.org/60b638e37/unhcr-global-trends-2020.
9. Lindert J, Carta MG, Schäfer I, Mollica RF. Refugees mental health—a public mental health challenge. Eur J Pub Health. 2016;26:374–5. https://doi.org/10.1093/eurpub/ckw010.
10. Silove D, Ventevogel P, Rees S. The contemporary refugee crisis: an overview of mental health challenges. World Psychiatry. 2017;16:130–9. https://doi.org/10.1002/wps.20438.
11. Wylie L, Van Meyel R, Harder H, Sukhera J, Luc C, Ganjavi H, et al. Assessing trauma in a transcultural context: challenges in mental health care with immigrants and refugees. Public Health Rev. 2018;39:22. https://doi.org/10.1186/s40985-018-0102-y.
12. Bajbouj M, Panneck P, Winter S-M, Ajami C, Alabdullah J, Benedikt Burger M, et al. A central clearing clinic to provide mental health services for refugees in Germany. Front Public Health. 2021;9:635474. https://doi.org/10.3389/fpubh.2021.635474.

13. Müller M, Khamis D, Srivastava D, Exadaktylos AK, Pfortmueller CA. Understanding refugees' health. Semin Neurol. 2018;38:152–62. https://doi.org/10.1055/s-0038-1649337.
14. Steel JL, Dunlavy AC, Harding CE, Theorell T. The psychological consequences of pre-emigration trauma and post-migration stress in refugees and immigrants from Africa. J Immigr Minor Health. 2017;19:523–32. https://doi.org/10.1007/s10903-016-0478-z.
15. Turrini G, Purgato M, Ballette F, Nosè M, Ostuzzi G, Barbui C. Common mental disorders in asylum seekers and refugees: umbrella review of prevalence and intervention studies. Int J Ment Heal Syst. 2017;11:51. https://doi.org/10.1186/s13033-017-0156-0.
16. Henkelmann J-R, de Best S, Deckers C, Jensen K, Shahab M, Elzinga B, et al. Anxiety, depression and post-traumatic stress disorder in refugees resettling in high-income countries: systematic review and meta-analysis. BJPsych Open. 2020;6:e68. https://doi.org/10.1192/bjo.2020.54.
17. Blackmore R, Boyle JA, Fazel M, Ranasinha S, Gray KM, Fitzgerald G, et al. The prevalence of mental illness in refugees and asylum seekers: a systematic review and meta-analysis. PLoS Med. 2020;17:e1003337. https://doi.org/10.1371/journal.pmed.1003337.
18. Hoell A, Kourmpeli E, Salize HJ, Heinz A, Padberg F, Habel U, et al. Prevalence of depressive symptoms and symptoms of post-traumatic stress disorder among newly arrived refugees and asylum seekers in Germany: systematic review and meta-analysis. BJPsych Open. 2021;7:e93. https://doi.org/10.1192/bjo.2021.54.
19. Satinsky E, Fuhr DC, Woodward A, Sondorp E, Roberts B. Mental health care utilisation and access among refugees and asylum seekers in Europe: a systematic review. Health Policy. 2019;123:851–63. https://doi.org/10.1016/j.healthpol.2019.02.007.
20. Scheppers E, van Dongen E, Dekker J, Geertzen J, Dekker J. Potential barriers to the use of health services among ethnic minorities: a review. Fam Pract. 2006;23:325–48. https://doi.org/10.1093/fampra/cmi113.
21. Kiselev N, Morina N, Schick M, Watzke B, Schnyder U, Pfaltz MC. Barriers to access to outpatient mental health care for refugees and asylum seekers in Switzerland: the therapist's view. BMC Psychiatry. 2020;20:1–14. https://doi.org/10.1186/s12888-020-02783-x.
22. van der Boor CF, White R. Barriers to accessing and negotiating mental health services in asylum seeking and refugee populations: the application of the candidacy framework. J Immigr Minor Health. 2020;22:156–74. https://doi.org/10.1007/s10903-019-00929-y.
23. Byrow Y, Pajak R, Specker P, Nickerson A. Perceptions of mental health and perceived barriers to mental health help-seeking amongst refugees: a systematic review. Clin Psychol Rev. 2020;75:101812. https://doi.org/10.1016/j.cpr.2019.101812.
24. Patel V, Chowdhary N, Rahman A, Verdeli H. Improving access to psychological treatments: lessons from developing countries. Behav Res Ther. 2011;49:523–8. https://doi.org/10.1016/j.brat.2011.06.012.
25. Trilesnik B, Altunoz U, Wesolowski J, Eckhoff L, Ozkan I, Loos K, et al. Implementing a need-adapted stepped-care model for mental health of refugees: preliminary data of the state-funded project "Refukey". Front Psych. 2019;10:688. https://doi.org/10.3389/fpsyt.2019.00688.
26. Bernal G, Jiménez-Chafey MI, Domenech Rodríguez MM. Cultural adaptation of treatments: a resource for considering culture in evidence-based practice. Prof Psychol Res Pract. 2009;40:361–8. https://doi.org/10.1037/a0016401.
27. Schnyder U, Bryant RA, Ehlers A, Foa EB, Hasan A, Mwiti G, et al. Culture-sensitive psychotraumatology. Eur J Psychotraumatol. 2016;7:31179.
28. Spanhel K, Hovestadt E, Lehr D, et al. Engaging refugees with a culturally adapted digital intervention to improve sleep: a randomized controlled pilot trial. Front Psychiatry. 2022;13:832196. Published 2022 Feb 23. https://doi.org/10.3389/fpsyt.2022.832196.
29. Andersson G, Titov N, Dear BF, Rozental A, Carlbring P. Internet-delivered psychological treatments: from innovation to implementation. World Psychiatry. 2019;18:20–8. https://doi.org/10.1002/wps.20610.

30. Rigabert A, Motrico E, Moreno-Peral P, Resurrección DM, Conejo-Cerón S, Cuijpers P, et al. Effectiveness of online psychological and psychoeducational interventions to prevent depression: systematic review and meta-analysis of randomized controlled trials. Clin Psychol Rev. 2020;82:101931. https://doi.org/10.1016/j.cpr.2020.101931.
31. Karyotaki E, Efthimiou O, Miguel C, Bermpohl FMG, Furukawa TA, Cuijpers P, et al. Internet-based cognitive behavioral therapy for depression: a systematic review and individual patient data network meta-analysis. JAMA Psychiatry. 2021;78:361–71.
32. Roehr S, Jung FU, Pabst A, Grochtdreis T, Dams J, Nagl M, et al. A self-help app for Syrian refugees with posttraumatic stress (Sanadak): randomized controlled trial. JMIR Mhealth Uhealth. 2021;9:e24807. https://doi.org/10.2196/24807.
33. Lindegaard T, Seaton F, Halaj A, Berg M, Kashoush F, Barchini R, et al. Internet-based cognitive behavioural therapy for depression and anxiety among Arabic-speaking individuals in Sweden: a pilot randomized controlled trial. Cogn Behav Ther. 2020;50:47–66. https://doi.org/10.1080/16506073.2020.1771414.
34. Heim E, Abi Ramia J, Abi Hana R, Burchert S, Carswell K, Cornelisz I, et al. Step-by-step: feasibility randomised controlled trial of a mobile-based intervention for depression among populations affected by adversity in Lebanon. Internet Interv. 2021;24:100380. https://doi.org/10.1016/j.invent.2021.100380.
35. Tay AK, Miah MAA, Khan S, Badrudduza M, Morgan K, Balasundaram S, et al. Theoretical background, first stage development and adaptation of a novel Integrative Adapt Therapy (IAT) for refugees. Epidemiol Psychiatr Sci. 2019;29:e47. https://doi.org/10.1017/S2045796019000416.
36. Koch T, Ehring T, Liedl A. Effectiveness of a transdiagnostic group intervention to enhance emotion regulation in young Afghan refugees: a pilot randomized controlled study. Behav Res Ther. 2020;132:103689. https://doi.org/10.1016/j.brat.2020.103689.
37. Murray LK, Haroz E, Dorsey S, Kane J, Bolton PA, Pullmann MD. Understanding mechanisms of change: an unpacking study of the evidence-based common-elements treatment approach (CETA) in low and middle income countries. Behav Res Ther. 2020;130:103430. https://doi.org/10.1016/j.brat.2019.103430.
38. Morina N, Kuenburg A, Schnyder U, Bryant RA, Nickerson A, Schick M. The association of post-traumatic and postmigration stress with pain and other somatic symptoms: an explorative analysis in traumatized refugees and asylum seekers. Pain Med. 2018;19:50–9. https://doi.org/10.1093/pm/pnx005.
39. Hinton DE, Otto MW. Symptom presentation and symptom meaning among traumatized Cambodian refugees: relevance to a somatically focused cognitive-behavior therapy. Cogn Behav Pract. 2006;13:249–60. https://doi.org/10.1016/j.cbpra.2006.04.006.
40. Rohlof HG, Knipscheer JW, Kleber RJ. Somatization in refugees: a review. Soc Psychiatry Psychiatr Epidemiol. 2014;49:1793–804. https://doi.org/10.1007/s00127-014-0877.
41. Al-Smadi AM, Tawalbeh LI, Gammoh OS, Ashour A, Tayfur M, Attarian H. The prevalence and the predictors of insomnia among refugees. J Health Psychol. 2019;24:1125–33. https://doi.org/10.1177/1359105316687631.
42. Lies J, Drummond SPA, Jobson L. Longitudinal investigation of the relationships between trauma exposure, post-migration stress, sleep disturbance, and mental health in Syrian refugees. Eur J Psychotraumatol. 2020;11:1825166. https://doi.org/10.1080/20008198.2020.1825166.
43. Jamil H, Hakim-Larson J, Farrag M, Kafaji T, Jamil LH, Hammad A. Medical complaints among Iraqi American refugees with mental disorders. J Immigr Health. 2005;7:145–52. https://doi.org/10.1007/s10903-005-3671-z.
44. Baglioni C, Nanovska S, Regen W, Spiegelhalder K, Feige B, Nissen C, et al. Sleep and mental disorders: a meta-analysis of polysomnographic research. Psychol Bull. 2016;142:969–90. https://doi.org/10.1037/bul0000053.
45. Spoormaker VI, Montgomery P. Disturbed sleep in post-traumatic stress disorder: secondary symptom or core feature? Sleep Med Rev. 2008;12:169–84er. (2021) 144:103922. https://doi.org/10.1016/j.brat.2021.103922.

46. Cheng P, Kalmbach DA, Tallent G, Joseph CLM, Espie CA, Drake CL. Depression prevention via digital cognitive behavioral therapy for insomnia: a randomized controlled trial. Sleep. 2019;42:zsz150. https://doi.org/10.1093/sleep/zsz150.
47. Stott R, Pimm J, Emsley R, Miller CB, Espie CA. Does adjunctive digital CBT for insomnia improve clinical outcomes in an improving access to psychological therapies service? Behav Res Ther. 2021;144:103922. https://doi.org/10.1016/j.brat.2021.103922.
48. Christensen H, Batterham PJ, Gosling JA, Ritterband LM, Griffiths KM, Thorndike FP, et al. Effectiveness of an online insomnia program (SHUTi) for prevention of depressive episodes (the GoodNight Study): a randomised controlled trial. Lancet Psychiatry. 2016;3:333–41. https://doi.org/10.1016/S2215-0366(15)00536-2.
49. Harvey AG, Dong L, Hein K, Yu SH, Martinez AJ, Gumport NB, et al. A randomized controlled trial of the transdiagnostic intervention for sleep and circadian dysfunction (TranS-C) to improve serious mental illness outcomes in a community setting. J Consult Clin Psychol. 2021;89:537–50. https://doi.org/10.1037/ccp0000650.
50. Spanhel K, Balci S, Feldhahn F, Bengel J, Baumeister H, Sander LB. Cultural adaptation of internet- and mobile-based interventions for mental disorders: a systematic review. NPJ Digit Med. 2021;4:128. https://doi.org/10.1038/s41746-021-00498-1.
51. Hall GCN, Ibaraki AY, Huang ER, Marti CN, Stice E. A meta-analysis of cultural adaptations of psychological interventions. Behav Ther. 2016;47:993–1014. https://doi.org/10.1016/j.beth.2016.09.005.
52. Anik E, West RM, Cardno AG, Mir G. Culturally adapted psychotherapies for depressed adults: a systematic review and meta-analysis. J Affect Disord. 2021;278:296–310. https://doi.org/10.1016/j.jad.2020.09.051.
53. Harper Shehadeh MJ, Heim E, Chowdhary N, Maercker A, Albanese E. Cultural adaptation of minimally guided interventions for common mental disorders: a systematic review and meta-analysis. JMIR Ment Heal. 2016;3:e44. https://doi.org/10.2196/mental.5776.
54. Abi Ramia J, Harper Shehadeh M, Kheir W, Zoghbi E, Watts S, Heim E, et al. Community cognitive interviewing to inform local adaptations of an e-mental health intervention in Lebanon. Glob Ment Heal. 2018;5:e39. https://doi.org/10.1017/gmh.2018.29.
55. Nygren T, Berg M, Sarkohi A, Andersson G. Development of an internet-based cognitive behavioral therapy self-help program for Arabic-speaking immigrants: mixed-methods study. JMIR Res Protoc. 2018;7:e11872. https://doi.org/10.2196/11872.
56. Burchert S, Alkneme MS, Bird M, Carswell K, Cuijpers P, Hansen P, et al. User-centered app adaptation of a low-intensity e-mental health intervention for Syrian refugees. Front Psych. 2019;9:663. https://doi.org/10.3389/fpsyt.2018.00663.
57. Harper Shehadeh MJ, Abi Ramia J, Cuijpers P, El Chammay R, Heim E, Kheir W, et al. Step-by-Step, an e-mental health intervention for depression: a mixed methods pilot study from Lebanon. Front Psych. 2020;10:986. https://doi.org/10.3389/fpsyt.2019.00986.
58. Bauer AM, Alegría M. Impact of patient language proficiency and interpreter service use on the quality of psychiatric care: a systematic review. Psychiatr Serv. 2010;61(8):765–73. https://doi.org/10.1176/ps.2010.61.8.765. PMID: 20675834; PMCID: PMC2946248.
59. Marcos LR, Alpert M, Urcuyo L, et al. The effect of interview language on the evaluation of psychopathology in Spanish-American schizophrenic patients. Am J Psychiatry. 1973;130:549–53.
60. Price CS, Cuellar I. Effects of language and related variables on the expression of psychopathology in Mexican American psychiatric patients. Hisp J Behav Sci. 1981;3:145–60.
61. Haasen C, Yagdiran O, Mass R, et al. Potential for misdiagnosis among Turkish migrants with psychotic disorders: a clinical controlled study in Germany. Acta Psychiatr Scand. 2000;101:125–9.
62. Sentell T, Shumway M, Snowden L. Access to mental health treatment by English language proficiency and race/ethnicity. J Gen Intern Med. 2007;22:289–93.
63. Flores G. Language barriers to health care in the United States. N Engl J Med. 2006;355:229–31.

64. Kaplan SH, Gandek B, Greenfield S, et al. Patient and visit characteristics related to physicians' participatory decision-making style. Results from the Medical Outcomes Study. Med Care. 1995;33:1176–87.
65. Cooper-Patrick L, Gallo JJ, Gonzales JJ, et al. Race, gender, and partnership in the patient-physician relationship. JAMA. 1999;282(6):583–9.
66. Cooper LA, Roter DL, Johnson RL, et al. Patient-centered communication, ratings of care, and concordance of patient and physician race. Ann Intern Med. 2003;139:907–15.
67. Sundquist J, Winkleby MA. Cardiovascular risk factors in Mexican American adults: a transcultural analysis of NHANES III, 1988–1994. Am J Public Health. 1999;89:723–30.
68. Saha S, Arbelaez JJ, Cooper LA. Patient-physician relationships and racial disparities in the quality of health care. Am J Public Health. 2003;93:1713–9.
69. Ferguson WJ, Candib LM. Culture, language and the doctor-patient relationship. Fam Med. 2002;34(5):353–61.
70. McGlade MS, Saha S, Dahlstrom ME. The Latina paradox: an opportunity for restructuring prenatal care delivery. Am J Public Health. 2004;94:2062–5.
71. Perez-Stable EJ. Language access and Latino healthcare disparities. Med Care. 2007;45:1009–11.
72. Spiegel JP. Cultural aspects of transference and countertransference revisited. J Am Acad Psychoanal. 1976;4:447–67.
73. Mucic D, Hilty DM, Yellowlees PM. e-Mental health toward cross-cultural populations worldwide. In: Mucic D, Hilty DM, editors. e-Mental health. Cham: Springer; 2016. p. 77–91.
74. Eytan A, Bischoff A, Rrustemi I, et al. Screening of mental disorders in asylum-seekers from Kosovo. Aust N Z J Psychiatry. 2002;36:499–503.
75. Bischoff A, Bovier PA, Rrustemi I, Gariazzo F, Eytan A, Loutan L. Language barriers between nurses and asylum seekers: their impact on symptom reporting and referral. Soc Sci Med. 2003;57(3):503–12.
76. Marcos LR. Effects of interpreters on the evaluation of psychopathology in non-English-speaking patients. Am J Psychiatry. 1979;136:171–4.
77. Drennan G, Swartz L. The paradoxical use of interpreting in psychiatry. Soc Sci Med. 2002;54:1853–66.
78. Price J. Foreign language interpreting in psychiatric practice. Aust N Z J Psychiatry. 1975;9:263–7.
79. Elderkin-Thompson V, Silver RC, Waitzkin H. When nurses double as interpreters: a study of Spanish-speaking patients in a US primary care setting. Soc Sci Med. 2001;52:1343–58.
80. Farooq S, Fear C, Oyebode F. An investigation of the adequacy of psychiatric interviews conducted through an interpreter. Psychiatr Bull. 1997;21:209–13.
81. Zayas L, Cabassa L, Perez MC, et al. Using interpreters in diagnostic research and practice: Pilot results and recommendations. J Clin Psychiatry. 2007;68:924–8.
82. Carrasquillo O, Orav EJ, Brennan TA, Burstin HR. Impact of language barriers on patient satisfaction in an emergency department. J Gen Intern Med. 1999;14:82–7.
83. Bowen S. Language barriers in access to health care. Ottawa: Health Canada; 2001.
84. Perez-Stable EJ. Language access and Latino health care disparities. Med Care. 2007;45:1009–11.
85. Karliner LS, Jacobs EA, Chen AH, et al. Do professional interpreters improve clinical care for patients with limited English proficiency? A systematic review of the literature. Health Serv Res. 2007;42(2):727–54.
86. Ton H, Koike A, Hales RE, et al. A qualitative needs assessment for development of a cultural consultation service. Transcult Psychiatry. 2005;42:491–504.
87. Jerrell JM. Effect of ethnic matching of young clients and mental health staff. Cult Divers Ment Health. 1998;4:297–302.
88. Jefee-Bahloul H. Telemental health in middle east: overcoming the barriers. Front Public Health. 2014;2:86. https://doi.org/10.3389/fpubh.2014.00086.
89. Samuels A. International telepsychiatry: a link between New Zealand and Australia. Aust N Z J Psychiatry. 1999;33:284–6.

90. Harley J. Economic evaluation of a tertiary telepsychiatry service to an island. J Telemed Telecare. 2006;12(7H):354–7.
91. Rathod S, Pinninti N, Irfan M, Gorczynski P, Rathod P, Gega L, Naeem F. Mental health service provision in low- and middle-income countries. Health Serv Insights. 2017;10:1178632917694350.
92. Suresh K, Bhui K. Ethnic minority patients' access to mental health services. Psychiatry. 2006;5:413–6.
93. Gary FA. Stigma: barrier to mental health care among ethnic minorities. Issues Ment Health Nurs. 2005;26:979–99.
94. Knifton L, Gervais M, Newbigging K, et al. Community conversation: addressing mental health stigma with ethnic minority communities. Soc Psychiatry Psychiatr Epidemiol. 2010;45:497–504.
95. Leong FTL, Kalibatseva Z. Cross-cultural barriers to mental health services in the United States. Cerebrum. 2011;2011:5.
96. Acarturk C, Konuk E, Cetinkaya M, Senay I, Sijbrandij M, Cuijpers P, Aker T. EMDR for Syrian refugees with posttraumatic stress disorder symptoms: results of a pilot randomized controlled trial. Eur J Psychotraumatol. 2015;6:27414.
97. Birtel MD, Mitchell BL. Cross-cultural differences in depression between White British and South Asians: causal attributions, stigma by association, discriminatory potential. Psychol Psychother Theory Res Pract. 2023;96:101–16. https://doi.org/10.1111/papt.12428.
98. Schouten BC, Meeuwesen L. Cultural differences in medical communication: a review of the literature. Patient Educ Couns. 2006;64(1–3):21–34.
99. Schouten BC, Meeuwesen L, Harmsen HAM. GPs' interactional styles in consultations with Dutch and ethnic minority patients. J Immigr Minor Health. 2009;11(6):468–75.
100. Shore JH, Savin DM, Novins D, Manson SM. Cultural aspects of telepsychiatry. J Telemed Telecare. 2006;12(3):116–21. https://doi.org/10.1258/135763306776738602.
101. Tolmac J, Hodes M. Ethnic variation among adolescent psychiatric in-patients with psychotic disorders. Br J Psychiatry. 2004;184:428–31.
102. Betancourt JR, Green AR, Carrillo JE, Ananeh-Firempong O II. Defining cultural competence: a practical framework for addressing racial/ethnic disparities in health and health care. Public Health Reports. 2003;118(4):293–302. https://doi.org/10.1093/phr/118.4.293.
103. Brooks TR. Pitfalls in communication with Hispanic and African-American patients: do translators help or harm? J Natl Med Assoc. 1992;84(11):941.
104. Levesque J, Harris MF, Russell G. Patient-centred access to health care: conceptualising access at the interface of health systems and populations. Int J Equity Health. 2013;12:18. https://doi.org/10.1186/1475-9276-12-18.
105. Coombs NC, Meriwether WE, Caringi J, Newcomer SR. Barriers to healthcare access among U.S. adults with mental health challenges: a population-based study. SSM Popul Health. 2021;15:100847. https://doi.org/10.1016/j.ssmph.2021.100847.
106. CDC Health Disparities & Inequalities Report (CHDIR) - Minority Health - CDC. Centers for Disease Control and Prevention. https://www.cdc.gov/minorityhealth/chdireport.html. Published November 26, 2013.
107. Wilbur K, Snyder C, Essary AC, Reddy S, Will KK, Saxon M. Developing workforce diversity in the health professions: a social justice perspective. Health Professions Education. 2020;6(2):222–9.
108. Brua C. Role-blurring and ethical grey zones associated with lay interpreters: three case studies. Commun Med. 2008;5(1):73.
109. Sarver J, Baker DW. Effect of language barriers on follow-up appointments after an emergency department visit. J Gen Intern Med. 2000;15:256–64.
110. Miranda J, McGuire TG, Williams DR, et al. Mental health in the context of health disparities. Am J Psychiatry. 2008;165:1102–8.
111. Freeman GK, Rai H, Walker JJ, et al. Non-English speakers consulting with the GP in their own language: a cross-sectional survey. Br J Gen Pract. 2002;52:36–8.

112. Bogic M, Njoku A, Priebe S. Long-term mental health of war-refugees: a systematic literature review. BMC Int Health Hum Rights. 2015;15:29. https://doi.org/10.1186/s12914-015-0064-9.
113. Fazel M, Wheeler J, Danesh J. Prevalence of serious mental disorder in 7000 refugees resettled in western countries: a systematic review. Lancet. 2005;365(9467):1309–14. S0140-6736(05)61027-6 [pii]. https://doi.org/10.1016/S0140-6736(05)61027-6.
114. Steel Z, Chey T, Silove D, Marnane C, Bryant RA, van Ommeren M. Association of torture and other potentially traumatic events with mental health outcomes among populations exposed to mass conflict and displacement: a systematic review and meta-analysis. JAMA. 2009;302(5):537–49. 302/5/537 [pii]. https://doi.org/10.1001/jama.2009.1132.
115. Myers CR. Using telehealth to remediate rural mental health and healthcare disparities. Issues Ment Health Nurs. 2019;40:233–9. https://doi.org/10.1080/01612840.2018.1499157.
116. Bakker A, Riper H, Olff M. E-health applications in the field of traumatic stress. Eur J Psychotraumatol. 2020;11(1):1762317.
117. Cox CM, Kenardy JA, Hendrikz JK. A randomized controlled trial of a web-based early intervention for children and their parents following unintentional injury. J Pediatr Psychol. 2010;35(6):581–92.
118. Marsac ML, Kassam-Adams N, Hildenbrand AK, Kohser KL, Winston FK. After the injury: initial evaluation of a web-based intervention for parents of injured children. Health Educ Res. 2011;26(1):1–12.
119. Ruggiero KJ, Price M, Adams Z, Stauffacher K, McCauley J, Danielson CK, et al. Web intervention for adolescents affected by disaster: population-based randomized controlled trial. J Am Acad Child Adolesc Psychiatry. 2015;54(9):709–17.
120. Marsac ML, Hildenbrand AK, Kohser KL, Winston FK, Li Y, Kassam-Adams N. Preventing posttraumatic stress following pediatric injury: a randomized controlled trial of a web-based psycho-educational intervention for parents. J Pediatr Psychol. 2013;38(10):1101–11.
121. Mouthaan J, Sijbrandij M, de Vries GJ, Reitsma JB, van de Schoot R, Goslings JC, et al. Internet-based early intervention to prevent posttraumatic stress disorder in injury patients: randomized controlled trial. J Med Internet Res. 2013;15(8):e165.
122. Asselbergs J, Sijbrandij M, Hoogendoorn E, Cuijpers P, Olie L, Oved K, et al. Development and testing of TraumaGameplay: an iterative experimental approach using the trauma film paradigm. Eur J Psychotraumatol. 2018;9(1):1424447.
123. Kassam-Adams N, Marsac ML, Kohser KL, Kenardy J, March S, Winston FK. Pilot randomized controlled trial of a novel web-based intervention to prevent posttraumatic stress in children following medical events. J Pediatr Psychol. 2016;41(1):138–48.
124. Olff M, Amstadter A, Armour C, Birkeland MS, Bui E, Cloitre M, et al. A decennial review of psychotraumatology: what did we learn and where are we going? Eur J Psychotraumatol. 2019;10(1):1672948.
125. van Buschbach S, van der Meer CAI, Dijkman L, Olff M, Bakker A. Web-based peer support education program for health care professionals. Jt Comm J Qual Patient Saf. 2020;11(3):227–31.
126. Rizzo A, Shilling R. Clinical virtual reality tools to advance the prevention, assessment, and treatment of PTSD. Eur J Psychotraumatol. 2017;8(Suppl 5):1414560.
127. van der Meer C, Bakker A, Schrieken BAL, Hoofwijk MC, Olff M. Screening for trauma-related symptoms via a smartphone app: the validity of smart assessment on your mobile in referred police officers. Int J Methods Psychiatr Res. 2017;26(3):e1579.
128. Litwack SD, Jackson CE, Chen M, Sloan DM, Hatgis C, Litz BT, Marx BP. Validation of the use of video teleconferencing technology in the assessment of PTSD. Psychol Serv. 2014;11(3):290–4.
129. Kuhn E, Greene C, Hoffman J, Nguyen T, Wald L, Schmidt J, et al. Preliminary evaluation of PTSD coach, a smartphone app for post-traumatic stress symptoms. Mil Med. 2014;179(1):12–8.

130. Van der Meer C, Bakker A, Van Zuiden M, Lok A, Olff M. Help in hand after traumatic events: a randomized controlled trial in health care professionals on the efficacy, usability, and user satisfaction of a self-help app to reduce trauma-related symptoms. Eur J Psychotraumatol. 2020;11(1):1717155.
131. Germain V, Marchand A, Bouchard S, Drouin MS, Guay S. Effectiveness of cognitive behavioural therapy administered by videoconference for posttraumatic stress disorder. Cogn Behav Ther. 2009;38(1):42–53.
132. van Gelderen MJ, Nijdam MJ, Vermetten E. An innovative framework for delivering psychotherapy to patients with treatment-resistant posttraumatic stress disorder: rationale for interactive motion-assisted therapy. Front Psychiatry. 2018;6:176.
133. Reger GM, Koenen-Woods P, Zetocha K, Smolenski DJ, Holloway KM, Rothbaum BO, et al. Randomized controlled trial of prolonged exposure using imaginal exposure vs. virtual reality exposure in active duty soldiers with deployment-related posttraumatic stress disorder (PTSD). J Consult Clin Psychol. 2016;84(11):946–59.
134. Olff M. Mobile mental health: a challenging research agenda. Eur J Psychotraumatol. 2015;6(1):27882.
135. Price M, Yuen EK, Goetter EM, Herbert JD, Forman EM, Acierno R, Ruggiero KJ. mHealth: a mechanism to deliver more accessible, more effective mental health care. Clin Psychol Psychother. 2014;21(5):427–36.
136. Ashwick R, Turgoose D, Murphy D. Exploring the acceptability of delivering Cognitive Processing Therapy (CPT) to UK veterans with PTSD over Skype: a qualitative study. Eur J Psychotraumatol. 2019;10(1):1573128.
137. Cernvall M, Sveen J, Bergh Johannesson K, Arnberg F. A pilot study of user satisfaction and perceived helpfulness of the Swedish version of the mobile app PTSD coach. Eur J Psychotraumatol. 2018;9(Suppl 1):1472990.
138. Smith KV, Thew GR, Graham B. Conducting ethical internet-based research with vulnerable populations: a qualitative study of bereaved participants' experiences of online questionnaires. Eur J Psychotraumatol. 2018;9(Suppl 1):1506231.
139. Price M, Van Stolk-Cooke K, Legrand AC, Brier ZMF, Ward HL, Connor JP, Gratton J, Freeman K, Skalka C. Implementing assessments via mobile during the acute posttrauma period: feasibility, acceptability and strategies to improve response rates. Eur J Psychotraumatol. 2018;9(Suppl 1):1500822. https://doi.org/10.1080/20008198.2018.1500822.
140. Knaevelsrud C, Brand J, Lange A, Ruwaard J, Wagner B. Web-based psychotherapy for posttraumatic stress disorder in war-traumatized Arab patients: randomized controlled trial. J Med Internet Res. 2015;17(3):e71. https://doi.org/10.2196/jmir.3582.
141. Lange A, van de Ven J-P, Schrieken B, Emmelkamp PM. Interapy, treatment of posttraumatic stress through the Internet: a controlled trial. J Behav Ther Exp Psychiatry. 2001;32(2):73–90.
142. Nickerson A, Bryant RA, Steel Z, Silove D, Brooks R. The impact of fear for family on mental health in a resettled Iraqi refugee community. J Psychiatr Res. 2010;44(4):229–35. https://doi.org/10.1016/j.jpsychires.2009.08.006. Epub 2009 Oct 28.
143. Cerda GM, Hilty DM, Hales RE, et al. Use of telemedicine with ethnic groups. Psychiatr Serv. 1999;50(10):1364.
144. Mucic D. Telepsychiatry in Denmark: mental health care in rural and remote areas. J e-Health Technol Appl. 2007;5(3):426.
145. Moreno FA, Chong J, Dumbauld J, et al. Use of standard webcam and Internet equipment for telepsychiatry treatment of depression among underserved Hispanics. Psychiatr Serv. 2012;63(12):1213–7.
146. Nieves JE, Stack KM. Hispanics and telepsychiatry. Psychiatr Serv. 2007;58(6):877.
147. Chong J, Moreno F. Feasibility and acceptability of clinic-based telepsychiatry for low-income Hispanic primary care patients. Telemed J E Health. 2012;18(4):297–30, and Asians.
148. Ye J, Shim R, Lukaszewski T, et al. Telepsychiatry services for Korean immigrants. Telemed E Health. 2012;18(10):797–802.

149. Yeung A, Martinson M, Baer L, et al. The effectiveness of telepsychiatry-based culturally sensitive collaborative treatment for depressed Chinese American immigrants: a randomized controlled trial. J Clin Psychiatry. 2016;77(8):e996–e1002.
150. Yeung A, Johnson DP, Trinh N-H, et al. Feasibility and effectiveness of telepsychiatry services for Chinese immigrants in a nursing home. Telemed J E Health. 2009;15(4):336–41.
151. Park HY, Kim JY, Koo HY, et al. Evaluation of a telehealth counseling program for expatriates. Telemed J E Health. 2019;25(8):693–700.
152. Shore JH, Brooks E, Savin D, Orton H, Grigsby J, Manson SM. Acceptability of telepsychiatry in American Indians. Tel e-Health. 2008;14(5):461–6.
153. Weiner MF, Rossetti HC, Harrah K. Videoconference diagnosis and management of Choctaw Indian dementia patients. Alzheimers Dementia. 2011;7(6):562–6.
154. Mucic D. Transcultural telepsychiatry and its impact on patient satisfaction. J Telemed Telecare. 2010;16(5):237–42.
155. Lopez AM, Cruz M, Lazarus S, et al. Case report: use of American sign language in telepsychiatry consultation. Tel e-Health. 2004;10(3):389–91.
156. Stewart RW, Orengo-Aguayo RE, Cohen JA, et al. A pilot study of trauma-focused cognitive–behavioral therapy delivered via telehealth technology. Child Maltreat. 2017;22(4):324–33. https://doi.org/10.1177/1077559517725403.
157. Pekmezaris R, Schwartz RM, Taylor TN, et al. A qualitative analysis to optimize a telemonitoring intervention for heart failure patients from disparity communities. BMC Med Inform Decis Mak. 2016;16:75. https://doi.org/10.1186/s12911-016-0300-9.
158. Truong M, Yeganeh L, Cook O, Crawford K, Wong P, Allen J. Using telehealth consultations for healthcare provision to patients from non-indigenous racial/ethnic minorities: a systematic review. J Am Med Inform Assoc. 2022;29(5):970–82. https://doi.org/10.1093/jamia/ocac015.
159. Bagchi AD, Melamed B, Yeniyurt S, et al. Telemedicine delivery for urban seniors with low computer literacy: a pilot study. Online J Nurs Inform. 2018;22(2):1–13.
160. Schulz TR, Richards M, Gasko H, Lohrey J, et al. Telehealth: experience of the first 120 consultations delivered from a new Refugee Telehealth clinic. Intern Med J. 2014;44(10):981–5.
161. Aisenberg E, Dwight-Johnson M, O'Brien M, et al. Building a community-academic partnership: implementing a community-based trial of telephone cognitive behavioral therapy for rural Latinos. Depress Res Treat. 2012;2012:257858.
162. Dwight-Johnson M, Aisenberg E, Golinelli D, et al. Telephone-based cognitive-behavioral therapy for Latino patients living in rural areas: a randomized pilot study. Psychiatr Serv. 2011;62(8):936–42.
163. Jang Y, Chiriboga DA, Molinari V, et al. Telecounseling for the linguistically isolated: a pilot study with older Korean immigrants. Gerontologist. 2014;54(2):290–6. https://doi.org/10.1093/geront/gns196.
164. Kerrigan V, McGrath SY, Majoni SW, et al. From "stuck" to satisfied: Aboriginal people's experience of culturally safe care with interpreters in a Northern Territory hospital. BMC Health Serv Res. 2021;21(1):1–13.
165. Ortega G, Rodriguez JA, Maurer LR, et al. Telemedicine, COVID-19, and disparities: policy implications. Health Policy Technol. 2020;9(3):368–71.
166. Yellowlees PM, Odor A, Patrice K, et al. PsychVACS: a system for asynchronous telepsychiatry. Telemed J E Health. 2011;17(4):299–303.
167. Yellowlees PM, Odor A, Iosif A, et al. Transcultural psychiatry made simple: asynchronous telepsychiatry as an approach to providing culturally relevant care. Tel e-Health. 2013;19(4):1–6.
168. Butler TN, Yellowlees P. Cost analysis of store-and-forward telepsychiatry as a consultation model for primary care. Tel e-Health. 2012;18(1):74–7.
169. www.denlilleprins.org.
170. Hilty DM, Yellowlees PM, Tarui N, et al. Mental health services for California American Indians: usual service options and a description of telepsychiatric consultation to select sites. In: Ramesh M, Shahram K, editors. Telemedicine. Rijeka: InTech Europe; 2013. p. 75–104.

171. Shore JH, Manson SM. A developmental model for rural telepsychiatry. Psychiatr Serv. 2005;56:976–80.
172. Leung AYM, Bo A, Hsiao H-Y, et al. Health literacy issues in the care of Chinese American immigrants with diabetes: a qualitative study. BMJ Open. 2014;4(11):e005294. https://doi.org/10.1136/bmjopen-2014-005294.
173. Martin A, Grudziecki J. DigEuLit: concepts and tools for digital literacy development. Innov Teach Learn Inf Comput Sci. 2006;5(4):249–67.
174. Sivaraman M, Fahmie TA. A systematic review of cultural adaptations in the global application of ABA-based telehealth services. J Appl Behav Anal. 2020;53(4):1838–55. https://doi.org/10.1002/jaba.763.
175. Fleming T, Creedy DK, West R. Cultural safety continuing professional development for midwifery academics: an integrative literature review. Women Birth. 2019;32(4):318–26. https://doi.org/10.1016/j.wombi.2018.10.001.
176. Sachs JW, Graven P, Gold JA, Kassakian SZ. Disparities in telephone and video telehealth engagement during the COVID-19 pandemic. JAMIA Open. 2021;4(3):ooab056.
177. Goel MS, Brown TL, Williams A, et al. Disparities in enrollment and use of an electronic patient portal. J Gen Intern Med. 2011;26(10):1112–6.
178. Narayan S, Mok H, Ho K, Kealy D. "I don't think they're as culturally sensitive": a mixed-method study exploring e-mental health use among culturally diverse populations. J Ment Health. 2023;32(1):241–7. https://doi.org/10.1080/09638237.2022.2091762. Epub 2022 Jun 30.
179. Lim RF, Lu F. Culture and psychiatric education. Acad Psychiatry. 2008;32:269–71.
180. Smedley B, Stith A, Nelson A, editors. Unequal treatment: confronting racial and ethnic disparities in health care. Washington, DC: National Academies Press; 2003.
181. Smedley BD, Butler AS, Bristow LR, editors. In the nation's compelling interest: ensuring diversity in the health care workforce. Washington, DC: Institute of Medicine (IOM) of The National Academies; 2004. http://www.nap.edu/books/030909125X/html.
182. Purnell LD. Transcultural health care: a culturally competent approach, vol. 4. Philadelphia: FA Davis Company; 2012.
183. Napier AD, Ancarno C, Butler B, et al. Culture and health. Lancet. 2014;384:1607–39. https://doi.org/10.1016/S0140-6736(14)61603-2.
184. Paez KA, Allen JK, Beach MC, et al. Physician cultural competence and patient ratings of the patient-physician relationship. J Gen Intern Med. 2009;24:495–8. https://doi.org/10.1007/s11606-009-0919-7.
185. Roncoroni J, Tucker CM, Wall W. Patient perceived cultural sensitivity of clinic environment and its association with patient satisfaction with care and treatment adherence. Am J Lifestyle Med. 2014;8:421–9. https://doi.org/10.1177/1559827614521760.
186. Berger JT. Culture and ethnicity in clinical care. Arch Intern Med. 1998;158:2085–90.
187. Hilty DM, Evangelatos G, Valasquez A, et al. Telebehavioral health for rural culturally diverse populations: approaches for clinical services, competencies and administration. J Tech Behav Sci. 2018;3:206–20. https://doi.org/10.1007/s41347-018-0054-6.
188. Hilty DM, Maheu M, Drude K, et al. Telebehavioral health, telemental health, e-therapy and e-health competencies: the need for an interdisciplinary framework. J Tech Behav Sci. 2017;2:171–89.
189. Hilty DM, Crawford A, Teshima J, et al. A framework for telepsychiatric training and e-health: competency-based education, evaluation and implications. Int Rev Psychiatry. 2015;27:569.
190. Hilty DM, Zalpuri I, Stubbe D, et al. Social media/networking as part of e-behavioral health and psychiatric education: competencies, teaching methods, and implications. J Tech Behav Sci. 2018;3:268–93.
191. Zalpuri I, Liu H, Stubbe D, et al. A competency-based framework for social media for trainees, faculty and others. Acad Psychiatry. 2018;42:808–17.
192. Hilty DM, Chan S, Torous J, et al. A telehealth framework for mobile health, smartphones and apps: competencies, training and faculty development. J Tech Behav Sci. 2019;4:106–23.

193. Hilty DM, Chan S, Torous J, et al. A competency-based framework for psych/behavioral health apps for trainees, faculty, programs and health systems. Psych Clin N Am. 2019;42:513–34.
194. Hilty DM, Chan S, Torous JB, Luo J, Boland RJ. A framework for competencies for the use of mobile technologies in psychiatry and medicine: scoping review. JMIR Mhealth Uhealth. 2020;8(2):e12229.
195. Maheu MM, Drude K, Hertlein K, et al. A framework for interprofessional telebehavioral health competencies: implementation and challenges moving forward. Acad Psychiatry. 2018;42:825–33.
196. Hilty DM, Gentry MT, McKean AJ, Cowan KE, Lim RF, Lu FG. Telehealth for rural diverse populations: telebehavioral and cultural competencies, clinical outcomes and administrative approaches. MHealth. 2020;6:20.
197. Hilty DM, Chan S, Torous J, Luo J, Boland R. Role of technology in professional development. Psychiatr Clin N Am. 2019;42:493–512.
198. Hilty DM, Torous J, Parish M, Chan S, Xiong G, Scher L, Yellowlees PM. A literature review comparing clinicians' approaches and skills to in-person, synchronous and asynchronous care: moving toward asynchronous competencies to ensure quality care. Telemed J E Health. 2020;27. https://doi.org/10.1089/tmj.2020.0054.
199. Proctor E, Silmere H, Raghavan R, Hovmand P, Aarons G, Bunger A, Griffey R, Hensley M. Outcomes for implementation research: conceptual distinctions, measurement challenges, and research agenda. Admin Pol Ment Health. 2011;38(2):65–76. https://doi.org/10.1007/s10488-010-0319-7.
200. Gargon E, Gurung B, Medley N, Altman D, Blazeby J, Clarke M, Williamson P. Choosing important health outcomes for comparative effectiveness research: a systematic review. Value Health. 2014;17(7):A435.
201. Curran GM, Bauer M, Mittman B, Pyne JM, Stetler C. Effectiveness-implementation hybrid designs: combining elements of clinical effectiveness and implementation research to enhance public health impact. Med Care. 2012;50(3):217–26.
202. Ekblad S, Manicavasagar V, Silove D, et al. The use of international videoconferencing as a strategy for teaching medical students about transcultural psychiatry. Transcult Psychiatry. 2004;41:120–9.
203. Fishkin R, Fishkin L, Leli U, et al. Psychodynamic treatment, training, and supervision using internet-based technologies. J Am Acad Psychoanal Dyn Psychiatry. 2011;39:155–68.
204. Mucic D. International telepsychiatry: a study of patient acceptability. J Telemed Telecare. 2008;14:241–3.
205. Werner P. Willingness to use telemedicine for psychiatric care. Telemed J E Health. 2004;10:286–93.
206. Gagnon MP, Orruño E, Asua J, Abdeljelil AB, Emparanza J. Using a modified technology acceptance model to evaluate healthcare professionals' adoption of a new telemonitoring system. Telemed e-Health. 2012;18(1):54–9.
207. Elbert NJ, van Os-Medendorp H, van Renselaar W, Ekeland AG, Hakkaart-van Roijen L, Raat H. Effectiveness and cost-effectiveness of eHealth interventions in somatic diseases: a systematic review of systematic reviews and meta-analyses. J Med Internet Res. 2014;16(4):e110. https://doi.org/10.2196/jmir.2790.
208. Rosser BA, Vowles KE, Keogh E, Eccleston C, Mountain GA. Technologically-assisted behaviour change: a systematic review of studies of novel technologies for the management of chronic illness. J Telemed Telecare. 2011;17(6):323–32. https://doi.org/10.1258/jtt.2011.110306.
209. Nair A, Venkataraman V. Telemedicine in psychiatry: a review. Indian J Psychiatry. 2016;58(2):117–26. https://doi.org/10.4103/0019-5545.183783.
210. Brennan PF, Strombom I. Improving health care by understanding patient preferences: the role of computer technology. J Am Med Inf Assoc. 1998;5(3):257–62. https://doi.org/10.1136/jamia.1998.0050257.

211. Baumeister H, Reichler L, Munzinger M, Lin J. The impact of guidance on internet-based mental health interventions—a systematic review. Internet Interv. 2014;1(4):205–15. https://doi.org/10.1016/j.invent.2014.08.003.
212. Venkatesh V, Davis FD. A theoretical extension of the technology acceptance model: four longitudinal field studies. Manag Sci. 2000;46(2):186–204. https://doi.org/10.1287/mnsc.46.2.186.11926.
213. Wu JH, Wang SC. What drives mobile commerce? An empirical evaluation of the revised technology acceptance model. Inf Manag. 2005;42(5):719–29. https://doi.org/10.1016/j.im.2004.07.001.
214. Davis FD. Perceived usefulness, perceived ease of use, and user acceptance of information technology. MIS Q. 1989;13(3):319–40. https://doi.org/10.2307/24900.
215. Monthuy-Blanc J, Bouchard S, Malano C, et al. Factors influencing mental health providers' intention to use telepsychotherapy in First Nations communities. Transcult Psychiatry. 2013;50(2):323–43.
216. Dingwall KM, et al. Like drawing into sand: acceptability, feasibility, and appropriateness of a new e-mental health resource for service providers working with Aboriginal and Torres Strait Islander People. Aus Psychol. 2015;50(1):60.
217. Mucic D. Telepsychiatry pilot-project in Denmark videoconference by distance by ethnic specialists to immigrants/refugees. WCPRR. 2007;2(1):3–9.
218. Melaka A, Edirippulige S. Psych-technology: a systematic review of the telepsychiatry literature. Centre for Online Health. Annu Rep. 2009.
219. Kirmayer LJ. Psychotherapy and the cultural concept of the person. Transcult Psychiatry. 2007;44(2):232–57. https://doi.org/10.1177/1363461507077195v.
220. Kirmayer LJ. Rethinking cultural competence. Transcult Psychiatry. 2012;49(2):149–64. https://doi.org/10.1177/1363461512444673.
221. World Health Organization. Migrants and refugees say COVID-19 has dramatically worsened their lives. 2020. https://www.who.int/news-room/feature-stories/detail/migrants-and-refugees-say-COVID-19-has-dramatically-worsened-their-lives.

Part III

Integrating Technology Into the Clinical Practice

Telepsychiatry: From "Telepathy" to the Mainstream

9

Davor Mucić, Donald M. Hilty, and Jay Shore

TELEPSYCHIATRY
TRADITIONAL SERVICE WITH
MODERN APPROACH

D. Mucić (✉)
The Little Prince Psychiatric Centre, Copenhagen, Denmark
e-mail: davor@denlilleprins.org

D. M. Hilty
Department of Psychiatry and Behavioral Sciences, Keck School of Medicine University of Southern California, Los Angeles, CA, USA
e-mail: hilty@med.usc.edu

J. Shore
Psychiatry and Public Health, University of Colorado, Anschutz, Aurora, CO, USA
e-mail: jay.shore@cuanschutz.edu

D. Mucić, D. M. Hilty (eds.), *Digital Mental Health*,
https://doi.org/10.1007/978-3-031-59936-1_9

Abstract

Telepsychiatry, recognized as the most established and comprehensively evaluated application within digital mental health modalities, has a rich documentation of use. Nonetheless, the full spectrum of telepsychiatry's capabilities remains underutilized, often attributed to the inertia within mental health care systems that impedes the incorporation of novel technologies into established clinical practices. A deeper exploration into its historical context, operational benefits, and constraints, along with the diverse array of applications and its capacity to facilitate remote assessments and treatments, is imperative. Such an exploration would invariably enhance our comprehension and, consequently, catalyze the integration of telepsychiatry into routine clinical services. An increased familiarity with telepsychiatry's functionalities promises to expand its deployment in everyday mental health care, optimizing patient outcomes through the strategic leverage of remote care technologies.

9.1 Introduction

Although telepsychiatry has been known since 1959, the general knowledge of the vast majority of experts in the world about the wide spectrum of its possibilities was modest... until the coronavirus disease 2019 (COVID-19) pandemic outbreak. In the late 1990s, when the first author of this chapter promoted the cross-cultural model of telepsychiatry, colleagues often asked whether telepsychiatry had anything to do with telepathy. The question/joke reflected the reality characterized by practicing traditional psychiatry as we were globally unfamiliar with the videoconference in daily clinical practice. In the twenty-first century, as Skype and subsequent video platforms became freely available on our computers and mobile phones, we slowly began to adopt videoconferencing as a way of communication... in our daily lives. However, professionals have not yet used videoconferencing for the diagnosis and treatment of mental patients on a larger scale. Just as the life stories of war refugees are divided into "life before and life after the war," the history of psychiatry is also divided into the time before and the time after the discovery of telepsychiatry. We are slowly but surely becoming aware of that.

This chapter aims to broaden the horizons and inform both therapists and potential patients about the essence of telepsychiatry, its advantages and disadvantages, and possible future development opportunities.

9.2 Definition and Brief History of Telepsychiatry

The term "telepsychiatry" includes real-time or delayed (i.e., synchronous or asynchronous) remote consultations through various media (virtual platforms, telephone, e-mail, and messaging or texting applications) [1–4]. However, the use of real-time interactive videoconferencing and telephone are the most frequent ways to link mental health care providers with the users at separate locations.

Telepsychiatry was originally created to meet the mental health needs of individuals in remote, rural, or hard-to-reach regions [5–13]. The telephone was invented in 1900, and for more than 50 years it was a crucial instrument for medical communication. However, in Nebraska, a two-way closed-circuit television system was employed for medical and educational purposes with a concentration on psychiatry in the 1956, which is when the first stories of telepsychiatry were made public. With the ability to send audio both ways, the educational network was extended to Iowa, North Dakota, and South Dakota in 1957. Beginning in 1959, simultaneous audio and video transmission led to advancements in consultation, diagnostic evaluation, and even group treatment (telepsychiatry program). "Closed-circuit television has been introduced into the field of mental hygiene as a medium for the administration of therapy to a mass audience. The present evidence indicates that the use of this type of television may promote the development of new and more effective methods for the treatment of the mentally ill" [14]. However, at the same time, the Store and Forward model, i.e., asynchronous telepsychiatry, was tested for teaching in psychiatry [15]. Four years later, the potential of telepsychiatry "as a means of extending mental health services to areas that are remote from psychiatric centers" was described [16]. Namely, videoconferences were used in 1961 to conduct group psychotherapy for adults. In the following years, it was also used for educational purposes [17–19]. Since 1960, it has been possible to get mental health care remotely, either by phone or video [20, 21].

Most of these early use cases were built due to concern over reaching rural patients but by the late 1960s urban centers were rapidly adopting the technology and adjusting it to fit their own specific needs. At a health center at Logan International Airport in 1969, Massachusetts General Hospital offered psychiatric consultations to adults and kids. Telepsychiatry expanded into most diagnostic and therapeutic contacts during the 1970s and 1980s as it became more typical.

The first microwave relay that allowed for direct consultation at the patient's location was financed in 1968 by the National Institute of Mental Health. The Dartmouth Department of Psychiatry made this achievement into a small-town associate hospital. The technological interface also made it possible for clinicians to use the device independently. Psychiatrists at the Massachusetts General Hospital utilized closed-circuit television to examine patients at the adjacent airport [22].

In this project/study, the word "telepsychiatry" was used for the first time, and remote-controlled pan, tilt, and zoom cameras were used. When the Mount Sinai School of Medicine was connected to a child guidance clinic in New York City shortly after, telepsychiatry was employed among children and adolescents [23].

Telepsychiatry was very occasionally utilized in the 1960s and 1970s despite its initial effectiveness and subsequent claims of its applicability and acceptance. Technology advancements in the late 1980s and early 1990s, which decreased the cost of equipment, along with increasing support from governmental organizations, resulted in an expansion in programs in North America and Australia [5–8, 24–26]. Up until the 1990s, the field developed slowly, but new technologies opened the door for additional growth and development. The ability to provide services to remote and underserved communities has been the main driving force, with continued extension to other underprivileged populations. By the late 1990s, it had grown further throughout the globe, especially in the USA, Canada, Australia, and eventually in Europe. Among the telepsychiatry pioneers in Europe were Scandinavian countries known for their large and sparsely populated geographical areas. The history of telepsychiatry in Denmark, which cannot boast of vast and sparsely populated areas, is particularly interesting. However, the reasons for its development in this smallest Scandinavian country were not caused by great geographical but cultural distances. Namely, the first cross-cultural model of telepsychiatry was launched in Denmark at the beginning of twenty-first century [27]. The main objective was the assessment and/or treatment of ethnic minorities with limited knowledge of the Danish language via telepsychiatry by bilingual clinicians, i.e., clinicians who speak the patient's native language. In this way, the use of translators was avoided. Moreover, the first ever international telepsychiatry service was launched in Denmark in 2005, linking bilingual clinics located in Sweden and Greenland with ethnic patients in Denmark [28]. Pioneering projects resulted in the establishment of a National Telepsychiatry Center in 2011. Today, Denmark is one of the countries with the most developed and regulated telepsychiatry systems in the European Union (EU).

Telepsychiatry research had started on how it compared to in-person care in terms of ease of access to care and capacity to overcome geographic barriers. By the 2000s, research and practitioners in the field started to view telepsychiatry as beneficial but slightly distinct from in-person care. The first guidelines for telepsychiatry were published in 2010 for the American Telemedicine Association (ATA) [29]. Telepsychiatry has since its initiation helped overcome the limitations of traditional service delivery methods for remote communities by providing a broad range of high-quality services typically available only in specialist centers. This has created equitable access and empowered users in remote areas while also reducing the cost of care provision by saving time and travel expenses for clinicians, health care professionals, and users. Lastly, it has provided support for mental health professionals working in remote environments.

9.3 Diagnostic Reliability and Clinical Outcomes

In order to establish telepsychiatry as an effective model of psychiatric treatment, it was necessary to compare its accuracy in recognizing and diagnosing psychiatric disorders, as well as how it directly compares to in-person psychiatry in other areas of importance, including clinical outcomes. The efficiency of telepsychiatry has been assessed related to accessibility to care, quality of care (i.e., outcomes, reliability, satisfaction, and comparison with in-person care), costs, education, empowerment, and other factors that influence effectiveness (e.g., technology and administrative coordination) [30, 31]. Telepsychiatry was reliable in diagnosing common psychiatric disorders equivalent to in-person consultations, albeit with a wide variety of diagnostic measures being used across different studies [32–35]. Telepsychiatry has been shown effective for diagnosis and assessment across many populations (e.g., adult, child, geriatric, and ethnic), for psychiatric disorders in many settings (e.g., emergency and home health), and been found to be comparable to in-person care. It has been used with a variety of models of care (i.e., collaborative care, asynchronous, mobile, and telemonitoring) with equally positive outcomes [26, 32, 36]. No distinctions between the in-person and telepsychiatry groups were identified in a study assessing the effect of telepsychiatry in neuropsychiatric testing using the Spanish counterparts of a common neuropsychiatric test battery. Moreover, dozens of clinician scales have been shown as reliable and valid [26]. Already early research demonstrated that the psychiatric interview conducted over videoconferencing is reliable for diagnostic assessment and treatment recommendations [37]. Diagnoses were reliably made by telepsychiatry, and patient acceptance of such interviews was high [38].

Back at 1995, McLaren et al. evaluated the use of interactive television in an acute psychiatric service in the UK and found it to be technically adequate and compatible with the performance of a wide range of clinical tasks in psychiatry [39]. Furthermore, there is evidence that telepsychiatry may improve treatment adherence in patients with depression, bipolar disorder, and schizophrenia [40]. Especially patients with mood disorders are more likely to attend video appointments than those with other diseases [41]. In particular, for patients with depression, telepsychiatry may enhance quality-of-life ratings and avoid relapses and recurrences [32]. This reliability did, however, remain consistent for a wide variety of mental illnesses, including intellectual disabilities, substance misuse disorders and cognitive impairments, as well as assessments of risk [32, 42, 43].

When we talk about telepsychiatry today, we usually think of using a real-time audio–video connection. However, phone in telepsychiatry has often been used especially after failed attempts to use video or when patients were not equipped to use video devices [44].

Phone therapy for depression is shown to be more effective than no-treatment or treatment-as-usual [45–48]. Anxiety treatments delivered over phone are at least moderately effective for reducing symptoms relative to no treatment and treatment as usual [49]. It is easy to understand why phones predominated in the video realm. As compared to video, phone services provide less of a technology obstacle and are more generally available equipment with lower connection costs [50, 51]. Accordingly, this expands access to care especially for certain groups such as race-ethnic minorities, those using English as a second-language, those with low-broadband access (often in rural areas), and people without insurance and older patients. All of them have higher phone usage compared to video [52–58].

The use of telepsychiatry not only benefited clinicians and patients but there were also broader consequences, such as a decrease in restrictive practice and bed occupancy [59–61]. The telepsychiatry patients had less than half the hospital admissions and length of stay than the control group [62]. It appears that by offering patients the choice of telepsychiatry versus traditional face-to-face appointments, end outcome measures are unlikely to change. For some groups of patients, e.g., children and adolescents on the autism spectrum, adults with disabling anxiety (e.g., panic or post-traumatic stress disorder; veterans), telepsychiatry may be preferable to in-person [26].

Accordingly, concerns about telepsychiatry, such as being inferior to in-person provided care, have not been demonstrated [63].

9.4 Advantages and Limitations of Telepsychiatry

There are both advantages and disadvantages of using videoconferencing for mental health care. There are also procedures (rules and regulations) that health care providers must follow when providing this sort of service. The benefits and drawbacks of telepsychiatry procedures as seen by mental health practitioners and patients have been examined in the recent survey [64].

In comparison to face-to-face care, video telehealth does improve patient access by lowering travel expenses, enabling more flexible scheduling, and enabling people with mobility challenges to connect from home [65]. More than 70% of the cost of time and travel for a patient and provider for a standard in-patient visit can be saved through the use of remote visits in rural and remote areas [66, 67]. Hospitals that outsource for mental health services via telepsychiatry instead of maintaining an on-site, salaried psychiatrist may also experience cost savings as well as better meeting the cultural and specialty needs of their specific patient population [68, 69].

Telepsychiatry is far more cost-effective alternative to in-person behavioral health within a rural population [70, 71]. Reaching historically marginalized communities via phone and video allows access to therapy with specialists and initiatives that might not be available locally [49, 72–74]. For patients, convenience is a major benefit of telepsychiatry, i.e., both video and/or phone. Patients frequently mention convenience as one of the top benefits of telehealth, particularly the ability to avoid traffic, parking, and scheduling issues [75–77]. Moreover, patients report convenience because sessions are more likely to start on time than in-person sessions, which occasionally started late [78]. A significant advantage of remote care is that patients who experience anxiety or have physical limitations can communicate with health care professionals via phone or video rather than having to visit clinical settings that can be emotionally or physically stressful [77]. While phone, video, and in-person care are all effective modes of care, phone and video are more convenient to patients. Video offers important visual information and can give providers a unique window into patients' homes, as appropriate. Phone, however, is more broadly accessible and may come with fewer technological issues [79]. Further, telepsychiatry can help people with mental health conditions like Obsessive-Compulsive Disorder (OCD), and social withdrawal (e.g., hikikomori), or those who cannot go out or use public transport to continue their therapy from home [80, 81].

It is interesting to note that Mishkind et al. [82] discovered a decline in no-show rates for video consultation sessions from more than 16.1% prior to COVID-19 restrictions to 7.8% afterward. This finding may be related to the higher perceived barriers to in-person services, but at least it shows that many patients found the services to be acceptable during a medical emergency, i.e., COVID19 lockdown. Patients usually used video consultations because it was difficult for them to visit a mental health facility or see a professional in person. Patients indicated that video-conferencing was convenient and often the only choice for obtaining therapy, e.g., owing to COVID-19 constraints [83, 84]. They made a point of stressing how much time they could save. This was thought to be especially important for individuals who lived the farthest from services, as well as for those for whom the sessions would likely be brief due to the trade-off between therapy and transportation [85–88]. Telepsychiatry is thought to be less expensive and less time-consuming than in-person care and less expensive (e.g., no travel-related expenses). While the initial hardware cost and the availability of an Internet connection were perceived as potential drawbacks [89], nowadays we mainly speak about the use of video platforms on patients' smartphones and/or laptops, i.e., the expenses related to the equipment are not anymore as significant as before. Patients find telepsychiatry sessions as beneficial as direct meetings with their psychiatrist and would use it again. There were no instances of telepsychiatry being associated with adverse reactions in patients from remote communities with inadequate exposure to modern mainstream culture and Internet [31]. Moreover, telepsychiatry reduces risks during travel to psychiatric centers. Telepsychiatry enables larger choice of therapists and may have an impact on reduction of stigma [8]. Individuals in rural areas who need mental health care face a lot of obstacles because of the stigma surrounding it. In tiny rural towns, privacy, and secrecy may be perceived as limited. In such environments, there is frequently a lack of understanding of mental illness and a lack of perceived need for mental health care, which might discourage people from seeking treatment [89]. The anonymity offered by telepsychiatry might lessen the stigma and feelings of embarrassment related to receiving mental health care [90].

There is a number of potential benefits of telepsychiatry with regard to psychiatrist *stress and burnout*. Telepsychiatry does not only improve patient access to and satisfaction with mental health services but also gives providers increased flexibility in their practice. Psychiatrists are at risk of experiencing burnout due to emotional stressors related to the nature of the clinical work, occupational hazards, changing nature of service delivery, and increasing administrative pressures [91]. Burnout may be a key factor contributing to psychiatrists working less, pursuing less acute cases, and leading to worsened outcomes for patients and the psychiatrists themselves [92]. One possible way telepsychiatry may reduce burnout is through creating an increased sense of control over the psychiatrist's schedule [91]. Reduction in commuting time results in more time for rest, self-care, family time, and social activities, all of which have been demonstrated to significantly lower the risk of burnout [93]. In addition, telepsychiatrists may decide to use the time that would otherwise be spent traveling for documentation and other administrative tasks, potentially reducing some of the ongoing stress associated with patient care. Telepsychiatry may improve safety by reducing some risks associated with the practice that can be unpleasant and lead to fatigue. Violence at working place is more common in psychiatry than in other specialities. Videoconferencing helps to mitigate some of the risks connected with working in psychiatry, such as the threat posed by aggressive or violent patients and the challenge of totally distancing oneself from the emotional strain of in-person patient meetings [93]. Given that telepsychiatrists could provide a backup for colleagues working in crisis preventive or emergency behavioral health settings, telepsychiatry may also reduce burnout among in-person clinicians [94].

However, the risks of social and professional isolation, the difficulty of completely separating work from home, the potential for a sense of alienation from the actual workplace, and a potential increase in household responsibilities when working from home are some of the notable difficulties faced by telepsychiatrists [95]. Therefore, telepsychiatrists may feel social and professional isolation, especially if they are working remotely full-time while still providing clinical services and interacting with patients or support workers. While little is known about the occupational effects of telepsychiatry on the health and well-being of psychiatrists, the literature demonstrates notable correlations between increased sedentary behavior and reported levels of burnout as well as the increased risk of developing obesity, type II diabetes, cardiovascular disease, and cancer [96]. Other concerns for telepsychiatrists include blurring the separation of work from home life and possible pressure to work longer hours or check e-mail after hours [95].

The limited ability to perform a somatic examination, particularly in clinically unsupervised settings, can be a problem unless good collaboration is established with the patient's general practitioner who can perform it on request. Further, sometimes it may be challenging to build a strong rapport in short-term telepsychiatry use [8]. Accordingly, some health care providers suggested having the first session be in-person communication and the future sessions be conducted online [97]. In contrast to in-person practice, the long-term use of telepsychiatry may make it harder to build a strong rapport or may degrade the quality of one that has already been created. Targeting patients with whom a strong rapport has been properly built in during in-person practice may be prudent when considering the use of long-term telepsychiatry [98]. During the remote sessions the patients noticed that therapists were wary of going too far into delicate emotions or traumatic experiences on camera. The providers claimed that it was because they were less able to accurately gauge their patients' emotional states and were afraid of abandoning them in an unsettled state if a technical malfunction occurred in the middle of a crucial talk [99].

Clinicians may experience legal problems if they practice in places with significantly diverse laws, customs, and structures unless more specific rules are developed. There are legal ramifications connected to jurisdiction and licensure when providing telepsychiatric care, and the provision of care must be limited to the province or state in which the practitioner is licensed. Another legal issue is identity fraud and confirmation of identification. Involuntary admissions and cooperative agreements with law enforcement, health, and social agencies to assist them have ramifications as well. The risk of not being able to react quickly to mental emergencies is unavoidable in the end. Therefore, recommendations from the APA and WPA Telepsychiatry Guidelines specifically address this risk, advising clinicians to make sure the patient is consistently located during sessions, has access to emergency contact information (a friend or family member of the patient), and is aware of available local resources in case of emergency, e.g., police and emergency medical services [100, 101].

Finally, an evidence base needs to be developed for any future unintended consequences associated with virtual care. Time spent in front of a screen can have a negative effect on the cognitive and executive functioning primarily of telepsychiatrists, especially those who work full-time via videoconferencing.

9.5 Patient and Clinician Satisfaction

Patient and provider satisfaction are two of the most widely studied outcomes related to telepsychiatry. The most consistently reported findings are the high levels of satisfaction and acceptance among patients. These have been found in virtually every study assessing patient satisfaction with telepsychiatric services, with up to 75–100% of the users reporting considerable satisfaction with telepsychiatric care [102]. High satisfaction has been noted for all patient populations (children, adults, elderly, ethnic minorities, and prison populations) and all kinds of psychiatric diagnoses. Moreover, patients report effective communication, believe it is as useful as in-person interventions, and express willingness to use it again [31, 103, 104].

Providing high care quality includes the care above the patients' expectations which accordingly maintain a high level of service [105]. To ensure a high quality of telepsychiatry services, health care systems should maintain availability, accessibility, timeliness, privacy, and confidentiality of service and caring. Moreover, they should offer responsive communication, accuracy, and reliability, as well as the improvement of patient quality of life [106].

Patients' expectations for the kind of interaction they will be having via videoconferencing seem to influence their attitudes. Some patients stated that they preferred in-person sessions to video sessions because they believed that the latter was less personalized because it was harder to discern non-verbal cues [100]. In contrary, other patients have reported preferring virtual consultations because of the ease of discussing sensitive topics, and certain patient groups have reported finding telepsychiatry more comfortable to engage with, such as individuals with autism spectrum disorder, Tourette's and those who generally find it to more difficult engage with in-person consultations [32]. Patient satisfaction was found to be particularly high among children and adolescents, possibly because of the familiarity with technology among this age group. Some studies found that children found the experience of the virtual consultation less threatening than an in-person consultation [32].

It seems that video consultations are less helpful for patients who present more complex symptoms, and vice versa for individuals with simpler problems. Some patients may not be able to communicate as effectively over the video, which would make the encounter more difficult [100].

In general, patients seem content as they emphasize the shorter wait times, greater flexibility, and decreased need for travel [3, 107–111]. Telepsychiatry has been found to increase access to specialized services, e.g., child and adolescent, veterans, and elderly, resulting in greater access to treatment and less distress for patients and their families [35, 112, 113].

However, provider satisfaction is not as consistent as patient satisfaction, with studies reporting both low and high satisfaction rates [32]. Provider skepticism is major cause of limited acceptance. Before the COVID-19 outbreak, providers' perceptions of phone use in mental health-related clinical practicing were noticeably negative [114]. But the perception of video-link was not much better. Moreover, it is interesting to note that positive telepsychiatry outcomes went against the professional expectation [115–121]. Among various barriers to telepsychiatric services, negative attitudes of clinicians and institutions are the most significant after controlling for other factors such as reimbursement and regulatory issues [122]. Clinicians may express dissatisfaction with telepsychiatry due to several factors, including apprehensions about building rapport and creating a positive therapeutic relationship with patients, discomfort with technology, insufficient training, and the belief that telepsychiatry could exacerbate their clinical workload, rather than reduce it [123–125]. Although professionals' concerns regarding safety remain a prominent issue, various reviews have demonstrated that telepsychiatry is safe, even in unsupervised settings, i.e., home-telepsychiatry, and does not produce any negative outcomes [126, 127].

Concerns about security of the systems overlaps with issues of confidentiality, privacy, and consent of patients [128]. It is common for physicians employing telepsychiatry to encounter or report any type of technology-related issue [129–136]. Along with concerns about a lack of technological expertise, clinicians are also concerned about how to translate the doctor–patient connection to the screen [31, 115–121, 128, 137–140]. However, after incorporating it into their practice, many clinicians change their attitudes and perceive telepsychiatry as a useful tool for psychiatric consultations [11, 59, 107, 141–152].

Although patient and provider satisfaction are important outcomes for telepsychiatry research to take into account, they might not always be accurate measures of clinical efficacy. A patient may, for instance, express great satisfaction with a telepsychiatry session while not necessarily benefiting from the care they got. The nature and severity of the mental health condition as well as the quality and accessibility of telepsychiatric services may also have an impact on patient satisfaction [12, 153, 154]. Furthermore, telepsychiatry patient satisfaction does not always reflect a preference for this type of treatment. Patients opt for telepsychiatry when it reduces travel, waiting times, absence from work, and costs, and when it enhances their sense of autonomy [128]. Patients generally still prefer in-person interactions for their mental health, despite the fact that telepsychiatry is practical and economical.

9.6 Doctor–Patient Relationship: Closeness Despite Distance

To diagnose and treat mental health disorders effectively, psychiatry depends on a strong patient–provider alliance that facilitates communication and helps practitioners recognize any changes in behavior or signs of mental health distress, which can be less apparent and less identifiable through typical diagnostic tools, and often present differently within the same diagnosis. Since many patients who need psychiatric care often require more individualized care, which involves the establishment of a strong patient–provider alliance in order to optimally benefit from treatment, in-person, private, and discrete interactions (whether individual, family, or group-based therapy) have long been the standard for mental health care [155]. Studies of doctor–patient communication in telepsychiatry are evenly divided between post-encounter surveys of consultation participants and qualitative investigations using observation, interviews, case reports, questionnaires, and content analysis. Virtually all were published after 1994 [156].

In order to build a strong therapeutic relationship, several prerequisites must be met. The office, a regular appointment duration and a regular schedule are instrumental in creating a positive environment and the therapeutic frame. The frame is the foundation or structure that promotes security, trust and confidentiality to explore and discuss anything. Accordingly, both in-person and remote care require a clinical environment that is private, professional, and warm—this includes good seating (e.g., ergonomic support), adequate lighting (e.g., for facial illumination), secure/private entries, and soundproofing. If a clinician uses more than one site of care (e.g., their primary location, their home, and/or a part-time office), the spaces should be professionally comparable in terms of layout and design. Planning ahead is essential to make sure the home room is clinically conducive if it is used for other purposes (e.g., no one else is there, no interruptions). A sign indicating the need for relative silence, avoiding disruptions, and using alternate locations for travel, such to that found in a mental health office in a busy primary care clinic, may be helpful. In terms of scheduling, it might be preferable to cancel or reschedule a potential appointment rather than attempt to provide care in an unfavorable setting (e.g., while driving or parking a car on the side of the road) or from a separate office that might be disruptive.

Some professionals expressed worry that the absence of in-person communication in telepsychiatry might impede the formation of a strong therapeutic alliance, which is frequently described as an emotional connection between the patient and the therapist as well as cooperation and agreement between the two parties on the objectives and tasks of the therapy [157]. Digital technologies offer additional methods of human communication, enabling social connections between different communities, cultures, and continents. In addition to being an important part of general social and communication skills, non-verbal decoding has also been linked to better interpersonal outcomes [158], is simple to measure using validated, reliable, and standardized objective measures, and can be improved with practice and feedback training [159]. Common for many patients and mental health care professionals is the fact that they have gained experience with video consultations due to the COVID-19 restrictions, and they may have developed videoconferencing-specific communication skills as a result. These skills will help them better express their emotions and, as a result, give the impression that they are in a more intimate setting. Therapists did say that experience made it simpler for them to interact with their patients [160].

Mutual engagement may also be affected by technology, but even low-cost telepsychiatry facilitates a "social presence" for participants to share a virtual space, get to know one another and to discuss complex issues [161]. The extent to which media facilitate the transfer of information varies. This is known as "richness," and it is based on four factors: feedback, numerous cues, a range of languages, and individual focus. In general, it is believed that oral and synchronous media are richer than asynchronous and asynchronous media, respectively. The clarity, responsiveness, and comfort of communication—which is typically defined as the transmission of ideas, emotions, and information between individuals through speech or other means—can be impacted by technology. Telepsychiatry and other technologies on a spectrum are used to simulate real-time experiences related to feelings, perception, images, and interaction. Clinicians use behavioral health techniques such as questioning, investigating fundamental concerns, spotting inconsistencies, and using reflection to explain issues and order fundamental values. The clinician places the patient's wishes, requirements, and preferences first. The ultimate objective is to establish a setting that supports therapeutic engagement and emotional well-being for everybody involved. If technology is employed, analysis of its effects on care and its potential applications (e.g., video and text) might assist determine when it might be useful. The therapeutic alliance formed during videoconferencing provided psychotherapy does not appear to affect treatment outcomes, but agreement on therapeutic tasks and goals does. As a result, more patients may discover that even though they feel the sessions are less personal, they can still be professional and sufficient [162].

Both the experience of telepsychiatry and the manner in which care is provided vary. The personalities, disorders, ages, cultures, languages, and psychosocial histories of patients vary. Furthermore, health care settings differ: primary care and mental health clinics; emergency rooms; patient, group, and nursing homes; shelters; hospices; schools; forensic labs; prisons; workplaces; public health centers; and academic institutions. Finally, different services have different levels of intimacy, breadth, and scope of interactions when it comes to evaluation, triage, assessment, and direct care/treatment/management. However, patients may feel a more powerful therapeutic bond during in-person sessions. Depending on whether they have previously visited with their psychiatrist in person or if all appointments, including the initial evaluation, have taken place virtually, they might also have different expectations. Additionally, those who have little familiarity with videoconferencing technology (e.g., elderly patients or patients from culturally isolated populations) could prefer in-person consultations and might even find telepsychiatry stressful [163]. In contrary, patients who are socially and geographically isolated report great benefits from telepsychiatry, with 90% of patients being comfortable with their telepsychiatry treatment and 84.5% believing it was as helpful as in-person, i.e., direct physical presence [31].

There is a consistent moderate relationship between positive therapeutic alliance and successful treatment outcomes [163]. Therapeutic alliance did not differ *diagnostically* between patients receiving telepsychiatry services compared to those receiving in-person psychiatric services [164]. While patients perceive video as similar to in-person care, they also highlight technological issues associated with video [78]. Indeed, poor audio quality may impact the interaction. Studies found that telehealth services were not effective in providing emotional support as patients' satisfaction with health care was constrained by low audio-visual quality [165]. Videoconferencing technologies may allow access to vocal cues, but may limit the ability to engage in mutual eye gaze or perceive body movements and gestures [166]. The therapeutic relationship and one's ability to demonstrate empathy may be impacted by difficulties hearing and interpreting the other person's speech [26, 115, 167]. Broken audio may be as limiting virtually; for example, when attempting a sensitive conversation, broken audio may be as disruptive as loud building work outside a clinic room would be in real life [32]. Technological disturbances are most often tolerated but not pervasive ones. This is relevant to consider when adopting new technologies for practice. Given that patients are more accepting of video consultations when they know their therapist introducing new videoconferencing services might be most suitable for patients who are already familiar with their therapist until the service is properly integrated and all technological challenges are solved [100]. Remote doctor–patient interactions may potentially have significant ethical and legal ramifications. Patients frequently worry about their privacy and security, which in the modern health care setting mostly refers to unauthorized access to computerized medical records [168]. Patients frequently report high comfort by communicating via real-time video link and that the sessions were private in the sense that the information they gave to the therapist was kept private [169]. But privacy is a broad concept that encompasses not only informational privacy (i.e., the disclosure of personal files and data), but also psychological privacy (i.e., the disclosure of private attitudes, beliefs, and feelings), social privacy (i.e., the control over social contacts), and physical privacy (i.e., the control over physical accessibility) [170]. When using two-way, interactive video instead of traditional in-person interactions, the nature of these interactions may be different. Video consultations frequently involve numerous clinicians and technologists, unlike in-person meetings.

Hannah Zeavin's "The Distance Cure" [48] explores the therapeutic validity of telepsychiatry by examining historical practices of psychiatry and psychoanalysis conducted without in-person sessions. From Sigmund Freud's analyses via written correspondence to call-in radio shows and suicide hotlines, the book delves into the evolution of remote mental health care. The author argues that different forms of media enable various types of togetherness fantasies that are, ultimately, variations of the same mental process rather than viewing teletherapy as "more distant" than in-person therapy. No intimate experience, regardless of how it is mediated (FaceTiming, letters, being in the same room), is more "real" than another. Studies report that between telephone and in-person groups, patients' assessments of therapists' helpfulness and empathy were comparable [171–173]. Similarly, patient satisfaction and ratings on the quality of relationships were comparable for video and in-person care [74, 173, 174]. In circumstances where a patient may have the option to use either phone or video, and prefers phone, we advise providers to first and foremost consider the clinical safety of the patient [79]. Rather than patient preference, factors such as the type of service being offered (psychotherapy, medication management, and case management), the specific mental health issues and medical circumstances of the patient (including practice standards associated with prescription of certain medications, such as opioids or benzodiazepines), and other state-specific standards of practice, should all inform a provider's decision on whether to use phone or video [79]. No significant differences in the therapeutic alliance between patients receiving telepsychiatric care and those receiving in-person care demonstrates that an important aspect of patient–provider interaction in psychiatry can still exist even over videoconferencing, i.e., *closeness despite the distance.*

9.7 Resistance, Barriers, Challenges

Telepsychiatry has benefits, but it is not a "One-Size-Fits-All" solution, i.e., not everyone can benefit from it. For instance, patients with schizophrenia are known to have a cognitive impairment, which may make it difficult for them to participate in telepsychiatry [175]. The main challenges of telepsychiatry include: uncertainty of required information and communication technology infrastructure, lack of standards (data exchange security, safety, and privacy), lack of regulatory body, reimbursement and insurance claims, accreditation of service provider, and licensing of health care professionals, a lack of efficacy studies, inconsistent availability of enough bandwidth, device simplicity and a lack of readily available technical help, and high equipment costs. Lack of specific procedures for managing behaviors such as self-harm or other adverse events during consultations may lead to institutional or individual liability which may cause clinicians to be reluctant to use telepsychiatry [144]. However, the main barrier is reluctance among clinicians and lack of professional guidance [32], particularly guidelines for dealing with medical errors [176] as well as a lack of telepsychiatry training and education at all levels of the psychiatrist's career. Studies have questioned the limitations of telepsychiatry when there was no professional guidance and regulations. It is important to note that the limited existing regulations were mostly developed in the wake of the COVID-19 outbreak and are often vaguely worded [177–180]. There are still valid worries that telepsychiatry might be utilized to fill rota gaps (i.e., when a hospital or department is unable to cover the working shift pattern required to manage patients due to the lack of available doctors), overwork professionals, and not do anything to solve chronic staffing difficulties across the mental health profession. Reimbursement rules either forbade coverage of telehealth consultations or only seldom permitted reimbursement [181, 182]. Therefore, there is a need to establish a clear structure guiding payment and claims for telepsychiatry services [183].

Although telepsychiatry service is convenient for patients, the many barriers from clinicians' perspectives are concerning, because they serve as "gatekeepers" for implementation and sustainability of telepsychiatry services. This suggests that solutions to overcome barriers must start by addressing the concerns of clinicians and enhancing clinical workflow [184]. Historically, professional reluctance to accept telepsychiatry has been centered around the building of rapport and therapeutic relationships [185]. However, in-depth research into patients' experiences with, e.g., using the telephone for mental health care shows evidence that it is possible to build rapport even over the telephone...but first and foremost with proper provider training [76]. A psychiatrist's effective appointment involves identifying mental health problems, diagnosing disorders, and creating a treatment plan while building up and maintaining a therapeutic relationship [186]. But if assessments take place outside of their immediate area, where they might not be familiar with the policy, safeguarding, and prescription guidelines, clinicians are reluctant to participate [114, 116, 119, 187]. When faced with remote assessment and/or treatment modalities, many health professionals expressed reluctance because they believed that telepsychiatry provided lower quality care [188, 189], and negatively impacted care outcomes [142, 143, 190–195].

In reality, patients have been more receptive to the use of telepsychiatry than psychiatrists, who have frequently been quick to dismiss the possibility of remote therapeutic interactions. With the advent of web-based videoconferencing systems and safe and secure Internet transmission, demand for telemental health diagnosis and treatment has increased. From the patients' perspective, technical access, which refers to having access to Internet services and Internet-enabled devices, reliable connectivity and access to technology have an impact on how widely telehealth services are used, especially in low- and middle-income nations [196]. Furthermore, patients may be exposed to the risk of data leakage, being overheard in their own home/environment or through compromised security [197]. The risk of data breaches and threats to patient confidentiality and privacy exists because virtual care is inherently fraught with risk [198].

To reduce the danger of data breaches, experts recommend using virtual platforms with firewalls, adware and malware protection, and data encryption built in [199]. Furthermore, it is crucial to provide effective consent procedures. Patients should be fully informed of the risks to their privacy and confidentiality during this procedure, as well as the limitations of the security measures in place to avoid breaches. Patients should be advised to have consultations in a private setting because sensitive information may be seen by anyone nearby. Privacy might indeed be an issue, especially if/when patients did not always have access to private locations where they could openly talk with the telepsychiatrist and express their intimate thoughts and worries [200].

Some authors argue that, from the perspective of the psychiatrist, during remote meetings with the patient, the possibility of looking directly into the eyes, tracking facial expressions and body language, and access to assessment of traces of self-harm, among other things, may be lacking [176]. When it comes to psychotherapy, of course, most patients prefer to meet with their mental health professional before their first psychotherapy video session, and their enthusiasm for trying video sessions increases after getting to know the therapist [159]. However, to some patients, video sessions are the only contact option, and in these circumstances, the hurdles to access therapy mixed with the patient's mental health needs trump the patient's wish to meet the therapist beforehand [99]. But because of the numerous barriers to mainstream acceptance, therapists are hesitant to incorporate video consultations into their treatment plans [184]. Moreover, some authors conclude that "creating a complete assessment of the patient makes exclusive remote therapy impossible under current conditions" [176]. Such a statement is understandable when viewed in the light of the inability to read the patient's body language. Current video platforms lack remote control of the video camera, which limits body language observations. However, using remote-controlled video equipment in clinically supervised settings significantly improves the ability to read body language. It can even be easier than in person because of the ability to zoom in so close to the patient's eyes, making it possible to predict when the patient is about to burst into tears. If we get so close to the patient in person, we will undoubtedly be seriously misunderstood.

Based on all above mentioned, the vast majority of professionals still view in-person interactions as the gold standard, while distant technologies are seen as a "necessary evil" that must be used to increase access and address the national deficit of in-person providers in the workforce [201]. Accordingly, some believe that telepsychiatry should be limited to follow-up consultations and known patients, perceiving telepsychiatry as a form of complementing the diagnosis and treatment process [176]. Overall, acceptance of telepsychiatry is affected by obstacles in getting to the clinic and meeting the doctor in person [99]. Telepsychiatry services are more acceptable the more obstacles there are. The COVID-19 pandemic has proven to be a significant barrier to in-person sessions, forcing mental health professionals to virtualize their services. All patients, regardless of location or their socioeconomic background, have been impacted by this. Due to COVID-19 pandemic, regulations regarding the use of telepsychiatry for a patient's initial visit have been relaxed. As a result, in 16 out of 17 regions [Australia, Brazil, Canada (Ontario), China, Denmark, Egypt, Germany, India, Italy, Japan, South Africa, South Korea, Spain (Madrid), Taiwan, Turkey, the UK (England), and the USA (New York)], involved in the recent survey [202], except Italy, telepsychiatry is now allowed for a patient's first visit. Diagnostic reliability, satisfactory clinical outcomes and patient satisfaction linked to telepsychiatry justify its continued use. Benefits that cannot be attained by in-person treatment alone will surely be acquired by using telepsychiatry in accordance with the patient's wishes and medical condition while keeping in mind the necessity to establish a good rapport. However, it is crucial to understand that while virtual platforms may increase access to care for some people, others might not be able to benefit from them [203]. Accessibility (e.g., having access to the Internet and smart telepsychiatry homes), user ability, provider competency, and language and cultural appropriateness are only a few of the challenges facing the successful adoption of telepsychiatry services [203]. If services are mostly provided digitally, people who are homeless can also be disproportionately excluded from receiving the proper treatment and interventions. Older people could have less experience using virtual platforms. To overcome these issues, telepsychiatry services must be developed in a collaborative manner with service users, clinicians, researchers, and policymakers in order to be inclusive and fulfill the different requirements of the population.

9.8 Telepsychiatry Guidelines

- In 2011, Cash wrote: "Telepsychiatry, if done well, can benefit patients. It also presents significant risks for the unwary" [204]. Acquainting ourselves with the guidelines for the proper use of telepsychiatry would help to solve the challenges and potential risks in the practice of remote care. One of the most widely recognized sets of guidelines is the American Telemedicine Association (ATA)—American Psychiatric Association (APA) Practice Guidelines for Telemental Health, which provide a comprehensive framework for the use of telepsychiatry [100]. In addition, telepsychiatry guidelines have also been developed for specific populations or settings/clinical applications. Including:
- Use in rural areas [205].
- Child and adolescent psychiatry [206].
- Ethical use of telemedicine and telehealth [207].
- Telemedicine, including telepsychiatry [208].
- Use in disaster response and recovery, emphasizing the need for cultural competence and sensitivity to trauma and stress [207].
- Patients at risk for suicide [209].

Guidelines for telepsychiatry have also been developed in, e.g., India [210], Australia [211], Canada [212], Denmark [213, 214], Poland [215], and the UK [216]. The American Psychiatric Association (APA) supports videoconferencing as an effective way to provide psychiatric health care, offering a resource called the Telepsychiatry Toolkit to educate providers about telepsychiatry [217]. Despite the progress with technology and the innovation during the pandemic, a set of guidelines is needed at a global level to unify key themes and address challenges related to clinical considerations, ethical and legal considerations, and technological requirements. To address these challenges, the World Psychiatric Association (WPA) has developed *Telepsychiatry Global Guidelines* [101]. The WPA Global Telepsychiatry Guidelines cover a wide range of essential elements, such as clinical practice, ethical considerations, technological challenges, education and training, research, and specific populations and settings, with an emphasis on international and cross-cultural dimensions.

9.9 Telepsychiatry Applications

It has been suggested to create a program outline that includes determining the telepsychiatry services to be provided, defining the patient population and clinicians involved, specifying the necessary space, training, technology support, staff, standard operating procedures, regulatory and monitoring processes, as well as sustainability requirements [100]. The chosen videoconferencing application must meet the necessary standards for quality, reliability, security, and backup processes before making a final decision.

Once all above mentioned prerequisites are met, videoconferencing can be used for clinical or patient care purposes, as well as for non-clinical applications such as administrative activities, learning activities, and research [11, 218, 219]. Telepsychiatry is routinely used for educational purposes, providing access to remote educational events and serving as a platform for web-based learning. Clinical management and psychotherapy supervision are major educational uses of telepsychiatry. Additionally, telepsychiatry can support various administrative and managerial functions, reducing costs, time, and travel associated with these tasks [24]. Assessment, diagnosis, pharmacological and psychological therapies, follow-up, and home-based care are just a few of the patient care services included in telepsychiatry. The formulation of clinical treatment plans, case management, crisis intervention, neuropsychological testing, legal assistance, forensic examinations, liaison services for other medical disciplines, and nursing care are additional services that telepsychiatry can offer. Both inpatient and outpatient treatment, emergency services, forensic settings, community settings, nursing homes, assisted living facilities, prisons, schools, and the homes of users, i.e., home-telepsychiatry, are among the sites for these services, which are equally varied. Rather than being limited to outpatient clinics, as is frequently believed, telepsychiatry might be utilized in a variety of mental health services and for a wide spectrum of patients who would not be able to access face-to-face consultations, e.g., inmates in correctional institutions, prisons [220, 221], and emergency departments [12, 59, 62, 140, 222, 223].

Successful telepsychiatric intervention models and modules for rural primary care provide/obtain: (1) mutual incentive for primary care and specialty partners (e.g., improved quality of care); (2) commitment from physicians, staff, and administration to pursue telemedicine and alternate modes of consultation; (3) systematic or multiple interventions that meet the needs of the site; (4) a system approach for the primary care system to monitor the flow of patients and measure outcomes; and (5) consultants who are able to bridge the differing philosophies that may be unique to rural primary care and urban academic settings and to specific cultural groups [224, 225].

A telebehavioral consultation model appears well-advised to develop skills for the primary care provider (e.g., triage, diagnosis, new or adjusted treatment plans) and since other models (e.g., managing the patient) are time intensive for the specialist [226, 227]. Distance consultation reduces provider isolation, provides case-based learning [228] as part of an ongoing relationship [226]. Examples are:

- In-person and telephone doctor-to-doctor "curbside" consultations. "Curbside" consultations are the most informal type of specialist consult. They occur when the physician consultant does not see the patient or review the patient's chart.
- Telephone or e-mail doctor-to-doctor "curbside" consultations.
- Case review with primary care providers.
- One-time cultural consultation, and distance neurocognitive assessment.

These interventions have helped patients receive adequate doses of antidepressants, and recover from depression [226, 229].

Finally, the patient population for telepsychiatry services can range from children to adults, the elderly, and special populations like prison inmates or military personnel. Mental health professionals, nurses, health workers, and educators can also utilize telepsychiatry [6, 11, 13, 120, 219].

9.10 Telepsychiatry in Clinical Practice

Telepsychiatry can be beneficial for providing mental health care in a variety of settings. When we talk about the clinical practice of telepsychiatry, we distinguish between clinically supervised and clinically unsupervised settings.

Clinically supervised settings: are patient locations where other medical or support staff are available in real-time to support the telepsychiatry sessions, e.g., hospitals, elderly homes, prisons, GP clinics, and rehabilitation institutions. In order to prevent the unintended consequences of using technology in mental health care, it is crucial to develop emergency protocols, including explaining roles and responsibilities in potential emergency situations. Outside clinic hours emergency coverage and guidelines for determining when other staff and resources should be brought in to help manage emergency situations are important to determine and inform the patient about. Clinicians should be aware of safety issues related to any patients displaying strong affective or behavioral states and, upon conclusion of a session, must understand how patients might then interact with remote site staff.

Many of the challenges faced by clinically supervised settings, e.g., hospital-based telepsychiatry, are similar to those faced by outpatient telepsychiatry, including ensuring that clinicians have the appropriate licenses to practice remotely, developing training programs to improve clinicians' skills, obtaining patient consent for participation, and using secure platforms that comply with privacy laws.

The increase in the number of patients who need psychiatric services is happening in parallel with the shortage of psychiatrists caused, among other things, by the aging of the psychiatric workforce [230, 231]. Accordingly, up to 60% of patients only receive care from GPs although they are not trained to diagnose and treat the vast majority of mental health conditions [232]. Workforce shortage is present in nursing homes as well, where the number of geriatric psychiatry fellows is steadily declining [233]. Therefore, many nursing homes will not have available on-site services of a geriatric psychiatric provider. Rural and medically underserved areas are also experiencing a shortage of psychiatric practitioners. Only 28% of psychiatrists were employed in hospitals, according to a 2019 national poll, and a 2018 research estimated that 54% of US counties lacked any psychiatrists [234]. These areas face many obstacles to receiving adequate psychiatric services due to difficulties related to availability of psychiatric practitioners, health care affordability, transportation, stigma, and long-distances between patients and providers [235]. Illness of hospital staff, travel restrictions, and absences from work due to concerns about contracting or transmitting COVID-19 only made the situation worse. By enabling clinicians to give remote care to hospitalized patients and increasing access to specialists, such as child, addiction, or geriatric psychiatrists, telepsychiatry could help to alleviate these shortages [236].

Mental health experts can provide psychiatric care in most hospital settings as long as personnel can set up safe technologies, like portable video communication equipment. There have been encouraging findings from small studies using telepsychiatry for inpatient psychiatry units, inpatient medical and surgical services, and emergency departments [237]. Studies revealed that telepsychiatry decreased patient flow-related outcomes in acute in-patient settings [92, 238–240]. Telepsychiatry may not only assist hospital personnel in providing remote care during the "lockdowns" caused by pandemics and/or natural disasters by enabling doctors to work remotely, but it may also draw in new groups of mental health experts who might not have otherwise considered working in these settings, i.e., serve as a potential solution for workforce shortages [92].

Hospital-based telepsychiatry has the potential of increasing access to care in a variety of settings and services. The research that is currently available has mostly focused on these services in academic medical centers and rural settings. Recent study has explored telepsychiatry models that could support the continuum of care related to hospitalizations such as the assessment of psychotropic regimens for nursing home residents [241]. Modifications of conventional audio–video telepsychiatry, such as integration with interpreter services, will be necessary to accommodate the needs of patients with sensory impairments and language barriers [242]. However, more knowledge is still required in order for doctors to design secure, moral, and economical systems in addition to better understanding the specific challenges and advantages of hospital-based telepsychiatry.

Clinically unsupervised settings: are patient locations where other medical or support staff are not readily available in real-time to support the telepsychiatry sessions, e.g., private home ("home-telepsychiatry"), working office, and so forth. This approach can be useful due to its potential to increase access to mental health care, particularly for individuals with limited mobility, those residing in rural or underserved areas, and during public health crises like the COVID-19 pandemic, natural disasters, and wars.

- There are several advantages of "home-telepsychiatry": Improved access to care that would not otherwise be available (e.g., in rural areas) and bring care to where the patient is.
- Early detection and prevention are improved through improved access to relevant expertise.
- Reducing delays in care.
- Improve continuity of care and follow-up as the patient may, e.g., travel on vacation but still maintain the treatment course. This is especially important for patients in regular psychotherapy.
- Reduce the need for time off work, childcare services, etc. to access in-person consultations.
- Reduced risk of consultation cancellation or absence, i.e., increased adherence to treatment.

- Prevention of infection or transmission of infectious diseases to others while waiting in crowded waiting rooms.
- Reduction of potential transport barriers that may occur due to:
  - Lack of transportation or
  - The need for long drives or
  - Phobia related to the transportation
  - Reducing the no-show rate and the risk of missing appointments. People with a "relaxed" attitude toward alcohol and drugs can run the risk of driving drunk or "high" and causing serious harm to themselves and others
- Reduction of the stigma barrier, since the patient is not seen in the environment against which he/she is stigmatized.
- Impact on climate changes. No driving = no CO_2 emission.

The majority of patient group respondents claimed that since they could attend the sessions in the comfort of their home or place of employment, telepsychiatry was more convenient than in-person (or "physical") sessions. Home-telepsychiatry can contribute to reducing the stigma associated with seeking mental health services by providing care in a familiar and comfortable environment. Remote-visits are a great option for patients who are either unable or unwilling to seek in-person care, e.g., Veterans' for whom telepsychiatry improves access to clinical care, decreases expenses and time for travel, and improves their quality by offering care in their own homes. Videoconferencing-delivered evidence-based PTSD therapies are practical and feasible and equally successful as in-person clinic-based therapy, including patient satisfaction and symptom improvement [75].

Furthermore, telepsychiatry is utilizing treatment coverage for opioid addiction in the privacy of the patients' home [243]. Telepsychiatry interviews can serve as the sole mode of contact between a patient and their psychiatrist, particularly in rural areas where distance can be a challenge. Additionally, telepsychiatry interviews can be used in combination with in-person visits. Hybrid telepsychiatry (i.e., supplemental to in person visits) is a reasonable option for homebound elderly patients living in urban areas and less expensive than nursing home admission [244]. All communication with the patient should follow clear policies describing the boundaries around ways in which patients can communicate with a provider and which content is appropriate to share over different technology platforms.

A novel "virtual hybrid hospital at home" program called Advanced Care at Home (ACH) has been implemented in Mayo Clinic in Florida (USA) in 2020. This model allows virtual providers in a command center to care for high-acuity patients in the home setting through collaboration with a vendor-mediated supply chain. Overall, data show that the providers adapted well to this new model of care, with 80% or more of providers giving positive scores to all three areas analyzed: providers' perception of quality and safety, providers' perception of decision-making and teamwork, and whether providers found working in ACH rewarding [245].

To be practiced responsibly, home-telepsychiatry requires thoughtful elucidation of key challenges, limitations, and possible solutions.

9.11 Limitations Related to Home-Telepsychiatry

1. Limited opportunity for somatic examination.
2. Limited ability to read the body language.
3. "Mirror image" displayed by the built-in camera, i.e., what is actually on the left is displayed on the right and vice versa.
4. The risk that the patient records the session and publishes it on the Internet.
5. Low bandwidth/unstable Internet connection affecting sound and picture quality.

Suggestions on how to deal with the above limitations are as follows:

Ad 1. Patients whom we see for the first time via video, i.e., we do not know them before, should be referred to a general practitioner for a physical examination. In this way, we also improve cooperation with GP. If the patient experiences acute somatic problems and reports them to us during the telepsychiatry session, we can contact the emergency room and refer the patient for an urgent examination.

Ad. 2 The built-in camera on mobile devices does not have the capacity to pan, tilt, or zoom, making it difficult to read the patient's body language. The only reliable method for capturing body language during telepsychiatry sessions is the use of still expensive stand-alone camera equipment with pan-tilt-zoom capabilities. As equipment costs decline over time, it will become more feasible to enhance video performance in home telepsychiatry settings.

Ad 3. The patient's T-shirt's letter inversion usually alerts us to mirror images. As long as the therapist is aware of this occurrence, mirroring the picture is not a big barrier. But if not, it could have a big impact, e.g., when a patient initially presents right-side paresis that actually is a left-side paresis from a recent stroke. Because of this, it is crucial to consider the mirroring effect while analyzing body language. Mirroring can be turned off on most mobile video apps.

Ad 4. It is important to inform the patient before each telepsychiatry session that recording is not permitted and obtain their consent by having them sign a document before the first session. The consent document should specify details such as the voluntary nature of participation and the prohibition on recording and publicly releasing the sessions by any of the involved parties.

Ad 5. Electric power failure or disrupted Internet connection are unpredictable obstacles. In order to avoid potential complications we must have prepared a backup plan that involves other real-time communication equipment (typically telephone). Eventually, it may be necessary to reschedule the consultation.

In addition to the above mentioned to address the disadvantages of home-telepsychiatry, several complementary strategies can be applied. However, most of the following is applicable to telepsychiatry in general:

- Bridging the digital divide: As of 2019, approximately one-quarter of individuals in the USA still lack fixed home broadband [246]. To overcome technological barriers, patients should provide with affordable and reliable Internet access, appropriate devices, and the necessary technical skills. Programs such as tablet loan initiatives and identifying Wi-Fi hot spots have assisted patients with connecting to virtual care. Additionally, community outreach programs have also helped patients with technical difficulties [247–249].

- Providing Wi-Fi hot spots and publicly available kiosks for patients to improve patient accessibility would be helpful. However, this would not necessarily address the travel issue for some patients, and additional steps would need to be taken to ensure Health Insurance Portability and Accountability Act compliance as well [250].
- Ensuring privacy and confidentiality: Clinicians and patients should use secure, encrypted videoconferencing systems, private areas in the home, and/or headphones to prevent outsiders from listening in on their interactions [251].
- Improving rapport and communication: Mental health practitioners ought to receive training on how to establish rapport and speak clearly during video consultations. This may entail empathetic listening techniques, active participation in verbal and non-verbal feedback, and handling any technical difficulties that can obstruct the therapeutic procedure [252].
- Establishing best practices and guidelines for home telepsychiatry should be a priority for regulatory organizations and professional associations, and should include suggestions for proper patient selection, assessment and treatment protocols, and ethical issues [253].
- Resolving issues with licensing and reimbursement: Remote and telehealth services should be regulated, reimbursed, and treated with parity to that of services provided to patients in person [254, 255]. Health care leaders suggest that both supervised and unsupervised telepsychiatry provision should adhere to the same standards of patient information documentation, maintenance, and transmission as traditional face-to-face patient encounters [256, 257].

Finally, all communication with the patient should follow clear policies describing the boundaries around ways in which patients can communicate with a provider and which content is appropriate to share over different technology platforms. Patients are expected to participate in the therapeutic process more actively and cooperatively in unsupervised telepsychiatry settings than in other settings. Utilizing tools like smartphones, laptops, or desktop computers with built-in video applications is part of this. Videoconferencing applications used for home-telepsychiatry, although the same is true for telepsychiatry in general, must be compatible with most devices and operating systems and follow national and regional legislation in that area [99]. Patients also need to cooperate with safety management procedures and make sure they have access to a private, quiet area. These precautions could include having family members, relatives, spouses, or other people who can help the patient if necessary in situ as support. In case of sudden homicide or suicide threats or behavior, it is important to know the patient's location and have contact details for the nearest emergency medical facility and police station.

In light of the above mentioned, it is important that telepsychiatry providers consider the suitability of a home-telepsychiatry service for each individual patient. The major issues to consider are:

- Their history regarding cooperativeness with treatment professionals.
- Their current and past difficulties with substance abuse.
- Their history of violence or self-injurious behavior.
- The geographic distance to the nearest emergency medical facility.
- The efficacy of the patient's support system.

When providing a telepsychiatry service in clinically unsupervised settings, it is critical to identify where the patient is located should the following situations occur:

- Patient requires referral to the nearest mental health institution or to a local psychiatrist for in-person consultation.
- To inform the local police/ambulance services for emergency intervention to save a patient's life (attempted suicide) or someone else's life (homicidal attempt).
- Mandatory reporting of certain diseases is tied to the jurisdiction where the patient is receiving services and may be a requirement under the law.

Furthermore, it is also important to consider what access to videoconferencing equipment the patients have in their home, and whether it is possible, justifiable, and efficient to lend equipment to patients with insufficient equipment for a period.

9.12 Potential Solutions to Overcome Barriers

Since the COVID-19 pandemic outbreak, telepsychiatry has grown exponentially, with virtual platforms now being used to provide patient care. The COVID-19 has made telepsychiatry's potential clear and has sped up policymakers' efforts to advance it and eliminate obstacles [258, 259]. The United States' liberalization of privacy laws, improvement of reimbursement and prescribing regulations have all contributed to the uptake of virtual care [260]. Similar to the USA, Canada has changed its legislation and included COVID-19-specific billing codes to make virtual care more accessible to patients of all medical specialties [261]. These changes are certainly to be commended, but they are not enough. In order to address telepsychiatry underutilization by providers and limited patient access, the following initiatives are recommended [262]:

- *Recognition of the larger responsibilities of academic health sciences centers.* There is a disproportionate concentration of psychiatrists, both specialists and subspecialists, within the confines of these centers, and they typically have a mandate to share their expertise within their province beyond their immediate catchment area. Telepsychiatry provides an efficient and effective way to fulfill that mandate.
- *Enhancement of existing technology.* Telepsychiatry services are provided principally through televideo studios or portable televideo units; technology exists to make it accessible through the computers of every psychiatrist, removing another

barrier. Younger psychiatrists—who have statistically opted out of telepsychiatry—use technology with apps and iPhones, not studios and portable units.

- *Better coordination of services.* Given the potential of telepsychiatry to bridge the geographic divide, a more thoughtful approach is needed, especially in light of the paucity of utilization. This begs for a strategy that has defined clinical priorities, geographic rationales, and measured outcomes.
- *Meaningful integration into residency training.* If our trainees see telepsychiatry as a routine part of clinical care that they observe and deliver, they are hopefully more likely to integrate it into their own practice on graduation. This needs to involve more than the educational tourism of an afternoon spent observing telepsychiatry assessment. Training in telepsychiatry should be incorporated into the psychiatry residency experience. Indeed, detailed pedagogical documents reflect still-aspirational goals for such training [116, 263].

Existing guidelines on telepsychiatry are relevant and applicable, but it is important for practitioners and researchers to stay informed about ongoing developments in the field. More studies are required to determine the efficacy of telepsychiatry in diverse clinical settings and patient populations. Moreover, there is a need for further investigation to identify the most effective approaches for implementing and assessing telepsychiatry programs, emphasizing the importance of continuous innovation and adaptation [264]. Ensuring that all patients have access to high-quality mental health care will require the development of culturally sensitive and contextually appropriate telepsychiatry programs. However, they may need to be adapted to meet the specific needs of different countries and regions. It is why the development of country-specific guidelines highlights the importance of tailoring best practices and ethical standards to meet the unique needs and cultural contexts of different regions. Moreover, a survey of the use of guidelines can provide important insights into how they are implemented and the impact they have on telepsychiatry programs worldwide. This information can be used to improve the guidelines and promote the adoption of evidence-based practices in telepsychiatry.

It is important to recognize that telepsychiatry is a versatile field that incorporates a range of technologies to enhance access to mental health care and overcome barriers such as distance, limited resources, and stigma. Providing telepsychiatry without prior training and/or education can have several downsides, including:

1. Increased risk of errors: Mental health professionals who are not trained in telepsychiatry may make errors or overlook important considerations, such as ensuring the confidentiality and security of patient information. We continue to observe instances, even today but especially under the pandemic, where telepsychiatry is being conducted through platforms (e.g., Skype or WhatsApp) that may not comply with privacy and security regulations in certain countries.
2. Lower quality of care: Without prior training, mental health professionals may not have the necessary skills and knowledge to provide high-quality telepsychiatry services. This could result in lower patient satisfaction and outcomes.

3. Legal and ethical implications: Providing telepsychiatry without proper training and education could raise legal and ethical concerns, such as violating patient confidentiality or failing to provide adequate informed consent.
4. Stigma toward telepsychiatry: Poor quality telepsychiatry services could contribute to negative attitudes and stigma toward the use of technology in mental health care.

Overall, providing telepsychiatry without prior training and education can have negative impacts on both mental health professionals and patients. It is therefore essential that mental health professionals receive adequate education and training in telepsychiatry to ensure safe and effective delivery of services. There are several reasons that emphasize the urgent need for regular digital mental health Continuing Medical Education (CME) courses at international conferences, the inclusion of telemental health in the faculty curriculum, and continuous training in this field throughout the education of psychiatry residents.

Firstly, it can help mental health professionals to stay up-to-date with the latest developments and best practices in telepsychiatry, including advancements in technology and changes in regulations. This can improve the quality of care provided to patients and ensure that mental health professionals are practicing in a safe and effective manner.

Secondly, continuous telepsychiatry education can help to address the potential knowledge gaps and skill deficits that mental health professionals may have when it comes to telepsychiatry. This can lead to increased confidence and competence in providing telepsychiatry services, which can improve patient outcomes and satisfaction.

Finally, offering education/training in telepsychiatry can signal to mental health professionals and the broader health care community that telepsychiatry is a legitimate and important mode of delivering mental health care. This can help to increase awareness and acceptance of telepsychiatry, which can ultimately lead to greater access to mental health care for patients.

Unfortunately, the vast majority of psychiatry training curricula globally do not currently include education and training in telepsychiatry, which has lagged behind its use. To increase the familiarity of professionals with telepsychiatry and its use in daily clinical work, telepsychiatry practice could benefit from standardized training. Training in best practices appears to be essential to the development of a sustainable and well-functioning telepsychiatry network [99]. The certification in telepsychiatry, as a measure to ensure that the introduction of telepsychiatry services was carried out in a safe and effective manner, has been proposed [265] and is supported by the authors of this chapter. One perspective in the debate surrounding mandatory education/training is that it can help ensure that mental health professionals have the necessary knowledge and skills to practice telepsychiatry safely and effectively.

However, there are also arguments against making education/training in telepsychiatry mandatory. For instance, mandating could potentially contribute to an increase in stigma toward the use of technology in mental health care. Additionally, it may impose additional demands on mental health professionals who are already facing time and resource constraints.

Encouraging and incentivizing mental health professionals to participate in CME courses and other forms of education/training in telepsychiatry could be another effective approach. It can be done via national and international psychiatric associations, which can play a crucial role in promoting and providing education and training in core competencies in telepsychiatry. This includes disseminating guidelines, providing training and support, and advocating for policies that support the integration of telepsychiatry into mental health care delivery. By taking a leadership role in this area, psychiatric associations can help to ensure that mental health professionals have the knowledge and skills necessary to provide safe, effective, and culturally responsive telepsychiatry services to patients.

9.13 Conclusions and Future Directions

Telepsychiatry has the potential to significantly improve the quality of care for individuals who might not otherwise be able to access conventional psychiatric services. It encourages patient empowerment, equal access, and high levels of satisfaction. Telepsychiatry is successful in many ways on par with in-person treatment. Numerous obstacles, including methodological problems, technological constraints, clinician or provider resistance, safety, security, and confidentiality worries, regulatory difficulties, and ethical and legal concerns, prevent the routine clinical use of telepsychiatry. The sustainability and advantages of incorporating telepsychiatric services into current mental health care systems are also not well supported by the available data. Hybrid models that combine remote and in-person types of service delivery have been suggested long ago [266]. Accordingly, telepsychiatry is usually used in conjunction with conventional forms of service delivery. The evidence related to telepsychiatry is much more extensive than presented in this chapter and more research will certainly be conducted as telepsychiatry broadens its application, adding to the body of evidence supporting claims that it is just as effective as in-person psychiatry. Expanding and researching telepsychiatry will help those who have difficulty getting access to mental health care and close a gap in our health care system. Future studies should show which type of assessments and/or treatments are most appropriate for telepsychiatry and how to enhance the precision, effectiveness, and user experience of these evaluations. Despite the fact that it is obvious that telepsychiatry is equivalent to in-person psychiatry, more research is required to identify the characteristics that promote its usage and to create plans for integrating telepsychiatry services into the larger health care delivery system. Telepsychiatry is poised to evolve as technology, clinical applications, and care models continue to develop. Encouraging the use of telepsychiatry through incentives can further promote this evolution.

As telepsychiatry continues to transform health care, it has the potential to increase capacity for interactions with patients and their families within but also across the country borders. The creation of international telepsychiatry services that will permit the exchange of professional expertise and the assessment and/or treatment of patients from a distance is anticipated as a result of the development of new technological devices and telecommunication technologies. Changes frequently occurs spontaneously. We witnessed that during the COVID-19 outbreak. But once created, significant changes are unable to endure via continuous improvisations. Education, training, the support of policymakers related to the unification of licensing and reimbursement rules are crucial to the realization of the global spread of telepsychiatry regardless of national borders.

References

1. Shore JH, Manson SM. A developmental model for rural telepsychiatry. Psychiatr Serv. 2005;56(8):976–80. https://doi.org/10.1176/appi.ps.56.8.976.
2. Myers K, Cain S. Practice parameter for telepsychiatry with children and adolescents. J Am Acad Child Adolesc Psychiatry. 2008;47(12):1468–83.
3. Norman S. The use of telemedicine in psychiatry. J Psychiatr Ment Health Nurs. 2006;13(6):771–7.
4. O'Keefe M, White K, Jennings JC. Asynchronous telepsychiatry: a systematic review. J Telemed Telecare. 2021;27(3):137–45.
5. Vaitheswaran S, Crockett P, Wilson S, Millar H. Telemental health: videoconferencing in mental health services. Adv Psychiatr Treat. 2012;18:392–8.
6. Grady B. Promises and limitations of telepsychiatry in rural adult mental health care. World Psychiatry. 2012;11:199–201.
7. Deslich S, Stec B, Tomblin S, Coustasse A. Telepsychiatry in the 21(st) century: transforming healthcare with technology. Perspect Health Inf Manag. 2013;10:1f.
8. Shore JH. Telepsychiatry: videoconferencing in the delivery of psychiatric care. Am J Psychiatry. 2013;170:256–62.
9. Chipps J, Ramlall S, Mars M. Practice guidelines for videoconference-based telepsychiatry in South Africa. Afr J Psychiatry (Johannesbg). 2012;15:271–82.
10. Antonacci DJ, Bloch RM, Saeed SA, Yildirim Y, Talley J. Empirical evidence on the use and effectiveness of telepsychiatry via videoconferencing: implications for forensic and correctional psychiatry. Behav Sci Law. 2008;26:253–69.
11. Richardson LK, Frueh BC, Grubaugh AL, Egede L, Elhai JD. Current directions in videoconferencing tele-mental health research. Clin Psychol (New York). 2009;16:323–38.
12. Hilty DM, Marks SL, Urness D, Yellowlees PM, Nesbitt TS. Clinical and educational telepsychiatry applications: a review. Can J Psychiatr. 2004;49:12–23.
13. Chipps J, Brysiewicz P, Mars M. Effectiveness and feasibility of telepsychiatry in resource constrained environments? A systematic review of the evidence. Afr J Psychiatry (Johannesbg). 2012;15:235–43.
14. Tucker H, Lewis RB, Martin GL, et al. Television therapy: effectiveness of closed-circuit television as a medium for therapy in the mentally ill. AMA Arch Neurol Psychiatry. 1957;77(1):57–69.
15. Wilmer HA. Television: technical and artistic aspects of videotape in psychiatric teaching. J Nerv Ment Dis. 1967;144(3):207–23. N Y State J Med. 1958 Dec 1;58(23):3831–8.
16. Wittson CL, Affleck DC, Johnson V. Two-way television in group therapy. Ment Hosp. 1961;12:22–3.
17. Holmes DJ. Closed circuit television in teaching psychiatry. Med Bull (Ann Arbor). 1961;27:330–6.
18. Krystal H. Postgraduate teaching in psychiatry combining television and FM-radio with seminars (a report of a demonstration project and survey). Psychosomatics. 1962;3:188–92. https://doi.org/10.1016/s0033-3182(62)72701-5.
19. Gibbard BA. Closed circuit television in a psychiatric training centre: a preliminary report. Laval Med. 1969;40(9):929–32.

20. Bashshur R, Shannon GW. History of telemedicine: evolution, context, and transformation. New Rochelle, NY: Mary Ann Liebert; 2009.
21. Shore J. The evolution and history of telepsychiatry and its impact on psychiatric care: current implications for psychiatrists and psychiatric organizations. Int Rev Psychiatry. 2015;27(6):469–75.
22. Dwyer TF. Telepsychiatry: psychiatric consultation by interactive television. Am J Psychiatry. 1973;130(8):865–9.
23. Straker N, Mostyn P, Marshall C. The use of two-way TV in bringing mental health services to the inner city. Am J Psychiatry. 1976;133:1202–5.
24. Millar HR. Telemental health in Scotland. Aberdeen: Scottish Centre for Telehealth; 2009. http://www.sctt.scot.nhs.uk/pdf/mentalhealth.pdf.
25. Rudolf JN. Effectiveness of telepsychiatry: an integrative literature review. Thesis, Master of Nursing, Montana State University Bozeman, Montana. 2011. http://scholarworks.montana.edu/xmlui/bitstream/handle/1/2164/RudolfJ0511.pdf?sequence=1.
26. Hilty DM, Ferrer DC, Parish MB, Johnston B, Callahan EJ, Yellowlees PM. The effectiveness of telemental health: a 2013 review. Telemed J E Health. 2013;19:444–5.
27. Mucic D. Telepsychiatry Pilot Project in Denmark. World Cult Psychiatry Res Rev. 2007;2:3–9.
28. Mucic D. International Telepsychiatry, patient acceptability study. J Telemed Telecare. 2008;14:241–3.
29. Yellowlees P, Shore J, Roberts L. American Telemedicine Association: practice guidelines for videoconferencing-based telemental health: October 2009. Telemed J E Health. 2010;16:1074–89.
30. Hilty DM, Liu W, Marks SL, Callahan EJ. The effectiveness of telepsychiatry: a brief review. CPA Bull. 2003;35(5):10–7.
31. Campbell R, O'Gorman J, Cernovsky ZZ. Reactions of psychiatric patients to telepsychiatry. Ment Illn. 2015;7(2):54.
32. Sharma G, Devan K. The effectiveness of telepsychiatry: thematic review. BJPsych Bull. 2023;47(2):82–9. https://doi.org/10.1192/bjb.2021.115.
33. Seidel RW, Kilgus MD. Agreement between telepsychiatry assessment and face-to-face assessment for emergency department psychiatry patients. J Telemed Telecare. 2014;20(2):59–62.
34. Moreno FA, Chong J, Dumbauld J, Humke M, Byreddy S. Use of standard webcam and Internet equipment for telepsychiatry treatment of depression among underserved Hispanics. Psychiatr Serv. 2012;63(12):1213–7.
35. Ruskin PE, Silver-Aylaian M, Kling MA, Reed SA, Bradham DD, Hebel JR, et al. Treatment outcomes in depression: comparison of remote treatment through telepsychiatry to in-person treatment. Am J Psychiatry. 2004;161(8):1471–6.
36. Vahia IV, Ng B, Camacho A, Cardenas V, Cherner M, Depp CA, et al. Telepsychiatry for neurocognitive testing in older rural Latino adults. Am J Geriatr Psychiatry. 2015;23(7):666–70.
37. Hawker F, Kavanagh S, Yellowlees P, Kalucy RS. Telepsychiatry in South Australia. J Telemed Telecare. 1998;4:187–94.
38. Baigent MF, Lloyd CJ, Kavanagh SJ, et al. Telepsychiatry: 'tele' yes, but what about the 'psychiatry'? J Telemed Telecare. 1997;3(Suppl 1):12–4.
39. McLaren P, Ball CJ, Summerfield AB, et al. An evaluation of the use of interactive television in an acute psychiatric service. J Telemed Telecare. 1995;1:79–85.
40. Basit SA, Mathews N, Kunik ME. Telemedicine interventions for medication adherence in mental illness: a systematic review. Gen Hosp Psychiatry. 2020;62:28–36.
41. Valentine LM, Donofry SD, Sexton MB. Demographic and psychiatric predictors of engagement in psychotherapy services conducted via clinical video telehealth. J Telemed Telecare. 2020;26(1–2):113–8.
42. Zheng W, Nickasch M, Lander L, Wen S, Xiao M, Marshalek P, et al. Treatment outcome comparison between telepsychiatry and face-to-face buprenorphine Medication-Assisted Treatment (MAT) for opioid use disorder: a 2-year retrospective data analysis. J Addict Med. 2017;11(2):138.

43. Tarp K, Bojesen AB, Mejldal A, Nielsen AS. Effectiveness of optional videoconferencing-based treatment of alcohol use disorders: randomized controlled trial. JMIR Ment Health. 2017;4(3):e38.
44. Mitchell JE, Crosby RD, Wonderlich SA, Crow S, Lancaster K, Simonich H, et al. A randomized trial comparing the efficacy of cognitive-behavioral therapy for bulimia nervosa delivered via telemedicine versus face-to-face. Behav Res Ther. 2008;46(5):581–92.
45. Corruble E, Swartz HA, Bottai T, Vaiva G, Bayle F, Llorca P-M, et al. Telephone-administered psychotherapy in combination with antidepressant medication for the acute treatment of major depressive disorder. J Affect Disord. 2016;190:6–11. https://doi.org/10.1016/j.jad.2015.07.052.
46. Simon GE, Ludman EJ, Tutty S, Operskalski B, Von Korff M. Telephone psychotherapy and telephone care management for primary care patients starting antidepressant treatment: a randomized controlled trial. JAMA. 2004;292(8):935–42. https://doi.org/10.1001/jama.292.8.935.
47. Ngai F-W, Wong PW-C, Leung K-Y, Chai P-H, Chung K-F. The effect of telephone-based cognitive-behavioral therapy on postnatal depression: a randomized controlled trial. Psychother Psychosom. 2015;84(5):294–303.
48. Fann JR, Bombardier CH, Vannoy S, Dyer J, Ludman E, Dikmen S, et al. Telephone and in-person cognitive behavioral therapy for major depression after traumatic brain injury: a randomized controlled trial. J Neurotrauma. 2015;32(1):45–57. https://doi.org/10.1089/neu.2014.3423.
49. Coughtrey AE, Pistrang N. The effectiveness of telephone-delivered psychological therapies for depression and anxiety: a systematic review. J Telemed Telecare. 2018;24(2):65–74.
50. Brenes GA, Ingram CW, Danhauer SC. Benefits and challenges of conducting psychotherapy by telephone. Prof Psychol Res Pract. 2011;42(6):543. https://doi.org/10.1037/a0026135.
51. Jacobs JC, Blonigen DM, Kimerling R, Slightam C, Gregory AJ, Gurmessa T, et al. Increasing mental health care access, continuity, and efficiency for veterans through telehealth with video tablets. Psychiatr Serv. 2019;70(11):976–82.
52. Schifeling CH, Shanbhag P, Johnson A, Atwater RC, Koljack C, Parnes BL, et al. Disparities in video and telephone visits among older adults during the COVID-19 pandemic: cross-sectional analysis. JMIR Aging. 2020;3(2):e23176.
53. Jaklevic MC. Telephone visits surge during the pandemic, but will they last? JAMA. 2020;324(16):1593–5.
54. Rodriguez JA, Betancourt JR, Sequist TD, Ganguli I. Differences in the use of telephone and video telemedicine visits during the COVID-19 pandemic. Am J Manag Care. 2021;27(1):21–6.
55. Chen J, Li KY, Andino J, Hill CE, Ng S, Steppe E, et al. Predictors of audio-only versus video telehealth visits during the COVID-19 pandemic. J Gen Intern Med. 2022;37(5):1138–44.
56. Drake C, Lian T, Cameron B, Medynskaya K, Bosworth HB, Shah K. Understanding telemedicine's "new normal": variations in telemedicine use by specialty line and patient demographics. Telemed J E Health. 2022;28(1):51–9. https://doi.org/10.1089/tmj.2021.0041.
57. Karimi M, Lee EC, Couture SJ, Gonzales A, Grigorescu V, Smith SR, De Lew N, Sommers BD. National survey trends in telehealth use in 2021: disparities in utilization and audio vs. video services. Off Assist Sec Plann Evaluat; 2022.
58. Uscher-Pines L, Jones M, Sousa J, Predmore Z, Ober A. The doctor will call me maybe: the uncertain future of audio-only visits and why we need them to address disparities. Health Aff Blog; 2021.
59. Ellington E, Repique R, John R. Telemental health adoption can change psychiatric-mental health nursing practice. J Am Psychiatr Nurses Assoc. 2013;19:222–4.
60. Fishkind AB, Cuyler RN. The role of telepsychiatry. In: Zun LS, Chepenik LG, Mallory MNS, editors. Behavioral emergencies for the emergency physician. Cambridge: Cambridge University Press; 2013. p. 303–7.
61. Godleski L, Darkins A, Peters J. Outcomes of 98,609 US Department of Veterans Affairs patients enrolled in telemental health services, 2006–2010. Psychiatr Serv. 2012;63(4):383–5.

62. Narasimhan M, Druss BG, Hockenberry JM, Royer J, Weiss P, Glick G, Magill J. Impact of a telepsychiatry program at emergency departments statewide on the quality, utilization, and costs of mental health services. Psychiatr Serv. 2015;66(11):1167–72.
63. Raney L, Bergman D, Torous J, Hasselberg M. Digitally driven integrated primary care and behavioral health: how technology can expand access to effective treatment. Curr Psychiatry Rep. 2017;19(11):86.
64. Basavarajappa C, Grover S, Dalal PK, Avasthi A, Kumar CN, Manjunatha N, Sahoo S, Saha G, Mehra A, Singh OP, Tripathi A, Gangadhar BN, Math SB. Perceived advantages and disadvantages of telepsychiatry—an online survey of psychiatrists in India. Indian J Psychiatry. 2022;64(1):93–7. https://doi.org/10.4103/indianjpsychiatry.indianjpsychiatry_332_21. Epub 2022 Jan 21. Erratum in: Indian J Psychiatry. 2022 Mar-Apr;64(2):221.
65. Jacobs JC, Hu J, Slightam C, Gregory A, Zulman DM. Virtual savings: patient-reported time and money savings from a VA National Telehealth Tablet Initiative. Telemed J E Health. 2020;26(9):1178–83. https://doi.org/10.1089/tmj.2019.0179.
66. Harley J. Economic evaluation of a tertiary telepsychiatry service to an island. J Telemed Telecare. 2006;12(7):354–7.
67. Spaulding R, Belz N, DeLurgio S, Williams AR. Cost savings of telemedicine utilization for child psychiatry in a rural Kansas community. Telemed J E Health. 2010;16(8):867–71.
68. Whitacre BE, Hartman PS, Boggs SA, Schott V. A community perspective on quantifying the economic impact of teleradiology and telepsychiatry. J Rural Health. 2009;25(2):194–7.
69. Waugh M, Voyles D, Thomas MR. Telepsychiatry: benefits and costs in a changing healthcare environment. Int Rev Psychiatry. 2015;27(6):558–68.
70. Shore JH, Brooks E, Savin DM, Manson SM, Libby AM. An economic evaluation of telehealth data collection with rural populations. Psychiatr Serv. 2007;58(6):830–5.
71. Bashshur RL, Shannon GW, Bashshur N, Yellowlees PM. The empirical evidence for telemedicine interventions in mental disorders. Telemed J E Health. 2016;22(2):87–113.
72. Choi NG, Marti CN, Bruce ML, Hegel MT, Wilson NL, Kunik ME. Six-month postintervention depression and disability outcomes of in-home telehealth problem-solving therapy for depressed, low-income homebound older adults. Depress Anxiety. 2014;31(8):653–61. https://doi.org/10.1002/da.22242.
73. Patel SY, Huskamp HA, Busch AB, Mehrotra A. Telemental health and US rural–urban differences in specialty mental health use, 2010–2017. Am J Public Health. 2020;110(9):1308–14. https://doi.org/10.2105/AJPH.2020.305657.
74. Egede LE, Acierno R, Knapp RG, Lejuez C, Hernandez-Tejada M, Payne EH, et al. Psychotherapy for depression in older veterans via telemedicine: a randomised, open-label, non-inferiority trial. Lancet Psychiatry. 2015;2(8):693–701. https://doi.org/10.1016/S2215-0366(15)00122-4.
75. Whealin JM, King L, Shore P, Spira JL. Diverse veterans' pre- and post-intervention perceptions of home telemental health for posttraumatic stress disorder delivered via tablet. Int J Psychiatry Med. 2017;52(1):3–20. https://doi.org/10.1177/0091217417703291.
76. Rushton K, Ardern K, Hopkin E, Welsh C, Gellatly J, Faija C, et al. 'I didn't know what to expect': exploring patient perspectives to identify targets for change to improve telephone-delivered psychological interventions. BMC Psychiatry. 2020;20(1):1–13.
77. Slightam C, Gregory AJ, Hu J, Jacobs J, Gurmessa T, Kimerling R, et al. Patient perceptions of video visits using veterans affairs telehealth tablets: survey study. J Med Internet Res. 2020;22(4):e15682.
78. Guinart D, Marcy P, Hauser M, Dwyer M, Kane JM. Mental health care providers' attitudes toward telepsychiatry: a systemwide, multisite survey during the COVID-19 pandemic. Psychiatr Serv. 2021;72:704–7.
79. Chen PV, Helm A, Caloudas SG, Ecker A, Day G, Hogan J, Lindsay J. Evidence of phone vs video-conferencing for mental health treatments: a review of the literature. Curr Psychiatry Rep. 2022;24(10):529–39. https://doi.org/10.1007/s11920-022-01359-8. Epub 2022 Sep 2.
80. Aboujaoude E, Salame W, Naim L. Telemental health: a status update. World Psychiatry. 2015;14:223–30.

81. Rooksby M, Furuhashi T, McLeod HJ. Hikikomori: a hidden mental health need following the COVID-19 pandemic. World Psychiatry. 2020;19:399.
82. Mishkind MC, Shore JH, Bishop K, et al. Rapid conversion to telemental health services in response to COVID-19: experiences of two outpatient mental health clinics. Telemed J E Health. 2021;27:778–84.
83. Frayn M, Fojtu C, Juarascio A. COVID-19 and binge eating: patient perception of eating disorder symptoms, tele-therapy, and treatment implications. Curr Psychol. 2021;40:6249–58.
84. Leukhardt A, Heider M, Reboly K, et al. Videobasierte behandlungen in der psychodynamischen psychotherapie in zeiten der COVID-19-pandemie. Interviewstudie mit psychotherapeut*innen und patient*innen [Video-based treatment in psychodynamic psychotherapy in times of the COVID-19 pandemic. Interview study with patients and psychotherapists]. Psychotherapeut. 2021;66:398–405.
85. Ashwick R, Turgoose D, Murphy D. Exploring the acceptability of delivering cognitive processing therapy (CPT) to UK veterans with PTSD over skype: a qualitative study. Eur J Psychotraumatol. 2019;10:1573128.
86. Christensen LF, Wilson R, Hansen JP, et al. A qualitative study of patients' and providers' experiences with the use of videoconferences by older adults with depression. Int J Ment Health Nurs. 2021;30:427–39.
87. Hensel JM, Yang R, Vigod SN, et al. Videoconferencing at home for psychotherapy in the postpartum period: identifying drivers of successful engagement and important therapeutic conditions for meaningful use. Couns Psychother Res. 2021;21:535–44.
88. Tarp K, Nielsen AS. Patient perspectives on videoconferencing-based treatment for alcohol use disorders. Alcohol Treat Q. 2017;35:344–58.
89. Bryant K, Greer-Williams N, Willis N, Hartwig M. Barriers to diagnosis and treatment of depression: voices from a rural African-American Faith Community. J Nat Black Nurses Assoc. 2013;24(1):31–8.
90. Rajgopal A, Li CR, Shah S, Sundar Budhathoki S. The use of telehealth to overcome barriers to mental health services faced by young people from Afro-Caribbean backgrounds in England during the COVID-19 pandemic. J Glob Health. 2021;11:03040. https://doi.org/10.7189/jogh.11.03040.
91. Vogt EL, Mahmoud H, Elhaj O. Telepsychiatry: implications for psychiatrist burnout and well-being. Psychiatr Serv. 2019;70(5):422–4. https://doi.org/10.1176/appi.ps.201800465.
92. Gardner JS, Plaven BE, Yellowlees P, Shore JH. Remote telepsychiatry workforce: a solution to psychiatry's workforce issues. Curr Psychiatry Rep. 2020;22(2):8. https://doi.org/10.1007/s11920-020-1128-7.
93. Maslach C, Leiter MP. Understanding the burnout experience: recent research and its implications for psychiatry. World Psychiatry. 2016;15:103–11.
94. Adler AB, Adrian AL, Hemphill M, et al. Professional stress and burnout in US military medical personnel deployed to Afghanistan. Mil Med. 2017;182:e1669–76.
95. Allen TD, Golden TD, Shockley KM. How effective is telecommuting? Assessing the status of our scientific findings. Psychol Sci Public Interest. 2015;16:40–68.
96. Salvagioni DAJ, Melanda FN, Mesas AE, et al. Physical, psychological and occupational consequences of job burnout: a systematic review of prospective studies. PLoS One. 2017;12:e0185781.
97. Wyler H, Liebrenz M, Ajdacic-Gross V, Seifritz E, Young S, Burger P, et al. Treatment provision for adults with ADHD during the COVID-19 pandemic: an exploratory study on patient and therapist experience with on-site sessions using face masks vs. telepsychiatric sessions. BMC Psychiatry. 2021;21(1):237.
98. Kinoshita S, Kishimoto T. Advantages and disadvantages of the long-term use of telepsychiatry. Ir J Psychol Med. 2023;40(3):538–9. https://doi.org/10.1017/ipm.2022.21.
99. Møller AM, Christensen LF, Hansen JP, Andersen PT. Patients' acceptance of video consultations in the mental health services—a systematic review and synthesis of qualitative research. Digit Health. 2022;8:20552076221075148. https://doi.org/10.1177/20552076221075148.

100. Shore JH, Yellowlees P, Caudill R, Johnston B, Turvey C, Mishkind M, et al. Best practices in videoconferencing-based telemental health April 2018. Telemed J E Health. 2018;24:827–32. https://doi.org/10.1089/tmj.2018.0237.
101. WPA Telepsychiatry Global Guidelines. 2021. https://www.wpanet.org/_files/ugd/842ec8_ffbb5cd0d874414383cffeee34b511ec.pdf.
102. Chakrabarti S. Usefulness of telepsychiatry: a critical evaluation of videoconferencing-based approaches. World J Psychiatry. 2015;5(3):286–304.
103. Mucic D. Transcultural telepsychiatry and its impact on patient satisfaction. J Telemed Telecare. 2010;16:237–42.
104. Mosadeghrad AM. Factors affecting medical service quality. Iran J Public Health. 2014;43:210–20.
105. McConnochie KM. Webside manner: a key to high-quality primary care telemedicine for all. Telemed J E Health. 2019;25:1007–11. https://doi.org/10.1089/tmj.2018.0274.
106. Chong J, Moreno F. Feasibility and acceptability of clinic-based telepsychiatry for low-income Hispanic primary care patients. Telemed J E Health. 2012;18:297–304.
107. Gelber H. The experience in Victoria with telepsychiatry for the child and adolescent mental health service. J Telemed Telecare. 2001;7:32–4.
108. Ferrer DC, Yellowlees PM. Telepsychiatry: licensing and professional boundary concerns. Virtual Mentor. 2012;14:477–82.
109. Bahloul HJ, Mani N. International telepsychiatry: a review of what has been published. J Telemed Telecare. 2013;19:293–4.
110. Hulsbosch AM, Nugter MA, Tamis P, Kroon H. Videoconferencing in a mental health service in The Netherlands: a randomized controlled trial on patient satisfaction and clinical outcomes for outpatients with severe mental illness. J Telemed Telecare. 2017;23:513–20.
111. Weiner M, Rossetti H, Harrah K. Videoconference diagnosis and management of Choctaw Indian dementia patients. Alzheimers Dement. 2011;7:562–6.
112. Nelson EL, Barnard M, Cain S. Treating childhood depression over videoconferencing. Telemed J E Health. 2003;9:49–55.
113. Faija CL, Connell J, Welsh C, Ardern K, Hopkin E, Gellatly J, et al. What influences practitioners' readiness to deliver psychological interventions by telephone? A qualitative study of behaviour change using the theoretical domains framework. BMC Psychiatry. 2020;20(1):1–16. https://doi.org/10.1186/s12888-020-02761-3.
114. Whitten P, Kuwahara E. A multi-phase telepsychiatry programme in Michigan: organizational factors affecting utilization and user perceptions. J Telemed Telecare. 2004;10:254–61.
115. Graham MA. Telepsychiatry in Appalachia. Am Behav Sci. 1996;39:602–15. https://doi.org/10.1177/0002764296039005007.
116. Hilty DM, Crawford A, Teshima J, Chan S, Sunderji N, Yellowlees PM, et al. A framework for telepsychiatric training and e-health: competency-based education, evaluation and implications. Int Rev Psychiatry. 2015;27:569–92.
117. Hubley S, Lynch SB, Schneck C, Thomas M, Shore J. Review of key telepsychiatry outcomes. World J Psychiatry. 2016;22:269–82.
118. Karlinsky H. Psychiatry, technology, and the corn fields of Iowa. Can J Psychiatry. 2004;49:1–3.
119. Lal S, Abdel-Baki A, Sujanani S, Bourbeau F, Sahed I, Whitehead J. Perspectives of young adults on receiving telepsychiatry services in an urban early intervention program for first-episode psychosis: a cross-sectional, descriptive survey study. Front Psychiatry. 2020;11:117.
120. Malhotra S, Chakrabarti S, Shah R. Telepsychiatry: promise, potential, and challenges. Indian J Psychiatry. 2013;55(1):3–11.
121. Hailey D, Roine R, Ohinmaa A. The effectiveness of telemental health applications: a review. Can J Psychiatr. 2008;53:769–78.
122. Hailey D, Ohinmaa A, Roine R. Limitations in the routine use of telepsychiatry. J Telemed Telecare. 2009;15:28–31.
123. Brooks E, Turvey C, Augusterfer EF. Provider barriers to telemental health: obstacles overcome, obstacles remaining. Telemed J E Health. 2013;19:433–7.

124. Simms DC, Gibson K, O'Donnell S. To use or not to use: clinicians' perceptions of telemental health. Can Psychol. 2011;52:41–51.
125. Luxton DD, Sirotin AP, Mishkind MC. Safety of telemental healthcare delivered to clinically unsupervised settings: a systematic review. Telemed J E Health. 2010;16:705–11.
126. Kramer GM, Mishkinda MC, Luxton DD, Shore JH. Managing risk and protecting privacy in telemental health: an overview of legal, regulatory, and risk-management issues. In: Myers K, Turvey CL, editors. Telemental health. Clinical, technical, and administrative foundations for evidence-based practice. Amsterdam: Elsevier; 2013. p. 83–107.
127. Savin D, Garry MT, Zuccaro P, Novins D. Telepsychiatry for treating rural American Indian youth. J Am Acad Child Adolesc Psychiatry. 2006;45:484–8.
128. Whealin JM, Seibert-Hatalsky LA, Willett Howell J, Tsai J. E-mental health preferences of veterans with and without probable posttraumatic stress disorder. J Rehabil Res Dev. 2015;52(6):725.
129. Moirangthem S, Rao S, Kumar CN, Narayana M, Raviprakash N, Math SB. Telepsychiatry as an economically better model for reaching the unreached: a retrospective report from South India. Indian J Psychol Med. 2017;39:271–5.
130. Munro CC, Hynan LS, Grosch M, Parikh M, Weiner MF. Teleneuropsychology: evidence for video teleconference-based neuropsychological assessment. J Int Neuropsychol Soc. 2014;20:1028–33.
131. O'Brien M, McNicholas F. The use of telepsychiatry during COVID-19 and beyond. Ir J Psychol Med. 2020;37(4):250–5.
132. Paing WW, Weller RA, Welsh B, Foster T, Birnkrant JM, Weller EB. Telemedicine in children and adolescents. Curr Psychiatry Rep. 2009;11:114–9.
133. Ramalho R, Adiukwu F, Gashi Bytyçi D, El Hayek S, Gonzalez Diaz JM, Larnaout A, et al. Telepsychiatry and healthcare access inequities during the COVID-19 pandemic. Asian J Psychiatry. 2020;53:102234.
134. Rothchild E. Telepsychiatry: why do it? Psychiatr Ann. 1999;29:394–401.
135. Ye J, Shim R, Lukaszewski T, Yun K, Kim SH, Ruth G. Telepsychiatry services for Korean immigrants. Telemed J E Health. 2012;18:797–802.
136. Jefee-Bahloul H. Telemental health in the Middle East: overcoming the barriers. Front Public Health. 2014;2:86.
137. Jones RM, Leonard S, Birmingham L. Setting up a telepsychiatry service. Psychiatr Bull. 2006;30:464–7.
138. Benyakorn S. Implementing telepsychiatry in Thailand benefits and challenges. J Med Assoc Thail. 2016;99:S260–6.
139. Buist A, Coman G, Silvas A, Burrows G. An evaluation of the telepsychiatry programme in Victoria, Australia. J Telemed Telecare. 2000;6:216–21.
140. Hensel J, Graham R, Isaak C, Ahmed N, Sareen J, Bolton J. A novel emergency telepsychiatry program in a Canadian Urban setting: identifying and addressing perceived barriers for successful implementation. [Un nouveau programme de télépsychiatrie d'urgence en milieu urbain Canadien: identifier et aborder les obstacles perçus d'une mise en œuvre réussie.]. Can J Psychiatry. 2020;65:559–67.
141. Elford DR, White H, St John K, Maddigan B, Ghandi M, Bowering R. A prospective satisfaction study and cost analysis of a pilot child telepsychiatry service in Newfoundland. J Telemed Telecare. 2001;7:73–81.
142. Gibson K, O'Donnell S, Coulson H, Kakepetum-Schultz T. Mental health professionals' perspectives of telemental health with remote and rural first nations communities. J Telemed Telecare. 2011;17:263–7.
143. Behere PB, Mansharamani HD, Kumar K. Telepsychiatry: reaching the unreached. Indian J Med Res. 2017;146:150–2.
144. Sales CP, McSweeney L, Saleem Y, Khalifa N. The use of telepsychiatry within forensic practice: a literature review on the use of videolink—a ten-year follow-up. J Forensic Psychiatry Psychol. 2018;29:387–402.

145. Gloff NE, LeNoue SR, Novins DK, Myers K. Telemental health for children and adolescents. Int Rev Psychiatry. 2015;27:513–24.
146. Hilty DM, Bourgeois JA, Nesbitt TS, Hales RE. Cost issues with telepsychiatry in the United States. Psychiatr Bull. 2004;28:6–8.
147. Vernig PM. Telemental health: digital disruption and the opportunity to expand care. J Am Psychiatr Nurses Assoc. 2016;22:73–5.
148. van Wynsberghe A, Gastmans C. Telepsychiatry and the meaning of in-person contact: a preliminary ethical appraisal. Med Health Care Philos. 2009;12:469–76.
149. Boydell KM, Hodgins M, Pignatiello A, Teshima J, Edwards H, Willis D. Using technology to deliver mental health services to children and youth: a scoping review. J Can Acad Child Adolesc Psychiatry. 2014;23:87–99.
150. Mielonen M, Ohinmaa A, Moring J, Isohanni M. Videoconferencing in telepsychiatry. J Technol Hum Serv. 2002;20:183–99.
151. Mettner J. The doctor is in another town: telepsychiatry brings care to people in rural Minnesota. Minn Med. 2013;96:22–5.
152. Thompson DA, Leimig R, Gower G, Winsett RP. Assessment of depressive symptoms during post-transplant follow-up care performed via telehealth. Telemed J E Health. 2009;15:700–6.
153. Richardson LK. "Can you see what I am saying?" An action-research, mixed methods evaluation of telepsychology in rural Western Australia. Murdoch: Murdoch University; 2012.
154. Zilcha-Mano S, Dinger U, McCarthy KS, Barber JP. Does alliance predict symptoms throughout treatment, or is it the other way around? J Consult Clin Psychol. 2014;82(6):931.
155. Wootton R, Yellowlees P, McLaren P, editors. Telepsychiatry and e-mental health. Oxfordshire: Taylor & Francis; 2003. ISBN: 9781853157882.
156. Lopez A, Schwenk S, Schneck CD, Griffin RJ, Mishkind MC. Technology-based mental health treatment and the impact on the therapeutic alliance. Curr Psychiatry Rep. 2019;21(8):76.
157. Hall JA, Andrzejewski SA, Yopchick JE. Psychosocial correlates of interpersonal sensitivity: a meta-analysis. J Nonverbal Behav. 2009;33:149–80. https://doi.org/10.1007/s10919-009-0070-5.
158. Schlegel K, Vicaria IM, Isaacowitz DM, Hall JA. Effectiveness of a short audiovisual emotion recognition training program in adults. Motiv Emot. 2017;41:646–60. https://doi.org/10.1007/s11031-017-9631-9.
159. Gullslett MK, Kristiansen E, Nilsen ER. Therapists' experiences of video consultation in specialized mental health services during the COVID-19 pandemic: qualitative interview study. JMIR Hum Factors. 2021;8:e23150.
160. Kaigwa LC, Njenga F, Ongeri L, Nguithi A, Mugane M, Mbugua GM, Anundo J, Kimari MZ, Onono M. Implementation of telepsychiatry in Kenya: acceptability study. BJPsych Open. 2022;8(3):e85. https://doi.org/10.1192/bjo.2022.53.
161. Marcotte-Beaumier G, Bouchard S, Gosselin P, et al. The role of intolerance of uncertainty and working alliance in the outcome of cognitive behavioral therapy for generalized anxiety disorder delivered by videoconference: mediation analysis. JMIR Ment Health. 2021;8:e24541.
162. Ardito RB, Rabellino D. Therapeutic alliance and outcome of psychotherapy: historical excursus, measurements, and prospects for research. Front Psychol. 2011;2:270.
163. Morgan RD, Patrick AR, Magaletta PR. Does the use of telemental health alter the treatment experience? Inmates' perceptions of telemental health versus face-to-face treatment modalities. J Consult Clin Psychol. 2008;76(1):158.
164. Orlando JF, Beard M, Kumar S. Systematic review of patient and caregivers' satisfaction with telehealth videoconferencing as a mode of service delivery in managing patients' health. PLoS One. 2019;14(8):e0221848.
165. Neureiter K, Fuchsberger V, Murer M, Tscheligi M. Hands and eyes: how eye contact is linked to gestures in video conferencing. In: Mackay WE, Brewster SA, Bødker S, editors. Proceedings of the CHI'13 extended abstracts on human factors in computing systems. New York, NY: Association for Computing Machinery; 2013. p. 127–132.

166. Shulman M, John M, Kane JM. Home-based outpatient telepsychiatry to improve adherence with treatment appointments: a pilot study. Psychiatr Serv. 2017;68:743–6.
167. Starr P. Health and the right to privacy. Am J Law Med. 1999;25:193–201.
168. Jenkins-Guarnieri MA, Pruitt LD, Luxton DD, Johnson K. Patient perceptions of telemental health: systematic review of direct comparisons to in-person psychotherapeutic treatments. Telemed J E Health. 2015;21:652–60.
169. Parrot R, Burgoon JK, Burgoon M, LePoire BA. Privacy between physicians and patients: more than a matter of confidentiality. Soc Sci Med. 1989;29:1381–5.
170. Zeavin H. The distance cure: a history of teletherapy. Cambridge, MA: The MIT Press; 2021. ISBN: 978-0-262-04592-6, xviii + 301 pp.
171. Dobkin RD, Mann SL, Gara MA, Interian A, Rodriguez KM, Menza M. Telephone-based cognitive behavioral therapy for depression in Parkinson disease: a randomized controlled trial. Neurology. 2020;94(16):e1764–73. https://doi.org/10.1212/WNL.0000000000009292.
172. Stiles-Shields C, Kwasny MJ, Cai X, Mohr DC. Therapeutic alliance in face-to-face and telephone-administered cognitive behavioral therapy. J Consult Clin Psychol. 2014;82(2):349–54. https://doi.org/10.1037/a0035554.
173. Luxton DD, Pruitt LD, Wagner A, Smolenski DJ, Jenkins-Guarnieri MA, Gahm G. Home-based telebehavioral health for US military personnel and veterans with depression: a randomized controlled trial. J Consult Clin Psychol. 2016;84(11):923. https://doi.org/10.1037/ccp0000135.
174. Watts S, Marchand A, Bouchard S, Gosselin P, Langlois F, Belleville G, et al. Telepsychotherapy for generalized anxiety disorder: impact on the working alliance. J Psychother Integr. 2020;30(2):208. https://doi.org/10.1037/int0000223.
175. Husain MO, Chaudhry IB, Thomasson R, Kiran T, Bassett P, Husain MI, et al. Cognitive function in early psychosis patients from a lower middle-income country. Int J Psychiatry Clin Pract. 2018;22:13–8. https://doi.org/10.1080/13651501.2017.1341987.
176. Kister K, et al. Are we ready for telepsychiatry? Benefits and challenges of digital psychotherapy. Curr Probl Psychiatry. 2023;24:52–67.
177. General Medical Council. Remote consultations. 2019. https://www.gmc-uk.org/ethical-guidance/ethical-hub/remote-consultations.
178. British Medical Association. COVID-19: video consultations and homeworking. 2021. https://www.bma.org.uk/advice-and-support/covid-19/adapting-to-covid/covid-19-video-consultations-and-homeworking.
179. NHS England. Specialty guides for patient management during the coronavirus pandemic (Publication 001559). 2020. https://www.nice.org.uk/media/default/about/covid-19/specialty-guides/specialty-guide-virtual-working-and-coronavirus.pdf.
180. Royal College of Psychiatrists. Digital—COVID-19 guidance for clinicians. 2020. https://www.rcpsych.ac.uk/about-us/responding-to-covid-19/responding-to-covid-19-guidance-for-clinicians/digital-covid-19-guidance-for-clinicians.
181. Dorsey ER, Topol EJ. State of telehealth. N Engl J Med. 2016;375(2):154–61.
182. Daschle T, Dorsey ER. The return of the house call. Am Coll Phys. 2015;162:587–8.
183. Lepkowsky CM. Telehealth reimbursement allows access to mental health care during COVID-19. Am J Geriatr Psychiatry. 2020;28:898–9.
184. Cowan KE, McKean AJ, Gentry MT, Hilty DM. Barriers to use of telepsychiatry: clinicians as gatekeepers. Mayo Clin Proc. 2019;94(12):2510–23. https://doi.org/10.1016/j.mayocp.2019.04.018.
185. Torous J, Wykes T. Opportunities from the coronavirus disease 2019 pandemic for transforming psychiatric care with telehealth. JAMA Psychiatry. 2020;77:1205. https://doi.org/10.1001/jamapsychiatry.2020.1640.
186. Lakdawala PD. Doctor-patient relationship in psychiatry. Mens Sana Monogr. 2015;13(1):82.
187. Kaftarian E. Lessons learned in prison and jail-based telepsychiatry. Curr Psychiatry Rep. 2019;21:15.

188. Ertelt TW, Crosby RD, Marino JM, Mitchell JE, Lancaster K, Crow SJ. Therapeutic factors affecting the cognitive behavioral treatment of bulimia nervosa via telemedicine versus face-to-face delivery. Int J Eat Disord. 2011;44(8):687–91.
189. Simpson S, Reid C. Telepsychology in Australia: 20/20 vision. Aust J Rural Health. 2014;22(6):306–9.
190. Gammon D, Bergvik S, Bergmo T, Pedersen S. Videoconferencing in psychiatry: a survey of use in northern Norway. J Telemed Telecare. 1996;2:192–8.
191. Batastini AB, McDonald BR, Morgan RD. Videoteleconferencing in forensic and correctional practice. In: Myers K, Turvey CL, editors. Telemental health: clinical, technical, and administrative foundations for evidence-based practice. Amsterdam: Elsevier; 2013. p. 251–71.
192. Agarwal PP, Manjunatha N, Gowda GS, Kumar MNG, Shanthaveeranna N, Kumar CN, et al. Collaborative tele-neuropsychiatry consultation services for patients in central prisons. J Neurosci Rural Pract. 2019;10:101–5.
193. Chipps J, Ramlall S, Madigoe T, King H, Mars M. Developing telepsychiatry services in KwaZulu-Natal—an action research study. Afr J Psychiatry. 2012;15:255–63.
194. Myers K. Telepsychiatry: time to connect. J Am Acad Child Adolesc Psychiatry. 2013;52:217–9.
195. Valdagno M, Goracci A, di Volo S, Fagiolini A. Telepsychiatry: new perspectives and open issues. CNS Spectr. 2014;19:479–81.
196. Combi C, Pozzani G, Pozzi G. Telemedicine for developing countries. A survey and some design issues. Appl Clin Inform. 2016;7:1025–50.
197. He D, Naveed M, Gunter CA, Nahrstedt K. Security concerns in android mHealth apps. AMIA Annu Symp Proc. 2014;2014:645–54.
198. Lustgarten SD, Garrison YL, Sinnard MT, Flynn AW. Digital privacy in mental healthcare: current issues and recommendations for technology use. Curr Opin Psychol. 2020;36:25–31. https://doi.org/10.1016/j.copsyc.2020.03.012.
199. Barnett JE. The ethical practice of psychotherapy: clearly within our reach. Psychotherapy. 2019;56:431–40. https://doi.org/10.1037/pst0000272.
200. Watzlaf VJM, Dealmeida DR, Zhou L, Hartman LM. Protocol for a systematic review of telehealth privacy and security research to identify best practices. Int J Telerehabil. 2015;7:15–22.
201. Uscher-Pines L, Raja P, Qureshi N, Huskamp HA, Busch AB, Mehrotra A. Use of tele–mental health in conjunction with in-person care: a qualitative exploration of implementation models. Psychiatr Serv. 2020;71(5):419–26.
202. Kinoshita S, Cortright K, Crawford A, Mizuno Y, Yoshida K, Hilty D, Guinart D, Torous J, Correll CU, Castle DJ, Rocha D, Yang Y, Xiang YT, Kølbæk P, Dines D, ElShami M, Jain P, Kallivayalil R, Solmi M, Favaro A, Veronese N, Seedat S, Shin S, Salazar de Pablo G, Chang CH, Su KP, Karas H, Kane JM, Yellowlees P, Kishimoto T. Changes in telepsychiatry regulations during the COVID-19 pandemic: 17 countries and regions' approaches to an evolving healthcare landscape. Psychol Med. 2022;52(13):2606–13. https://doi.org/10.1017/S0033291720004584.
203. Strudwick G, Impey D, Torous J, Krausz RM, Wiljer D. Advancing E-mental health in Canada: report from a multistakeholder meeting. JMIR Ment Health. 2020;7:e19360. https://doi.org/10.2196/19360.
204. Cash CD. Telepsychiatry and risk management. Innov Clin Neurosci. 2011;8(9):26–30.
205. Substance Abuse and Mental Health Services Administration. Using telehealth to expand access to essential health services in rural areas; 2017.
206. American Academy of Child and Adolescent Psychiatry. Guidelines for the practice of telepsychiatry with children and adolescents. 2017. https://www.aacap.org/AACAP/Clinical_Practice_Center/Business_of_Practice/Telepsychiatry/Telepsychiatry_Guide_and_Pol.aspx.
207. Maheu MM, Drude KP, Hertlein KM, Lipschutz R, Wall KM, Long R. Telebehavioral health guidelines for disasters: a call to action. J Technol Behav Sci. 2018;3(3):156–69.
208. American Medical Association. AMA telehealth quick guide. 2016. https://www.ama-assn.org/practice-management/digital/ama-telehealth-quick-guide.

209. Department of Veterans Affairs & Department of Defense. Clinical practice guideline for the assessment and management of patients at risk for suicide; 2019.
210. Ministry of Health & Family Welfare, Government of India. Telemedicine practice guidelines. 2020. https://www.mohfw.gov.in/pdf/Telemedicine.pdf.
211. Royal Australian and New Zealand College of Psychiatrists. Professional practice guideline 19 telehealth in psychiatry. 2021. https://www.ranzcp.org/getmedia/aaec525c-f2da-4b98-b10f-76175ae494e2/ppg-19-telehealth-in-psychiatry.pdf.
212. Practice Guidelines for Video-based Telehealth Services. BC Children's Hospital. 2014. http://www.bcchildrens.ca/mental-health-services-site/Documents/Practice%20Guidelines%20for%20Video-based%20Telehealth%20Services-2014.pdf.
213. Helverskov T, Nielsen AS, Bendixen IK, Folker MP. Retningslinje for Videokonsultationer i Psykiatrien i Region Syddanmark, 1. og 2. udgave. 1st and 2nd ed. 2021.
214. Nielsen AC, et al. Vejledning til anvendel. 2020. http://www.bcchildrens.ca/mental-health-services-site/Documents/Practice%20Guidelines%20for%20Video-based%20Telehealth%20Services-2014.pdf. se af video i ambulant behandling i Region Hovedstadens Psykiatri. https://www.fagperson.psykiatrien.rm.dk/siteassets/04-til-ansatte-og-samarbejdspartnere/generelle-informationer/videomoder/2022.05_video-vejledning_v15_webtilgangelig.pdf.
215. Krzystanek M, Matuszczyk M, Przybyło J, Dudek D, Gałecki P, Bieńkowski P, Szafrański T, Samochowiec J. Letter to the editor. The Polish standard of teleconsultation in psychiatry. Psychiatr Pol. 2021;55(6):1473–7. https://doi.org/10.12740/PP/142523.
216. Private and Independent Practice Specialist Interest Group for Psychiatrists. PIPSIG guidelines for the use of telepsychiatry. London: Royal College of Psychiatrists; 2013. https://www.rcpsych.ac.uk/docs/default-source/members/sigs/private-and-independent-practice-pipsig/pipsig-telepsychiatry-guidelines-revised-mar16.pdf?sfvrsn=30d4c605_2.
217. American Psychiatric Association (APA). Telepsychiatry toolkit. 2021. https://www.psychiatry.org/psychiatrists/practice/telepsychiatry/toolkit.
218. American Telemedicine Association. Practice guidelines. 2020. https://www.americantelemed.org/resource_categories/practice-guidelines/.
219. Pineau G, Moqadem K, St-Hilaire C, Levac E, Hamel B, Bergeron H, Obadia A, Caron L. Telehealth: clinical guidelines and technological standards for telepsychiatry. http://www.isfteh.org/files/media/68a2b452fb83e00f41219a6cbd075f27.pdf.
220. Hariman K, Ventriglio A, Bhugra D. The future of digital psychiatry. Curr Psychiatry Rep. 2019;13:88.
221. Deslich SA, Thistlethwaite T, Coustasse A. Telepsychiatry in correctional facilities: using technology to improve access and decrease costs of mental health care in underserved populations. Perm J. 2013;17(3):80–6.
222. Southard EP, Neufeld JD, Laws S. Telemental health evaluations enhance access and efficiency in a critical access hospital emergency department. Telemed J E Health. 2014;20(7):664–8.
223. Hilty DM, Johnston B, McCarron RM. How e-mental health adds to traditional outpatient and newer models of integrated care for patients, providers, and systems. In: Mucic D, Hilty DM, editors. e-Mental health. Berlin: Springer International Publishing; 2016. p. 129–49.
224. Hilty DM, Gentry MT, McKean AJ, Cowan KE, Lim RF, Lu FG. Telehealth for rural diverse populations: telebehavioral and cultural competencies, clinical outcomes and administrative approaches. Mhealth. 2020;6:20. https://doi.org/10.21037/mhealth.2019.10.04.
225. Hilty DM, Rabinowitz TR, McCarron RM, et al. Telepsychiatry and e-mental health models leverage stepped, collaborative, and integrated services to primary care. Psychosomatics. 2018;59:227–50.
226. Hilty DM, Nesbitt T, Kuenneth TS, et al. Rural versus suburban primary care needs, utilization, and satisfaction with telepsychiatric consultation. J Rural Health. 2007;23:163–5.
227. Katon W, Von Korff M, Lin E, et al. Collaborative management to achieve treatment guidelines impact on depression in primary care. JAMA. 1995;273:1026–31.
228. Greenberg WE, Paulsen RH. Moving into the neighborhood: preparing residents to participate in a primary care environment. Harv Rev Psychiatry. 1996;4:107–9.

229. Simon GE. Randomized trial of monitoring, feedback, and management of care by telephone to improve treatment of depression in primary care. Br Med J. 2000;320:550–4.
230. National Council Medical Director Institute. The psychiatric shortage: causes and solutions. 2017. https://www.thenationalcouncil.org/wp-content/uploads/2017/03/Psychiatric-Shortage_National-Council-.pdf.
231. Moran M. No. of seniors matching into psychiatry takes large leap. Psychiatr News. 2017;52:1. https://doi.org/10.1176/appi.pn.2017.4b8.
232. Butler DJ, Fons D, Fisher T, Sanders J, Bodenhamer S, Owen JR, Gunderson M. A review of the benefits and limitations of a primary care-embedded psychiatric consultation service in a medically underserved setting. Int J Psychiatry Med. 2018;53(5–6):415–26.
233. Lee WC, Sumaya CV. Geriatric workforce capacity: a pending crisis for nursing home residents. Front Public Health. 2013;1:24.
234. Beck AJ, Page C, Buche J, et al. Estimating the distribution of the US Psychiatric Subspecialist Workforce. Ann Arbor, MI: University of Michigan School of Public Health Behavioral Health Workforce Research Center; 2018. http://www.behavioralhealthworkforce.org/wp-content/uploads/2019/02/Y3-FA2-P2-Psych-Sub_Full-Report-FINAL2.19.2019.pdf.
235. Brenes GA, Danhauer SC, Lyles MF, Hogan PE, Miller ME. Barriers to mental health treatment in rural older adults. Am J Geriatr Psychiatry. 2015;23(11):1172–8.
236. Hilty DM, Seritan AL, Rabinowitz T. Telemedicine and IT: use of digital technology on inpatient units. In: Fenn HH, Hategan A, Bourgeois JA, editors. Inpatient geriatric psychiatry. Cham: Springer International Publishing; 2019.
237. Salmoiraghi A, Hussain S. A systematic review of the use of telepsychiatry in acute settings. J Psychiatr Pract. 2015;21:389–93.
238. Butterfield A. Telepsychiatric evaluation and consultation in emergency care settings. Child Adolesc Psychiatr Clin North Am. 2018;27:467–78.
239. Koblauch H, Reinhardt SM, Lissau WJ, Jensen P. The effect of telepsychiatric modalities on reduction of readmissions in psychiatric settings: a systematic review. J Telemed Telecare. 2018;24:31–6.
240. Hilty DM, Sunderji N, Suo S, Chan S, McCarron RM. Telepsychiatry and other technologies for integrated care: evidence base, best practice models and competencies. Int Rev Psychiatry. 2018;30:292–309.
241. Kimmel RJ, Toor R. Telepsychiatry by a public, academic medical center for inpatient consults at an unaffiliated, community hospital. Psychosomatics. 2019;60:468–73.
242. Morris NP, Hirschtritt ME. Telepsychiatry, hospitals, and the COVID-19 pandemic. Psychiatr Serv. 2020;71(12):1309–12. https://doi.org/10.1176/appi.ps.202000216. Epub 2020 Sep 16. PMID: 32933415.
243. Mahmoud H, Vogt E. Telepsychiatry: an innovative approach to addressing the opioid crisis. J Behav Health Serv Res. 2019;46(4):680–5. https://doi.org/10.1007/s11414-018-9611-1.
244. Amirsadri A, Burns J, Pizzuti A, Arfken CL. Home-based telepsychiatry in US urban area. Case Rep Psychiatry. 2017;2017:6296423. https://doi.org/10.1155/2017/6296423. Epub 2017 May 29.
245. Maniaci MJ, Maita K, Torres-Guzman RA, Avila FR, Garcia JP, Eldaly A, Forte AJ, Matcha GV, Pagan RJ, Paulson MR. Provider evaluation of a novel virtual hybrid hospital at home model. Int J Gen Med. 2022;15:1909–18. https://doi.org/10.2147/IJGM.S354101.
246. Pew Research Center. Demographics of internet and home broadband usage in the United States. Published June 12, 2019. Accessed 9 Mar 2021. https://www.pewresearch.org/internet/fact-sheet/internet-broadband/.
247. Zulman DM, Wong EP, Slightam C, et al. Making connections: nationwide implementation of video telehealth tablets to address access barriers in veterans. JAMIA Open. 2019;2(3):323–9.
248. Block L, Ruane K. The future of state telehealth policy. Published 2020. Accessed 9 Mar 2021. https://www.nga.org/wp-content/uploads/2020/11/The-Future-of-State-Telehealth-Policy.pdf.

249. Nouri SS, Khoong EC, Lyles CR, Karliner LS. Addressing equity in telemedicine for chronic disease management during the COVID-19 pandemic. Published May 4, 2020. Accessed 4 Mar 2021.
250. Eyrich NW, Andino JJ, Fessell DP. Bridging the digital divide to avoid leaving the most vulnerable behind. JAMA Surg. 2021;156(8):703–4. https://doi.org/10.1001/jamasurg.2021.1143.
251. Sabin JE, Skimming K. A framework of ethics for telepsychiatry practice. Int Rev Psychiatry. 2015;27(6):490–5. https://doi.org/10.3109/09540261.2015.1094034. Epub 2015 Oct 23.
252. Chaet D, Clearfield R, Sabin JE, Skimming K, Council on Ethical and Judicial Affairs American Medical Association. Ethical practice in telehealth and telemedicine. J Gen Intern Med. 2017;32(10):1136–40. https://doi.org/10.1007/s11606-017-4082-2. Epub 2017 Jun 26.
253. https://familymedicine.uw.edu/wp-content/uploads/2020/06/Telemedicine-Best-Practice-Guidelines-1.pdf.
254. Riplinger L. AHIMA public policy statement on telehealth. J AHIMA. American Association of Nurse Practitioners (AANP), Board of Directors "Position Statement: Telehealth." 2019. https://www.aanp.org/advocacy/advocacy-resource/position-statements/telehealth.
255. American Telemedicine Association (ATA). Health. virtually. Everywhere. 2020. https://www.americantelemed.org/policies/ata-policy-principles/.
256. Federation of State Medicine Boards (FSMB). Model policy for the appropriate use of telemedicine technologies in the practice of medicine. 2014. www.fsmb.org.
257. Curfman AL, Hackell JM, Herendeen NE, et al. AAP Section on Telehealth Care, Committee on Practice and Ambulatory Medicine, Committee on Pediatric Workforce "Telehealth: improving access to and quality of pediatric health care". Pediatrics. 2021;148(3):e2021053129.
258. Kannarkat JT, Smith NN, McLeod-Bryant SA. Mobilization of telepsychiatry in response to COVID-19-moving toward 21(st) century access to care. Adm Policy Ment Health. 2020;47:489–91.
259. United Nations. Policy brief: COVID-19 and the need for action on mental health. https://unsdg.un.org/sites/default/files/2020-05/UN-Policy-Brief-COVID-19-and-mental-health.pdf.
260. Torous J, Jan Myrick K, Rauseo-Ricupero N, Firth J. Digital mental health and COVID-19: using technology today to accelerate the curve on access and quality tomorrow. JMIR Ment Health. 2020;7:e18848. https://doi.org/10.2196/18848.
261. Ontario Ministry of Health and Ministry of Long-Term Care. Changes to the schedule of benefits for physician services (schedule) in response to COVID-19 influenza pandemic; 2020.
262. Goldbloom D, Gratzer D. Telepsychiatry 2.0. Can J Psychiatry. 2017;62(10):688–9. https://doi.org/10.1177/0706743717714469.
263. Saeed SA, Johnson TL, Bagga M, et al. Training residents in the use of telepsychiatry: review of the literature and a proposed elective. Psychiatr Q. 2017;88(2):271–83.
264. Shore JH, Hilty DM. Telepsychiatry and health technologies: a guide for mental health professionals. Washington, DC: American Psychiatric Publishing; 2019.
265. Baird MB, Whitney L, Caedo CE. Experiences and attitudes among psychiatric mental health advanced practice nurses in the use of telemental health: results of an online survey. J Am Psychiatr Nurses Assoc. 2018;24(3):235–40.
266. Hyler SE, Gangure DP, Batchelder ST. Can telepsychiatry replace in-person psychiatric assessments? A review and meta-analysis of comparison studies. CNS Spectr. 2005;10:403–13.

How Digital Mental Health Adds to Traditional Outpatient and Newer Models of Integrated Care for Patients, Providers, and Systems

10

Robert M. McCarron, Donald M. Hilty, and Krzysztof Krysta

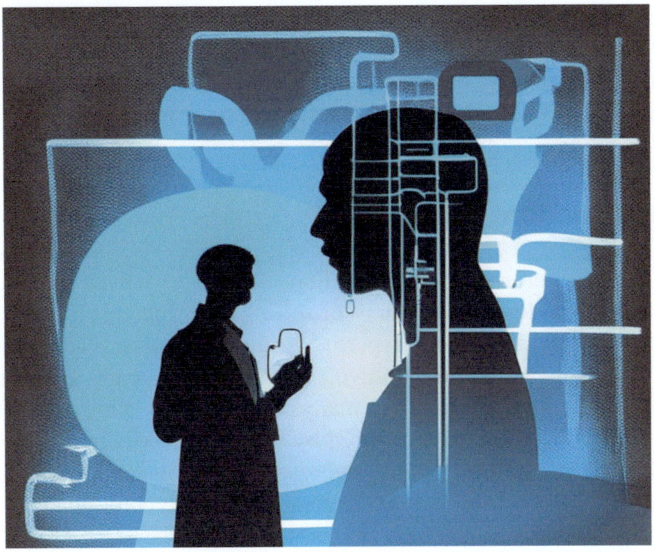

R. M. McCarron
Department of Anesthesiology and Pain Medicine, University of California, Sacramento, CA, USA
e-mail: robert.mccarron@ucdmc.ucdavis.edu

D. M. Hilty
Department of Psychiatry and Behavioral Sciences, Keck School of Medicine University of Southern California, Los Angeles, CA, USA
e-mail: donald.hilty@uhsinc.com; hilty@med.usc.edu

K. Krysta (✉)
Department and Clinic of Psychiatric Rehabilitation, Faculty of Medical Sciences in Katowice, Medical University in Katowice, Katowice, Poland
e-mail: krysta@mp.pl

D. Mucić, D. M. Hilty (eds.), *Digital Mental Health*,
https://doi.org/10.1007/978-3-031-59936-1_10

Abstract

Contemporary healthcare promotes a patient-centered approach, integrates health/mental healthcare, emphasizes interdisciplinary teamwork, and adopts innovations such as communications technology. Telemedicine (including telepsychiatry) adds versatility to service delivery by improving access to care, leveraging expertise of key disciplines to the point-of-service, and disseminating education. Key disciplines in integrated care that provide mental health services into primary care are the psychiatrists, mid-level professionals, and nurses. These clinicians provide clinical, administrative, and care coordination expertise or oversight. A more recent addition to this integrated team is the care navigator who essentially coordinates care across all other team members and the patients. Overall, telemedicine, cross-training, stepped care roles, and use of clinically "versatile" clinicians— all of these help to fill "holes" in services for patients. Evidence-based treatment becomes more accessible, better disseminated, and in "real-time" with the use of health technologies. Best practices for clinical care, education, and program development are needed for integrated care and e-health.

10.1 Introduction

Healthcare is being confronted with questions on how to deliver quality, affordable, and timely care to patients in a variety of settings [1]. Increased clinical operating efficiency gets the clinician with expertise to the point-of-service and emphasizes teamwork for clinical, administrative, and informal care coordination (see Table 10.1). Specifically, this involves many disciplines working at the "top of one's license." For psychiatry, this is facilitated by having non-MD mental health professionals seeing the less complex cases and reserving the psychiatrist's direct clinical time judiciously; this may include management of more complicated cases or providing clinical oversight and review of cases seen by others. Psychiatric disorders/illnesses significantly impact primary care, as those with psychiatric illness (e.g., schizophrenia, bipolar disorder, and recurrent major depression) have higher mortality primarily due to socioeconomic factors, poor access to effective primary/preventative care, and the burden of chronic health conditions [2].

One of the best options for integrated care appears to be using telemedicine/telepsychiatry for clinical care, education, and other interventions [3]. In its sixth decade, telepsychiatry has increased access to care in urban, suburban, and rural settings—with patient, clinicians, and healthcare systems very satisfied with it for a wide variety of services and cultures [3, 4]. Telepsychiatry has been shown effective for diagnosis and assessment across many populations (e.g., adult, child, geriatric, and ethnic), for psychiatric disorders in many settings (e.g., emergency, home health), and has been found to be comparable to in-person care. It has been used with a variety of models of care (i.e., collaborative care, asynchronous, mobile, and telemonitoring) with equally positive outcomes [3]. Telehealth has been shown to

Table 10.1 Healthcare innovation and evolution: the changing ecosystem

Stressors/changes/ trends to healthcare and "global" parties involved	Changes, trends, and stressors in the healthcare ecosystem	Challenges moving from traditional practice to a new model/ecosystem of healthcare
$		
% GNP	1/6 of the GNP is more than other countries spend, not sustainable, and contains duplication/ inefficiency/waste	Change is the primary obstacle, assuming that a new paradigm could be agreed upon and integration could occur
Recession and unbalanced budget	Economic times are not good and most likely, over time, more "pressure" will arise	Short-term costs, fear, and loss of existing frameworks will be used as reasons to not change
National leadership		
Accountability	Leaders want more accountability from providers and institutions Medicine leaves itself vulnerable by "blind spots" (e.g., lack of self-policing, COIs) and an ineffective, unintegrated lobby	Fiefdoms, systems in isolation and even private practices are being assailed The "rich" get richer and the "poor" get poorer at least in research and AHC grants
Control vs. free market tension	The current system has "ballooned" as much as it can, it will deflate, parties will "leave" due to inadequate profits and reform will cut costs, and technology goes "around" current obstacles for those with means	Cost will be cut in a "good" or "worse" ways = > there is incentive to look at this for patients, payees, and payors? Obama care will re-sort populations e-health will re-distribute care
Decrease disparities	Many Americans support better access and the costs of SES determinants (e.g., lack of education) for uninsured are more obvious	Many parties' dissatisfaction will unite toward reform; ACA and 2014; communities are mobilizing
Payors/reimbursement		
Metrics are changing or need to shift	Reimbursement based on non-outcomes (e.g., a trainee providing care, service delivered) do not result in the "best" outcomes	The movement for quality, affordability, access, portability, safety, and other indices is strong
MD-centered to patient-centered		
What should be the unifying or organizing model of service delivery?	The AHC or clinic model of care works for only a few, not efficient, costly, and not patient-centered	How do we partner with patients to share decisions (better), work with communities, and define goals based on populations?
Parameters of "good" care are?	Systems were set up on "best" care models what were defined by AHCs or specialties, not always tested in all populations and not accessible to many	The "best" care by "best" provider "Fast," timely, portable Cheap/inexpensive or affordable Culturally and linguistically sensitive

(continued)

Table 10.1 (continued)

Stressors/changes/ trends to healthcare and "global" parties involved	Changes, trends, and stressors in the healthcare ecosystem	Challenges moving from traditional practice to a new model/ecosystem of healthcare
Provider/team satisfaction		
How do we define it and what are our values?	"Traditional" metrics were "good" care, expert-based (now EBM), training the new generation, making scientific advances and knowledge My career is not everything to me?	Additions or reform questions: How can I see impact better, enjoy what I do, be helpful to high utilizers or those with differences, make a good living, be independent and team up?
AHC-centered to patient-or community-centered systems		
What is the difference, really? We already work to help patients, right?	We (AHCs) "know" best and are the leaders—Why do we need help? Why do things have to change? Do our skills need to change? Translational research is a "good" idea but not for everything Of course we want quality and safe care…we do that already	If we do include others, who should they be and what do we have to change? How to "stay" a doctor and shift from knowledge → skills → leadership and improvisation We have to do translational education, clinical care, and administration too? How do I learn to collect different data, enter it, analyze it, and measure outcomes?
Transformed training: Quality, safe		
Other		
	Medicine moves slowly to maintain the patient-doctor relationship, ensure validity of diagnosis and treatments, and preserve the profession	How do we… Use technology for integration and access Vertically and horizontally integrate care Make care transparent and predictable Shift evaluation to a primary role Maintain privacy, confidentiality, and such

assist healthcare professionals by providing timely access to specialty care [5, 6] and also for education/lifelong learning opportunities [7, 8].

Integrated care provides an approach to psychiatric illness in a general medical setting, and though not quite as well known, providing general medical care in a primary psychiatric clinical setting (i.e., "reverse integration"). The *seven core characteristics/levels* of integrated care include first, responsibility, decision-making, and oversight of patient care; this is true for the entire interdisciplinary team from physicians to care coordinators. A second characteristic is the co-location of services, both literally and/or virtually—that applies to both inpatient and outpatient sector care. Characteristics three to five are integrated funding, evaluation, and outcome measurement. We contend that two additional characteristics are needed: sixth, an e-platform, and seventh, reimbursement. Reimbursement is variable in the United States as it may align (e.g., a capitated or sole "Medicare" population) or not align (i.e., mixed populations) with one or more payers.

This chapter will help the reader to: (1) Use a patient-centered, integrated approach to facilitate quality, access, and affordable care, in general, and for comorbid conditions (e.g., depression/diabetes); (2) Learn how telehealth is a versatile option for stepped and integrated care models; and (3) Evaluate role definitions, telehealth, and integrated care training needs, cross-training and interdisciplinary teamwork that help with integrated care.

10.2 Patient-Centered and Integrated Care: The Participants, Quality Care, and Evaluation

Integrated models of care (IMCs) are patient-centered and usually have a psychiatrist as a consultant with co-location of psychiatric and medical services [9]. IMC improves *medical* outcomes in primary care settings, [10] via mental health (MH) case managers, [11, 12] in terms of patient functional improvement, [13] reduced disability days, [14] increased quality-adjusted life years, [15] and increased adherence to medication [14] when compared with other models of care. IMC psychiatric outcomes may include improved global assessment of function (GAF), geriatric depression scale (GDS) scores, or mini-mental status examination (MMSE) scores.

Patients are generally stratified in quadrants—with the setting pre-determining those quadrants. In outpatient care, there are four quadrants [16]:

- I: low medical and mental health (MH),
- II: low medical and high MH,
- III: low MH and high medical, and.
- IV: high for both.

In the medical inpatient setting, the quadrants are:

- I: medium-to-high psychiatric acuity and none-to-low medical acuity,
- II: medium-to-high medical acuity and none-to-low psychiatric acuity,
- III: medium-to-high psychiatric acuity and low-to-medium medical acuity, and.
- IV: medium-to-high psychiatric acuity and medium-to-high [17].

Poor outcomes for patients with psychiatric and medical comorbidity have been alarming. In addition to the poor medical outcomes mentioned above, patients with major depression are also at higher risk of medical illnesses, such as diabetes mellitus and ischemic heart disease [18, 19] and there may be increased risk of diabetes, metabolic syndrome, cardiovascular disease, and stroke associated with atypical antipsychotics [20]. A recent review measured the outcomes in the literature, systematically, in terms of the participants, description of the IMC, interventions, and outcomes [21].

Outcomes can be stratified by who is designated the primary service and the secondary consultant, which is usually the model except for fully integrated units. The history and recent trends in the literature are best summarized as:

- Medical outpatient: historically, it went from the 1980s with no/little psychiatric/MH care, to "curbside" consultations, [22] to one-time psychiatric consultation one-time usually off-site, to consultation on-site, to 1995 with a collaborative care model, [23] to the late 1990s with a telepsychiatry consultation & disease management; [24, 25] email and phone consultation [26] to traditional integrated behavioral health on site (above) and now collaborative care by telepsychiatry [25, 27].
- Medical inpatient: historically, it went from no/little psychiatric/MH care, to "curbside" consultations, one-time psychiatric consultation or ongoing, to liaison for education role and support and eventually to medical-psychiatric units; only recently has a collaborative care model been applied to the inpatient setting.
- Psychiatric outpatient setting: historically, it went from none/little, to "curbside" consultations, one-time medical evaluation/consultation usually off-site, but very rarely to consultation or a collaborative care model; no reverse integration by telepsychiatry consultation has been described to date.
- Psychiatric inpatient/hospital setting: historically, it went from none/little, to "curbside" consultations, one-time medical evaluation in the emergency room (ER; either "medical clearance" or medicine consultation in psychiatry ER) or at admission, but very rarely to consultation or a collaborative care model; no reverse integration by telepsychiatry consultation has been described to date. Ironically, dietetics/nutrition is often co-located on the unit, and an additional medical initial or PRN evaluation may occur.

In addition to traditional psychiatric consultation to medicine or primary care and integrated or joint units, there are: (1) multidisciplinary joint treatment by a geriatric team in addition to the usual care on a general medicine ward; [28] (2) a "Type IV" integrated medicine and psychiatry treatment program with the provisions of an acute medicine as well as a psychiatric ward. Administered through the department of internal medicine; [17] and a (3) nurse-led mental health liaison service in addition to usual care in internal medicine [29].

10.2.1 Program Evaluation and Leadership

Program evaluation has become increasingly important to meet program, patient, provider, and externally driven (Joint Commission, reimbursement) needs. Its roots therefore are founded in a clinical care, business, quality improvement, and organizational leadership. Alignment of participants' missions from the top to the bottom cannot be overstated—is there support for infrastructure, short-and long-term planning, competency development for participants, adequate funding, and fitness? Good evaluation of outcomes related to telemental health (TMH) begins with a program and its fitness: organization, function (e.g., adaptability, change management), leadership (i.e., vision, operations), and team members (e.g., interdisciplinary with overlapping roles or cross-training), experience with growth, and many other parameters. Programmatic changes are based on the evaluation of all participants and an iterative feedback loop.

Contemporary program evaluation—and the integration of mental health and medical services—represents a substantial philosophical shift for many. Adding an e-services component increases versatility but also adds complexity [30, 31]. The potential for misunderstanding among large teams is tremendous unless a shared mental model of expectations, roles, and outcomes is created [32]. For integrated care, questions are the starting place and the point to return to, since few programs are built proactively to do this work. Questions fall into four main domains:

- Leadership and decision-making: Is there a common goal? Is there joint responsibility? Are the medical and MH sides well represented and collaborative? This is from the big (i.e., program design) to the small (when to discharge, clinical goals).
- Structure: How are the services co-located-physically/virtual? Is the reporting among the clinical, administrative, and other academic/practice bodies well aligned?
- Stepped care with a range of in-person and e-service options: Do folks practice at “the top of their license”? Can the patient access care in many ways or places? Is telemedicine facilitating or delivering the services/expertise efficiently?
- Are outcomes for clinical services (i.e., medically-and MH-based), team players’ education/training, [33] and program goals in harmony and measurable?

10.3 Telemedicine and TMH: How It Can Help Integrate Care

E-platforms have traditionally distributed academic networks of like-minded researchers and clinicians into regional health information organizations (RHIOs). These RHIOs: empower consumers and clinicians in day-to-day healthcare delivery by improving access to evidence-based information at the point of care; facilitate the delivery of a wider range of health services, particularly to primary and community care; provide accurate data to support research and clinical policy and governance arrangements; and ensure a sustainable, secure, reliable electronic environment, underpinned by strong, policy-driven privacy protection [33]. Previously, the single most important technical innovation was broadband distribution, which enables high-quality videoconferencing, multi-media-based applications, and other options, particularly doctor’s desk. The contemporary e-platform adds the EMR, integration of in-person, and TMH care administration (i.e., scheduling, documentation, payment, and other), enhanced patient-to doctor or system engagement/communication (e.g., HIPAA-compliant email "into" the EMR (e.g., Relay Health), and leveraging the expertise at a distance (phone, email, video, asynchronous, and other methods).

Telemental health (TMH) models of clinical care and education have pros and cons, [3, 35, 36] including their level of overall intensity, cost, feasibility, and depth of the relationship between the TMH provider, the PCP, and the patient. *Low-intensity* models include tele-education, formal case review, and in-person, telephone, or email doctor-to-doctor "curbside" consultations. A systematic approach was a multi-specialty phone and email teleconsultation system for adults and children with developmental disabilities [37]. *Moderate-intensity* models include an integrated program of mental health screening, therapy on site, and telepsychiatric consultation (phone, email, or video), with continuing medical education (CME) and training on screening questionnaires [38, 39] or asynchronous telepsychiatry (ATP) to primary care in English and Spanish-speaking patients in primary care [4, 40, 41]. High-*intensity* models are typically the ones previously mentioned involving collaborative care [27, 42–44] (Table 10.2).

Stepped care models may be the most cost-effective models in a health system where the effectiveness of the intervention is maximized by making the best use of resources adequately available at the right time [44, 45]. The stepped care model seems to be a logical approach from both clinical and economic perspectives and several countries; [46] England and New Zealand have implemented guidelines for the stepped care model for managing common mental disorders, including depression and anxiety. The first trial on 170 older adults recruited in primary care found the stepped care program halved the incidence of depression and anxiety disorders from 24% to 12% in 12 months [47] with demonstrated cost-effectiveness [48] and the positive effects were sustained at 24 months [49].

The patient-centered medical home (PCMH) is a concept founded on the presence of inadequate treatment in primary care and/or an inability to access needed services [50]. Under the oversight of the primary care provider, PCMH allows telepsychiatric input at home and has been shown to improve patient care and health [51, 52]. Desk-mounted video systems offer great convenience for therapy to cancer patients to avoid travel, but the cost used to be prohibitive for most consumers [51, 52].

HealthLinkNow, in the United States, with funding from the Center for Medicaid and Medicare Innovation, has integrated telepsychiatry services into multiple primary care clinics across three states. This PCMH model employs care navigators (CNs) who are key to coordination for patients, primary care providers, and psychiatrists. These CNs also provide training on telemedicine and electronic health records (psychiatrist use) and personal health records (patients use)—all of this is done remotely. The CNs do the initial patient intakes and follow-up with patients after consultations to promote adherence to the treatment plan.

There are populations, settings, and other issues that add complexity. One consideration is geographic, with rural/remote populations, though these are better online with broadband pipelines now. Another is the urban underserved, who face obstacles of lack of money, transportation, healthcare coverage, and "easy" access

Table 10.2 Training/education for synchronous and asynchronous telepsychiatry to primary care: competencies, goals, and objectives

Outline of annual curriculum
1. *Basic* skills, knowledge, and attitudes. Areas: Clinical; psychosomatic medicine-based; other subspecialty applications; culture; and technology
2. *Advanced* skills, knowledge, and attitudes. Areas: Problem analysis; feedback; depression; and difficult situations
3. *Additional* advanced skills, knowledge, and attitudes and *consultation* skills. Areas: Management of complex clinical cases; stepped care; planning for system limitations; and self-identification of strengths and weaknesses
4. Advanced skills, knowledge, and attitudes. Areas: Cultural formation and clinical consultation with other providers
Overview of needs for mental health services
Skill objectives
Overview of models, training, and services by telepsychiatry
Model of services
Sample training clinic model for residents and students
1. Services provided
2. Psychiatric (regular) clinical
3. Medical
4. Psychosomatic medicine or consultation-liaison
5. Subspecialty basics
6. Technology
Knowledge objectives
1. Primary care
2. Regular areas
3. Subspecialty basics
4. Technology
5. Alternative treatments
Attitude objectives
6.1 administrative objectives leadership 6.2 documentation
Teaching and learning objectives: Faculty, fellows, residents, mss, and interdisciplinary team members
Readings
1. Primary care
2. Psychiatric disorders
3. System issues
4. Subspecialty-related
5. Technology and communication
6. Other

to in-person or telemedicine access points (going ten blocks without a bus is no easier than 2 miles via three buses). Culturally diverse populations of many ethnicities, cultures, and languages—even sign language—have been aided [3, 30, 53]. Caution is merited for using relatives or untrained interpreters, who may miscommunicate medical complaints [54] or de-emphasize information [55]. Other special settings and populations also include involuntary, inpatient, and incarcerated; the old and young; and those in emergency rooms, schools, or other settings.

10.4 The Interdisciplinary Team: Role Definitions, Training Needs, Cross-Training, and Adapting to New Stepped and Integrated Care Models

10.4.1 Overview

One place to start with this discussion is considering a 3-dimensional cube with 3 axes: *team member/provider of care, method of service delivery, and medical/MH complexity*. The *team member/provider of care* would be a range of care coordinators or point persons of contact for basic entry into care. This could mean fielding emails from patients, checking in with patients at the clinic, or data management staff. On the other end of the spectrum would be your psychiatrist /family physician/ internist complemented by additional specialists. The members in-between would be medical assistants, licensed vocational nurses, registered nurses, nurse practitioners, physician assistants (i.e., mid-level providers who are readily available and manage basic and some advanced clinical problems), and MH clinicians. The *method of service delivery* would include a range of web site to in-person to tele-transported expertise, starting with education websites, brochures, kiosks, and local support networks/groups (e.g., Depression and Bipolar Support Alliance or American Diabetes Association) to in-person individual or group education with a coordinator (e.g., diabetes or depression/grief group), to tele-based groups (e.g., for those in a remote area or with an uncommon illness), to video capture and data stored/organized in a "digital packet" then forwarded to an expert for review (i.e., asynchronous telepsychiatry), and to the top synchronous teleconsultant evaluation and/or management tier (i.e., the Rolls Royce of technology). The *medical/MH complexity* may predetermine where the patient enters the above axes and where in the cube he/she spends the most time (i.e., the least ill as a small bottom cube and the most ill in a top smaller cube), proportionally, in the total 3-dimensional cube.

10.4.2 Best Practice for Integrated Care: Depression and Diabetes (or Heart Disease or Other Conditions)

10.4.2.1 ID Info

A 49-year-old Native American male with diabetes, obesity, and alcohol use presents to the rural clinic with obesity, "I need medication" and a mother that reports "he eats too many sweets." He was referred to a telepsychiatric consultation at an academic center 175 miles away.

10.4.2.2 Background

Patients with diabetes mellitus (DM) have high rates of psychiatric disorders, particularly depression, with a 14% mean range of 8.5–27%, [56] with higher rates in Native Americans [57]. Depression contributes to poor adherence to diabetic regimens, feelings of helplessness related to chronic illness, and poor outcomes. DM and mental illness cause significant disability and increase risk for one another, as well as other disorders like coronary artery disease (CAD) [18, 58–60]. Patients with co-morbid depression and diabetes fare worse than those with diabetes who are not depressed. Depressed patients with diabetes are less adherent to self-care regimens. Moreover, depression is associated with poorer glycemic control [61, 62] and increased cardiovascular risk factors [63]. Depression is also associated with increased complications from diabetes such as retinopathy, nephropathy higher rates of disability, dementia, and mortality [64].

10.4.2.3 HPI

This patient has been seen, as has his entire family, at the reservation's internal medicine service as an adult, and he was described as "irritable, angry...and lacking hope." A substance abuse counselor is concerned about him drinking "3-4 beers per day." He was referred to an adjacent city's psychiatrist (45 miles; 70 min away from the coast) but did not go. He is referred to a psychosomatic medicine service via telemedicine 140 miles away.

10.4.2.4 Evaluation

A psychiatrist met with all parties—the patient/mother first and then the PCP came in, with a discussion of depression as a new diagnosis and alcohol use that was maladaptive.

10.4.2.5 Treatment Options

1. "Regular" care.
   (a) Substance treatment with family attending.
   (b) Dietary consultation for patient and family, including itemized groceries (good and bad), co-shopping, and meal plans.
   (c) One-time telepsychiatric consultation leading to an antidepressant treatment and access to brief CBT; both are effective for depression and may lower Hg1Ac levels [65].
   (d) Diabetic and weight education, website, and support group in neighboring city.
2. Better" integrated care.
   (a) Administrative: ignoring limitation for one doctor visit per day (federal reimbursement) → internist and teleconsultant same day. The PCP and psychiatrist can work with the patient to address the depression and how it directly contributes to both the alcohol misuse and the uncontrolled diabe-

tes, The psychiatrist can model targeted motivational interviewing techniques that can be used in the PC setting,
(b) Transportation to healthcare visits locally and to neighboring city.
(c) Joint (or juxtaposed) tele-endocrinology and—psychiatric consultations for integrated data, decision-making, and follow-up planning.
(d) Multisite, nurse-based diabetic coordinator support group by telemedicine (within or across cultures; in English).

10.4.3 Best Practice for Integrated Care: Training/Education for Integrated Care

Training/education programs vary in their approach (from low to higher levels in parentheses) in terms of: the center of the learning process (curriculum to patient-or learner); outcomes (knowledge, attitudes, and skills); individual vs. teamwork (spontaneous vs. shared mental models); teaching methods (case/practice vs. lecture/didactic), and perhaps most-importantly level of supervision for feedback, encouragement of reflection, and developing lifelong habits.

"Good" integrated training uses milestone-based learning with didactics temporally mirroring clinical experiences, when possible, and combined training is an outcome to shoot for [66]. This pedagogical approach is longitudinal in nature, ideally beginning in postgraduate year one or two (PGY-1 or 2) and extending through PGY-4. It has an online curriculum with modules on integrated and collaborative care and the curriculum shifts from core medical topics in year 2 (key systems, geriatrics, pain, and some prevention) to MH topics in year 3 (epidemiology, collaborative care, integrated care models) to year 4 (being a consultant, team-based learning, brief therapies, and advocacy skills).

Telehealth has increased both education of, and service delivery by, rural doctors and nurses. A review of the effectiveness of videoconference-based tele-education for medical and nursing education showed high satisfaction with videoconferencing education and that it is equivalent or better than in-person education knowledge acquisition and integration [67]. Clinically, the evidence base is growing on nursing interventions like coaching via telehealth [68]. Simulated patients at a distance are used to teach general clinical skills, how to work as part of a team, how to gain experience in previously unfamiliar work settings, and how to get on the same page across disciplines (i.e., how to develop mental models) for the care of a patient [30, 31].

10.4.4 Project Consultation: Program Development and Improvement Via Organizational Consultation (See Appendix)

10.4.4.1 Overview

The director of a rural health Network of 10 clinics that shared resources sought help from an academic medical center to access a telepsychiatry service. The original idea, primarily, was to use the service as a part of MH care for the clinics. It was thought this would boost the likelihood to obtain funding from external agencies, as part of a community-wide project.

10.4.4.2 Original Plan

The original proposal was a good start and well researched in terms of rural health, underserved populations, and mental health services (see Appendix). It had a list of services to be provided: in-person on-site and telepsychiatric consultation. There was no budget for evaluation.

10.4.4.3 Evaluation/Consultation

The consultant suggested an evaluation plan/budget and re-write the project description three times, before arriving at a plan for direct services, training/education, community collaboration, and an evaluation budget (see Appendix). Specifically, it had outcomes for patients, PCP skills, and administrative/clinic functions.

10.5 Summary/Results

Most services were delivered either on-site—such as mental health screenings using questionnaires, therapy through "warm" handoffs, and educational sessions for staff at all levels—or remotely, through telepsychiatric consultations, data collection and analysis, and written summaries.

- The rural health network used the consultation to:
  - Improve health service delivery and outcomes, [37, 38]
  - Recruitment MH providers and PCPs to site,
  - Employ screening, diagnostic, and outcome questionnaires/clinician-administered short scales (e.g., Child Behavioral Checklist or CBCL),
  - Learning integrated care principles, and.
- Four academic publications occurred and other reports were disseminated, including the case mix population of patients served by telepsychiatry and another specific to children.

10.6 Virtual Care in Consultation-Liaison Psychiatric Services

The COVID-19 pandemic has had far-reaching implications on mental health services globally. As the pandemic unfolded, healthcare providers, including physicians and liaison psychiatrists, experienced unprecedented changes in their working conditions and mental health status. A cross-sectional study by Telles Correia et al. (2022) evaluated the impact of the pandemic on doctors in general hospitals and liaison psychiatrists across Europe. The authors found that the pandemic necessitated novel patient consultation methods, resulting in a rise in telehealth practices, including consultations via patients' mobile phones, video cameras, microphones installed in wards, internal hospital phone lines, and interviews with the doctor responsible for the patient [69].

Similarly, a significant shift toward telepsychiatry was witnessed in perinatal care, an area typically characterized by limited access to mental health resources. Gopalan et al. (2021) explored the efficacy of telepsychiatry consultations in a rural hospital's labor and delivery unit. Their findings, based on a year's worth of electronic medical records data, suggested that telehealth consultations successfully engaged at-risk mothers in psychiatric treatment, primarily addressing depression, anxiety, and medication management. This research underscores the critical need for enhancing access to telepsychiatry for rural, perinatal populations, particularly in light of the accelerated adoption of telemedicine due to the COVID-19 pandemic [70].

Beran and Sowa's (2021) study offers further insight into the transformation of consultation-liaison (C-L) psychiatric services during the pandemic. Their research focused on the structural changes in clinical services, the impacts on consultation volumes, and the experiences of psychiatric trainees and attending physicians during the transition to virtual care. Notably, they found that despite a decrease in the average weekly consultation volume and charges during the pandemic, both attending physicians and trainees reported moderate or high comfort and satisfaction with telephone and video consultations. Importantly, the transition to virtual care did not negatively impact trainee satisfaction with supervision, learning, and their consult psychiatry experience [71]. This body of research collectively provides evidence for the feasibility and effectiveness of rapidly implementing virtual care in consultation-liaison psychiatric services without negatively impacting the learning experience of trainees and overall patient care.

10.7 Discussion and Conclusions

Contemporary healthcare is a patient-centered approach and integrates health and mental healthcare. TMH facilitates this process by leveraging the expertise of key disciplines to the point-of-service. It is mostly used to provide mental healthcare in the medical setting, and it has not been used much to provide medical care in mental health settings. Good programs emphasize teamwork and have clinical, administrative, and care coordination oversight.

There is little doubt that integrated care with integration on the seven levels described above—responsibility (decision-making, oversight of patient care), co-location of services, funding, evaluation plan, outcome measurement, an e-platform, and reimbursement—is the new "gold standard" for patient-centered care. This model for quality care must undergo further integration with the patient/consumer movement, academic health center (AHC), and community missions. A salient question becomes, "Is it easier to deconstruct and rebuild the traditional academic health center "culture" and structure, or build a new AHC that is more progressive (e.g., Mayo Clinic model)?"

A question also remains on where to go from there, in terms of minimal standards for medical and psychiatric care dependent on the setting and who provides the care? Outpatient psychiatric clinics "should" have VS, weight, and other staples of medical clinics; inpatient ones need medical clearance, medical co-management, and specialty consultation—rarely is that the case, though. In terms of who provides what care, is there a way to reasonably update PCP training in MH/psychiatry (e.g., ½ proctored/supervised tracks like a fellowship rather than full-time ones that disrupt clinical and other life arrangements)? Or, could a psychiatrist provide basic medical care (e.g., screening, education, prescribing for routine or chronic but stable conditions (e.g., hypertension) as part of a theoretically three-tiered medical acuity system?

And, what are the training best practices of the future? Will training evolve from separate undergraduate medical education (UME) to graduate medical education (GME), and lifelong continuing medical education (CME) streams—linked by throwing the participants in clinical settings—to a more purposeful framework that emphasizes team care, with shared models, team-based learning and practicing at the top of the license? Will tele-education leverage resources better, will simulation be more of a fundamental method, and how much will we practice before performing examinations/procedures/other work with patients?

Acknowledgments American Telemedicine Association Telemental Health Interest Group.

Appendix A Appendix: Program Development and Improvement Via Organizational Consultation

Overview

The director of a rural health Network of 10 clinics that shared resources sought help from an academic medical center to access a telepsychiatry service. The original idea, primarily, was to use the service as a part of MH care for the clinics. It was thought this would boost the likelihood to obtain funding from external agencies, as part of a community-wide project.

Logistics

- Assessment of initial proposal. The proposal was a good start and well researched in terms of rural health, underserved populations, mental health services, and a plan of services to be covered. There was no budget for evaluation. The original proposal was outlined as follows:
- The consultant suggested an evaluation plan/budget and rewrite the project description three times, before arriving at the following outline.

Project component	Objective	Outcome
Direct service delivery	Provide 7000 h of mental health services at seven primary care sites in NSRHN region (28 h a month clinical, 4 h on data) per site. Mid-level provider 1 day a week	Increase assessment for mental illness by 50% at each site. Decrease depression via treatment in 65% of diagnosed consumers accepting care
Telepsychiatry consultation	Provide 600 h of psychiatrist services via on-site care and telemedicine	Assure high-quality assessment and knowledgeable prescription of psychotropic medication for diagnosed consumers in need of medication

Project components	Objectives	Outcomes
1. Direct service delivery	50% more consumers at six primary care clinics will be screened for behavioral illness	Increased identification and treatment of behavioral health problems
	Consumers treated for depression will show a 25% reduction in depression	Increased consumer health and Well-being
	90–100% of the consumers who are receiving inadequate psychotropic medication doses will be identified so that interventions can take place	Improved consumer behavioral health outcomes
	25% improvement in consumer satisfaction with primary behavioral healthcare services	Increased consumer health and Well-being
2. Training and technical assistance	Increase by 25% primary care providers' knowledge and skills in assessment, diagnosis, and treatment of mental illness	Improved service delivery and increased consumer access to behavioral healthcare services delivered at their primary care clinic
	Increase by 25% the knowledge and understanding of all clinic staff about how to integrate behavioral health into primary care practices	Full integration of behavioral healthcare services into six primary care clinic sites
	Development of integrated care protocols, policies and procedures, and use of outcomes data to inform quality improvement activities at each site	Full integration of behavioral healthcare services into six primary care clinic sites
3. Collaborate along the continuum of BH/MH services	Identify and document the entire continuum of care in each county	Improved knowledge of available care for consumers
	Hold a minimum of 10 interdisciplinary team meetings for didactics, case-based discussions, and collaboration on difficult cases. Teams will solicit consumer and front-line provider recommendations to alleviate barriers to care	Improved referral relationships, case management, and better informed service providers along the behavioral healthcare continuum

Project components	Objectives	Outcomes
4. Policy development	Make recommendations to decision makers based on outcome data and clinical provider and consumer identified barriers	Increased awareness of service delivery barriers and identification of policies to improve access to care
	Develop options to address service delivery concerns	Improved systems of care. Increased access to consumer-focused, collaborative services

The final evaluation plan was formatted into three groups:

1. Patients: objectives, methods, and outcomes for diagnosis, treatment of depression, and satisfaction.
2. PCPs: skills and knowledge objectives, methods, and outcomes.
3. Administrative/clinic function: (a) integrated care protocols, policies, and procedures, and use of outcomes data to inform quality improvement activities at each site; (b) documentation of the continuum of care in each county; (c) interdisciplinary team meetings for didactics, case-based discussions and collaboration on difficult cases; and (d) policy development.

Summary/Results of Project

- Several services were provided both on-site—including mental health screenings using questionnaires, therapy through "warm" handoffs, and staff education across all levels—and remotely, through telepsychiatric consultations, data collection and analysis, and written reports.
- The rural health network used the consultation for the following:
  - Improve health service delivery and outcomes [38, 39].
  - Recruitment MH providers and PCPs to site.
  - Employ screening, diagnostic and outcome questionnaires/clinician-administered short scales (e.g., Child Behavioral Checklist or CBCL).
  - Learning integrated care principles.
- Four academic publications occurred and other reports were disseminated, including the case mix population of patients served by telepsychiatry and another specific to children.

References

1. Akinci F, Patel PM. Quality improvement in healthcare delivery utilizing the patient-centered medical home model. Hosp Topics. 2014;92(4):96–104.
2. Druss BG, Zhao L, Von Esenwein S, et al. Understanding excess mortality in persons with mental illness: 17-year follow up of a nationally representative US survey. Med Care. 2011;49:599–604.

3. Hilty DM, Ferrer D, Parish MB, et al. The effectiveness of telemental health: a 2013 review. Tel J e-Health. 2013;19(6):444–54.
4. Yellowlees PM, Odor A, Iosif A, et al. Transcultural psychiatry made simple: asynchronous telepsychiatry as an approach to providing culturally relevant care. Tel e-Health. 2013;19(4):1–6.
5. Phillips BC. Healthcare reform and the future of nursing and nurse practitioner. Nurse practitioners business blog, 2010. 15 Mar 2015. https://npbusiness.org/health-care-reform-future-nursing-nurse-practitioners/?
6. Health and Human Services. The 2008 report to the secretary: rural health and human services issues: twentieth anniversary Report. 15 Mar 2015. ftp://ftp.hrsa.gov/ruralhealth/committee/NACreport2008.pdf.
7. Hilty DM, Yellowlees PM, Nesbitt TS. Evolution of telepsychiatry to rural sites: change over time in types of referral and PCP knowledge, skill, and satisfaction. Gen Hosp Psychiatry. 2006;28(5):367–73.
8. Hilty DM, Nesbitt TS, Kuenneth TA, et al. Telepsychiatric consultation to primary care: rural vs. suburban needs, utilization and provider satisfaction. J Rural Health. 2007;23(2):163–5.
9. Druss BG, Rohrbaugh RM, Levinson CM, et al. Integrated medical care for patients with serious psychiatric illness: a randomized trial. Arch Gen Psychiatry. 2001;58:861.
10. Dobscha SK, Corson K, Perrin NA, et al. Collaborative care for chronic pain in primary care. JAMA J Am Med Assoc. 2009;301:1242–51.
11. Unützer J, Katon W, Callahan CM, et al. Collaborative care management of late-life depression in the primary care setting. JAMA J Am Med Assoc. 2002;288:2836–4285.
12. Bower P, Gilbody S. Managing common mental health disorders in primary care: conceptual models and evidence base. Br Med J. 2005;330:839–42.
13. Katon WJ, Seelig M. Population-based care of depression: team care approaches to improving outcomes. J Occup Environ Med. 2008;50:459–67.
14. Simon GE, Katon WJ, Lin EHB, et al. Cost-effectiveness of systematic depression treatment among people with diabetes mellitus. Arch Gen Psychiatry. 2007;64:65–72.
15. Wang PS, Patrick A, Avorn J, et al. The costs and benefits of enhanced depression care to employers. Arch Gen Psychiatry. 2006;63:1345.
16. Davis MH, Everett A, Kathol R, et al. American Psychiatric Association ad hoc work group report on the integration of psychiatry and primary care, 2011. 15 Mar 2015. http://naapimha.org/wordpress/media/Integration-of-Psychiatry-and-Primary-Care.pdf.
17. Kishi Y, Kathol RG. Integrating medical and psychiatric treatment in an inpatient medical setting: the type IV program. Psychosomatics. 1999;40:345.
18. Mezuk B, Eaton W, Albrecht S, et al. Depression and type 2 diabetes over the lifespan. Diabetes Care. 2008;31:2383–90.
19. Van der Kooy K, van Hout H, Marwijk H, et al. Depression and the risk for cardiovascular diseases: systematic review and meta-analysis. Int J Geriatr Psychiatry. 2007;22:613–26.
20. American Diabetes Association. American Psychiatric Association, American Association of Clinical Endocrinologists, north American Association for the Study of obesity and diabetes: consensus development conference on antipsychotic drugs and obesity and diabetes. Diabetes Care. 2004;27:596–601.
21. Hussain M, Seitz D. Integrated models of care for medical inpatients with psychiatric disorders: a systematic review. Psychosomatics. 2014;55(4):315–25.
22. Manian FA, Janssen DA. Curbside consultations. JAMA. 1996;275:145–6.
23. Katon W, Von Korff M, Lin E, et al. Collaborative management to achieve depression treatment guidelines. J Clin Psychiatry. 1997;58(Suppl 1):20–4.
24. Hilty DM, Servis ME, Nesbitt TS, et al. The use of telemedicine to provide consultation-liaison service to the primary care setting. Psychiatr Ann. 1999;29:421–7.
25. Hilty DM, Marks SL, Wegeland JE, et al. A randomized controlled trial of disease management modules, including telepsychiatric care, for depression in rural primary care. Psychiatry. 2007;4(2):58–65.
26. Hilty DM, Yellowlees PM, Cobb HC, et al. Use of secure e-mail and telephone psychiatric consultations to accelerate rural health care delivery. J Tel e-Health. 2006;12(4):490–5.

27. Fortney JC, Pyne JM, Mouden SP, et al. Practice-based versus telemedicine-based collaborative care for depression in rural federally qualified health centers: a pragmatic randomized comparative effectiveness trial. Am J Psychiatry. 2013;170(4):414–25.
28. Slaets J, Kauffmann R, Duivenvoorden H, et al. A randomized trial of geriatric liaison intervention in elderly medical inpatients. Psychosom Med. 1997;59:585–91.
29. Baldwin R, Pratt H, Goring H, Marriott A, Roberts C. Does a nurse-led mental health liaison service for older people reduce psychiatric morbidity in acute general medical wards? A randomized controlled trial. Age Ageing. 2004;33:472–8.
30. Hilty DM, Yellowlees PM, Nasatir SEH, et al. Program evaluation and practical, step-by-step program modification in telemental health. In: Behavioral Telehealth series volume 1-clinical video conferencing: program development and practice. Cham: Springer; 2014. p. 105–34.
31. Rutledge CM, Haney T, Bordelon M, et al. Telehealth: preparing advanced practice nurses to address healthcare needs in rural and underserved populations. Int J Nurs Educ Schol. 2014;11(1):1–9.
32. Ross S, Allen N. Examining the convergent validity of shared mental model measures. Behav Res. 2012;44:1052–62.
33. Armstrong EG, Mackey M, Spear SJ. Medical education as a process management problem. Acad Med. 2004;79(8):721–8.
34. Hilty DM, Yellowlees PM, Cobb HC, et al. Models of telepsychiatric consultation-liaison service to rural primary care. Psychosomatics. 2006;47(2):152–7.
35. Hilty DM, Marks SL, Urness D, et al. Clinical and educational applications of telepsychiatry: a review. Can J Psychiatr. 2004;49(1):12–23.
36. Hilty DM, Ingraham RL, Yang RP, et al. Multispecialty phone and email consultation to primary care providers for patients with developmental disabilities in rural California. J Telemed E-Health. 2004;10:413–21.
37. Neufeld JD, Bourgeois JA, Hilty DM, et al. The e-mental health consult service: providing enhanced primary care mental health services through telemedicine. Psychosomatics. 2007;48:135–41.
38. Yellowlees PM, Hilty DM, Marks SL, et al. A retrospective analysis of child and adolescent e-mental health. J Am Acad Child Adol Psychiatr. 2008;47(1):1–5.
39. Yellowlees PM, Odor A, Patrice K, et al. PsychVACS: a system for asynchronous telepsychiatry. J Tel e-Health. 2011;17(4):299–303.
40. Butler TN, Yellowlees P. Cost analysis of store-and-forward telepsychiatry as a consultation model for primary care. Telemed J E Health. 2012;18(1):74–7.
41. Richardson L, McCauley E, Katon W. Collaborative care for adolescent depression: a pilot study. Gen Hosp Psychiat. 2009;31:36–45.
42. Myers KM. Effectiveness of a telehealth service delivery model for treating attention-deficit hyperactivity disorder: results of a community-based randomized controlled trial. J Am Acad Child Adolesc Psychiatry. 2015;54:263.
43. Haaga DA. Introduction to the special section on stepped care models in psychotherapy. J Consult Clin Psychol. 2000;68:547–8.
44. van't Veer-Tazelaar N, van Marwijk H, et al. Prevention of anxiety and depression in the age group of 75 years and over: a randomized controlled trial testing the feasibility and effectiveness of a generic stepped care program among elderly community residents at high risk of developing anxiety and depression versus usual care. BMC Public Health. 2006;1:186.
45. NICE. NICE Clinical Guidelines 90 and 91 Depression: Treatment and management of depression in adults, including adults with a chronic physical health problem. 2009. 15 Mar 2015. http://www.nice.org.uk/nicemedia/live/12329/45890/45890.pdf.
46. van't Veer-Tazelaar PJ, van Marwijk HW, van Oppen P, et al. Stepped-care prevention of anxiety and depression in late life: a randomized controlled trial. Arch Gen Psychiatry. 2009;66:297–304.
47. van't Veer-Tazelaar P, Smit F, van Hout H, van Oppen P, van der Horst H, et al. Cost-effectiveness of a stepped care intervention to prevent depression and anxiety in late life: randomized trial. Br J Psychiatry. 2010;196:319–25.

48. van't Veer-Tazelaar PJ, van HWJ M, van Oppen P, et al. Prevention of late-life anxiety and depression has sustained effects over 24 months: a pragmatic randomized trial. Am J Geriatr Psychiatry. 2011;19:230–9.
49. Rosenthal TC. The medical home: Growing evidence to support a new approach to primary care. J Am Board Fam Med. 2008;21(5):427–40.
50. Hollingsworth JM, Saint S, Hayward RA, et al. Specialty care and the patient-centered medical home. Med Care. 2011;49(1):4–9.
51. Cluver JS, Schuyler D, Frueh BC, et al. Remote psychotherapy for terminally ill cancer patients. J Tel Telecare. 2005;11:157–9.
52. Yellowlees PM, Shore JH, Roberts L, et al. Practice guidelines for videoconferencing-based Telemental health. Tel e-Health. 2010;16(10):1074–89.
53. Brooks TR. Pitfalls in communication with Hispanic and African-American patients: do translators help or harm? J Nat Med Assoc. 1992;84(11):941.
54. Brua C. Role-blurring and ethical grey zones associated with lay interpreters: three case studies. Commun Med. 2008;5(1):73.
55. Gavard JA, Lustman PJ, Clouse RE. Prevalence of depression in adults with diabetes: an epidemiological evaluation. Diabetes Care. 1993;16(8):1167–78.
56. Thackeray R, Merrill RM, Neiger BL. Disparities in diabetes management practice between racial and ethnic groups in the United States. Diab Educator. 2004;30(4):665–74.
57. Wells K, Stewart A, Hays R, et al. The functioning and well being of depressed patients: results from the medical outcomes study. JAMA. 1989;262:914–9.
58. Campayo A, de Jonge P, Roy JF, et al. Depressive disorder and incident diabetes mellitus: the effect of characteristics of depression. Am J Psychiatry. 2010;167:580–8.
59. Carnethon MR, Biggs ML, Barzilay JI, et al. Longitudinal association between depressive symptoms and incident type 2 diabetes mellitus in older adults: the cardiovascular health study. Arch Intern Med. 2007;167(8):802–7.
60. Lustman PJ, Anderson RJ, Freedland KE, et al. Depression and poor glycemic control: a meta-analytic review of the literature. Diabetes Care. 2000;23:934–42.
61. Katon W, Lyles CR, Parker MM, et al. Association of depression with increased risk of dementia in patients with type 2 diabetes: the diabetes and aging study. Arch Gen Psychiatry. 2012;69:410–7.
62. Katon WJ, Von Korff M, Lin EH, et al. The pathways study: a randomized trial of collaborative care in patients with diabetes and depression. Arch Gen Psychiatry. 2004;61:1042–9.
63. Rustad JK, Musselman DL, Nemeroff CB. The relationship of depression and diabetes: pathophysiological and treatment implications. Psychoneuroendocrinology. 2011;36:1276–86.
64. Lustman PJ, Griffith LS, Freedland KE, et al. Cognitive behavior therapy for depression in type 2 diabetes mellitus. A randomized, controlled trial. Ann Intern Med. 1998;129(8):613–21.
65. McCarron RM, Bourgeois JA, Chwastiak LA, et al. Integrated medicine and psychiatry (IMAP) curriculum for psychiatry residency training: a model designed to meet growing mental health workforce needs. Acad Psychiatry. 2015;39:461.
66. Chipps J, Brysiewicz P, Mars M. A systematic review of the effectiveness of videoconference-based tele-education for medical and nursing education. Worldviews Evid-Based Nurs. 2012;9(2):78–87.
67. Young H, Miyamoto S, Ward D, et al. Sustained effects of a nurse coaching intervention via telehealth to improve health behavior change in diabetes. Tel e-Health. 2014;20(9):828–34.
68. Telles Correia D, Novais F, Mattei G. Impact of the COVID-19 pandemic on general hospital physicians work and mental health: an international cross sectional study. Eur Psychiatry. 2022;65(S1):S44.
69. Gopalan P, Auster L, Brockman I, Shenai N. Consultation-liaison telepsychiatry on an inpatient obstetrical labor and delivery unit. J Acad Consult Liaison Psychiatry. 2021;62:577–81.
70. Beran C, Sowa NA. Adaptation of an academic inpatient consultation-liaison psychiatry service during the SARS-CoV-2 pandemic: effects on clinical practice and trainee supervision. J Acad Consult Liaison Psychiatry. 2021;62:186–92.

Social Media and Clinical Practice: What Stays the Same, What Changes, and How to Plan Ahead?

11

Donald M. Hilty, Myo Thwin Myint, Kristoffer Calvert Strauss, Pamela E. Hoffman, and Dorothy Stubbe

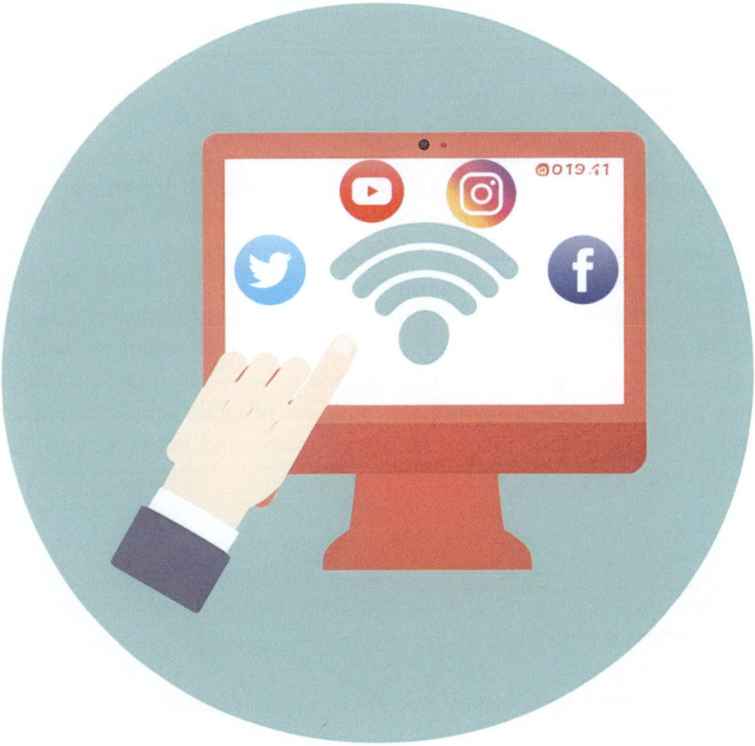

D. M. Hilty (✉)
Department of Psychiatry and Behavioral Sciences, Keck School of Medicine University of Southern California, Los Angeles, CA, USA
e-mail: donald.hilty@uhsinc.com; hilty@med.usc.edu

D. Mucić, D. M. Hilty (eds.), *Digital Mental Health*,
https://doi.org/10.1007/978-3-031-59936-1_11

Abstract

While the patient-centered healthcare movement, like traditional medicine movements, aims to deliver quality, affordable, and timely care in a variety of settings, the consumer movement on new technologies is passing it by with emerging technologies and new ways of communicating with others (text, e-mail, Twitter, and Facebook). This chapter builds on what we know about telemental health, technology, and communication progress over the past 50 years in maintaining the tenets of "good" quality care, adjusting slightly to telemedicine models, and considering more significant adjustments for the use of social media. The areas of challenges include privacy and confidentiality health and personal practice, having "good" interpersonal/clinical boundaries, awareness of what information is out there about you, and discussing clear expectations about online communication between doctors and patients as part of the informed consent process. Guidelines, strategies, and tips for the clinician are offered.

11.1 Introduction

Today's youth are using technology in a variety of ways, from texting and tweeting, to chatting, online gaming, and posting through a variety of Internet portals. Of US adults and those aged 18–29%, respectively, 88% and 99% use the Internet, 73% and 77% use home broadband [1]. As of 2018, approximately 95% of American adults have a cell phone, and 77% have a smartphone [1]. In particular, social media or networking, Internet, and smartphone usage continues to grow at alarming rates without apparent boundaries, stretching across countries, cultures, and levels of technical skill. Social media is usually defined as web-based and mobile services that allow people to share a connection, monitor progress, and create/manipulate text, audio, photos, and or video [2]. Social media and networking options like

M. T. Myint
Triple Board Graduate and Child & Adolescent Psychiatry Fellowship Programs, Tulane University School of Medicine, New Orleans, LA, USA
e-mail: mmyint@tulane.edu

K. C. Strauss
Department of Psychiatry and Behavioral Sciences, Stanford University School of Medicine, Stanford, CA, USA
e-mail: strauss k@stanford.edu

P. E. Hoffman
Yale School of Medicine, New Haven, CT, USA
e-mail: pamela.hoffman@yale.edu

D. Stubbe
Child Study Center and Child and Adolescent Psychiatry and Program Director of Residency Training, Yale School of Medicine, New Haven, CT, USA
e-mail: dorothy.stubbe@yale.edu

Twitter[R] and Facebook[R] are common among the Digital Native (Z), Millennial (Y), and X Generations.

Children, adolescents, and young adults under 25 years of age (i.e., youth) are raised in an increasingly digitalized society, with technology as an integral part of daily life [1]. Social media (SM) is currently used for professional-to-professional (P2P), professional-to-consumer (P2C), consumer-to-consumer (C2C), and consumer-to-professional (C2P) purposes. SM is very attractive to youth as it is portable and offers ever-changing, immersive, diverse, individualized social engagement [3]. Social networks (e.g., Facebook, Twitter, and LinkedIn), media sharing networks (e.g., Instagram, Snapchat, and YouTube), discussion forums (e.g., Reddit, Quora, and Digg) and bookmarking and content curation networks (e.g., Pinterest, Flipboard) are used by youth, with YouTube (81%) and FB (69%) dominating the online landscape, respectively [1].

There are many current hazards to the technology explosion—for patients, trainees, and faculty. Patients may access misinformation about diagnoses and treatments [4]. Confidentiality, privacy, and professional boundaries may be easily breached. Youth are vulnerable in many ways and may need supervision with SM due to limited ability to self-regulate, vulnerability to peer pressure, and susceptibility to sharing personal information [5]. Teens both acknowledge SM's role in helping build their social connections and expose them to a diverse world and cite concerns around the social pressure SM generates [6]. Most (65%) parents worry their kids spend too much time in front of screens and its impact on mental and physical health, safety, well-being, social development, and family dynamics [7]. The Children's Online Privacy Protection Rule (COPPA) has effectively guided participants since 2000, *if and when* those 13 years or less adhere to parental/guardian permission [8]. Trainees and clinicians require competency-based education related to this topic [9]. Mid and advanced career faculty, often referred to as "digital immigrants," may be technologically ill-informed [10], and most have not yet applied andragogy (adult learning theories) to the topics of Internet use, social media, and professionalism. Therefore, we have a paradox and a crisis: faculty may trail trainees with regard to hands-on experience and expertise with technology and they may require faculty development training to keep current with the benefits and potential pitfalls of media [11].

This chapter will help the reader to consider ... (objectives/aims)

1. Explore the intersection of clinical care, social media, and other technologies (e.g., relationship, communication) and help clinicians differentiate between normal and problematic use;
2. Summarize findings of the relationship between SM use in children/adolescents/young adults and psychopathology and mental/behavioral health conditions or problems (e.g., suicide, cyberbullying, sexting); and.

Highlight the Importance of Clinical Boundaries, Privacy, Confidentiality, and Others, so that Clinicians Have a Basic Approach to Engage, Screen, and Treat Patients

11.2 The Intersection of Communication, Technology, and Mh Care

11.2.1 The Evolution of Psychiatric Practice

The biopsychosocial model put the presenting problem in the context of the patient's life and identifying determinants of the symptoms/psychopathology [12]; more importantly it was a compromise between the biomedical and analytic groups. We explore beliefs, norms, and values, and to a greater degree than most in medicine, the ethnic, culture and language issues that affect health. The culture of the patient includes symptoms, presentation, meaning, causation, family factors, coping styles, treatment seeking, mistrust, stigma, immigration, and overall health status. Oftentimes, in order to better understand a patient's perspective, we need to hear them tell their story in his own words. Stories, though subjective, are well described in their role in healing, conveying abstract meaning (myths), moving people to change, and teaching learners to apply knowledge and learn skills

Time-tested "quality" care in psychiatry is mostly attributed to the patient-doctor engagement, the therapeutic relationship, shared decision-making, and biopsychosocial treatment. Shared decision-making equalizes the informational and power symmetry between doctors and patients—both parties share information and develop consensus in a decision [13]. Psychiatry is a good model of early and contemporary shared decision-making. When patients were allowed to choose between different treatment options for depression rather than being randomly allocated to treatment groups, patients chose psychotherapy more often than pharmacotherapy with no significant difference in patient satisfaction or outcomes. Cognitive psychology and psychiatry have illuminated perceptual biases: why we think as we think, when our decisions are prone to error, and how to reduce those errors [14]. Our work with patients encourages reflection, tolerating ambiguity, and dealing with the unexpected.

The expanding use of social media and advances in digital connectivity dictate that we must, once again, contemplate how best to account for and integrate new trends in technology with existing clinical practice. Social networking has been defined as "web-based services that allow individuals to (1) construct a public or semi-public profile within a bounded system, (2) articulate a list of other users with whom they share a connection, and (3) view and traverse their list of connections and those made by others within the system" [2]. Much as with the integration of TMH into existing psychiatric practice over the past 50 years, the ultimate goal of providing high-quality care to patients may include social media, but we must be mindful of components and principles of effective mental health care, which we can ill-afford to compromise.

The importance of the therapeutic alliance in successful treatment is well established across disciplines. In mental health treatment, the relationship between the provider and patient is unlike any other in one's personal life. Efforts to establish rapport, but with consistent attention to boundaries, allow the provider to be seen, not as a friend (importantly), but as a professional to whom patients can feel confident revealing themselves [15]. Effective communication facilitates such disclosure. When the parameters of the therapeutic frame are significantly and repeatedly blurred, the trust that previously long-held secrets will be handled appropriately and with benefit to treatment begins to erode. The introduction of social media and other digital communications brings with them multiple opportunities to unintentionally jeopardize this process.

The impact of new technology on how we go about formulating an assessment and plan should also be considered (Table 11.1). For example, the components of a thorough formulation, including the biopsychosocial model, should remain the same. Questions arise, however, from increasingly facilitated access to information on our patients through social media applications and the ability to quickly search the Internet for data. At what point does the obligation to thoroughly inform our understandings begin to conflict with a patient's right to privacy? How do we define that data which is "fair game" and that which should remain privileged? We must also protect patient autonomy and ensure that limitations imparted by new modalities of communication do not infringe upon the principles of collaboration and informed consent. Finally, treatment planning which includes any new technology must still account for patient safety, appropriate follow-up, and attention to the management of emergency situations. Provider access to a patient's SM could assist in identifying suicidal ideation and/or acts, but there are ethical and privacy concerns (patients fail to disclose risk factors to physicians, despite sharing them with the public on SM platforms such as Facebook and Twitter) [16].

11.2.2 Verbal and Nonverbal Communication

The assessment of telepsychiatry's impact on the doctor-patient relationship is complicated by the many types of patients, settings, and practice styles for which it is employed. Patient types vary by disorder, age, culture, and setting. A critical variable in communication is telemedicine's ability to simulate real-time experiences in terms of image and interaction. Another concept that bears on communication is "presence" [17]. Presence is defined as "... the fact or condition of being at the specified or understood place." In a physical environment, informational cues are incorporated without conscious awareness (e.g., a patient is seen walking in a reticent way). Participants need to be aware that the virtual environment created by telemedicine may be missing cues from the in-person physical environment.

Internet use can have positive effects, when in moderation, social aspects of being a member of a community may help maintain peer connections [18], and games may have benefits for youth with social anxiety or adults with sedentary lifestyles [19]. Some Internet activities improve results on tests and increase motivation for learning among young people [20]. Active SM (i.e., directed, person-to-person exchanges) use increases bonding social capital, bridges social capital, and decreases loneliness; passive use does not [3]. With regard to college students, studies examined the relationship of SM with well-being [21], fear of missing out (FOMO) [22], attachment and social capital [23], and social closeness based on

Table 11.1 Assessment of social media use by youth and young adults: questions for families and providers

Areas/questions	Prompts or specifics	Follow-up questions
Normalize and screen for use of electronics and devices • Which do you use? • How much time per day?	Teens spend an average of 6–8 h daily Options Mobile phone Computer/tablet Gaming systems (X-box, Wii, PlayStation) TV Other	• Which do you use the most? • Which is your favorite? • Compared with the average teen, about how much screen time do you have daily?
Screen for social networking accounts/ profile which is your favorite? Why? • Are you "friends" with your parents or siblings? • Do your parents limit your time? – Day time – Overnight • Do your parents have your passwords?	Facebook Twitter Instagram YouTube Tumblr Google plus Pinterest e-mail Snapchat Video sharing platforms Chat rooms MySpace Other	• Do you use media to deal with stress? – HOW often? # hours/day? • Does media use cause you stress, and if so, how? • What do you post? – Photos, posts, phone, school, city, birthdate? – Videos: What kind? – Have you ever posted or received inappropriate photos? – Have you ever posted something online that caused problems for you, a friend, or a family member? • How many friends do you have? – Do you personally know all of the friends on your social media? • Relationships – How have you used privacy settings? – Have you lied about your age to gain access to websites/online accounts? – Have you interacted with strangers online, and if so, do you use your real name?
Screen for positive aspects of internet and media use	Which specific sites have been helpful to you?	• Have you gotten health or mental health information online? • Have you used self-help sites? • Have you made friends or gotten closer to a friend online? • Have you used apps for wellness? • Have you ever helped a friend who felt suicidal online or via text/chat?

(continued)

Table 11.1 (continued)

Areas/questions	Prompts or specifics	Follow-up questions
Screen for problematic use	Problematic and risky internet use screening scale (PRIUSS) screen (see text of paper for description) or CAGE approach: 1. Have you ever felt you should *cut down* on your internet use? 2. Have others *annoyed* you by criticizing your internet use 3. Have you ever felt bad or *guilty* because of your internet use? 4. Do you need to look at the internet first thing in the morning (*eye-opener*)?	• How often are you online rather than going to sleep at night? • Have you visited sites with sensitive topics? – Weapons? – Porn? – Sites that promote suicide, anorexia, or other things your parents might worry about? • Have you ever had any bad experiences online? • Are there any internet sites that you visit that you don't want your parents to know about?
Screen for risky behavior	Meeting others on-line that you don't know Bullying or harassed Pranks or jokes that go wrong Saying/typing things you ordinarily would not Posting videos, photos, and other things Visiting sites with violent themes Sexting	• Have you interacted with strangers online, and if so, do you use your real name and ID info? • Have you planned to meet up with someone you met on the internet? • Have you ever been bullied or harassed online? Or have you bullied or harassed others online? • Have you played jokes or pranks that came off the wrong way? • Have you said or agreed with things that blew up and/or regretted it (e.g., race/ethnicity, gender/sex, other)? • Have you posted photos, videos, or other things that you regret or do not want friends/parents) to see? • Have you visited sites that focus on suicide, death, or violence? • Have you ever sexted?

activity [24]. A secure attachment was positively associated with online bonding, bridging, and all capital and offline bridging capital; an avoidant attachment was negatively associated with online bonding capital [23]. Interacting with other users (e.g., commenting on updates) helps users feel closer to other people and predicts positive emotional states after Facebook use.

In adult samples, clinical populations seek social support, engagement, or a connection with mental health services. Online modalities help boost social support for cancer survivors, new mothers' well-being, and older adults' connection with family and friends. Studies show that 33% of military personnel may prefer a technology-based platform for mental health care to talking with a counselor in-person [25]. Web-based behavioral treatments have also been demonstrated to be effective and desirable in the treatment of substance use disorders (SUD) [26]. Ease of use, concerns about medical record privacy, and other factors entice those with substance abuse, schizophrenia, autism spectrum disorder, and affective disorders [27–29] to gain mental health services via the Internet. The APA policy statement on SM suggests that psychiatrists discuss the pros/cons of SM use, monitor the impact of digital footprints on life and patient care, caution on engaging in SM due to adverse impacts, reflection about healthy and potentially risky behaviors, and policies on expected rules of engagement (e.g., content), alternative appropriate pathways for urgent/emergent issues (e.g., suicidal ideation) [29].

11.3 Social Media Studies

11.3.1 Clinical Populations and Disorders

A review of 78 studies of SM with outcomes in clinical populations and disorders with a mean age was 18.4 years (median 18) and included adolescents (49) and young adults (28), found more Caucasian patients than any other groups and over 50% + females [30]. The most common SM studied were Facebook (37), Twitter (10), Instagram (5), MySpace (2), and YouTube (2); they came from the countries US (43), Asia (5), UK (3), Canada (3), Australia (3), and other Europe (16). The most studied disorders were depression (49) and anxiety (21).

Cross-sectional and longitudinal studies of SM use and depression found that shorter periods of SM use (< 3 h) particularly with purposeful or active engagement are associated with better mood and psychological well-being, whereas longer SM use predicts depression (and often anxiety) or poorer psychological function—and partly due to sleep disruptions [31]. These studies are also consistent with one prospective study, which suggests a threshold effect above 3 h that has a negative impact for many though not all users—low-stable (80% at 3–4 h/day/item); high-decreasing (12.3% at 4–5 h/day/item), and low-increasing (7.3% at 3 to nearly 5 h/day).

Sometimes depression predicts SM use [32, 33] and it reduces perception of support [34]. Specifically, Twitter use may reduce depressive thoughts and symptoms, but only for people with low initial levels of in-person social support, and conveying positive sentiment predicted a reduction in depressive thoughts and feelings irrespective of people's level of in-person social support [35]. Depressive signals were observable in tweets made that predict future depression [36]. Instagram *browsing* was related to increases in adolescents' depressed mood later [37].

The type of media use may also be important. Hours spent on SM and Internet use were more strongly associated with self-harm behaviors, depressive symptoms, low life satisfaction, and low self-esteem than hours spent on electronic gaming and TV watching [38]. In addition, girls generally demonstrated stronger associations between screen media time and mental health indicators than boys (e.g., heavy Internet users were 166% more likely to have clinically relevant levels of depressive symptoms than low users among girls, compared to 75% more likely among boys). A cross-sectional study showed that Facebook number of friends is positively correlated, while Facebook peer interaction is negatively associated, with cortisol levels [39]. These results provide preliminary evidence that Facebook behaviors are associated with diurnal cortisol concentrations in adolescents; Instagram use was marginally positively associated with depressive symptoms, and positive social comparison was significantly negatively associated with depressive symptoms [40].

Studies of anxiety disorders are similar to findings in depression studies, as greater social anxiety symptoms were mediated by spending more time on Facebook and passively using Facebook (i.e., viewing other profiles without interacting) [41]. In a study with 3 focus groups of those with anxiety disorders, 6 themes emerged: seeking approval; fearing judgment; escalating interpersonal issues; wanting privacy; negotiating self and social identity; and connecting and disconnecting [42]. A qualitative study revealed 3 types of negative use including "oversharing" (frequent updates or too much personal information), "stressed posting" (sharing negative updates), and encountering "triggering posts" [43]. Both social anxiety and need for social assurance had a significant positive association with problematic use of or fear of missing out [30, 44].

11.3.2 Clinical Problems like Suicide, Cyberbullying, Sexting and Other Behaviors

The review of 34 studies on clinical problems such as cyberbullying, sexting, and posts on suicide most commonly included Facebook (10), Twitter (8), Instagram (5), YouTube (3), and MySpace (2). Studies were conducted in the US (15), UK (6), other Europe (4), Asia (4), Canada (3), and Australia (2) [30]. Excessive SM, depression, suicide, and school burnout are strongly related. One longitudinal study found that excess SM use causes psychological distress and suicide attempts [45]. Emotional engagement, school burnout, and depression contribute to excessive SM use. Similarly, students with burnout are at higher risk for depression and excessive use. Excessive use leads to later school burnout and school burnout leads to later excessive use. Suicidal individuals endorsed significantly less belongingness and significantly higher burdensomeness; a higher proportion of achievement-related words appears protective.

AI/machine learning (ML) analysis of SM content was better than self-report measures for predicting suicide and para-suicidal events, using suicide-related tweets and natural language processing algorithms of Sina Weibo [30]. People who are at high suicidal risk can be easily differentiated from those who are not by ML (LIWC, decision tree, and cross-validation analyses) [46]. Suicidal individuals endorsed significantly less belongingness and significantly higher burdensomeness; ML algorithms accurately identify the clinically significant suicidal rate in 92% of cases (sensitivity: 53%, specificity: 97%, positive predictive value: 75%, negative predictive value: 93%); a higher proportion of achievement-related words appears protective. There are differences between those who have attempted to take their life and matched controls due to quantifiable signals of suicide attempt in tweets.

The relationship of depression, self-esteem, and cyberbullying has been evaluated. A study of 8–13 year olds evaluated if cyber victimization is prospectively related to negative self-cognitions and depressive symptoms beyond other types of victimization [35]. The majority of participants reported experiencing at least some degree of peer victimization at either wave 1 or wave 2 (physical = 68.1%; relational = 89.8%; verbal = 87.9%; property-related = 65.8%; cyber = 63.1%). Victimization was correlated with negative cognition and depressive symptoms; it predicted depressive symptoms; age and gender were not predictors of cyber victimization or depression. Another study found that problematic SM use is weakly correlated with depression ($r = 0.22$), gender ($r = -0.15$), age ($r = -0.13$), GB ($r = -0.10$), and self-esteem ($r = -0.11$) [47]. Depression is associated with problematic SM use and indirectly predicted cyberbullying perpetration (associations weak). Experiences of LGBT users included both help for coping and cyberbullying leading to depression, stress, and SI [48].

Bystander responses to suicidal behavior and cyberbullying are in sharp contrast. Only 33.6% of participants left a positive, supportive comment on at least one of two suicide posts. Content severity, experience with a loved one's suicide attempts, and use of Facebook to meet people were predictive of providing positive comments [49]. Positive bystander responses (PBRs) were higher in cyberbullying than in traditional bullying incidents [50]. Females exhibited more PBRs across both types of bullying. Bullying severity impacted PBRs, in that PBRs increased across mild, moderate, and severe incidents, consistent across traditional and cyberbullying. PBRs related to cyberbullying include: (1) seek help from a teacher or parent; (2) seek help from peers or friends; (3) direct intervention; and (4) provide comfort or emotional support.

11.4 Clinical Scenarios

11.4.1 Impact on the Therapeutic Relationship

Consider the hypothetical case of the therapist, who, while browsing her own Facebook account one evening, comes across a "friend request" from a current patient with whom she is engaged in therapy. The therapist must now consider the implications behind the request, choose whether or not to accept, and determine how best to respond to the patient regarding her decision. Does this request reflect a desire on the part of the patient to push the boundaries of the therapeutic frame, perhaps related to some aspect of his presenting problem or in response to an unfolding dynamic in session? [51] A recent study at Rouen University Hospital in France found that 73% of residents in multiple specialties had Facebook profiles, 6% of whom had friend requests from patients, 4 of which were accepted [52].

By avoiding dual relationships with patients, we establish that we are now, and even after therapy, only in the treating role. Patients are empowered to reveal shameful or painful details to their providers, in part through the trust that doing so will have little consequence on any outside relationship [53]. While we understand that a true friendship entails a more equal exchange of private information and confidences [15], patients may not have the same understanding. After all, the newly accepted provider now appears on the same list as the rest of the patient's friends and family. One can see how this sudden integration might impact the ability and willingness to self-disclose.

It is also worth noting the effect on the amount of information available to both parties following an affirmation of "friend" status. Many privacy settings on Facebook are dependent on this designation. That is to say, the ability to view pictures, wall-posts, send messages, and access various bits of personal information may be granted to "friends," while potentially forgetting the sheer range of acquaintances one has included in that same friends list (perhaps to include one's closest friends, one's family members, an old classmate with whom one no longer really associates, a friend of a friend one met at a function once). Aside from issues of privacy (to be discussed in short order), patients may now find themselves privy to many details of their providers' personal lives. While many argue that some self-disclosure on the part of the therapist can be useful when strategically applied, most agree that a great deal of disclosure is rarely advised and can become an obstacle [15]. For cases in which examining transference might be valuable to the treatment, the ability to maintain a somewhat neutral presence might be compromised.

11.4.2 Patient Privacy

Social media sites were not designed with protected doctor-patient interactions in mind, rather, they were designed for social networking. Hence, they are not equipped with the various protective measures, which are required of, for example, an electronic medical record [54]. At the same time, the provider has a responsibility to extend considerations of privacy to interactions with patients online. Something as simple as a patient forgetting to log off his profile could lead to a breach in confidentiality when a family member stumbles upon therapeutic communications. At a minimum, providers need to protect their electronic devices with the same level of security as their paper charts.

Considerations should also be made to local regulations with regard to storing and transmitting identifiable health information. In the United States, this would include assessing whether those communications are considered HIPAA-compliant. Regulations and/or risk-management policies may also dictate the need to document communications with patients. In this case, one must determine which information collected and disseminated online belongs in the patient's chart, and the patient must be made aware of those intentions.

Less-obvious issues relating to patient privacy might also arise. Acquaintances of the patient might wonder about the new connection with a known psychiatrist, or vice-versa, a therapist's friends might be able to deduce that the new addition (whose origin the therapist will not divulge upon asking) is indeed a patient. In rural communities with relatively few people, this may be an even bigger issue, especially if the patient expressly desires to keep her involvement in treatment a secret.

Finally, providers should ask themselves what information about the patient is ethically appropriate to access. After all, a new friend designation suddenly opens up the contents of many patients' accounts for perusal. Such a quandary applies to the notion of performing Internet searches on patients as well [55]. It has been suggested to divide information into the categories of public-public (that which was clearly designated for public consumption, including newspapers, opinion blogs, and public registries), public-private (that which might be available publicly, but which was clearly not intended for the general public, to include content commonly found in one's social media account), and private-private (that which is not easily publicly accessible and is not intended as such, to include a private face-to-face conversation or a private e-mail) [15]. While public-public information is generally considered acceptable to access, and private-private information is not, they illustrate the issue of public-private information with the example of walking past a patient's home with the intent to peek into their window. They argue that the failure of a patient to implement the intended privacy settings on a social media account (or in the above case, not having considered the implications of friending their provider) is akin to a patient neglecting to close the blinds on their window, and thus, still constitutes an intrusion on patient privacy [15].

11.4.3 Provider and Patient Privacy

While providers should strive to respect the privacy of their patients online, it is unlikely that most patients will employ the same standards in reverse. While the anonymity afforded to those who search for information about their providers makes quantifying such activities difficult, the expansion of sites featuring physician information and consensus from the literature suggests that this is common practice [52, 53]. Available information is seemingly endless and can include profession-related things like reviews from patients (accurate or not), educational background, professional affiliations, and one's CV, but also more personal items like one's political contributions, family genealogy, and even how much was paid for one's home. Since the average user views many pages of results per search term, it may be prudent for providers to search themselves and be familiar with at least the first few pages of results. Providers should also be aware that information voluntarily posted online is likely permanent and use discretion accordingly [56].

11.4.4 Professionalism and Provider Image

Many providers across the world, much like their patients, enjoy their own private social media accounts outside of work. Not all practitioners, however, routinely monitor their privacy settings (or set them in the first place) and some are shown engaging in behavior, which might influence the perceptions of others with regard to their character and, perhaps, their professions as a whole. A survey conducted in 2006 and 2007 of then-recent medical graduates in New Zealand found that 65% of graduates had Facebook accounts. Around 63% of those had implemented privacy settings, while 37% of those remaining (those who were readily visible to the public) revealed private details such as sexual orientation, religious views, and relationship status. Another 10% showed images of the users apparently intoxicated [56].

Another study in 2008 involving medical students at the University of Florida found that 68.3% of medical students and 12.8% of residents had Facebook accounts. A random subset of 10 profiles found that 7 included pictures involving alcohol and 3 had depictions of unprofessional conduct including drunkenness, foul language, overt sexuality, and patient-privacy violations. A small proportion of students had joined online Facebook groups with racially charged or sexist titles [57].

Finally, a survey including 78 US medical schools in 2009 yielded 60% who reported incidents of students posting unprofessional content online. Discriminatory language (48%), depiction of sexually suggestive material (38%), use of profanity (52%), and violations of patient privacy (13%) were among the incidents reported. Policies on online conduct already in place were reported by 38%, with another 11% actively developing them [58].

The understandable need for providers to live personal lives outside the public's eye can clash most unfortunately with the accessibility of information available online and the aforementioned patient desire to be informed about one's provider. Problems might even arise for those who choose not to contribute content. With the ability to "tag" other people in photos posted online, providers might learn they were featured in professionally unbecoming photographs long after many others have seen them [53]. Privacy settings may be insufficient to prevent such content from being seen by the particularly earnest or technologically savvy users [59].

Content found online can have far-reaching consequences. Some employers are beginning to utilize Internet and social media searches to screen potential candidates. There have been several news reports depicting medical board reprimands and even dismissals following patient privacy violations [60]. Another man found his career in jeopardy after the content was found linking him to illicit drug use and male prostitution [60]. Public sentiment seems to suggest that many take notice of what professionals post online and hold medical providers to a higher standard of conduct. While combing through the lay public's comments on a story about unprofessional online behavior by medical students, Greysen et al. found the comments

"Anybody who isn't smart enough to figure out what's OK to post on the Internet has absolutely no business being in charge of other people's health," and "As professionals, doctors, teachers, lawyers, etc., are held to a certain standard. If that's not your cup of tea, find a different job" [61].

On its face, being held to an expected level of decorum might seem unfair. Providers who lead stressful practices might feel constantly under the microscope without room for reprieve. Others might cite limits on free speech and self-expression. It is helpful, however, to consider the amount of deference afforded to physicians by many (with some cultures more than others) and the responsibility that might entail. People might look to a psychiatrist or therapist for cues on how to respond to a natural disaster or perhaps an interpersonal conflict. On the flip side, those with little contact with mental health providers might see certain conduct as affirming a particular stigma or personal belief (for example, that psychiatrists are simply pill-pushers who don't actually care about their patients individually). Or perhaps more disturbing, consider the parent of a child in need of mental health care, whose hesitancy to engage available resources is further heightened by witnessing crass and boorish behavior by a psychiatrist online.

The general consensus is mental health providers do have a duty to maintain a certain level of decorum and professionalism when in the public eye (a duty that is perhaps owed to the profession as a whole and to all those whose health might be otherwise negatively affected). With the nature and reach of social media, the concept of "in the public eye" may extend to anything, which is posted online, particularly when efforts to protect that information are either non-existent or fail. This notion is replicated in many institutional policies as well as in the American Medical Association's Policy on professionalism in the use of social media (Shore et al., 2011) [59]. The latter also dictates a physician's responsibility to identify and bring to their attention the unprofessional behavior of other providers.

11.4.5 Patient Safety

As stated previously, providers wishing to introduce new technologies into clinical practice must do so while continuing to account for the patient's safety, an appropriate plan for follow-up and monitoring, and a clear plan for responding to emergency situations. This would certainly hold true when engaging patients via social media (or via text messaging, chat platforms, e-mail, or any other form of digital communication for that matter). On Facebook, contacts have the ability to send messages directly to one another, and to post messages on another contact's personal page (or "wall"), which may then be seen by any audience member fitting the criteria of the page owner's privacy settings, and to also post "status updates" which are then displayed to other contacts in a running "newsfeed" on Facebook's homepage.

Consider a psychiatrist who has accepted contacts from several patients for the purpose of organizing an online medication group. Suppose one of her patients leaves a post on the psychiatrist's wall to the effect of "Thanks SO much for all your stupid advice. Don't worry, you won't ever hear from me again. By the time you read this, I will be dead!" Existing literature is lacking for clear guidelines on how to handle such an event [62]. What should the psychiatrist's response be in this case? What if the post had been left 2 days prior and the psychiatrist was not in the habit of routinely checking her personal page? Alternately, are the psychiatrist's responsibilities the same if the patient voiced suicidal thoughts in a status update that went unnoticed? It would certainly seem unreasonable to expect her to monitor all of her patient's personal pages (bringing into question again issues of patient privacy). It is also worth mentioning that the above scenario could conceivably occur while using both one's personal account and with a separate professional account, as suggested in the AMA Policy.

Other types of discovery may prove similarly problematic. In many jurisdictions, licensed providers are required by law to report suspicions of child abuse and neglect. If evidence of such presented itself via a patient's photo in the provider's newsfeed, it may be her professional responsibility to investigate further or report her concerns to the appropriate agency. Similarly, the Tarasoff law in the United States assigns psychiatrists a duty to help protect potential targets from harm when their patients issue threats of violence. Similarly to the threat of suicide, the psychiatrist would need to consider how best to respond and to do so in an emergent manner. To throw an additional element into the mix, can we be sure the person we are interacting with online is truly our patient and not an imposter with access to login information? [54].

These situations are not straightforward, and yet, it is prudent to consider them ahead of time (as much as possible), rather than scramble in the moment to determine the best course of action. At a minimum, it would seem that establishing clear expectations and rules for communication online with one's patients is essential before entering into such an arrangement. Things to cover might include the frequency at which the provider will check his or her account, the expected time frame for response, and what types of emergent information may be inappropriate to communicate online. In addition to a signed contract, a provider might reiterate the rules in print in strategic locations online. Of course, this still may not prevent an angry or attention-seeking patient from violating these rules and precipitating the same levels of distress and frustration nevertheless.

Drawing from previous sections of this chapter, other things to agree upon beforehand might be establishing what constitutes a boundary crossing or disruption of the frame, rules for things like "tagging" the provider in posts or pictures, and measures to protect privacy, such as agreements not to interact with people in each other's contact lists. A discussion about potential implications for the patient's privacy as well as the potential impact on the therapeutic relationship may also be apropos. Ultimately, the decision regarding how and if to implement social media into clinical practice is an individual one, based in part upon how the unique characteristics of one's practice, patient base, and intended online endeavor combine to inform the potential risks and benefits. Consultation from a trusted source would likely be worth the effort and highly advised.

11.5 Guidelines for Patient Care

11.5.1 Guidelines for Social Media Use, Particularly in Child and Adolescent Populations

Guidelines for SM include confidentiality, informed consent, risk management, competence, multiple relationships, professional conduct, security of information, personal use of SM, and regulatory board use of SM [63]. The American College of Physicians released a comprehensive overview of physician online professionalism, including the following recommendations [64], focusing on communication with patients, gathering information, online education, and other topics. Although numerous papers insist on the separation of personal and professional [59, 64], others have argued how difficult it can be to separate both types of presence online [65]. In fact, physicians should assume that one's private profile could be found.

The *Journal of Medical Internet Research* provided guidelines for healthcare providers to more proactively take advantage of social media based on a review of over 100 articles, websites, policies, and reports [66]: maintain professionalism, be authentic within the scope of practice, and follow general etiquette but adapt for professional care. Additional guidelines available for addressing youth patients and addressing privacy issues are based on ethics codes from the American Psychological Association, American Counseling Association, and the American Psychiatric Association [30].

Overall, the social media guidelines have several things in common (Table 11.2). These fall into four categories: (1) Follow standard privacy and confidentiality

Table 11.2 Existing social media guidelines: a summary of the common tenets

1. Providers should utilize all available privacy settings to protect personal information but should recognize that these settings may not be infallible
2. Every effort must be made to maintain patient confidentiality online while maintaining awareness of unique challenges the online setting may provide
3. Online searches for patient information should only be done in the interest of furthering patient care, and preferably with the patient's knowledge and consent
4. Providers should consider keeping personal and professional information in separate accounts
5. Providers should consider conducting routine searches for their own information to maintain awareness of available content and their online images
6. Providers should take care to maintain the same professional boundaries online as they would in face-to-face relationships
7. Providers and patients should establish clear expectations about online communication, including expected response time and protocols for planned absences
8. When unavailable, providers should arrange coverage for established online communications much as they would for their phone, pager, etc.
9. Providers should educate patients regarding the potential risks of connecting via social media and consider establishing a contract before entering such a relationship
10. Providers should establish clear protocols for managing emergencies that might arise in the course of a social media relationship
11. Many guidelines explicitly recommend against directly friending a patient online

practices for health and personal (i.e., including provider) information; (2) maintain "good" boundaries (e.g., don't "Friend" patients) and be aware of what information is out there about you (e.g., search self once-in-a-while); (3) establish clear expectations about online communication (modes, protocols, absences, emergencies); and (4) discuss all of the above with the patient as part of the informed consent process (e.g., reasons for additional searches).

11.6 Discussion

The evidence bases on patient-centered care, models of care, TMH—when coupled with the long-running tenets of good clinical care in the field of medicine—is a relatively decent platform for the clinician to approach new services and technological developments. In-person and TMH clinical guidelines focus on quality, affordable, and timely care in a variety of settings. Adult guidelines are the most mature, but child and adolescent guidelines are not far behind. A wide range of patients can be served, assessments can be carried out, and the technology/plant can be adjusted. Since the scope of practice in child and adolescent psychiatry involves children, adolescents, parents, and other family members, the complexity of care appears higher—more sources of data sources, more boundaries to attend to, a broader interdisciplinary team membership, and a variety of additional treatments.

The consumer movement on new technologies and ways of communicating with others (text, e-mail, Twitter, and Facebook)—which is being led by adolescents and young adults— compounds the complexity of the care issue described above. For those only treating adults or geriatric patients, though, this learning curve can help clinicians. Significant adjustments for the use of social media include the privacy and confidentiality of health and personal information, maintaining "good" interpersonal/clinical boundaries, being aware of what information is out there about you, and clearly discussing expectations about online communication as part of the informed consent process.

The evidence base will grow rapidly and many areas need development. First, tiering of evidence would be desirable, particularly in areas related to child and adolescent-specific assessments and treatments. Second, qualitative studies may be more important in this era due to the complexity involved with social media than quantitative measures. Third, we must ask "good" questions to continue apprising ourselves of developments as social media, Facebook and texting will impact a patient's illness, interpersonal communication, and relationships with healthcare professionals "on the fly." Guidelines or stances by professional bodies may help, but only if they remain up-to-date and do not follow a decade behind to deal with the fear of the unknown in taking positions. Some medical associations (e.g., Canadian) support the conservative use of social media; some oppose it (e.g., American) though the US community has an array of supporters; and others firmly oppose it (e.g., British) [67–69].

Research in SM is moving toward standardized methods, interventions, and evaluation measures. Studies are limited or have not looked at key issues like: (1)

sociodemographics and health, digital and language literacy; (2) clinical population state or trait; (3) passive consumption, broadcasting and directed purposeful or active engagement/communication; (3) quality of assessment (e.g., self-report questionnaires rather than clinician-administered instruments or structured assessments—without confirmation, verification, observation, and corroboration); (4) temporal dimensions of symptoms and assessment; (6) and/or longitudinal design and comparison groups. Broadly speaking, the reviews also did not always clarify the relationship between SM and behavioral health issues (i.e., associations, mediating versus causal relationships). Researchers and providers are capitalizing on AI and ML methods to advance data processing, stratify risk (e.g., suicide) and predict future negative outcomes. This will help with longitudinal correlation, prediction, and/or biomarking/digital phenotyping of patients' outcomes (e.g., depression during and after pregnancy). For example, SM provides the capability to collect, build, and model person-specific, intelligently filtered information presented in a timely manner to monitor, intervene, and follow trajectories for mood and suicide [30, 36, 46].

11.7 Conclusions

Technology both facilitates and affects current evidence-based care, sometimes for the better and sometimes for the worse, and providers need to stay abreast of changes in contemporary practice. Continuing education and discussing the many issues involved with patients and families, as well as peers, is suggested

Acknowledgments American Telemedicine Association, Telemental Health Interest Group

References

1. Pew Research Center. Teens, Social Media and Technology 2018. https://www.pewresearch.org/internet/2018/05/31/teens-social-media-technology-2018/. 2018.
2. Boyd DM, Ellison NB. Social network sites: definition, history, and scholarship. J Comput-Mediat Commun. 2007;13(1):210–30.
3. Orben A. Teenagers, screens and social media: a narrative review of reviews and key studies. Soc Psychiatry Psychiatr Epidemiol. 2020;55(4):407–14. https://doi.org/10.1007/s00127-019-01825-4.
4. Cheston CC, Flickinger TE, Chisolm MS. Social media use in medical education: a systematic review. Acad Med. 2013;88(6):893–901.
5. Madden M, Lenhart, A, Cortesy S, Gasser URS, Duggan M, Smith A et al. Teens, Social Media, and Privacy. https://www.pewresearch.org/internet/2013/05/21/teens-social-media-and-privacy/.
6. Anderson EL, Steen E, Stavropoulos V. Internet use and problematic internet use: a systematic review of longitudinal research trends in adolescence and emergent adulthood. Int J Adolesc Youth. 2017;22(4):430–54.
7. O'Keeffe GS. Social media: challenges and concerns for families. Pediatr Clin. 2016;63(5):841–9.

8. Federal Trade Commission. The Children's Online Privacy Protection Rule. 2013. https://www.ftc.gov/enforcement/rules/rulemaking-regulatory-reform-proceedings/childrens-online-privacy-protection-rule. 2013.
9. Zalpuri I, Liu HY, Stubbe D, Wrzosek M, et al. Social media and networking competencies for psychiatric education: skills, teaching methods, and implications. Acad Psychiatry. 2018;42(6):808–17. https://doi.org/10.1007/s40596-018-0983-6.
10. Prensky M. Digital natives, digital immigrants part 1. On the Horizon. 2001;9:1–6.
11. Deen SR, Withers A, Hellerstein DJ. Mental health practitioners' use and attitudes regarding the internet and social media. BJU Int. 2017;119(6):955–60.
12. Engle GL. The clinical application of the biopsychosocial model. Am J Psychiatry. 1980;137(5):535–44.
13. Hamann J, Leucht S, Kissling W. Shared decision making in psychiatry. Acta Psychiatr Scand. 2003;107(6):403–9.
14. Hebb DO. Distinctive features of learning in the higher animal. In: Delafresnaye JF, editor. Brain mechanisms and learning. London: Oxford University Press; 1961.
15. Frankish K, Ryan C, Harris A. Psychiatry and online social media: potential, pitfalls and ethical guidelines for psychiatrists and trainees. Australas Psychiatry. 2012;20:181–7.
16. Pourmand A, Roberson J, Caggiula A, et al. Social media and suicide: a review of technology-based epidemiology and risk assessment. Telemed J E Health. 2019;25(10):880–8. https://doi.org/10.1089/tmj.2018.0203.
17. Hilty DM, Randhawa K, Maheu M, et al. A review of telepresence, virtual reality and augmented reality applied to clinical care. J Tech Behav Sci. 2020;5:178–205.
18. Kowert R, Vogelgesang J, Festl R, et al. Psychosocial causes and consequences of online video game play. Comp Human Behav. 2015;45:51–8.
19. Glover J, Fritsch SL. Kids, anxiety and social media: a review. Child Adolesc Clin N Am. 2018;27:171–82.
20. Guan SSA, Subrahmanyam K. Youth internet use: risks and opportunities. Curr Opin Psychiatry. 2009;22:351–6.
21. Rasmussen E, Punyanunt-Carter N, La Freniere J, et al. The serially mediated relationship between emerging adults' social media use and mental well-being. Comput Hum Behav. 2020;102:206–13. https://doi.org/10.1016/j.chb.2019.08.019.
22. Hunt MG, Marx R, Lison C, Young J. No more FOMO: limiting social media decreases loneliness and depression. J Soc Clin Psychol. 2018;37(10):751–68.
23. Lin JH. The role of attachment style in Facebook use and social capital: evidence from university students and a national sample. Cyberpsychol Behav Soc Netw. 2015;18(3):173–80. https://doi.org/10.1089/cyber.2014.0341.
24. Neubaum G, Kra¨ mer NC. My friends right next to me: a laboratory investigation on predictors and consequences of experiencing social closeness on social networking sites. Cyber Psychol Behav Soc Netw. 2015;18:443–9.
25. Wilson JA, Onorati K, Mishkind M, et al. Soldier attitudes about technology-based approaches to mental health care. Cyberpsychol Behav. 2008;11(6):767–9.
26. Marsch LA, Guarino H, Acosta M, et al. Web-based behavioral treatment for substance use disorders as a partial replacement of standard methadone maintenance treatment. J Subst Abuse Treat. 2014;46(1):43–51.
27. Canadian Medical Association. Social media and Canadian physicians—issues and rules of engagement. 2015. https://www.cma.ca/socialmedia. 1 Aug 2023.
28. Välimäki M, Kannisto KA, Vahlberg T, Hätönen H, Adams CE. Short text messages to encourage adherence to medication and follow-up for people with psychosis (Mobile.Net): randomized controlled trial in finland. J Med Internet Res. 2017;19(7):e245. Published 2017 Jul 12. https://doi.org/10.2196/jmir.7028.
29. American Psychiatric Association position statement on the risks of adolescents' Online Activity. 2018. https://www.psychiatry.org/getattachment/fb0fcd5b-45d5-4177-9756-47a35f389048/Position-2018-Risk-of-Adolescents-Online-Activity.pdf.

30. Hilty DM, Stubbe DS, McKean AS, et al. A scoping review of social media in child, adolescents and young adults: research findings in depression, anxiety and other clinical challenges. BJPsych Open. 2023;9:e152.
31. Vernon L, Modecki KL, Barber BL. Tracking effects of problematic social networking on adolescent psychopathology: the mediating role of sleep disruptions. J Clin Child Adolesc Psychol. 2017;46(2):269–83. https://doi.org/10.1080/15374416.2016.1188702.
32. Gámez-Gaudix M. Depressive symptoms and problematic use among adolescents: analysis of the longitudinal relation-ships from the cognitive-behavioral model. Cyber Psychol Behav Soc Network. 2014;17:714–9.
33. Houghton S, Lawrence D, Hunter SC, et al. Reciprocal relationships between trajectories of depressive symptoms and screen media use during adolescence. J Youth Adolesc. 2018;47(11):2453–67. https://doi.org/10.1007/s10964-018-0901-y.
34. Park J, Lee DS, Shablack H, et al. When perceptions defy reality: the relationships between depression and actual and perceived Facebook social support. J Affect Disord. 2016;200:37–44. https://doi.org/10.1016/j.jad.2016.01.048.
35. Cole DA, Zelkowitz RL, Nick E, et al. Longitudinal and incremental relation of cybervictimization to negative self-cognitions and depressive symptoms in young adolescents. J Abnorm Child Psychol. 2016;44(7):1321–32. https://doi.org/10.1007/s10802-015-0123-7.
36. De Choudhury M, Counts S, Horvitz E, et al. Characterizing and predicting postpartum depression from shared Facebook data. In: Presented at: 17th ACM conference on Computer supported cooperative work & social computing—CSCW '14; Feb 15–19, 2014; Baltimore, MD, USA; 2014. p. 626–38. https://doi.org/10.1145/2531602.2531675.
37. Frison E, Eggermont S. Browsing, posting, and liking on Instagram: the reciprocal relationships between different types of Instagram use and adolescents' depressed mood. Cyber Psychol Behav Soc Network. 2017;20(10):603–9. https://doi.org/10.1089/cyber.2017.0156.
38. Twenge JM, Farley E. Not all screen time is created equal: associations with mental health vary by activity and gender (published online ahead of print, 2020 Aug 2). Soc Psychiatry Psychiatr Epidemiol. 2020;56:207. https://doi.org/10.1007/s00127-020-01906-9.
39. Morin-Major JK, Marin MF, Durand N, et al. Facebook behaviors associated with diurnal cortisol in adolescents: is befriending stressful? Psychoneuroendocrinology. 2016;63:238–46. https://doi.org/10.1016/j.psyneuen.2015.10.005.
40. Lup K, Trub L, Rosenthal L. Instagram #instasad?: exploring associations among instagram use, depressive symptoms, negative social comparison, and strangers followed. Cyberpsychol Behav Soc Netw. 2015;18(5):247–52. https://doi.org/10.1089/cyber.2014.0560.
41. Shaw AM, Timpano KR, Tran TB, et al. Correlates of Facebook usage patterns: the relationship between passive Facebook use, social anxiety symptoms, and brooding. Comput Hum Behav. 2015;48:575–80. https://doi.org/10.1016/j.chb.2015.02.003.
42. Calancie O, Ewing L, Narducci LD, et al. Exploring how social networking sites impact youth with anxiety: a qualitative study of Facebook stressors among adolescents with an anxiety disorder diagnosis. Cyberpsychol. 2017;11(4):Article 2. https://doi.org/10.5817/CP2017-4-2.
43. Radovic A, Gmelin T, Stein BD, et al. Depressed adolescents' positive and negative use of social media. J Adolesc. 2017;55:5–15. https://doi.org/10.1016/j.adolescence.2016.12.002.
44. Dempsey AE, O'Brien KD, Tiamiyu MF, et al. Fear of missing out (FoMO) and rumination mediate relations between social anxiety and problematic Facebook use. Addict Behav Rep. 2019;9:100150. Published 2019 Apr 12. https://doi.org/10.1016/j.abrep.2018.100150.
45. Salmela-Aro K, Upadyaya K, Hakkarainen K, et al. The dark side of internet use: two longitudinal studies of excessive internet use, depressive symptoms, school burnout and engagement among Finnish early and late adolescents. J Youth Adolesc. 2017;46(2):343–57. https://doi.org/10.1007/s10964-016-0494-2.
46. Braithwaite SR, Giraud-Carrier C, et al. Validating machine learning algorithms for twitter data against established measures of suicidality. JMIR Ment Health. 2016;3(2):e21. Published 2016 May 16. https://doi.org/10.2196/mental.4822.
47. Kırcaburun K, Kokkinos CM, Demetrovics Z, et al. Problematic online behaviors among adolescents and emerging adults: associations between cyberbullying perpetration, problematic social media use, and psychosocial factors. Int J Mental Health Addiction. 2019;17(4):891–908.

48. Escobar-Viera CG, Whitfield DL, Wessel CB, et al. For better or for worse? a systematic review of the evidence on social media use and depression among lesbian, gay, and bisexual minorities. JMIR Ment Health. 2018;5(3):e10496. Published 2018 Jul 23. https://doi.org/10.2196/10496.
49. Corbitt-Hall DJ, Gauthier JM, Troop-Gordon W. Suicidality disclosed online: using a simulated Facebook task to identify predictors of support giving to friends at risk of self-harm. Suicide Life Threat Behav. 2019;49(2):598–613. https://doi.org/10.1111/sltb.12461.
50. Macaulay PJR, Boulton MJ, Betts LR. Comparing early adolescents' positive bystander responses to cyberbullying and traditional bullying: the impact of severity and gender. J Technol Behav Sci. 2019;4:253–61. https://doi.org/10.1007/s41347-018-0082-2.
51. Gutheil TG, Gabbard GO. The concept of boundaries in clinical practice: theoretical and risk-management dimensions. Am J Psychiatry. 1993;150(2):188–96.
52. Moubarak G, Guiot A, Benhamou Y, et al. Facebook activity of residents and fellows and its impact on the doctor-patient relationship. J Med Ethics. 2011;37(2):101–4.
53. Gabbard GO, Kassaw KA, Perez-Garcia G. Professional boundaries in the era of the internet. Acad Psychiatry. 2011;35(3):168–74.
54. Yellowlees P, Nafiz N. The psychiatrist-patient relationship of the future: anytime, anywhere? Harv Rev Psychiatry. 2010 Mar-Apr;18(2):96–102.
55. Clinton BK, Silverman BC, Brendel DH. Patient-targeted googling: the ethics of searching online for patient information. Harv Rev Psychiatry. 2010;18(2):103–12.
56. MacDonald J, Sohn S, Ellis P. Privacy, professionalism and Facebook: a dilemma for young doctors. Med Educ. 2010 Aug;44(8):805–13.
57. Thompson LA, Dawson K, Ferdig R, et al. The intersection of online social networking with medical professionalism. J Gen Intern Med. 2008;23:954–7.
58. Chretien KC, Greysen SR, Chretien JP, et al. Online posting of unprofessional content by medical students. JAMA. 2009;302:1309–15.
59. Shore R, Halsey J, Shah K, et al. Report of the AMA Council on ethical and judicial affairs: professionalism in the use of social media. J Clin Ethics Summer. 2011;22(2):165–72.
60. Ginory A, Sabatier LM, Eth S. Addressing therapeutic boundaries in social networking. Psychiatry. 2012;75(1):40–8.
61. Greysen SR, Kind T, Chretien KC. Online professionalism and the mirror of social media. J Gen Intern Med. 2010;25(11):1227–9.
62. Myers KM, Lieberman D. Telemental health: responding to mandates for reform in primary healthcare. Tel e-Health. 2013;19(6):438–43.
63. Drude K, Messer-Engel K. The development of social media guidelines for psychologists and for regulatory use. J Technol Behav Sci. 2021;6(2):388–96. https://doi.org/10.1007/s41347-020-00176-1.
64. Farnan JM, Snyder Sulmasy L, et al. Online medical professionalism: patient and public relationships: policy statement from the American College of Physicians and the Federation of State Medical Boards. Ann Intern Med. 2013;158(8):620–7.
65. Behnke S. Ethics in the age of the internet. Monit Psychol. 2008;39(7):74.
66. Grajales FJ, Sheps S, Ho K, et al. Social media: a review and tutorial of applications in medicine and health care. J Med Internet Res. 2014;16(2):e13.
67. American Medical Association. Opinion 9.124—Professionalism in the use of social media. AMA Code of Medical Ethics 2011. 1 Aug 2023. http://www.ama-assn.org/ama/pub/physician-resources/medical-ethics/code-medical-ethics/opinion9124.page?
68. British Medical Association. Using social media: practical and ethical guidance for doctors and medical students. (2013-10-27). 1 Aug 2023. http://www.medschools.ac.uk/SiteCollectionDocuments/social_media_guidance_may2011.pdf.
69. Canadian Medical Association. Social media and Canadian physicians—issues and rules of engagement. 1 Aug 2023. http://www.cma.ca.libproxy.usc.edu/socialmedia.

Part IV

Updates on Patient Centered Digital Mental Health Treatments

Web-and Internet-Based Services: Education, Support, Self-Care, Formal, and Hybrid Treatment Approaches

12

Davor Mucić, Donald M. Hilty, Peter M. Yellowlees, and Marek Krzystanek

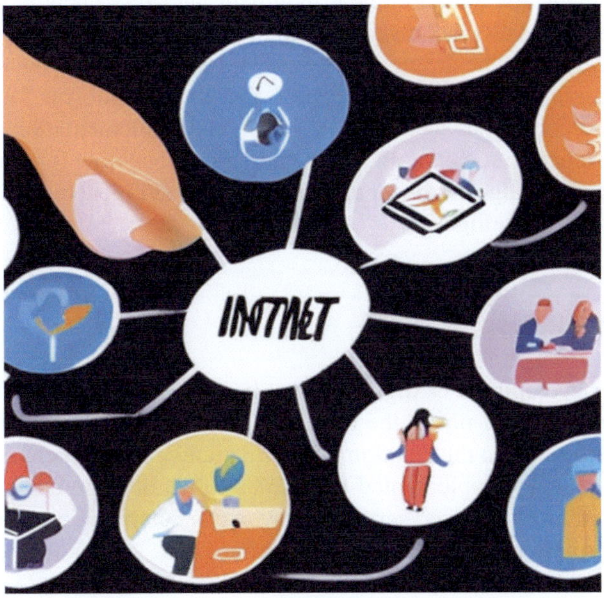

D. Mucić
The Little Prince Psychiatric Centre, Copenhagen, Denmark
e-mail: davor@denlilleprins.org

D. M. Hilty
Department of Psychiatry and Behavioral Sciences, Keck School of Medicine University of Southern California, Los Angeles, CA, USA
e-mail: donald.hilty@uhsinc.com; hilty@med.usc.edu

P. M. Yellowlees
Department of Psychiatry and Behavioral Sciences, UC Davis, Sacramento, CA, USA
e-mail: pmyellowlees@ucdavis.edu

D. Mucić, D. M. Hilty (eds.), *Digital Mental Health*,
https://doi.org/10.1007/978-3-031-59936-1_12

Abstract

Web-and Internet-based resources are remarkably popular with the public, patients, and providers as interventions over the last decades. Opportunities exist for health information, support groups, formal education programs, tools for self-directed lifestyle and illness management, obtaining advice/consultation, and self-or provider-directed treatments. Traditional treatments are more easily disseminated to the point-of-service. Modification of regular treatments is being developed, based on smartphone and web medical applications, and applying virtual reality/avatars from games into medicine. Digital mental health (DMH) innovations/new treatments for special populations are made possible, and hybrid models are now becoming more and more popular, creating the opportunity to develop a true personalized psychiatry and integration of medical data from treatment by psychiatrists and somatic physicians. Clinicians must become aware of, adapt, use sound clinical judgment, and serve new advisory roles to patients, as we are all challenged to keep the best of mental healthcare, yet make it more accessible. The development of DMH forces the introduction of mandatory training in the use of medical applications and platforms for both medical students and doctors, as well as the creation and implementation of recommendations of scientific societies and legal regulations, enabling further development of DMH based on algorithms for narrow artificial intelligence, and in the future—general artificial intelligence.

12.1 Introduction

The dynamic development of digital mental health (DMH) use accelerated during the pandemic, leading if not to the transformation of analog medicine into digital medicine, then at least to the creation of hybrid medicine, in which traditional inpatient therapy is being supplemented by various forms of remote telemedicine care [1]. MH-related Internet-based services may be characterized in several categories: (1) health information via sites; (2) support groups (i.e., general or specific topic) or participation in a "community"; (3) formal educational resources; (4) tools for self-directed assessment, lifestyle change, or decision-making on management of an illness (e.g., diabetes and depression); (5) one-time medical advice/consultation or general advice in a group led by a professional, often involving self-directed formal treatment; and (6) MH services with professionals (telemental health (DMH) care; Internet-based cognitive behavioral therapy (CBT), or another form of psychotherapy) [2–7]. The Internet overcomes obstacles: geographic distance from services; those with special needs (i.e., autism-spectrum and sensory and motor disabilities);

M. Krzystanek (✉)
Department and Clinic of Psychiatric Rehabilitation, Faculty of Medical Sciences in Katowice, Medical University in Katowice, Katowice, Poland
e-mail: m.krzystanek@sum.edu.pl

the housebound (i.e., physical or MH like panic disorder or phobias); and among/in particular generations (i.e., teenagers).

Thus, the Internet and World Wide Web have complemented regular MH care, added user-friendly additional care, and greater access and customization/personalization. During the pandemic, DMH largely replaced the provision of psychiatric and psychotherapeutic services impossible to obtain in stationary form, contributing to maintaining the continuity of treatment for patients and fulfilling a protective role for maintaining mental health services [1]. So the "content" or ranges of care is broader—and the "processes" to access services are more numerable. Patients' preferences for help-seeking, education, and treatments are becoming better known—at least to providers who evolve with practice trends and the new applications of technology. In the traditional provider-based healthcare system, providers and systems decide where, what, and how folks get care. In the person-or patient-centered system, folks just go where they want to go and access information and care. DMH has become a desirable alternative in a patient-centered health service system where patients can decide how to obtain health services. The wide introduction of DMH has also contributed to the development of community psychiatry, increasing patients' access to medical professionals. Similarly, in banking, people migrated to ATMs based on simple task completion and used tellers, as necessary. Many ask, "Is it that simple for MH issues, symptoms and disorders?" Ironically, a provocative comment regarding Internet addiction and its treatment via Internet-based approaches was, "It sounds like holding AA meetings in a bar."

We approach web-and Internet-based treatments in the following context, considering information on: (1) consumer use of the spectrum of online information; (2) traditional healthcare service trends; (3) innovations by programs that had to move forward to meet their patients' needs or to overcome obstacles (i.e., rural and military) and illness-specific factors (e.g., e-treatment or communication for those with post-traumatic stress disorder (PTSD); and finally (4) new technology-based methodologies that have initial, good application to clinical populations, usually from the field of DMH (i.e., virtual reality (VR), augmented VR, avatars, biosensors, other).

MH providers must meet the challenges and requirements that are emerging to fulfill the care-related requests brought about by this wave of change brought about by consumer preferences and technology. With the informal and self-directed service use increasing, one question is, "If the person or patient is in care, should this be overseen by a professional, and if so, how?" In addition, "Can we assume the person or patient will plug in and get where they need to go or find the best service for them?" It may be better for patients to use regular therapy, while others would benefit from the VR lab online video-meetings for socialization, dealing with fears, exposure to symptoms, and to "try on" different personalities or behavioral styles. MH providers, while curious, also contend with pre-existing pathologies or seemingly new pathologies related to the Internet (e.g., addiction, group suicide, and cyberbullying), disruptions of development, and high-profile community events (e.g., disasters or tragedies portrayed in the media).

The period of the pandemic contributed to the development of online applications for group video-meetings, which were adapted to individual and group therapeutic meetings in MH. The introduction of new forms of providing medical services gave rise to many new regulatory and legal problems and prompted scientific societies all over the world to formulate recommendations regarding DMH treatment [8, 9]. The essence of these recommendations is the creation by the MH provider of videoconferencing conditions that assure the same level of comfort and intimacy as a face-to-face meeting. Video-meetings conducted as part of DMH must take place in digitally secure medical applications that ensure the protection of medical data, and the patient must agree to conduct therapy remotely. Applications for online therapy should undergo a certification process in which scientific societies must participate, which will ensure the appropriate standard of medical services. Certification of videoconferencing telemedicine applications, as well as other medical applications, and then monitoring their effectiveness and safety of use have become new challenges that the healthcare system around the world must face today. An important issue is also the need to change the system of training students at medical universities and train them in the treatment and health monitoring using various forms of DMH.

We will paint a picture of what folks are doing, what seems to work, and some of the possibilities for helping patients in this chapter. We realize that while we seek options that are robust, standardized, or evidence-based, that we also have to attend to trends, pilots, and things that do not work. With the exception of extremes, we consider that the content and process of care by technology is probably not inherently good or bad. Those value judgments are important, but may have more to do with how technology is used, what it is used for, and whether health promotion is the ultimate outcome. The reader will learn about the pros and cons of:

1. The spectrum of web-and Internet-based health options for consumers (and patients), including health information, support groups, formal education programs, tools for self-directed lifestyle and illness management, options advice/consultation, and self-or provider-directed treatments (e.g., cognitive behavioral therapy (CBT), DMH care).
2. Web-and Internet-based treatments for patient care, including traditional treatments more easily disseminated, innovations/new treatments used in special populations, and hybrid models of care.
3. The present and the future of web-and Internet-based quasi-experimental treatments with that have initial, good application to clinical populations, usually from the field of MH informatics (e.g., VR, virtual reality exposure therapy (VRET), augmented reality, and avatar therapy).

12.2 Spectrum of Web-and Internet-Based Health Options for Consumers (and Patients and Providers)

Certain basic rules of healthcare shape this discussion—that is, how we approach low-cost and readily accessible health resources versus high-cost care (e.g., synchronous DMH). First, in any actual doctor/patient consultation, we know that across specialties about 80% of all consultations/visits for any doctor are generally straightforward [10]. The 80/20 rule, then, is a concept that essentially means about 20% of the patients use about 80% of resources in seeing doctors. This 80/20 phenomenon means that in healthcare we really need to concentrate on the simple transactions to be efficient and to free up the most highly trained professionals to undertake the more complicated transactions. Second, the complementarity principle simple states that computer programs do well what humans do badly, and vice versa; we should avoid duplication. Third, it may be easier to redesign a system before putting in a new technology, rather than trying to match a technology to a currently inefficient system.

It is certain that the Internet is an important and influential source of information for consumers, as according to a 2008 survey, about 80% of Americans rely on the Internet to find health information to make their healthcare decisions [11]. Globally, Africa, the Middle East, and Latin America are the fastest growing populations in terms of Internet usage [12]. In the United States, Internet use has grown dramatically over the past decade, with a jump from 44% of the population [13]. DMH, specifically, is one of the best-known areas [13]. Online health information varies in quality and readability [14–16], but it has been very popular by enhancing coping strategies, empowerment, and self-efficacy for patients, caregivers, and providers [17]. Users report reduced feelings of anxiety and isolation, enhanced connectedness in the doctor–patient relationship, and ability to make decisions on health-related behaviors [18–20].

Social networking has been defined as "web-based services that allow individuals to (1) construct a public or semi-public profile within a bounded system, (2) articulate a list of other users with whom they share a connection, and (3) view and traverse their list of connections and those made by others within the system." [21] While it may be part of the many categories below, it is covered more in other chapters, except for directly targeted patient programs.

12.2.1 Health Information

Who are these users of the Internet? [12, 13] Most are women (86% of women vs. 73% of men), seeking for information on diseases or medical problems, treatments or procedures, doctors or other health professionals, hospitals or other medical facilities, food safety or recalls, drug safety or recalls, and pregnancy and childbirth. Caregivers (a term used for adults who provide unpaid care to a parent, child, friend, or other loved ones) have access to the Internet at a high rate (79%) and of those, 88% look online for health information. Education affects use: 89% of those with a college degree vs. 70% with a high school degree vs. 38% with less. Income is a predictor: 95% of adults with household income $75,000+ vs. 57% with household income less than $30,000.

Health promotion strategies are typically at free-standing websites [22] and the impact of these has been reviewed [23]. Many patients migrate to sites like PatientsLikeMe (http://www.patientslikeme.com/), a consumer-driven site where individuals log on to connect with others in the community who are experiencing similar medical issues. Some options like role-playing game "Second Life" described below, which when used as an educational tool, may improve understanding of psychotic symptoms (i.e., auditory-and/or visual hallucinations) [24]. For some patients this is ideal: those with anxiety (e.g., phobias or panic disorder), trauma (e.g., military personnel with PTSD), geographic obstacles (e.g., rural or otherwise long travel), poor access to care (e.g., waiting time), or dislike of local services (e.g., seen as ineffective or of limited quality).

Young people with developmental challenges may have limited access to MH services. Web and social media are changing not only communication patterns especially for them, but also the way they are looking for help, sharing experiences, and learning new behaviors. Children and adolescents, comfortable with and reinforced by Internet-based chats and groups, may express ideas of self-harm, negative affective states, or pessimistic cognitions of other peers [25, 26]—all of this is good, if it duplicates telling others who will respond or help them; it is more concerning, though, if it is posted and not seen.

Common prejudice is that psychotic patients are not eligible for remote consultations and for the use of technology, in general. There is a combination of stimulus overflow, inability to deal with the abundance of information, difficulties with concentration, lack of energy, paranoia, and fear of symptom provocation. However, they succeed to use the Internet as a source of information related to their illness as well as for medication issues (e.g., to check medication side effects in the hope of finding better medication) [27–29]. Systems have been tested to provide symptom and mood regulation, medication adherence, social support, and sleep hygiene on a smartphone platform [30, 31], and sensors may predict mood or schizophrenia relapse with personalized early warning signs—such as isolation, movement inactivity, and unusual behavior [32].

Moreover, patients with psychotic symptoms may benefit from DMH even more than traditional way of treatment. Telemedicine treatment of a patient with schizophrenia who does not have to leave his comfort zone related to his place of residence and does not have to sit in the doctor's waiting room, exposing himself to potential distress and stigmatization, gives better results, especially in terms of emotional well-being and mood [33, 34]. Long-term use of such treatment may result in even better improvement in terms of treatment of other symptoms of schizophrenia and, what is very important, it is effective and does not cause deterioration in psychotic patients who, as it might seem, could potentially interpret their monitoring by the telemedicine system in a delusional manner. Fortunately, this is not the case. Similarly, schizotypal personality disorder patients have been found to be especially likely to use the Internet, with a particular interest in social interaction on the web [35].

12.2.2 Support Groups and Participation in a "Community"

Most support groups are for consumers and patients on the subject of health-related behaviors. Internet-mediated support groups can include specialized groups for individuals with disabilities or unique modes of experience [36]. Web-based support to individuals with stigmatizing or rare illness is extremely important as such groups are often socially isolated so that social networking websites represent a tool to build community [37]. Such support is particularly suitable and well accepted by stigmatized patients who appreciate the anonymity and easy access, enabling exchange of experiences as well as flow of information [38]. They may contribute to increase knowledge, change attitudes, and alter behavior. Many programs use a peer-to-peer forum to ask questions, tell stories, and share positive ideas; others include a healthcare provider.

Social networking sites may provide a stress buffering resource for those serving in the military who experienced adverse life events [39]. In military populations the fear of stigma among other concern reduces treatment seeking for MH issues [32, 40]. Technology-based approaches may increase MH care access for this population. One study found that 33% of soldiers who reported that they were not willing to talk to a counselor in person were willing to utilize at least one technology-based platform for mental healthcare [41]. Similarly, soldiers measured preferred using the iPhone over paper or computer due to its interface, portability, and convenience [42].

For ethnic minorities, there is more than one meaning to the use of the Internet. For the Aboriginal communities in Canada, it may represent a support medium through which the members communicate the Indigenous language and cultural traditions [43, 44]. The Internet became a medium for meetings between the generations to share and preserve traditional knowledge—indeed, this worked better than past processes to some degree.

Caregivers, too, may benefit using telecommunication technology. A review of Internet-based interventions for medical and MH disorders showed that approximately two-thirds of open or randomized controlled trials reduced stress and improved quality of life—at least significantly in terms of specific measured outcomes [17]. Family caregivers located in rural areas found e-health support to be beneficial in comparison with conventional caregiver support [45]. The interventions include interactive communities, bulletin board chatting, and therapy groups [17].

12.2.3 Formal Materials or Opportunities for Consumers, Patients, Caregivers, and Providers

Many consumers, patients, caregivers, and providers are seeking more than health information from websites, bulletin boards, webcasts, discussion boards, and chat rooms. They need or want more robust, structured programs (e.g., online classes, learning modules, videos, and skills training). Providers often shoot for professional education courses. Caregivers feel a need-to-know clinical tips, self-help coping strategies, and tips on advocacy—a review of Internet-based interventions for medical and MH disorders showed that approximately two-thirds of initiatives reduced stress and improved quality of life; some of these were of open or randomized controlled trials that measured outcomes [17]. Patient populations included MH (dementia, schizophrenia, and anorexia) and medical (older adults/aging, heart transplant, traumatic brain injury, hip fracture, cancer, and stroke). Caregivers' outcomes improved and they are satisfied and comfortable with support services delivered by cell phones [46].

Young people may benefit from web-based information, screening and assessment, and online treatment. Child and adolescents patients have been targeted over the last decade at schools, free-standing promotions in malls, at home via TV, and at primary care or MH specialist settings. A series of Internet interventions have been developed to provide broad MH promotion in children and adolescents: Kindertelefoon (www.kindertelefoon.nl), YooMagazine (www.Yoomagazine.net), Ciao, ReachOut (www.reach-out.org), and Walkalong (www.walkalong.ca). Increasing the frequency of personality disorders and mental disorders in the population of children and adolescents is another challenge for DMH. Young people who have grown up with the Internet and smartphones seem particularly vulnerable to the use of DMH for their medical education, health monitoring, and remote psychiatric and psychotherapeutic assistance, conducted with the consent of a parent or legal guardian. DMH can contribute in particular to increasing the accessibility of young people to intimate contact with a psychologist, psychotherapist, and even a psychiatrist without exposing them to stigmatization and hate in the peer environment. Hence the need to develop telemedicine platforms dedicated to psychological support for schools using DMH.

12.2.4 Tools for Self-Directed Habit, Lifestyle, or Illness Changes: Assessment and Treatment

These tools typically target good habits/health promotion, disease prevention, and informal management of symptoms or problems. Techniques might include use of a diary, a questionnaire, or a survey to provoke reflection or "stepping back" to re-evaluate one's assumptions in a conclusion. Exercise and substance (i.e., alcohol) logs are popular. Mood assessments like MoodyMe (https://itunes.apple.com/us/app/moody-me-mood-diary-tracker/id411567371?mt=8) are commonly used, as are those that map behavior patterns across time, including triggers, diet, sleep, and other related factors. Stress reduction care provision with a mobile phone app is increasing because of many potential users and economic impacts on community [47].

Various mobile applications especially those focusing on self-help in dealing with anxiety disorders, MH well-being, and stress reduction have been adjusted so that various patient groups may benefit of it also via respective mother tongue. One example is "Fear Fighter," a computer-guided self-exposure approach to treat phobia/panic developed at the end of last century [48]. Exposure therapy is effective for phobia/panic, but qualified and trained therapist resources are scarce. Both patients and clinicians achieve benefits by having better access, saving time, and enhancing healthcare efficiency [49]. The app also enables the patient to get necessary guidance/assistance whenever and wherever he/she needs it.

The range of initiatives for support caregivers includes hotlines for consultation on key decisions (i.e., decision support), psychosocial treatments like CBT (individual or group), problem solving training, coaching for positive parenting skills. Caregivers (and consumers) may benefit from Internet-or application-based assessment questionnaires to self-diagnose and refer (e.g., patient health questionnaire for depression; hospital anxiety and depression scale). A study of public social networking accounts of college students found that 25% of college students exhibited depressive symptoms based upon the Diagnostic and Statistical Manual of Mental Disorders (DSM) criteria, and 2.5% met the DSM criteria for major depressive disorder. Online reinforcement from their friends may have made them more likely to discuss their depressive symptoms publicly via social networking sites [50].

Support and self-help programs allow users to ask questions of health professionals while remaining anonymous. Self-help programs are designed to offer relevant treatment approach typically without guidance from the therapist. Such self-help interventions without therapist guidance are especially attractive for the users that are stigmatized (e.g., severe mentally ill or individuals with drinking problem) [51].

Combined work by the Telemedicine and Advanced Technology Research Center, the Military Operational Medicine Research Program, United States Army Medical Research and Materiel Command, the National Center for Telehealth and Technology, and the Department of Veterans Affairs has released apps for the general public in dedicated app stores [52]. One is called PTSD Coach [53]. It is designed to help veterans learn about and manage symptoms that commonly occur after trauma. While such apps are not designed to act as a substitute for treatment, this technology may become an important tool for managing and even initially detecting PTSD symptoms. They are used in many ways to support MH intervention including: symptom assessment, illness-specific education, treatment resource location, and tracking of treatment progress [54].

Some of the above options, while not considered "care," involve some oversight by providers for health (e.g., diabetes) and MH (e.g., depression). This usually involves bulletin boards with occasional comments or steering by professionals. For example, in an asynchronous chat group for education, the provider can use customized in bursts (e.g., sending a paper to read or a video to watch) based on the discussion to provide information, correct misunderstood concepts, and how to use a self-report measure. For one-time medical advice/consultation or general advice in a group led by a professional, sometimes the "best" outcome is a supportive referral to see a professional when things are not very simple or too many concurrent problems are at-hand.

12.3 Web-and Internet-Based Treatments for Patient Care: Traditional Treatments Easily Disseminated, Innovations/New Treatments, and Hybrid Models of Care

12.3.1 Traditional Treatments More Easily Accessed

Rapid eye movements are part of the Eye Movement Desensitization and Reprocessing approach typically used for treatment of a patient's suffering from an acute stress disorder. However, relevant experts are not to be found just like that, which is why a videoconference-mediated treatment has been tested with promising results [55].

DMH has contributed to development of "remote speech therapy," a Swedish innovation since 2010 and now well established in rural areas in Finland and Scotland, as well [56]. The aim of the project was to reduce therapists' travel time while enabling patients in rural communities to have better access to speech and language therapy services. School children living in remote communities had the opportunity to receive therapy sessions in their schools while the speech therapist was located at the healthcare center. Remote speech therapy was a precursor to the situation we currently have in the world after the pandemic crisis, when online therapy has become a medical standard permitted by law and only the patient chooses whether he wants to be treated stationary or remotely. This approach leads to the vision of neotechnological medicine, in which there will be no distinction between the doctor's intervention and the form of its implementation, and all activities of MH will be aimed at the prevention and treatment of mental disorders regardless of the form of providing health services.

12.3.2 Innovations or Additions to Regular Traditional Treatments

The least structured of these options is patient–doctor correspondence that is integrated with clinical care and the EHR. As the Internet increases level of knowledge and information amount regarding specific illness, the users may easily talk to their doctor regarding their specific conditions and potential treatment options [20]. Schizophrenic patients especially perceive the shift in hierarchy to a more equal relationship. In this respect, a specific advantage for patients with psychosis is not having to face another person, but still being able to gain information and interact with others without feeling devalued or unsafe [27].

One promising area is supporting patients in attendance to treatment, which is as important as motivational work prior to conducted treatment. Psychiatric treatments fail to produce intended outcomes when patients miss their appointments; about 50% of patients actively engage in recommended treatment regimens [57]. The reasons for non-engagement include stigma and absence of insight (denial). Each of these aspects may be influenced via direct or remote provision of education, motivation, and support to enhance attendance (i.e., treatment readiness), recognition of treatment benefits, and collaboration with care providers—all together, a positive psychiatric treatment history is more likely [58]. Recent patient-centered strategies to increase patient compliance are simple mail, telephone, or SMS reminders that have shown to be an effective way to support patient attendance to follow-up appointments [59, 60].

DMH can provide effective forms of improving compliance not only in the field of pharmacological therapy, but also in relation to improving adherence to non-pharmacological recommendations. Such telemedical active care is currently being implemented in Poland by one of the authors. It consists in using the same telemedical application by doctors and patients named "teleCZP," in which the doctor programs all pharmacological and non-pharmacological recommendations, while the application monitors the patient's health, reminds him of individual elements of therapy, monitors compliance with the recommendations, and reacts to non-compliance to therapy through the triage module, sending notifications to patient and for caregiver or other health provider. Thanks to DMH, similar medical applications can revolutionize the community psychiatry system because by collecting data for machine learning and deep learning algorithms, such application becomes an active but constantly supervised active participant in the treatment process, partially unburdening the doctor and the MH system and increasing the density of therapeutic interactions between visits to a psychiatrist. This form of DMH is an example of using of narrow artificial intelligence in MH.

Higher intensity interventions include synchronous DMH (covered in other chapters) and Internet-based CBT (ICBT), used most often for patients with depression and anxiety. Online MH interventions are as effective as traditional in-person therapy for disorders such as depression and anxiety (e.g., CBT for panic disorder and agoraphobia) [61–65]; effect sizes and recovery rates were comparable. Based on a 30-month follow-up study for treatment of social phobia, the long-term effects of in-person delivered CBT was comparable to ICBT [63]. ICBT appears to be effective, not surprisingly, when delivered in clinical practice by a qualified therapist [6, 66]. More specifically, Internet-based CT combined with monitoring by text messages (mobile cognitive therapy, mCT), and minimal therapist support (e-mail and telephone), is an effective approach of prevention of relapse in depression [65].

Once again, the military may be in the lead of Internet-based care options, with foci of remote screening and assessment, post-deployment adjustment, suicide prevention and management, and delivery of training/education [67]. Many personnel prefer to receive care at home—particularly those with anxiety, PTSD, and phobia—and those who prefer to avoid the stigma of entering a mental health facility [68]. A randomized trial of home-based DMH treatment for depression was equal or better than office-based care [69].

12.4 The Present and the Future: Innovative Treatments Used for Patients—Virtual Reality, Avatars, and Other Inventions

12.4.1 Overview

DMH gives us both an overview of novel assessment and treatment options, and a vision of the future. Technically, DMH is within this scope, but the field extends much further. Since MH assessment methods are time consuming and highly subjective, various automated MH assessment methods have been developed to improve efficiency as well as to provide more objective assessments [68]. Image and behavior analysis included facial expressions and gestures. Biosignals such as skin conductance, EEG, EMG, and EGA measurements have been used to monitor various physiological and psychological conditions. Language pattern and specifically discriminant word analyses are used in schizophrenia [70], while acoustic analysis is used for depression [71]. Online decision support is also common.

"Mental health care will soon involve clinicians logging onto online social networks: checking patients' online activity, evaluating patients' moods, administering surveys and determining if additional appointments are needed, adjusting medications, reviewing video of a significant event or issue uploaded by a patient, or even running software algorithms or other diagnostic tools to evaluate a patient's mental state though the language and information shared over social networking?" [72] This picture of MH treatment might seem a bit farfetched 15 years ago, but as online patient–provider interaction increases, and the popularity of social networks increases this image is slowly becoming reality. After logging in to the application, the doctor can check how the patient feels, how he takes medications, and how he implements the therapeutic plan. What is more, the application can initiate a self-diagnosis by the patient to assess whether he or she still meets the criteria for a given condition. The application, taking care of the patient, integrates treatment conducted by a psychiatrist, psychologist, psychotherapist, and psychiatric nurse. Thus, DMH has already changed the image of modern psychiatry.

12.4.2 Asynchronous Telepsychiatry (ATP)

ATP to primary care is feasible, valid, and reliable in English-and Spanish-speaking patients in primary care [73]. Similar methods are used in radiology, dermatology, ophthalmology, cardiology, and pathology. One ATP model uses a basic questionnaire for screening by the provider of the patient, video capture of that interview, and uploading of patient histories for a remote psychiatrist for review in a Health Insurance Portability and Accountability Act (HIPAA)-adherent manner [74]. Diagnosis and treatment recommendations are made and Primary Care Physician (PCPs) implement care successfully about 80% of the time and the model is cost-effective [75, 76]. DMH has opened the possibility of integrating data collected by doctors from various medical disciplines. Additionally, thanks to DMH, it is possible to integrate various therapies conducted simultaneously or sequentially by different doctors. This indicates the possibility of implementing the postulates of holistic medicine thanks to DMH.

12.4.3 Mobile Mood Diary

This application is like the paper daily diary, but on a smartphone platform. Employing CBT relies mainly on writing down daily activities, charting their moods and energy levels. Patients used to bring their recorded paper daily diary to discuss with the therapist on their weekly therapy sessions; some forgot or stop doing their CBT for whatever reason. A new application, especially for teenagers, is texting and typing on their smartphones. Psychiatrists find mobile mood diary greatly beneficial since they can look into graphs illustrating the patient's mood swings throughout the day [77]. Similarly, in DMH applications, patients can collect data on well-being, sleep quality, severity of other psychopathological symptoms, side effects, etc. These data can then be processed by machine learning or deep learning algorithms and can be returned to the doctor and patient in the form of therapeutic or lifestyle suggestions.

12.4.4 Virtual Reality (VR)

VR is a computer-generated reality that provides input to the user's sensory system and interacts with the user. It is usually defined as computer-simulated environment that can simulate physical presence in places in the real world or imagined worlds. In addition to visual canal stimulation, VR applications can also stimulate the auditory canal through speakers or headphones, and less often also use tactile, or olfactory stimulation. The goal of VR is to replace sensory stimuli from the real world and create an impression that a user is present in the virtual world. To interact with a user in real time, the VR system collects information about the user's position and head movements through sensors and input devices such as a head tracking system or a joystick. VR is the concept of being virtually, but not physically at a specific place, and several VR platforms have been developed in the past 20 years, mostly for games.

Medical applications using VR can be created both for a smartphone and for a desktop computer or dedicated end devices. Sensory stimuli are delivered to the brain either through VR glasses (it can be a smartphone with 3D frames or a head-mounted display (HMD)) or by projection-based systems such as CAVE systems (automatic virtual environment in a cave), i.e. a room with up to six projection sides. Mobile VR applications are easier to access and less costly, but the graphic resolution of the image is limited by the smartphone processor and battery life. Stationary devices do not have these limitations, but they cannot be used in every place and sometimes require the patient to go to a specially prepared space in a dedicated facility [78].

The virtual characters (avatar, virtual agent, and no avatar system) as well as virtual environments have been developed to practice dynamic and real-life social interactions in a safe environment [79]. The virtual character (avatar) is the graphical representation of the user or the user's alter ego in 3D form. People are known to psychologically identify with virtual representations that do not necessarily reflect their actual appearances [80]. Thus, in virtual worlds, people can explore different versions of their self and become someone else [81]. Moreover, the appearance of avatars can cause behavioral and attitudinal shifts that might positively influence current treatment or motivate individuals who were reluctant to that due to lack of insight or stigma [82–85]. However, when participating in violent games, avatars personalize risk by simulating harm to digital representations with which people directly identify; this may contribute to behavioral change into the physical world [86].

Virtual environments are either single user virtual environments (SVEs) or collaborative virtual environments (CVEs). In an SVE, a single user explores the virtual environment and responses from the environment or a virtual agent (avatar) must be preprogrammed. In a CVE, more than one user may inhabit the virtual environment at the same time (e.g., patient and the therapist or trainer) and can interact with each other in real-time via avatars. Users control their avatars independently and can communicate directly with each other, even when physically located in different places, through speech, movement, and gesture in the virtual space [20, 87–90]. CVEs have been used to examine and investigate the ability *to recognize* emotions [91], and also teaching students how *to manifest* their emotions and *understand* the emotions of other people [92]. One of the leading and most popular Internet-based VR applications is Second Life.

Second Life (http://secondlife.com/) allows providers and patients (represented by electronic virtual figures or avatars) to log on and meet on virtual "islands" or "clouds" (which are "private" virtual locations within the site) that can depict a variety of scenes including a virtual therapy office) [74]. It is open to the public and can be accessed free of charge. Fees are charged to purchase virtual "land" or server space, to use to build fantasy environments (i.e., stores, museums, or even go on a date). Virtual characters and environments represent a valuable tool for the supportive therapies and the training of social skills and non-verbal decoding (e.g., high-functioning autism), as they provide a safe, repeatable, and diversifiable learning environment [93].

In daily life ordinary mentally healthy individuals, as well as people with various MH conditions, participate in Internet-mediated electronic games. The use of the software controls that change the avatar's features (i.e., the height and weight, color of skin, eyes, hair, width of the nose, and other markers of racial identity) can have an immediate effect on the participant's sense of physical embodiment. Many participants strive for an accurate mirroring of their bodily appearance off screen but some explore radical alterations of self [94]. These choices and the degree to which an individual feels actually present in the virtual environment may be related to MH and well-being [95]. It has been reported that participants in online role-playing games who created an avatar reflecting the "ideal self" reported greater perceived interactivity in the virtual world than those who created a replica avatar mirroring the actual self [96].

An alternative to using avatars is generating an image in VR applications that the user would see while he was in a given environment. The use of avatars is a transfer of gaming standards to therapeutic applications, while VR applications without an avatar may allow for faster and easier immersion in the virtual reality environment, which is a condition for the effectiveness of the exposure [97, 98].

Another type of a VR platform is a fully immersive system, which uses software systems give the user a full immersion in the VR environment. This can take place in a virtual cave, which could be a six-walled room with multiple projectors transmitting images on these walls. Some systems require a specific visual aid such as 3-dimensional glasses while others can be used with only the naked eye. A similar concept of fully immersive VR environment is the use of specific glasses that has the 3-dimensional screen inside the device. These immersive technologies are relatively costly which makes it less accessible to many providers and patients for treatment [78].

A review of VR reports it has been used in the treatment of many MH conditions [74], including eating disorders, autism spectrum disorders, stress management, pain management, and diagnosis and treatment of neurological conditions such as stroke. As autism spectrum disorders are characterized by impairments in communication and reciprocal interaction [88], socio-communicative deficits are manifested via problems with spontaneously producing, understanding, and responding to non-verbal cues. Autistic individuals do not spontaneously attend to social information, and are thus less able to intuitively interact in social context [99].

One of the most effective and widely used applications in MH is VR exposure therapy (VRET), used in the treatment of phobia and trauma-related disorders like PTSD. Meta-analyzes of VRET in phobias confirm the effectiveness of VRET and its equivalence with in vivo exposure therapy [reviewed in 103]. VRET in agoraphobia and social phobia is effective when performed from 8 to 12 sessions, on average once a week for at least 15 min. In turn, the treatment of specific phobias is effective even in the form of one longer session, lasting 45–180 min. Head mounted displays are an effective technology for VRET. Increasing the frequency of sessions and adding drug therapy may shorten the overall treatment duration. Moreover, the effectiveness of VRET in phobias is greater without psychiatric comorbidity and on the condition of generating and maintaining in the patient a sense of immersion in the VR environment. Further studies should focus on the possibility of augmentation of pharmacological treatment with VRET, indications for combining in VR exposure with in vivo exposure, as well as the durability of VRET effects with possible maintenance therapy. In the future, it is also necessary to check the effectiveness of treatment protocols in which VRET is used more than once a week in terms of the possibility of reducing the total duration of treatment of phobias [100].

VRET may be a better tolerated form of exposure treatment than the in vivo exposure [101]. VRET can also be performed in a hybrid form—first in VR therapy and then in vivo therapy [102]. This way of conducting therapy can be especially recommended for patients who have very strong phobic symptoms and are not ready for in vivo exposure even in the company of a psychotherapist. There are very few studies on the other possibility of hybridizing VRET with a drug therapy. In one of them, it was shown that the combined use of VRET and Selective Serotonin Reuptake Inhibitor (SSRI) drugs brings better effectiveness in treating phobias than pharmacotherapy alone [103].

Guidelines specific to patient–provider communication or care provision or conducting therapy in online virtual environments such are available [74]:

1. Patients who are only receiving generic educational information on an open VR environment can be anonymous, and should not be tracked in any way. Any providers on that island should be fully identified, and should have named or numbered avatars that clearly identify who they are, and that link to published biographies.
2. Patients who wish to move to a secure VR environment for some form of virtual therapy, whether this is individual counseling or cognitive behavioral therapy should be treated in accordance with the following protocols to ensure high practice standards, and legal and ethical processes:
   (a) All patients should undergo an in-person or telemedicine assessment to evaluate patient safety and appropriateness for treatment with this modality, establish care, confirm their diagnosis, create a treatment plan, and discuss consent. This is particularly important in a potential emergency situation where therapists have to know the physical location of a patient, as per telemedicine guidelines, in order to call for help.
   (b) All patients should then sign a written consent form if required in the state in which they reside (which can be done electronically), be trained in how to use the virtual environment, be given a tour of the private island, and receive a copy of their diagnostic assessment and treatment plan.
   (c) HIPAA compliance of the virtual environment must be documented, verifiable and ensured prior to patient contact.
   (d) If patients and providers are federal employees, they can be treated in the virtual environment from any state by any provider. If the patient or the provider is not a federal employee, the treating provider must be licensed to practice in the state from which the patient logs in.
   (e) All providers will have fully authenticated avatars using their real names, and will have biographies published that link their professional identities to their avatars for patients to read.
   (f) Patients and providers will then schedule sessions on the private island for either counseling or cognitive behavioral therapy, or a combination of both.
   (g) Any major changes to the treatment plan, such as altered medications, should require an in-person telemedicine consultation.
   (h) Either the provider or patient may at any time either cease therapy, or request a telemedicine or in-person consultation to review progress.

12.4.5 Avatar Therapy

As mentioned above it was only a question of time when computerized technology combined with the Internet will be used to help in treatment of severe mentally conditions. Avatar therapy is a novel therapy based on a computer program developed within last few years by clinicians from University College in London. This approach has a potential to significantly reduce the frequency and intensity of the voices, their omnipotence and malevolence [95]. The treatment would have a schizophrenic patient select an avatar on a computer and create a virtual representation of the scary voices that previously existed solely in his/her imagination. The system then synchronizes the avatar's lips with its speech, enabling a therapist to speak to the patient through the avatar in real time. The therapist encourages the patient to oppose the voice and gradually teaches them to take control of their hallucinations.

Within this approach the clinician plays two roles, one as a supportive therapist and the other one as the persecutory avatar. As the session proceeds, the two roles merge and avatar successively agrees to stop disturbing the patient and instead begins to make a helpful suggestion in order to increase the patient's self-confidence. In accordance to this, the expression on avatar's face may be altered from menacing to neutral or even friendly smiling.

Each therapy session lasts 30 min, and afterward, the patient is given MP3 recordings of their session, so that they can listen on a music player or computer when an auditory hallucination strikes again. Significant reduction in depressive symptoms was detected at the 3-month follow-up; increased quality of life, likewise, was due to reduction in symptoms.

More research is needed in this area, including randomized trails, reliability/validity studies, and provider training.

12.5 Discussion and Conclusion

Web-and Internet-based resources are remarkably popular with the public, patient, and provider interventions over the last decades. Opportunities exist for health information, support groups, formal education programs, tools for self-directed lifestyle and illness management, obtaining advice/consultation, and self-or provider-directed treatments (e.g., CBT or DMH). Traditional treatments are more easily disseminated to the point-of-service. Modification of regular treatments are in process, based on medical smartphone and web applications and importing of VR/avatar from games into medicine, and innovations/new treatments for special populations are rolling out possible; hybrid models of care that combine in-person and the Internet care become part of everyday life of MH care. An additional possibility offered by new technologies is the implementation of solutions related to artificial intelligence. Medical data collected by medical applications can be processed by computational algorithms and can give feedback to both the patient and the doctor.

Hybrid treatment, using a combination of DMH medical applications with pharmacological treatment, can result in augmentation of treatment and increase its effectiveness. There are practically no limits to creating medical applications for the treatment of any mental disorder. The coming years must bring evaluation criteria, certification rules for medical applications, and their registration as digital therapeutics. These applications are already becoming medical devices reimbursed by public healthcare system.

Patients are empowered by increased access to information, providers, and exposures—in ways that can be adjusted to patient needs and comfort, with or without clinician supervision. These steps help patients initiate, participate, and steer their care. Clinicians have to become aware of, adapt to, use sound clinical judgment, and serve new advisory roles to patients, as we are all challenged to keep the best of MH care, yet make it more accessible. While the psychoanalytic notion that "the therapist is an empty slate" on which the patient is writing his/her own life-story is still true for some treatments, we now have a patient able to create his "virtual self" in form of avatar and interact within virtual environments, in order to deal with social anxiety, recognize and express emotions, and deal with stress through titrated exposures to heal past traumas. Even those with severe MH conditions appear to benefit. By focusing the therapy on the patient who uses medical application with personalized pharmacological and non-pharmacological recommendations, DMH makes it possible to implement personalized psychiatry, based on constantly updated real data from the use of the application by the patient.

DMH allows to cross the boundaries of psychiatry toward the integration of medical data from treatment by various specialists, including family doctors. Thus, DMH is also a starting point for the unification of medicine and the integration of somatic and mental treatment. DMH in the MH sector can be extremely attractive for family doctors, supporting diagnostics, decision making, monitoring, and stimulating the patient to pro-health behavior. Thanks to DMH, it will be possible to improve the still low compliance in relation to medical recommendations and increase the still unsatisfactory drug adherence [104].

The ability to integrate medical data opens a new problem of creating a unified medical record of patient's data collection, thanks to which it will be possible to integrate data between various medical applications and platforms. The authors see here a special role of national and international psychiatric societies, which influence the rules of certification of medical applications as well as the creation of regulations and legal tools forcing application developers to build them according to the rules, ensuring the possibility of creating a big database to be used by general artificial intelligence in the future.

However, potential disadvantages are waiting around the corner. Because of the increase in our use of technology and computer programs utilizing avatars, spending so much time in a virtual world (e.g., Second Life), a "contrast effect" is likely to occur [105, 106]. When participants are presented with attractive avatars and a world much better than the real one, the risk for massive "emigration" into virtual realities is likely to increase. Other problems persist, regarding the quality of information on Internet, its reliability, and confusion when sites are in conflict. Privacy and confidentiality concerns will continue to some degree. Patients' attitudes toward clinicians and MH care may shift, for the better or for the worse. It is critical that providers increase their awareness and understanding of web-based options to understand patients' concerns (e.g., events related to networking, interactions with others), to incorporate low-intensity but user-friendly approaches (e.g., health prevention strategies), and to offer new treatment approaches.

The challenge for medicine for the next decade is to determine the clinical effectiveness of new technologies and medical applications introduced to the MH market. Further studies of the usefulness of new technologies in the treatment of mental disorders should concern the effectiveness of medical applications using new technologies such as VR or artificial intelligence algorithms and the possibility of their integration with pharmacotherapy/psychotherapy and the effectiveness of hybrid therapies. Ultimately, the patient should choose the form of therapy, but the task of medicine is to formulate recommendations regarding the effectiveness and indications for new technologies in treatment. Further clinical trials are needed for this.

References

1. Mucic D, Shore JH, Hilty DM, Krysta K, Krzystanek M. Lessons learned or forgotten? Impacts of COVID-19 on the future direction of global (e-)mental health care. Curr Psychiatry Rep. 2021;23(12):86.
2. Celio AA, Winzelberg AJ, Wilfley DE, et al. Reducing risk factors for eating disorders: comparison of an internet-and a classroom-delivered psychoeducational program. J Consult Clin Psychol. 2000;68(4):650–7.
3. Ritterband LM, Thorndike F. Internet interventions or patient education web sites? J Med Internet Res. 2006;8(3):e18.
4. Christensen H, Griffiths K, Groves C, et al. Free range users and one hit wonders: community users of an internet-based cognitive behaviour therapy program. Aust NZ J Psychiatry. 2006;40(1):9–62.
5. Clarke G, Eubanks D, Reid E, et al. Overcoming depression on the internet (ODIN) (2): a randomized trial of a self-help depression skills program with reminders. J Med Internet Res. 2005;7(2):e16.
6. Andersson G, Carlbring P, Holmstrom A, et al. Internet-based self-help with therapist feedback and in vivo group exposure for social phobia: a randomized controlled trial. J Consult Clin Psychol. 2006;74(4):677–86.
7. Ljotsson B, Lundin C, Mitsell K, et al. Remote treatment of bulimia nervosa and binge eating disorder: a randomized trial of internet-assisted cognitive behavioural therapy. Behav Res Ther. 2007;45(4):649–61.
8. Mucic D. Telepsychiatry global guidelines. WPA. 2021. https://3ba346de-fde6-473f-b1da536498661f9c.filesusr.com/ugd/e172f3_19ce700c2a1f484b98efdcaf02c3c6ff.pdf.
9. Krzystanek M, Matuszczyk M, Przybyło J, Dudek D, Gałecki P, Bieńkowski P, Szafrański T, Samochowiec J. Letter to the editor. The polish standard of teleconsultation in psychiatry. Psychiatr Pol. 2021;55(6):1473–7.
10. Maghazil A, Yellowlees PM. Novel approaches to clinical care in mental health: from asynchronous telepsychiatry to virtual reality. In: Lech M, Song I, Yellowlees PM, et al., editors. Mental health informatics. London: Springer Publishing; 2014.
11. Elkin N. How America Searches: Health and Wellness. 2008. 7 Mar 2015. http://www.icrossing.com/sites/default/files/how-america-searches-health-and-wellness.pdf.
12. Internet World Stats. Internet users in the world-Distribution by world regions. 2011. 28 Feb 2015. http://www.internetworldstats.com/stats.htm.
13. Internet World Stats. United States of America: Internet usage and broadband usage report. 2011. 28 Feb 2015. http://www.internetworldstats.com/am/us.htm.

14. Ferreira-Lay P, Miller S. The quality of internet information on depression for lay people. Psychiatr Bull. 2008;32:170–3.
15. Kalk NJ, Pothier DD. Patient information on schizophrenia on the internet. Psychiatr Bull. 2008;32:409–11.
16. Nemoto K, Tachikawa H, Sodeyama N, et al. Quality of internet information referring to mental health and mental disorders in Japan. Psychiatry Clin Neurosci. 2007;61(3):243–8.
17. Hu C, Kung S, Rummans TA, et al. Reducing caregiver stress with internet-based interventions: a systematic review of open-label and randomized controlled trials. J Am Med Inform Assoc. 2014;22:e194. https://doi.org/10.1136/amiajnl-2014-002817.
18. Andersson G, Bergström J, Carlbring P, et al. The use of the internet in the treatment of anxiety disorders. Curr Opin Psychiatry. 2005;18(1):73–7.
19. Erwin BA, Turk CL, Heimberg RG, et al. The internet: home to a severe population of individuals with social anxiety disorder? J Anxiety Disord. 2004;18(5):629–46.
20. Murray E, Lo B, Pollack L, et al. The impact of health information on the internet on the physician-patient relationship: patient perceptions. Arch Intern Med. 2003;163(14):1727–34.
21. Boyd DM, Ellison NB. Social network sites: definition, history, and scholarship. J Comput-Mediat Commun. 2007;13(1):210–30.
22. Siemer PC. Telemental health and web-based applications in children and adolescents. Child Adolesc Psychiatr Clin N Am. 2011;20(1):135–53.
23. Laranjo L, Arguel A, Neves AL, et al. The influence of social networking sites on health behavior change: a systematic review and meta-analysis. J Am Med Inform Assoc. 2015;22(1):243–56.
24. Yellowlees PM, Cook JN. Education about hallucinations using an internet virtual reality system: a qualitative survey. Acad Psychiatry. 2006;30(6):534–9.
25. Griffiths KM, Calear AL, Banfield M. Systematic review on internet support groups (ISGs) and depression: what is known about depression ISGs? J Med Internet Res. 2009;11(3):e41. https://doi.org/10.2196/jmir.1303.
26. Griffiths KM, Calear AL, Banfield M. Systematic review on internet support groups (ISGs) and depression (1): do ISGs reduce depressive symptoms? J Med Internet Res. 2009;11(3):e40. https://doi.org/10.2196/jmir.1270.
27. Schrank B, Sibitz I, Unger A, et al. How use patients with schizophrenia the internet: qualitative study. J Med Internet Res. 2010;12(5):e70. https://doi.org/10.2196/jmir.1550.
28. Koivunen M, Välimäki M, Pitkänen A, et al. A preliminary usability evaluation of web-based portal application for patients with schizophrenia. J Psychiatr Ment Health Nurs. 2007;14(5):462–9.
29. Ahmed M. Computer-facilitated dialogue with patients who have schizophrenia. Psychiatr Serv. 2002;53(1):99–100.
30. Ben-Zeev D, Kaiser SM, Brenner CJ, et al. Development and usability testing of FOCUS: a smartphone system for self-management of schizophrenia. Psychiatr Rehabil J. 2013;36(4):289–96. PMID: 24015913.
31. Ben-Zeev D, Brenner CJ, Begale M, et al. Feasibility, acceptability, and preliminary efficacy of a smartphone intervention for schizophrenia. Schizophr Bull. 2014;40:1244.
32. Ben-Zeev D, Corrigan PW, Britt TW, et al. Stigma of mental illness and service use in the military. J Ment Health. 2012;21(3):264–73.
33. Krzystanek M, Krysta K, Borkowski M, Skałacka K, Przybyło J, Pałasz A, Mucic D, Martyniak E, Waszkiewicz N. The effect of smartphone-based cognitive training on the functional/cognitive markers of schizophrenia: a one-year randomized study. J Clin Med. 2020;9(11):3681.
34. Krzystanek M, Borkowski M, Skałacka K, Krysta K. A telemedicine platform to improve clinical parameters in paranoid schizophrenia patients: results of a one-year randomized study. Schizophr Res. 2019;204:389–96.
35. Mittal VA, Tessner KD, McMillan AL, et al. Elevated social internet use and schizotypal personality disorder in adolescents. Schizophr Res. 2007;94(1–3):50–7.

36. Antze P. On the pragmatics of empathy in the neurodiversity movement. In: Lambek M, editor. Ordinary ethics. New York, NY: Fordham University Press; 2010. p. 310–27.
37. Gowen K, Deschaine M, Gruttadara D, et al. Young adults with mental health conditions and social networking websites: seeking tools to build community. Psychiatr Rehab J. 2012;35(3):245–50.
38. Berger M, Wagner TH, Baker LC. Internet use and stigmatized illness. Soc Sci Med. 2005;61(8):1821–7.
39. Lewandowski J, Rosenberg BD, Jordan Parks M, et al. The effect of informal social support: face-to-face versus computer-mediated communication. Comput Hum Behav. 2011;27(5):1806–14.
40. Pietrzak R, Johnson D, Goldstein M, et al. Perceived stigma and barriers to mental health care utilization among oef-oif veterans. Psychiatr Serv. 2009;60(8):1118–22.
41. Wilson JA, Onorati K, Mishkind M, et al. Soldier attitudes about technology-based approaches to mental health care. Cyber Psychol Behav. 2008;11(6):767–9.
42. Bush NE, Skopp N, Smolenski D, et al. Behavioral screening measures delivered with a smartphone app: psychometric properties and user preference. J Nerv Ment Dis. 2013;201(11):991–5.
43. Alexander CJ, Adamson A, Daborn G, et al. Inuit cyberspace: the struggle for access for Inuit Qaujimajatuqangit. J Can Stud. 2009;43(2):220–49.
44. Adelson N, Olding M. Narrating aboriginality on-line: digital storytelling, identity and healing. J Community Informatics. 2013;9(2):85–90.
45. Blusi M, Dalin R, Jong M, et al. The benefits of e-health support for older family caregivers in rural areas. J Telemed Telecare. 2014;20(2):63–9.
46. Chi NC, Demiris G. A systematic review of telehealth tools and interventions to support family caregivers. J Telemed Telecare. 2015;21(1):37–44.
47. Luxton D, Hansen RN, Stanfill K, et al. Mobile app self-care versus in-office care for stress reduction: a cost minimization analysis. J Telemed Telecare. 2014;20(8):431–5.
48. Shaw SC, Marks IM, Toole S. Lessons from pilot tests of computer self help for agora/claustrophobia and panic. MD Comput. 1999;16:44–8.
49. Kenwright M, Liness S, Marks I, et al. Reducing demands on clinicians by offering computer-aided self-help for phobia/panic. Feasibility study. Brit J Psychiatry. 2001;179(5):456–9.
50. Moreno MA, Jelenchick LA, Egan KG, et al. Feeling bad on Facebook: depression disclosures by college students on a social networking site. Depress Anxiety. 2011;28(6):447–55.
51. Riper H, Kramer J, Smit F, et al. Web-based self-help for problem drinkers: a pragmatic randomized trial. Addiction. 2008;103(2):218–27.
52. US Department of Veterans Affairs. Department of Veterans Affairs (VA) Mobile Health Fact Sheet Final [Internet]. Department of Veterans Affairs, 2013. 28 Feb 2015. https://mobilehealth.va.gov/sites/default/files/files/VAMobileHealthFactSheet.pdf.
53. National Center for Telehealth and Technology. PTSD Coach [Internet]. PTSD Coach | t2health. 2013. 28 Feb 2015. http://www.t2.health.mil/apps/ptsd-coach.
54. Luxton DD, McCann RA, Bush NE, et al. mHealth for mental health: integrating smartphone technology in behavioral healthcare. Prof Psychol Res Practice. 2011;42(6):505–12.
55. Todder D, Kaplan Z. Rapid eye movements for acute stress disorder using video conference communication. Tel e-Health. 2007;13(4):461–4.
56. Wakeling M, Heaney D. Competitive health services in sparsely populated areas—eHealth applications across the urban-rural dimension. Report on Scotland pilots. 2011. 28 Feb 2015 https://www.ehealthservices.eu.
57. Agyapong VI, Rogers C, Machale S, et al. Factors predicting adherence with psychiatric follow-up appointments for patients assessed by the liaison psychiatric team in the emergency department. Int J Psychiatry Med. 2010;40:217–28.
58. Gonzalez J, Williams JW, Noël PH, et al. Adherence to mental health treatment in a primary care clinic. J Am Board Fam Pract. 2005;18:87–96.
59. Zanjani F, et al. Management of psychiatric appointments by telephone. J Telemed and Telecare. 2015;21(1):61.

60. Kunigiri G, Gajebasia N, Sallah D. Improving attendance in psychiatric outpatient clinics by using reminders. J Telemed Telecare. 2014;20(8):464–7.
61. Amstadter AB, Broman-Fulks J, Zinzow H, et al. Internet-based interventions for traumatic stress-related mental health problems: a review and suggestion for future research. Clin Psychol Rev. 2009;29(5):410–20.
62. Carlbring P, Ekselius L, Andersson G. Treatment of panic disorder via the internet: a randomized trial of CBT vs. applied relaxation. J Behav Ther Exp Psychiatry. 2003;34(2):129–40.
63. Carlbring P, Nordgren LB, Furmark T, et al. Long-term outcome of internet-delivered cognitive-behavioural therapy for social phobia: a 30-month follow-up. Behav Res Ther. 2009;47(10):848–50.
64. Kiropoulos LA, Klein B, Austin DW, et al. Is internet-based CBT for panic disorder and agoraphobia as effective as face-to-face CBT? J Anxiety Disord. 2008;22(8):1273–84.
65. Kok G, Bockting C, Berger H, et al. Mobile cognitive therapy: adherence and acceptability of an online intervention in remitted recurrently depressed patients. Internet Interv. 2014;1(2):65–73.
66. Andersson G, Hesser H, Veilord A, et al. Randomised controlled non-inferiority trial with 3-year follow-up of internet-delivered versus face-to-face group cognitive behavioural therapy for depression. J Affect Disord. 2013;151(3):986–94.
67. Doarn CR, Shore J, Ferguson S, et al. Challenges, solutions, and best practices in telemental health service delivery across the pacific rim-a summary. Telemed J E Health. 2012;18(8):654–60.
68. Diederich J, Song I. Mental health informatics: current approaches. In: Lech M, Song I, Yellowlees PM, et al., editors. Mental health informatics. London: Springer; 2014.
69. Luxton DD, Pruitt LD, O'Brien K, et al. Design and methodology of a randomized clinical trial of home-based telemental health treatment for U.S. military personnel and veterans with depression. Contemp Clin Trials. 2014;38(1):134–44.
70. Diederich J, Al-Ajmi A, Yellowlees P. Ex-ray: data mining and mental health. Appl Soft Comput J. 2007;7(3):923–8.
71. France DJ, Shiavi RG. Acoustical properties of speech as indicators of depression and suicidal risk. IEEE Trans Biomed Eng. 2000;47(7):829–37.
72. Parish MB, Yellowlees PM. The rise of person-centered health care and the influence of health informatics and social network applications on mental health care. In: Lech M, Song I, Yellowlees PM, et al., editors. Mental health informatics. London: Springer; 2014.
73. Yellowlees PM, Odor A, Patrice K, et al. Transcultural psychiatry made simple: asynchronous telepsychiatry as an approach to providing culturally relevant care. Tel e-Health. 2013;19(4):1–6.
74. Yellowlees PM, Holloway KM, Parish MB. Therapy in virtual environments—clinical and ethical issues. Telemed e-Health. 2012;18(7):558–64.
75. Yellowlees PM, Odor A, Patrice K, et al. PsychVACS: a system for asynchronous telepsychiatry. J Tel e-Health. 2011;17(4):299–303.
76. Butler TN, Yellowlees P. Cost analysis of store-and-forward telepsychiatry as a consultation model for primary care. Tel e-Health. 2012;18(1):74–7.
77. Trudeau M. Mental health apps: like a "therapist in your pocket" NPR Mental Health. 2010. 28 Feb 2015. http://www.npr.org/templates/story/story.php?storyId=127081326.
78. Krysta K, Wilczyński K, Paliga J, Szczęsna A, Wojciechowska M, Martyniak E, Krzystanek M. Implementation of the MOTEK CAREN system in behavioural therapy for patients with anxiety disorders. Psychiatr Danub. 2016;28(Suppl-1):116–20.
79. Krämer NC. Nonverbal communication. In: human behavior. In: Blascovich J, Hartel CR, editors. Military contexts. Washington, DC: The National Academies Press; 2008. p. 150–88.
80. Kim J. Two routes leading to conformity intention in computer-mediated groups: matching versus mismatching virtual representations. J Comput Mediat Commun. 2011;16:271–87.
81. Turkle S. Life on the screen: identity in the age of the internet. New York, NY: Simon & Schuster; 1995.

82. Yee N, Bailenson JN. The Proteus effect: the effect of transformed self-representation on behavior. Hum Commun Res. 2007;33:271–90.
83. Yee N, Bailenson JN. The difference between being and seeing: the relative contribution of self perception and priming to behavioral changes via digital self-representation. Media Psychol. 2009;2:195–209.
84. Groom V, Bailenson JN, Nass C. The influence of racial embodiment on racial bias in immersive virtual environments. Soc Influ. 2009;4:1–18.
85. Peck T, Seinfeld S, Aglioti M, et al. Putting yourself in the skin of a black avatar reduces implicit racial bias. Conscious Cogn. 2013;22:779–87.
86. Parks P, Cruz R, Ahn SJ. Don't hurt my avatar: the use and potential of digital self-representation in risk communication. Int J Robots Educ Art. 2014;4(2):11–20.
87. Schroeder R. Social Interaction in virtual environments: key issues, common themes, and a framework for research. In: Schroeder R, editor. The social life of avatars. New York, NY: Springer; 2002. p. 1–18.
88. Bellani M, Fornasari L, Chittaro L, et al. Virtual reality in autism: state of the art. Epidemiol Psychiatr Sci. 2011;20:235–8.
89. Millen L, Cobb S, Patel H. Participatory design approach with children with autism. Int J Disabil Hum Dev. 2011;10:289–94.
90. Parsons S, Cobb S. Who chooses what I need? Child voice and user-involvement in the development of learning technologies for children with autism. EPSRC Observatory for Responsible Innovation in ICT. 2013. 28 Feb 2015. http://torrii.responsible-innovation.org.uk/resource-detail/1445.
91. Fabri M, Moore DJ. Emotionally expressive avatars for chatting, learning and therapeutic intervention. In: Jacko JA, editor. Human-computer interaction. HCI intelligent multimodal interaction environments lecture notes in computer science. Berlin: Springer; 2007. p. 275–85.
92. Cheng Y, Ye J. Exploring the social competence of students with autism spectrum conditions in a collaborative virtual learning environment—the pilot study. Comput Educ. 2010;54:1068–77.
93. Georgescu AL, Kuzmanovic B, Roth D, et al. The use of virtual characters to assess and train non-verbal communication in high-functioning autism. Front Hum Neurosci. 2014;8:807.
94. Bloustien GF, Wood D. Face, authenticity, transformations and aesthetic in second life. Body Society. 2013;19(1):52–81.
95. Leff J, Williams G, Huckvale M, et al. Avatar therapy for persecutory auditory hallucinations: what is and how does it work? Psychosis. 2014;6(2):166–76.
96. Seung AJ. Avatars mirroring the actual self versus projecting the ideal self: the effects of self-priming on interactivity and immersion in an exergame, *Wii* fit. Cyber Psychol Behav. 2009;12(6):761–5.
97. Price M, Mehta N, Tone EB, Anderson PL. Does engagement with exposure yield better outcomes? Components of presence as a predictor of treatment response for virtual reality exposure therapy for social phobia. J Anxiety Disord. 2011;25(6):763–70. https://doi.org/10.1016/j.janxdis.2011.03.004. Epub 2011 Mar 15. PMID: 21515027; PMCID: PMC3401534.
98. Anderson P, Zimand E, Schmertz S, Ferrer M. Usability and utility of a computerized cognitive-behavioral self-help program for public speaking anxiety. Cogn Behav Pract. 2007;14:198–207. https://doi.org/10.1016/j.cbpra.2006.02.006.
99. Klin A, Jones W, Schultz R, et al. The enactive mind, or from actions to cognition: lessons from autism. Philos Philos Trans R Soc Lond B Biol Sci. 2003;358(1430):345–60.
100. Krzystanek M, Surma S, Stokrocka M, Romańczyk M, Przybyło J, Krzystanek N, Borkowski M. Tips for effective implementation of virtual reality exposure therapy in phobias-a systematic review. Front Psych. 2021;12:737351.
101. Moher D, Liberati A, Tetzlaff J, Altman DG, PRISMA Group. Preferred reporting items for systematic reviews and meta-analyses: the PRISMA statement. Ann Intern Med. 2009;151(4):264–169.

102. Botella C, Fernández-Álvarez J, Guillén V, García-Palacios A, Baños R. Recent Progress in virtual reality exposure therapy for phobias: a systematic review. Curr Psychiatry Rep. 2017;19(7):42.
103. Thomas BH, Ciliska D, Dobbins M, Micucci S. A process for systematically reviewing the literature: providing the research evidence for public health nursing interventions. Worldviews Evid-Based Nurs. 2004;1(3):176–84.
104. Krzystanek M, Krysta K, Skałacka K. Treatment compliance in the long-term paranoid schizophrenia telemedicine study. J Technol Behav Sci. 2017;2(2):84–7. https://doi.org/10.1007/s41347-017-0016-4. Epub 2017 May 18. PMID: 29082310; PMCID: PMC5640764.
105. Kenrick TD, Gutierres SE. Contrast effects and judgments of physical attractiveness: when beauty becomes a social problem. J Pers Soc Psychol. 1980;38(1):131–40.
106. Leding JK. The contrast effect with avatars. Comput Hum Behav. 2015;44:118–23.

Artificial Intelligence and Predictive Modeling in Mental Health

13

Donald M. Hilty, Yang Cheng, and David D. Luxton

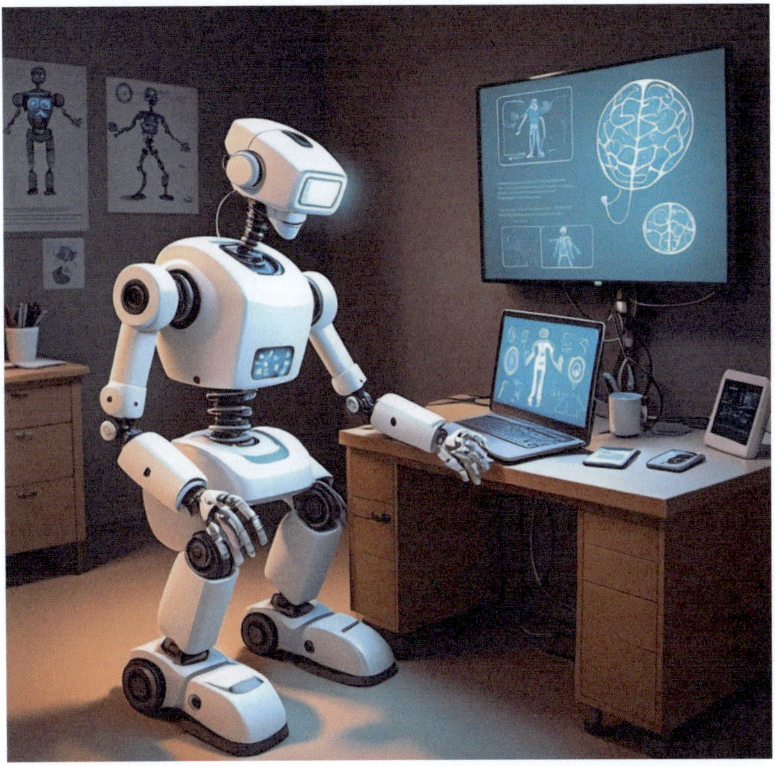

D. M. Hilty (✉)
Department of Psychiatry and Behavioral Sciences, Keck School of Medicine University of Southern California, Los Angeles, CA, USA
e-mail: donald.hilty@uhsinc.com; hilty@med.usc.edu

D. Mucić, D. M. Hilty (eds.), *Digital Mental Health*,
https://doi.org/10.1007/978-3-031-59936-1_13

Abstract

The widespread option of video, mobile health, electronic health records (EHR), and other technologies are increasingly based on advances in predictive modeling (PM), artificial intelligence (AI), and machine learning (ML) techniques. This technology is helping clinicians and health systems provide innovative and game-changing health care. PM and AI are used to improve care and decrease costs through a variety of mechanisms, such as early identification of patients requiring more intensive follow-up through readmission, post-operative complication risk modeling, and automation of diagnostic interpretation previously completed by humans. Wearable sensors facilitate collection of behavioral data, alerting, communicating/giving feedback, detecting change, monitoring symptoms, accessing information, and providing preventive and therapeutic interventions. There are gaps, still, in converting AI, ML, and PM processes to user-friendly experiences for patients and clinicians in United States and globally. Further research is needed in implementation and effectiveness of these technological approaches to health care, on clinical workflow (e.g., skills or competencies), professional development, and institutional changes in systems.

13.1 Introduction

The use of telehealth, mobile health, and remote patient monitoring during the COVID-19 pandemic has given users a vision of what is possible in the future to reshape the delivery of health care worldwide. Communication and clinical care is dramatically shifting—partly due to advances in artificial intelligence, machine learning, and predictive modeling. An era with in-time, continuous data collection and analytics to support clinical decision-making—for patients and clinicians. Advances in predictive modeling (PM), artificial intelligence (AI), and machine learning (ML) make health care data grow expotentially and can funnel it into electronic health records (EHR) for use [1]. As nations move toward health care payment and reimbursement systems based on the provision of a service *and* demonstration of quality care, it is important to show improved patient health outcomes as assessed by standardized outcome and process metrics. There is more interest in population health, economic cost analyses, and the linkage between health and

Y. Cheng
Department of Communication, Raleigh, NC, USA
e-mail: ycheng20@ncsu.edu

D. D. Luxton
Department of Psychiatry and Behavioral Sciences, University of Washington School of Medicine, Seattle, WA, USA

Department of Psychiatry & Behavioral Sciences, Seattle, WA, USA
e-mail: ddluxton@uw.edu

social progress, such that moving beyond symptom rating scales—good for clinicians to make adjustments to treatments, provide consultations, or make referrals—and general administrative outcomes are needed (e.g., no-show rates, the proportion of first-time patients presenting for follow-up, the percentage treatments completed over time).

The widespread implementation of electronic health records (EHRs) is allowing health care institutions to collect high-quality longitudinal data on large populations that can be linked to contextual data in complex networks of causation [2]. Advances in mobile devices (smartphones, tablets, and wearables) and sensor technologies also provide ability to collect behavioral data, alert users, communicate/give feedback, detect change, monitor symptoms, and provide preventive and therapeutic interventions [1, 3, 4] via algorithms [5, 6, 7]. Wearable sensor and remote patient monitoring technologies transform care by moving to a 24 × 7, longitudinal framework with in-time feedback based on the ecology (home, health, lifestyle, and social) of patients in natural settings [7] with automatic monitoring systems [1, 8, 9].

System management also plays a key role in health care and includes health information systems (IS), telemedicine, information technology (IT), facilities and clinics (e.g., labs, home health) and delivery structures (e.g., integrated networks). IT falls into three general categories: clinical information systems, administrative information and decision support systems, which are supported by advances in AI and can assist with clinical decision-making (i.e., clinical decision support (CDS)) to provide entirely new capabilities [1] at home, in life and in health care. Advances in sensing technologies and affective computing have enabled machines to analyze data for patterns in time and longitudinally, or at the bedside, to detect, assess, and respond to emotional states. Use of ML and pattern recognition is improving public and population health surveillance, and providing feedback and options for people, patients, clinicians and systems. Low-and middle-income countries have begun to formulate mental health performance indicators for domains such as needs, utilization, quality and financial risk protection [10], hoping that new and simpler collection of data, monitoring and documentation will improve outcomes [10, 11]. Iterative development with input has helped with prioritization, customization and coordination for health and governmental systems [11].

These technological developments have come at an opportune time, as there is significant interest in and commitment toward investment in analytics to improve care delivery and bend the cost curve. This dramatic shift in health care also creates a need for a collaboration between medicine, clinical informatics, and computer science.

The objectives of this chapter are to:

1. Provide an overview of AI technologies and how they are integrated into workflow;
2. Describe common clinical uses of PM via AI and ML in mental health, with consideration of user-and system-end practices and challenges (e.g., mobile phones and wearable sensors) in common populations (e.g., mood and anxiety disorders);

3. Offer an overview of types of chatbots for mental health treatment and delineate the main gratifications of using chatbots;
4. Provide a glimpse of shifts over the next 10 years and future directions, as well as discuss areas of research needed to further the translation into clinical practice; and.
5. Contextualize the need for patients, clinicians, and institutions to learn skills and for technology to be user-friendly.

13.2 Artificial Intelligence and Machine Learning: Key Concepts and Examples

The goal of AI is to build machines capable of performing tasks that require intelligence, such as reasoning, learning, planning, problem-solving, and perception [1]. AI is a interprofessional field encompassing computer science, engineering, psychology, philosophy, ethics, and more. AI technologies principally consist of computer software (computer programs), but also associated hardware and enabling technologies, such as sensors, cloud computing, virtual reality, and robotics [12]. ML is a branch of AI that aims to give computers the ability to learn without being explicitly programmed [1]. ML subfields and applications include statistical learning methods, neural networks, instance-based learning, genetic algorithms, data mining, image recognition, natural language processing (NLP), computational learning theory, inductive logic programming, and reinforcement learning [1].

ML models fall under two primary approaches: supervised and unsupervised. Supervised ML is when the program is trained on a pre-defined set of examples or sets, whereas unsupervised ML is when the program is provided with data, but must discover patterns and relationships in the data. A scoping review of ML applied to mental health found four main application domains in the literature: (1) detection and diagnosis; (2) prognosis, treatment, and support; (3) public health; and (4) research and clinical administration [13]. The most common mental health conditions addressed included depression, schizophrenia, and Alzheimer's disease. ML techniques used included support vector machines (SVM), decision trees, neural networks, latent Dirichlet allocation and clustering.

The capability of machines to interpret and process human (natural) language is called natural language processing (NLP), a sub-field of AI that combines computer science with linguistics (i.e., computational linguistics or statistical text classification). NLP has many practical uses for behavioral and mental health care. For instance, NLP combined with ML can allow for searches of EHRs to identify of patterns in patient data, assist with diagnosis, detect risks, and more (e.g., IBM's *Watson*) [14]. NLP and speech recognition software have also greatly improved how people interface with technology by providing a more natural, user-friendly, and transparent interaction experience [1]. For example, speech processing technology is used to help health professionals enter notes into EHRs to enhance clinical documentation accuracy and timeliness.

There are several shifts taking place in this new e-spectrum of care with new technologies entering life and health care—used in varying degrees by patients, clinicians, and health systems—and many more may be standard or readily elective circa 2040 (Table 13.1). These technological options may be organized or stratified into levels of care based on technology access (i.e., easy to less available), the type of interface (e.g., a human–computer vs. human–human interface via computer), capacity of the technology to engage (e.g., chatbot), other participants in care (e.g., caregiver and primary care provider), specialist time (i.e., psychiatrist or behavioral health clinician), the model of care and use of informatics or health system [15].

Table 13.1 Artificial intelligence e-behavioral health continuum of interventions for patients, families and clinicians

Source	User goals/Aims	Liabilities	Suggestions
User-friendly—Simple technology—Less interaction—Less regulated—Variable quality			
Publically available options			
Website information	Gain perspective, obtain standard and updated health information Good for somatic symptom disorders	Quality of information and lack of regulation Ease of access	Refer to sites by psychiatric and medical organizations Keep information simple
Support/chat groups	Patient: Education and perspective Caregivers: Tips and support on coping	Peer compatibility Information quality	Verify quality and those with a professional facilitator
Social media (SM) passive and active	Patient: Education and perspective Caregivers: Tips and support on coping	Privacy Little time for clinicians	Active participation is more therapeutic than passive surfing
Natural language processing (computational linguistics or statistical text classification)	Patient: Use for immediate crisis intervention tool Clinician: Have patient diaries, statements, clinical notes and background data analyzed	Coarse or non-specific outcomes that require more human time Errors Adaptation to each new area often required	Customize in a few areas for clinical use Generalize with artificial intelligence and use advanced machine learning techniques
Clinical care screening and engagement			
Education program for self-assessment	Person/patient: Education, tips Caregiver: Education, support, and advice	Some learners prefer in-person Ease of access Quality of information	Give assignments Clarify if knowledge vs. skill development
Telephone-based diagnostic systems	Person/patient/caregiver: Additional options, speed up diagnostic process Clinician: Reduces in-person time	Not user friendly—As not particularly warm—But effective	Prepare by setting expectations and emphasizing how it helps

(continued)

Table 13.1 (continued)

Source	User goals/Aims	Liabilities	Suggestions
e-base self report questionnaires fed into electronic health record	Person/patient/ caregiver: Additional option, taking action Clinician: Reduces in-person time	False positives and negatives, but nonetheless helpful Clinicians/team members may need training to score	Use common, easy to score ones like the patient health questionnaire Integrate automatic scoring
Patient–computer virtual, augmented, and mixed reality approaches (XR for all)			
XR applications to clinical populations	Digitally recreated simulations of real-world activities, often involving dynamic social and emotionally engaging stimuli for interaction and assessment	Lab setting design is not always able to create psychological realism Need a sensorally rich and perceptually realistic environment	Design with lab and field settings to facilitate natural interaction between the user, objects and the environment
Autonomous virtual human (VH) agents for clinical interviewing	Start the early steps for creating a treatment plan that would be followed on by a live clinician. Kiosk-based VH agent can leverage advances in sensing technology (e.g., cameras and microphones) Support and train social and safety skills	Impersonal, automated Gaps requiring human judgment, errors Creation and use of highly interactive, intelligent VHs for such clinical purposes is still in progress	Comparative evaluation across interviews Participants reported willingness to disclose, willingness to recommend and general satisfaction
Virtual affective agents and therapeutic games	Capable of affective interaction, such as expression of "emotions" and recognition of human emotions, based on emotional and social intelligence (e.g., awareness of social cues and user goals),	Computing diagnostic features requires solving all sorts of open problems in respective fields (e.g., computer vision, acoustic signal processing, digital signal processing, time series modeling, natural language understanding)	Engage people in provide highly immersive learning, training and therapeutic environments that can be customized to the user's specific learning needs or therapeutic goals
Chatbot and other robotic technologies	Affective human-computer interaction: Respond to the user's emotions and other stimuli; assessment of facial recognition	Working out autonomy, information exchange, how people and robots adapt/learn and how the task shapes interaction	Ensure respect, dignity, privacy and consent Avoid racist, sexist, and ableist morphologies

(continued)

Table 13.1 (continued)

Source	User goals/Aims	Liabilities	Suggestions
Automated mental state detection	Read-out" a person's mental state via verbal, behavior, body, and other data	Challenges from sensor inputs to diagnostic patterns Need supervised learning with supplemental annotations	Affective states and attentional lapses (i.e., lack of mindfulness) prototypes
Human behavior modeling and simulation (e.g., agent-based modeling and simulation) using motivation, state and action	Used for serious mental illness and addressing the needs of the most vulnerable populations in our society, based on comprehension, manageability and meaningfulness	A person's behavior is not always determined by their intention to perform the behavior and that this intention is, in turn, may not be a function of their attitude toward the behavior and subjective norms	Improvement on discriminative ability of traditional risk prediction models, which are little better than coin flipping at predicting readmissions
Brain computer interface (BCI): System that translates "brain signals into new kinds of outputs": Implantable and non-invasive	Exercise training devices for neurological disorders, usually: Wearable powered braces for daily use; range of motion and strength training devices for musculoskeletal disorders; assistance (e.g., exercise) with activities of daily living; and social or telepresence robots	Professionals believe it may interfere with, or be perceived by patients to interfere with, in-person communication between the provider and patient. Cultural acceptance: Some have more positive attitudes toward some robot morphologies compared to other cultures.	The interface determines: (1) what degree the user is separated from the physical world; (2) what stimuli are introduced and how; (3) artificial intelligence versus human control; and (4) the proportion of objective, quantifiable data collected
Customized human–human care interactions			
Consult with e-services clinician for self-care decisions	Person/patient/ caregiver: Additional options, perspective, context Clinician: Helps independent learners and requires less time with patient	Complexity: Not often as simple as do A or do B Scope of practice questions	Link with social work, hotline and/ or clinic, if needed Context with input from own clinician is better
Assisted self-care assessment and decision-making	Person/patient/ caregiver: Empowering as customized and supported Clinician: Effective to distribute skills	Asynchronous communication has limitations Context for decisions is lacking	Use clinicians in health system Integrate in electronic health record (EHR) and care team

(continued)

Table 13.1 (continued)

Source	User goals/Aims	Liabilities	Suggestions
Asynchronous video or one-time synchronous consultation	Person/patient/ caregiver: Good step to enable primary provider Clinician: Efficient use of time, help from others and empowers patients	Can primary provider use tips? They will work for which patients? Learning curve takes some time?	Build into the regular care continuum Provide training on how to do each step
Synchronous, telepsychiatry (TP)	Person/patient: Effective and is much more convenient Clinician: If patients like it, it is good	Has to be scheduled (and paid for) Workflow sometimes a little more demanding on clinician/team	Have technology, clerical and administrative support Training on clinical skills
Hybrid care: In-person & e-option (TP & e-option)	Person/patient: Options to connect Clinician: Preferred if gives options and workflow not cumbersome	Systems vary in quality, training, prioritization and quality improvement; time and $ costs	Develop integrated workflow for clinicians and administrators Facilitate positive e-culture
Systems for patients and clinicians via informatics system designs for care			
eConsult between primary care provider (PCP) and specialist in EHR	PCP (geriatrician, family medicine): Timely to visit and sent 'in time' Specialist: Simple questions (e.g., facts, steps to do) can be answered	May not work for difficult patient cases that require integration Time to clarify question, review chart and communicate plan	Monitor timeliness, follow up and quality; build into care workflow and culture of care Use video: Effective and easier
Asynchronous, between-session, patient-clinician contact (e.g., *app, text)*	Person/patient/ caregiver has minor question or needs a detail ➔ e-mail/text; tracking symptoms ➔ app Clinician: e-mail/text for quick, simple advice; apps good for monitoring	Align 1–2 apps with 1–2 purposes to focus Errors, miscommunications Time, documentation and privacy issues	Training for faculty and team Integrate into EHR for clinical decision support Use evidence-based app and evidence-based approach

(continued)

Table 13.1 (continued)

Source	User goals/Aims	Liabilities	Suggestions
24 X 7 ecological, in-time and multi-directional collection, integration, communication and decision support based on artificial intelligence, machine learning and predictive modeling	Person/patient: Options to reflect and make decisions in real time (e.g., behavior to improve mood or reduce stress via electrodermal activity) Clinician: Adds new workflow but better data for decision-making System: Benefits from context-aware systems that automatically detect when patients require assistance or intervention	Culture shift from traditional visit or TP care to in-time Work in teams with technology as a new 'team member' or digital navigators 'steer' Functional > structural	Train professionals in teams and shift faculty beyond health 'knowledge' experts to synthetic data leaders Define roles in teams and system for workflow
Digital phenotyping/ biomarkers and public/population health surveillance	Public health surveillance and population health integration Clinical and non-clinical populations to correlate multimodal sensor data, cognitions and depressive mood Early signs of relapse and intervention	Privacy concerns Quality and safety barriers to adoption Specificity to state and trait	Use large multi-centric databases is an essential element for development and validation
Workflow investment—Complex technology—More interaction—High quality—High clinician time			

Key (note: some items have more than one print style):

- Regular print = common options in most health care systems in 2020
- *Italics print* = options available in only some health care systems or parts of systems (e.g., Veterans Affairs)
- **Bold print** = options that will likely be integrated into health care system workflow in 2040

The contemporary spectrum of care *within* health systems typically involves telephone, secure e-mail, in-person, video, EHR, patient portals, and a few other options (e.g., use of apps). The range of low-(e.g., e-mail and phone), mid-(e.g., disease management and consultation care), and high-intensity (e.g., collaborative and hybrid care) options provides systems flexibility [15].

People and patients have already been using other technological options for health like the Internet, chat rooms, and social media that many clinicians see as *outside* of traditional care. Yet, social media is integral to some (e.g., adolescents and young adults) and therefore part of care, so clinicians need to systematically screen technology use and for what purpose(s) and risks (e.g., self-disclosure, cyberbullying, and privacy) are involved [16]. The field of data science has emerged as a way of addressing the growing scale of data, and the analytics and computational power it requires. This allows researchers to extract information from complex datasets in order to interpret data, detect patterns, and create predictive models for care. A specific segment of this work has focused on analyzing and detecting symptoms of mental disorders through status updates in social networking websites (e.g., risk for post-partum depression). Ethical issues have arisen, for example, related to privacy and other safeguards.

Computational approaches exist for determining optimal clinical decisions at a *single timepoint* from traditional statistical methods to data mining/ML methods, or leverage dynamical information and methods across *multiple decision timepoints* for sequential decision-making (i.e., *temporal modeling*) [1]. Research has shown the potential for using temporal modeling, such as Markovian models and reinforcement learning, to understand patterns of clinical change in patients over time in the health care domain. Such modeling can facilitate treatment planning and enhance clinical decision-making by providing more sophisticated CDS tools to both patients and providers. Clinical decision support (CDS) is not simply an alert, notification, or explicit care suggestion. It encompasses a variety of tools including, but not limited to: computerized alerts and reminders for clinicians and patients; clinical guidelines; condition-specific order sets; focused patient data reports and summaries; documentation templates; diagnostic support; and contextually relevant reference information.

The challenges are figuring out how all of this technology fits into the real-world clinical and research processes. Health is a dynamic, longitudinal process and real-world patients display individualized characteristics and symptoms that impact treatment effectiveness. Signal processing algorithms and ML algorithms (e.g., neural networks, random forests, SVM, and NLP) can provide more data-driven probabilistic inferences (e.g., IBM's Watson) [1]. To a degree, the randomized controlled trial (RCT) may no longer be the best approach to understanding causal relationships compared to AI, PM, and precision medicine [17]. Indeed, precision medicine is changing the paradigm of treatments based on evidence gathered in large populations of patients toward customization of health care tailored to the individual patient [18, 19].

13.3 Predictive Modeling

Advances in AI applications such as PM and ML techniques provide opportunities for making use of data to improve care and decrease costs through a variety of mechanisms, such as early identification of patients requiring more intensive follow-up through readmission and post-operative complication risk models, and automation of diagnostic interpretation previously completed by humans [2]. PM supplements clinical judgment when identifying risks associated with mental or behavioral illness. It employs computing power and statistical techniques to model complex processes with higher accuracy—for depression [20, 21], bipolar disorder [22, 23], and schizophrenia [24–26]. AI, ML, and PM also improve diagnostic "bench" research with functional magnetic resonance imaging (fMRI) applied to the bedside [27, 28]. Predictive models offer several notable benefits, including efficiently integrating data that may span years or come from multiple sources and in using objective data that do not rely on human subjectivity. While PM is particularly suited for large health care systems where patients interact with multiple providers in a variety of ways via EHRs, it may help reorganize health care by moving from health system/clinic/clinician-to person/patient-centered evaluation and treatment [3].

PM can be positioned under the broader umbrella term "statistical modeling." While traditional statistical approaches focus on explaining data in terms of causality or identify relations, PM strives to find the model that provides the most accurate predictions. Predictions are derived from so-called attributes or features that are derived from observations. These features are not unlike the variables utilized in traditional statistical approaches. Promising methods include predictive modeling techniques such as decision trees, Bayesian approaches, SVM and artificial neural networks. To use these methods for sequential data mental health applications, the data has to be pre-processed into meaningful variables that can then be used in PM. To succeed in leveraging the potential of predictive models for the purpose of developing effective interventions, each step requires goal setting, understanding data, construction and interpretation of the models, understanding user perception of these models, and finally deployment of the models developed. To fulfill all these requirements, interdisciplinary collaboration between clinical researchers and computer scientists is required.

Various learning techniques and types of target functions exist. There are many types of algorithms (Table 13.2) and these are commonly distinguished between: (1) probabilistic modeling methods such as Naïve Bayes classifiers; (2) divide-and-conquer modeling methods such as decision trees (e.g., random forest); (3) (extended) linear modeling methods such as generalized linear models (e.g., logistic regression), SVM or artificial neural networks; and (4) instance-based learning methods such as k-nearest neighbors (KNN) [29]. As an example, Naïve Bayes is a naïve probabilistic model to find the value that achieves the maximum probability computed from a conditional probability chain. This model is called naïve because it assumes all measured attributes are independent, though in the real world, data attributes are not always perfectly independent. With this assumption, conditional probabilities of attributes can be easily computed as long as all values of attributes are given.

Supervised learning is a so-called *bottom-up approach* as it is driven by the data. It is complemented by the *top-down* approach, which is knowledge-driven. In the latter approach, existing theories are formalized into computational models that connect theoretical concepts from a domain to executable code. An example of a SL setting is the case of classifying diseases of patients: each patient is a data instance, a patient's measured conditions are attributes and the patient's disease is a class. The

Table 13.2 The summary of characteristics of machine learning algorithms frequently used in the field of mental health

Algorithm	Advantage	Disadvantage
SVM	Working relatively accurate in general in practice	An appropriate kernel and careful data-preprocessing is required to precisely analyze complicated data
Random Forest	The algorithm itself automatically covers its previous weakness in dealing with some attributes by adding more weak learners	Difficult to interpret the relationship between attributes and the target Prediction speed can be relatively slow for a complex random forest
Naïve Bayes	Need relatively short time for training and prediction Can provide intermediate conditional probabilities of attributes	Unrealistic assumption: Independency of all attributes
KNN	Training process is not required	Relatively large additional data is required for even a small increase in the number of features to consider Relatively large additional data is required for even a small increase in the number of features to consider Highly dependent on the distance metric to be used

ML algorithm would employ attributes to predict a disease class. Given the measured data of a number of patients, the ML model can be built and then can be used to pre-screen patients' disease before medical professionals' diagnosis. To be specific, the SL algorithms require subjects with measured values for attributes and labels that represent their diagnosis. The real diagnosed labels supervise the ML model to be trained. Once a model completed its training, it can predict diagnosis labels of new patients with the measured attributes.

When applied to clinical interventions, most treatments have been designed with a "one-size-fits-all" approach, which is useful for some patients, but not helpful or even harmful for others. Analyses of clinical trials generally focus on summarizing overall average treatment effects without more deliberate investigation of which patients actually benefit. For example, if the number needed to treat using a new therapy is 50, then 50 individuals need to receive this treatment for 1 individual to benefit. But what characterizes the individual who benefits? Therapies can also both help and harm, successfully improving some outcomes while also placing patients at increased risk for other adverse events.

13.4 Machine Learning (ML) Techniques for Nosologic and Diagnostic Approaches

Applying ML techniques to MRI data has the potential to provide an objective-and evidence-based approach for identification and management of schizophrenia. ML MRI models have the potential to identify biological markers and delineate symptom clusters. An increasing number of studies have attempted to classify schizophrenia versus healthy controls based on functional alterations in resting-state brain patterns. Most earlier studies assessed patients already undergoing treatment, which means their fMRI scans were confounded with antipsychotic drug effects. Further, diagnostic models obtained from larger datasets (more than 100 subjects) typically have classification accuracies well below 80%. An ensemble algorithm with multiple parcellations for schizophrenia prediction—which stacks predictions from several single-source models, each based on features of regional activity and functional connectivity, over a range of different a priori parcellation schemes—outperformed earlier machine learning models with a classification accuracy of 87% (vs. chance accuracy of 53%) [28].

Pattern recognition methods applied to neuroimaging data represent a new and promising approach that could support clinicians in the diagnosis of mental disorders, using structural and functional MRI for the study of the neurobiological bases of schizophrenia [24]. Computerized methods are necessary to analyze large amounts of imaging data with great precision [27]. The most relevant information is extracted from the images, and then a model classification method is able to process this information in order to determine the probability of disease. The new approach uses ML techniques such as SVM (i.e., a high-dimensional, pattern recognition, and supervised learning algorithm), a multivariate pattern analysis, or a random forest. A review of studies noted accuracy of approximately 75% with structural MRI (sMRI) versus well above 90% with fMRI based on PM [27].

Generalized anxiety disorder (GAD) and major depressive disorder (MDD) are highly prevalent and impairing problems, but frequently go undetected, leading to substantial treatment delays. EHRs collect a great deal of biometric markers and patient characteristics that could foster the detection of GAD and MDD in primary care settings. One study approached the problem of predicting MDD and GAD using a novel ML pipeline to re-analyze data from an observational study [21]. After explicitly excluding all psychiatric information, 59 biomedical and demographic features from the general health survey and a set of engineered features were used for model training; the model's performance found an area under curve (AUC) of 0.73 (sensitivity: 0.66, specificity: 0.7) and 0.67 (sensitivity: 0.55, specificity: 0.7) for GAD, and MDD, respectively. Additionally, advanced techniques were used to illuminate which features had the greatest impact on prediction for each disease. The top predictive features for MDD were being satisfied with living conditions and having public health insurance. Post-traumatic stress may be predicted by using SVM [30]. A SVM-based recursive feature elimination was employed for feature selection, and SVM was used for predicting trajectory membership. Accuracy reported as the mean AUC was 0.64 only on the basis of background information, 0.82 on the basis of background and emergency department variables, 0.88 on the basis of data through 1 week, and 0.93 on the basis of data through 1 month.

Despite significant research conducted on suicide screening and assessment, systematic reviews suggest that predictive abilities have not improved in the past 50 years of research and the likelihood of an accurate prediction remains close to chance [31]. To address this challenge, several organizations have developed predictive models for suicide risk. The Durkheim Project [32] began as a Defense Advanced Research Projects Agency (DARPA)-sponsored study for estimating suicide-risk among U.S. military veterans, and entailed the collection of data from smartphone and social media use. The text and mobile device data was processed and then sent into a secure analytics network to be analyzed by ML processes that monitor the content and behavioral patterns that are statistically associated with suicidal behavior. The system allowed for identification of persons at heightened-risk, thus providing opportunity for immediate intervention [33]. Another example is the national prevention program known as Recovery Engagement and Coordination for Health-Veterans Enhanced Treatment (REACH VET)—for veterans identified as being at high risk for suicide. PM in youth presenting for outpatient services may help to predict self harm [34]. Out of 1962 young people, with PM, prediction of the top 25% of young people harming themselves moved from 51.6–56.2% to 82.1–84.4%. A suicide flag via ML for clinicians is also helpful if directly clinically relevant and actionable [35].

13.5 Mobile, Wearable Sensors, and Related Technologies

13.5.1 Overview

A variety of sensors and wearables are being used today and they are creating new options for patient care, clinician decision-making, and population health. These options reduce geographical, cost, and temporal barriers, and they also provide an opportunity to bring patients and clinical teams together for communication, support, and intervention. A scoping review of these technologies for mood and anxiety disorders [4] found smartphones (66.3%), wristbands or smartwatches (22.8%), and holters (6.5%) as the most common. The most common sensors (e.g., smartwatches, heart rate monitors, and smart glasses) were accelerometers (50.0%), phones (39.1%), global positioning systems (GPS) (35.9%), microphones (30.4%), actigraphs (25.0%), and electrocardiograms (ECG) (25.0%); implantable medical devices are used for other health conditions. The majority of studies (90%) used the Android operating system (OS), compared to the Apple iOS, which may be explained by the ease with the former for data capture, communication, and processing tasks to run in the background.

Sensors convert human biological data into digital signals for a microprocessor to interpret and transmit. Most studies use instruments relevant to their application domain, including questionnaires, ecologic momentary assessment (EMA), and clinician assessments. These are objective, accurate (although not always validated as such), and can validate self-report data (e.g., Fitbit). There was significant variation in the timing of validation measures, from one-time measures to many per day or pre-post assessments. For data processing, software applications that communicated with a remote server were used in most studies to save data for processing and, at times, provide within-study feedback to participants.

13.5.2 Evidence-Base for Sensors and Wearables

One major subset of studies focused on feedback in the form of applications that display graphs representing mental health status [4]. Many studies found that motivational messages (e.g., specific suggestion for action), tailored messages (e.g., specific to disease, stage of progress, demographic information, and treatment plan), and health professional contact enhanced therapeutic engagement are generally more effective than receiving numeric health measure feedback [36]. These individualized (or similar user) models appear more effective [37] than generalized models (e.g., generic message for a depression cohort). Individualized design of training and exercise programs may be helpful to maximize the improvements in performance and avoid risks.

Another area of research is related to validating diagnosis and/or determining predictors of outcomes. Within the depression studies, cell tower identification using GPS, screen active duration, and activity measurement have the strongest linkage with depression severity compared to distance traveled and short message service (SMS) text message received, whereas manic patients have longer calls, more messages sent and more travel [4]. For bipolar disorder, studies generally support the interpretation of sensed data by employing traditional measures or assessments for depression (e.g., Patient Health Questionnaire (PHQ)-8 or PHQ-9 self-report instruments) and clinician assessment/batteries [38].

Mood and anxiety studies use algorithms to interpret or predict participant's status (e.g., SVM, naïve Bayes classifiers, decision trees, random forests, linear regression, Bayesian networks, logistic regression, and other ML methods) [39]. Stress studies have involved adults, college students, health care professionals, and healthy volunteers, and measured stress with self-report questionnaires [40]. The College Sleep Project used multi-modal sensors (physiological, behavioral, environmental, and social) from smartphones to identify associations among and develop predictors for sleep behaviors, stress, mental health, and academic performance [41].

13.6 Chatbots and Mental Health

13.6.1 Overview

Chatbots refer to digital tools, designed to either replacing or complementing human support agents through the utilization of artificial intelligence (AI) and other automation technologies [42]. Over time, various chatbot platforms have been released, which included Apple Siri in 2011, Microsoft's Cortana, Google Assistant, and Amazon's Alexa. These chatbots, primarily integrated into mobile devices, have been widely applied to assist in multiple disciplines such as customer service, digital education, and e-health care through interactive conversations with their users.

In the field of mental health, the shortage of clinical professionals has hindered the widespread delivery of high-quality health care, while the demand for innovative technological solutions has been gradually increasing. As artificial intelligence technology has rapidly advanced, a variety of chatbots have been created to screen, diagnose, and treat mental health conditions. These chatbots not only serve as a supplement to the clinical workforce but also appeal to patients who may be reluctant to seek help from clinicians due to societal stigma [43]. According to the research conducted by Palanica et al. [44] and Vaidyam et al. [45] mental health chatbots can be classified into two categories: those specifically designed to address mental health disorders and those that cover general health issues, including mental illness. For instance, chatbots such as 3D WorldBuilder, Joy, Tess, Woebot, and Wysa specifically focus on mental illness treatment; bots such as Babylon Health, GYANT, HealthTap, and Mediktor operated on mobile apps could be applied for health in general [46]. The modalities and platforms of these chatbots have been continuously evolving, transitioning from text-based interactions to embodied 3D avatars. These mental health chatbots are available on various platforms, such as messaging apps of mobile devices, computer applications or web-based interfaces.

13.6.2 Gratifications of Using Chatbots for Mental Health

As the use of chatbots in health care communication continues to grow, researchers have conducted studies to examine gratifications of using chatbots for mental health. Compared to human mental health clinicians, chatbots offer immediate and personalized conversations, saving users both time and money. Scholars such as Cheng and Jiang, Fitzpatrick, and Kocaballi [47–50] have explored the impact of chatbots on mental health and found that users' social, utilitarian, technological, and hedonic gratifications can influence their engagement with these chatbots. Building upon these four categories of gratifications, we can categorize the gratufications of mental health chatbots into four dimensions: technology, hedonic, utilitarian, and social gratifications.

Technology gratifications refer to the ease of access and immediate conversation that chatbots provide, fulfilling users' technology-related gratifications. For individuals facing mental health issues, chatbots offer timely and interactive support, which has been shown to significantly improve user satisfaction [47]. In the aftermath of mass-shooting disasters, Cheng and Jiang [47] found that chatbots have a unique appeal to users due to their technological convenience. In critical situations, chatbots can offer immediate support by providing crisis helpline information, calming techniques, or guiding users through distressing moments until professional help can be obtained.

Hedonic gratification: Chatbots can provide emotional support to individuals experiencing mental health issues by engaging in empathetic conversations. These chatbots can adapt their responses to address users' emotions, encouraging users to manage their emotional well-being [51]. They can offer a listening ear, validate feelings, and provide encouragement. Additionally, mental health chatbots have demonstrated their effectiveness in reducing anxiety and depression through compassionate dialogues [49].

Utilitarian gratifications: Chatbots can offer essential information and intelligent solutions for resolving mental health issues. For instance, chatbots can be used for mental health assessments and screenings to identify potential disorders or symptoms; they can ask relevant questions and provide a preliminary evaluation based on the user's responses [43]. Chatbots can also deliver educational content about mental health conditions, treatment options, coping strategies, and self-help techniques. In addition, chatbots can help individuals monitor and track their mental well-being over time. Users can record their moods, thoughts, and activities, and the chatbot can provide insights, patterns, or alerts based on the collected data [43].

Social gratifications: Social companionship is a key social gratification, encompassing social interaction and social presence [47]. Mental health chatbots serve as companions, providing social support to users over extended periods. By fostering long-term social companionship, chatbots with advanced abilities can assist in delivering cognitive behavioral therapy (CBT)-based interventions by guiding users through structured exercises, helping them challenge negative thoughts, and reinforcing positive behaviors [43].

13.7 AI Opportunities and Challenges

A paradigm shift is occurring from passive use of health data by clinicians and consumers to interactive use in real-time is underway, and this creates a need and an opportunity for research and integration into care (Luxton, 2016) [1]. Information from sensors and devices increases awareness of a person's internal physical and emotional experience, thereby providing feedback for self-regulation. For example, for persons with an anxiety disorder, input from wearable devices can provide useful feedback in exposure-based treatment to promote learning, allow them to practice responses and monitor response to interventions. International standards pertain to design, pre-clinical validation and clinical validation of devices that include wearable sensors, and these vary widely from the European Union (E.U.) to the U.S [52]. Wearable medical devices are required to comply with IEC 62366–1:2015 standards that regulate the application of usability engineering to medical devices to achieve approval and two new E.U. regulations on medical devices that came into effect in 2020 are Regulations 2017/745 on medical devices and Regulation 2017/746 on in vitro diagnostic medical devices [53].

In addition, scholars have raised concerns about users becoming excessively attached to chatbots, potentially stemming from a distorted or parasocial relationship, which could be attributed to a patient's psychiatric illness [45]. Ethical considerations, including confidentiality and privacy, have also emerged as significant factors influencing the future of chatbots in mental health. For instance, research indicated that users' perceived privacy risk associated with chatbot usage negatively impacted their satisfaction and intention to continue using the chatbot [48]. Ethical issues such as safeguarding user information, ensuring data privacy, and addressing responsibility in the event of interactive accidents could significantly preclude the effectiveness of chatbot usage for mental health [47].

Therefore, future chatbots can be equipped with advanced natural language understanding capabilities, enabling them to listen empathically to users and deliver empathic and contextually relevant responses [51]. As chatbots become more prevalent in mental health support, addressing ethical considerations becomes crucial. Developers can focus on ensuring transparency about the nature of chatbot interactions, informing users when they are interacting with an AI system. Efforts should also be made to safeguard user data, maintain confidentiality, and adhere to strict privacy guidelines. While chatbots can provide valuable support, human oversight remains essential. Incorporating the expertise of mental health professionals in the development and monitoring of chatbot systems can ensure their ethical use. Collaboration between chatbots and human therapists or counselors can lead to a blended approach, where chatbots provide initial support and guidance, and humans offer deeper therapeutic interventions. Last but not least, chatbots can be designed to continuously learn and improve based on user feedback and real-time data. By analyzing user interactions and outcomes, chatbots can refine their responses and interventions, adapting to individual needs and staying up to date with the latest research in mental health.

Research opportunities and challenges can be broadly organized into 4 categories: (1) clinical health outcomes; (2) medico-legal, professional, and privacy policy issues; (3) outcome, evaluation, and other models; and (4) human–computer interaction (Table 13.3) [3, 4]. Methodological issues relate to user friendliness and scientific design. Mobile health interventions will likely succeed if they are seamlessly integrated into the patterns of people's daily lives and make minimal external demands. It is therefore important for developers of mobile and ambient technologies to apply the best practices in user experience and user-centered design in order to assure optimal function and effectiveness of these technologies. It is also important for health care professionals and organizations to be aware of these factors that may impact how their patients (and care providers) interact with these technologies. Usability is limited by users' getting distracted, connectivity issues, small screen sizes, low screen resolution, limited processing power, and difference in input devices (e.g., smaller buttons) that may cause errors.

System users are hoping for data from apps and mobile phones to be seamlessly returned to, and integrated in, the EHR to assist both clinicians and patients, but this has not been widely achieved, due in part to complex issues involved in the use of smartphone and other consumer technology in psychiatry. These issues include consumer technology usage, clinical utility, commercialization, and evolving consumer technology [54]. Based on a thorough review of the extant usability literature, the People at the Centre of Mobile Application Development (PACMAD) usability model has been proposed, which was designed to address the limitations of existing usability models when applied to mobile devices [55]. It places emphasis on factors associated with cognitive load. The seven attributes of this model are:

- *Effectiveness:* the user's ability to complete the intended task within the established context.
- *Efficacy:* the user's ability to complete the intended task "with speed and accuracy."

Table 13.3 Research opportunities and challenges for wearable sensors based on artificial intelligence and machine learning

Clinical health outcomes
• Extension of smartphone-based passive wearable sensors to new health and Well-being domains, such as caregiving • Development, implementation, and evaluation of clinician and trainee competency sets to ensure quality of care and research • Testing the integration of passive wearable sensors into clinical care, care coordination, and telehealth • Implementation of mobile health into interprofessional-based team-based care, with development of shared mental models and clarification of roles • Studies of passive wearable sensors for population health management, public health, and precision medicine • Comparative effectiveness studies of passive sensing-enabled, wearables, and RPM interventions on health outcomes, with adequate validation of measures • Research with a generalizable, adequate sample sizes for both short-and long-term impact
Outcome, evaluation, and other models
• Linkage of methods, monitoring, and interventions with health outcomes, quality of life measures, and economic cost analysis • Comparison of personalized and similar-user models with general models across several measured phenomena to assess the relative fitness of each model • Comparison of models between devices to see if significant differences exist • Focus on higher-level data and clinical interpretations (e.g., mood cycling) as the detection of lower-level data (e.g., activity duration) • Implementation of data analytics models that allow insight into symptom prediction and early intervention approaches
Human–computer interaction
• Analysis of cost effectiveness and efficacy of passive sensing on smartphones and wearables versus traditional methods such as paper-based logging
• Replication of studies with larger and more diverse samples • Integration with electronic health record and personal health record products in the contexts of personal health information management and clinical use of patient-generated data • Development and testing of clinician-facing interfaces to efficiently and effectively analyze and utilize passively acquired data • Research on the user-centered design, adoption and acceptance of technologies, and concerns about privacy • Use of artificial intelligence tools to improve and streamline analysis of data and provide outputs that are timely and meaningful with respect to patient care
Medico-legal, professional, and privacy policy issues
• Understanding privacy and data ownership concerns and preferences among potential end-users of smartphone-based passive sensing wearables • Specific technology topics for research on privacy include cross-application communication, cross-device communication, and health data aggregators • Development and testing of new privacy and security protocols as well as strategies for users to set custom privacy and security settings • Implementation of a legal framework to address privacy and data ownership in passive sensing on smartphones and wearables, especially for sensitive health domains such as mental health • Discussion of a legal framework to address failures in data protection strategies, taking into account consumers, clinicians, and researchers

- *Satisfaction:* the user's perception of "comfort and pleasantness" while engaging with the system.
- *Learnability:* how easily a user can gain proficiency with the given system.
- *Memorability:* the user's ability to retain how the system works even if the user has not used it frequently.
- *Errors:* the ability to complete any given task within the system without hitting into errors.
- *Cognitive load:* refers to a user's total amount of mental exertion required to use the specified system, such as a mobile application or website.

There remains a need for more research on the effectiveness of mobile health to improve health outcomes. Whether mobile health leads to better overall health outcomes and reduced disease burden is still unknown and premature adoption of untested mobile health technologies may detract from, rather than contribute to, what is needed for overall health improvement.

13.7.1 Ethical and Privacy Issues

There are ethical issues with AI technologies in behavioral and mental health care. The main issue to address should be the patients' safety, if smartphones are used for monitoring and treatment of a mood disorder [38]. Therefore, regular review of data and "warning signs" should be triggered by sensors [56]. While manufacturers and health care providers should consider such functions, these may fall outside the requirements offered by the Food and Drug Administration (FDA) in the United States and the European Union [52]. Key issues are the risks associated with over reliance on machines to make decisions and liability when machines make an error [1].

Ethical issues concern providing and obtaining adequate informed consent from participants, information quality in monitoring apps, personal privacy, and international legal and cultural differences [1, 57]. There are also privacy, data security, and ethical considerations (e.g., Health Insurance Portability and Accountability Act (HIPAA)) in the United States. Transmission of health information requires HIPAA compliance, data encryption, and other data security procedures, and theoretically this would include physiological data that could be used to identify a person. Mobile health may also create privacy issues associated with third parties (e.g., bystanders and family members) since mobile cameras and microphones that collect images and sounds from nonparticipants. All of these issues should be evaluated during the technology design process, so that appropriate encryption and data security features are built in [58].

13.7.2 Competencies for Clinicians Example (E.G., Wearable Sensors)

Competency-based education focuses on clinical skill development in addition to knowledge acquisition. An overview of competencies for synchronous and asynchronous competencies covered sets designed for video, mobile health, social media, wearable sensor technologies [59]. The slow integration of telehealth into clinical care and curricula may be a revealing story for sensors and wearables [60]. Sensor and wearable curricular approaches are similar to those for mobile health and asynchronous competencies [59, 61]. In addition to the sensors being the focus (i.e., content) of these competencies, sensors can shape the learning process, teaching learners, and simultaneously giving them experience (e.g., armband to measure proper hand washing via signal processing and ML).

AI-and ML-contextualized competencies for wearable sensors are outlined according to Accreditation Council of Graduate Medical Education domain of Patient Care is offered (Table 13.4), with the contextual information previously reviewed [4]. The proposed framework, domains vertically, learner levels horizontally, uses the six ACGME domains. Furthermore, the organizational/institutional competencies suggested for synchronous and asynchronous technology implantation [59, 60] complement EHR, CDS, and IS processes, by aligning work by training directors, faculty, department administrators, and health system leaders.

Institutional competencies have been suggested as many health systems are still working on basic clinical, technological, and administrative workflow, and may benefit from institutional level evaluation in order to implement new technologies. Institutional competencies include: (1) assess readiness; (2) create/hardwire the culture; (3) write policies and procedures; (4) establish the curriculum and competencies; (5) train learners and faculty; and (6) evaluate/manage change [59, 60]. Key participants include patients, trainees, faculty, and leaders; teams across professions and systems within the institution; and organizational leaders who set priorities and distribute resources. For integrating synchronous and asynchronous technologies, institutional competencies have been organized into focus areas: Patient-Centered Care; Evaluation and Outcomes; Teams, Professions, and Systems within Institutions; and the Institutional Structure, Process, and Administration [59]. Competencies for clinical care can help ensure quality, and faculty should role-model placing the patient's needs first and embracing technology for health care reform [62]. Further student and trainee learning opportunities should be developed in order support the practice of new skills.

Table 13.4 An outline of potential wearable sensor competencies based on artificial intelligence and organized by U.S. Accreditation Council of Graduate Medical Education domains

Area/Topic	Novice/Advanced Beginner (milestone levels 1–2)	Competent/Proficient (milestone levels 3–4)	Advanced/Expert (milestone level 5)
Patient care			
Patient assessment/ evaluation	Inquire about experience, comfort, trust	Conduct assessment of digital literacy and ease/ ambiance	Teach/develop evidence-based consent, medico-legal and policy issues
	Screen use of mobile phone, apps wearable sensors	Screen use of apps, Bluetooth, wearable (e.g., Fitbit and AirPods)	Optimize flexibility of IS, EHR, and CDS for patients and clinicians
	Screen for ability to text, install app, and use software	Assess quality and security of current/ potential data options	
Management and treatment planning	Make clear communications (e.g., text, notifications, and symbols)	Assess comfort with wearable in daily life (e.g., ease and fit with contact/water sports)	Weigh resources, culture and change
	Pilot/monitor/evaluate a technology learn about data feed to EHR	Select option based on preference, feasibility (e.g., text for EMA)	Disseminate best practices of informatics, AI, and PM
	Clarify data review "outside" regular hours	Supplement/replace manual process; match treatment objective with capability	Liaison for clinicians and IS administrators
			Advise on legal, billing & policy
Procedures	Encourage demonstrations to fit with purpose used	Customize approach, check settings and manage obstacles	Customize workflow
		Use continuum of automated data	Lead team to assess options
Decision-making, synthesis IS	Effectively locate regular wearable data in EHR	Adjust parameter(s) for decision-making and documentation	Teach pre-intra-platform data feeds into EHR
	Consider CDS tools of IS and EHR	Help others use tools (e.g., mood activity trigger for mania)	Evaluate clinician and patient tools/ algorithms
	Identify basic principles of effective CDS, decision science informatics tools	Weigh accelerometer, actigraphy, GPS sensor subtype (e.g., light, sound) options	Offer generic customized (e.g., demographic, treatment) tools

(continued)

Table 13.4 (continued)

Area/Topic	Novice/Advanced Beginner (milestone levels 1–2)	Competent/Proficient (milestone levels 3–4)	Advanced/Expert (milestone level 5)
Interpersonal communication skills			
Therapeutic relationships	Create non-judgmental space	Build rapport that fosters trust, respect understanding, including discussing problems managing conflict	Role model effective, continuous relationships
	Identify cultural, psychological social barriers to communication		Coach flexibility teamwork
Patient-centered care	Consider individual generational goals preferences	Listen clarify goals, values, preferences expectations to share decision-making	Seek family, cultural, language technology consultants for advice
	Simplify avoid technical jargon	Ensure timely documentation (e.g., registry)	Improve individual system care
IPE TBC	Learn the importance of TBC for care, learning communication	Build, re-design TBC via wearables IS	Teach IPE TBC via technology in terms of options, roles practices
		Emphasize clear concise communication	

app Application, *AI* Artificial Intelligence, *CDS* Clinical Decision Support, *EMA* Ecological Momentary Assessment, *EHR* Electronic Health Record, *IS* Information System, *IT* Information Technology, *IPE* Interprofessional Education, *ML* Machine Learning, *QI* Quality Improvement, *PM* Predictive Modeling, *SP* Smartphone, *TBC* Team-based Care

13.8 Discussion/Conclusions

Although the potential benefits of PM are clear, the mental health field does not yet have a set of "best practices" for implementing the results into clinical practice [31]. Once a predictive model is established, mental health systems are left with the task of intervening with individuals who may not actually be at risk (given that predictive models are not perfect), and depending on the goals of the program, many individuals identified by the predictive model will not have self-identified as having a need for intervention. Therefore, the clinical use of results from statistical models is challenging (e.g., REACH VET local mental health leaders collaborated to discuss potential clinical actions and best practices). For AI, new reporting guidelines have been developed to bridge the development-to-implementation gap in clinical artificial intelligence [63]. DECIDE-AI considered the complexity of human decision-making processes, differences between the development population and the target patient population and safety evaluation as users' decisions may not mirror the algorithm's recommendations.

Health care clinicians, systems, and governmental agencies across the world are trying to set individual patient, aggregate and population outcomes that can be evaluated by mental health data/indicators across medical settings. Effectiveness, implementation science, and translational approaches are suggested, with input from all stakeholders in health care settings [64, 65] for scalable psychological interventions for people in communities affected by adversity [66]. To implement interventions that are based on predictive learning, effective program leadership at the top is needed, along with local leader prioritization of the program, clear communication, and preparation of the clinical staff. Progressive businesses have integrated core business divisions—research and development, operations, marketing and finance—with an information technology (IT) division (i.e., a shared IT-business framework) to leverage knowledge and capital [67]. This paradigm has been applied to video to *organize* care with technology rather than *append* IT to health care (i.e., IT-business-health model) [68]. Clinician or learner-centered approaches—competencies—that parallel patient-centered ones are needed to ensure quality care as part of health care reform [9, 66].

The state of the evidence is rapidly improving with use of many technologies, standardized measures, and, importantly, high levels of patient engagement and enrollment, including a variety of international and culturally diverse populations (e.g., age, disorder, ethnicity, generation, geographic, military, etc.). Research in clinical health outcomes, medico-legal issues, evaluation, and human–computer interaction is suggested [3, 4]. Evaluation with implementation/effectiveness approaches is best combined with longitudinal, quality of life, and economic cost analysis dimensions [4, 69]. Future studies could investigate smartphone, biological and clinical data to identify markers of risk, diagnosis, state, stage, a treatment response and prognosis in different populations [4, 70]. More broadly, digital phenotyping or behavioral markers are being developed for both clinical and non-clinical populations to correlate multimodal sensor data, cognitions, and depressive mood. The creation of large multicentric databases is an essential element in the development and validation of artificial intelligence tools, particularly in the setting of deep learning [71].

There are gaps, still, in converting AI, ML, and PM processes to user-friendly experiences for patients and for the everyday clinician in the United States and across the globe. Only a few systems are using these as the primary assessment and/or treatment modality [72, 73]. The COVID-19 pandemic forced health care providers and systems to rapidly adapt their way of providing services—at least for telehealth (video and telephone). The attainment of technological capabilities and practical skills to assure competent, legal and ethical practice for video, though, is substantially different than the use of PM for Alzheimer's care [74]. PM re-raises some ethical concerns and social considerations potentially stemming from—among others—the risk of false classification, the dependence of the results on the assumptions, and from the statistical complexity. Thus, institutional movement on mobile health, wearable sensor, and informatics practices has not been rapid and it requires substantial planning and organizational change [59]. These issues and the complexity of AI, ML, and PM processes—and the misperception that these technologies are replacing humans instead of complementing our work—are not easy to communicate to an individual patient, leaders, and the general public.

References

1. Luxton DD. Artificial intelligence in behavioral health care. Boston, MA: Elsevier; 2016.
2. Edgcomb JB, Zima B. Machine learning, natural language processing, and the electronic health record: innovations in mental health services research. Psychiatr Serv. 2019;70(4):346–9. https://doi.org/10.1176/appi.ps.201800401.
3. Hilty DM, Armstrong CM, Luxton DD, et al. A scoping review of sensors, wearables and remote monitoring for behavioral health: uses, outcomes, clinical competencies and research directions. J Tech Behav Sci. 2021;6:278. https://doi.org/10.1007/s41347-021-00199-2.
4. Hilty DM, Armstrong CM, Stewart A, et al. A framework of sensor, wearable and remote patient monitoring competencies for clinical care and training: scoping review. J Tech Behav Sci. 2021;6:252. https://doi.org/10.1007/s41347-020-00190-3.
5. Cho G, Yim J, Choi Y, Ko J, Lee SH. Review of machine learning algorithms for diagnosing mental illness. Psychiatry Investig. 2019;16(4):262–9. https://doi.org/10.30773/pi.2018.12.21.2.
6. Watson J, Hutyra CA, Clancy SM, et al. Overcoming barriers to the adoption and implementation of predictive modeling and machine learning in clinical care: what can we learn from US academic medical centers? JAMIA Open. 2020;3(2):167–72. Published 2020 Apr 10. https://doi.org/10.1093/jamiaopen/ooz046.
7. Seko Y, Kidd S, Wiljer D, McKenzie K. Youth mental health interventions via mobile phones: a scoping review. Cyberpsychol Behav Soc Netw. 2014;17(9):591–602.
8. Ariga K, Makita T, Ito M, Mori T, et al. Review of advanced sensor devices employing nanoarchitectonics concepts. Beilstein J Nanotechnol. 2019;10:2014–30.
9. National Academy of Sciences, engineering, and medicine. Health and Medicine Division. 2020. http://www.nationalacademies.org/hmd/Global/Meetings.aspx.
10. Jordans M, Chisholm D, Semrau M, et al. Evaluation of performance and perceived utility of mental healthcare indicators in routine health information systems in five low-and middle-income countries. B J Psych Open. 2019;5(5):e70. https://doi.org/10.1192/bjo.2019.22.
11. Ahuja S, Hanlon C, Chisholm D, et al. Experience of implementing new mental health indicators within information systems in six low-and middle-income countries. B J Psych Open. 2019;5(5):e71. Published 2019 Aug 6. https://doi.org/10.1192/bjo.2019.29.
12. Luxton DD, Riek L. Artificial intelligence and robotics for rehabilitation. In: Brenner BS, Reid-Arndt E, et al., editors. Handbook of rehabilitation psychology. 3rd ed. Washington DC: American Psychological Association Books; 2019.
13. Shatte ABR, Hutchinson DM, Teague SJ. Machine learning in mental health: a scoping review of methods and applications. Psychol Med. 2019;49(9):1426–48. https://doi.org/10.1017/S0033291719000151.
14. Luxton DD. Should Watson be consulted for a second opinion? AMA J Ethics. 2019;21(2):E131–7. https://doi.org/10.1001/amajethics.2019.131.
15. Hilty DM, Rabinowitz TR, McCarron RM, et al. Telepsychiatry and e-mental health models leverage stepped, collaborative, and integrated services to primary care. Psychosomatics. 2018;59(3):227–50.
16. Bickman L. Improving mental health services: a 50-year journey from randomized experiments to artificial intelligence and precision mental health. Admin Pol Ment Health. 2020;47(5):795–843. https://doi.org/10.1007/s10488-020-01065-8.
17. Zalpuri I, Liu H, Stubbe D, et al. A competency-based framework for social media for trainees, faculty and others. Acad Psychiatry. 2018;42(6):808–17.

18. Love-Koh J, Peel A, Rejon-Parrilla JC, et al. The future of precision medicine: potential impacts for health technology assessment. PharmacoEconomics. 2018;36(12):1439–51. https://doi.org/10.1007/s4r0273-018-0686-6.
19. Manchia M, Pisanu C, Squassina A, Carpiniello B. Challenges and future prospects of precision medicine in psychiatry. Pharmacogenomics Pers Med. 2020;13:127–40. Published 2020 Apr 23. https://doi.org/10.2147/PGPM.S198225.
20. Pigoni A, Delvecchio G, Madonna D, Bressi C, Soares J, Brambilla P. Can machine learning help us in dealing with treatment resistant depression? A review. J Affect Disord. 2019;259:21–6. https://doi.org/10.1016/j.jad.2019.08.009.
21. Nemesure MD, Heinz MV, Huang R, et al. Predictive modeling of depression and anxiety using electronic health records and a novel machine learning approach with artificial intelligence. Sci Rep. 2021;11(1):1980. https://doi.org/10.1038/s41598-021-81368-4.
22. Librenza-Garcia D, Kotzian BJ, Yang J, et al. The impact of machine learning techniques in the study of bipolar disorder: a systematic review. Neurosci Biobehav Rev. 2017;80:538–54. https://doi.org/10.1016/j.neubiorev.2017.07.004.
23. Claude LA, Houenou J, Duchesnay E, Favre P. Will machine learning applied to neuroimaging in bipolar disorder help the clinician? A critical review and methodological suggestions. Bipolar Disord. 2020;22(4):334–55. https://doi.org/10.1111/bdi.12895.
24. Wolfers T, Buitelaar JK, Beckmann CF, Franke B, Marquand AF. From estimating activation locality to predicting disorder: a review of pattern recognition for neuroimaging-based psychiatric diagnostics. Neurosci Biobehav Rev. 2015;57:328–49. https://doi.org/10.1016/j.neubiorev.2015.08.001.
25. Kim YK, Na KS. Application of machine learning classification for structural brain MRI in mood disorders: critical review from a clinical perspective. Prog Neuro-Psychopharmacol Biol Psychiatry. 2018;80(Pt B):71–80. https://doi.org/10.1016/j.pnpbp.2017.06.024.
26. Mikolas P, Hlinka J, Skoch A, et al. Machine learning classification of first-episode schizophrenia spectrum disorders and controls using whole brain white matter fractional anisotropy. BMC Psychiatry. 2018;18(1):97. Published 2018 Apr 10. https://doi.org/10.1186/s12888-018-1678-y.
27. de Filippis R, Carbone EA, Gaetano R, et al. Machine learning techniques in a structural and functional MRI diagnostic approach in schizophrenia: a systematic review. Neuropsychiatr Dis Treat. 2019;15:1605–27. Published 2019 Jun 19. https://doi.org/10.2147/NDT.S202418.
28. Kalmady SV, Greiner R, Agrawal R, et al. Towards artificial intelligence in mental health by improving schizophrenia prediction with multiple brain parcellation ensemble-learning. NPJ Schizophr. 2019;5(1):2. Published 2019 Jan 18. https://doi.org/10.1038/s41537-018-0070-8.
29. Becker D, van Breda W, Funk B, Hoogendoorn M, Ruwaard J, Riper H. Predictive modeling in e-mental health: a common language framework. Internet Interv. 2018;12:57–67. Published 2018 Mar 8. https://doi.org/10.1016/j.invent.2018.03.002.
30. Galatzer-Levy IR, Ma S, Statnikov A, et al. Utilization of machine learning for prediction of post-traumatic stress: a re-examination of cortisol in the prediction and pathways to non-remitting PTSD. Transl. Psychiatry. 2017;7(3):e0. Published 2017 Mar 21. https://doi.org/10.1038/tp.2017.38.
31. Reger GM, McClure ML, Ruskin D, et al. Integrating predictive modeling into mental health care: an example in suicide prevention. Psychiatr Serv. 2019;70(1):71–4. https://doi.org/10.1176/appi.ps.201800242.
32. Poulin C, Thompson P, Bryan C. Public health surveillance: predictive analytics and big data. In: Luxton DD, editor. Artificial intelligence in behavioral and mental health care. New York: Elsevier/Academic Press; 2016.
33. Luxton DD, Poulin C. Advancing public health in the age of big data: methods, ethics, and recommendations. In: Goldschmidt L, Relova RM, editors. Patient-centered healthcare technology: the way to better health. London, UK: Institution of Engineering and Technology; 2020.
34. Iorfino F, Ho N, Carpenter JS, et al. Predicting self-harm within six months after initial presentation to youth mental health services: a machine learning study. PLoS One. 2020;15(12):e0243467. Published 2020 Dec 31. https://doi.org/10.1371/journal.pone.0243467.

35. Brown LA, Benhamou K, May AM, et al. Machine learning algorithms in suicide prevention: clinician interpretations as barriers to implementation. J Clin Psychiatry. 2020;81(3):19m12970. Published 2020 Apr 21. https://doi.org/10.4088/JCP.19m12970.
36. Ma Y, Xu B, Bai Y, et al. Infer daily mood using mobile phone sensing. Ad Hoc Sensor Wireless Network. 2014;20:133–52.
37. Wahle F, Kowatsch T, Fleisch E, et al. Mobile sensing and support for people with depression: a pilot trial in the wild. JMIR Mhealth Uhealth. 2016;4(3):e111. https://doi.org/10.2196/mhealth.5960.
38. Faurholt-Jepsen M, Munkholm K, Frost M, et al. Electronic self-monitoring of mood using IT platforms in adult patients with bipolar disorder: a systematic review of the validity and evidence. BMC Psychiatry. 2016a;16(1):7. https://doi.org/10.1186/s12888-016-0713-0.
39. Elgendi M, Menon C. Assessing anxiety disorders using wearable devices: challenges and future directions. Brain Sci. 2019;9(3):50. https://doi.org/10.3390/brainsci9030050.
40. Seppälä J, De Vita I, Jämsä T, et al. Mobile phone and wearable sensor-based mhealth approaches for psychiatric disorders and symptoms: systematic review. JMIR Ment Health. 2019;6(2):e9819. https://doi.org/10.2196/mental.9819.
41. Sano A, Phillips AJ, Yu AZ, et al. Recognizing academic performance, sleep quality, stress level, and mental health using personality traits, wearable sensors and mobile phones. Int Conf Wearable Implant Body Sens Netw. 2015;2015:2015. https://doi.org/10.1109/BSN.2015.7299420.
42. Basumallick C. What is a chatbot? Meaning, working, types, and examples. https://www.spiceworks.com/tech/artificial-intelligence/articles/what-is-chatbot/.
43. Abd-Alrazaq AA, Alajlani M, Alalwan AA, Bewick BM, Gardner P, Househ M. An overview of the features of chatbots in mental health: a scoping review. Int J Med Inform. 2019;132:103978. https://doi.org/10.1016/j.ijmedinf.2019.103978.
44. Palanica A, Flaschner P, Thommandram A, et al. Physicians' perceptions of chatbots in health care: cross-sectional web-based survey. J Med Internet Res. 2019;21(4):e12887. https://doi.org/10.2196/12887.
45. Vaidyam AN, Wisniewski H, Halamka JD, et al. Chatbots and conversational agents in mental health: a review of the psychiatric landscape. Can J Psychiatry. 2019;64(7):456–64. https://doi.org/10.1177/0706743719828977.
46. Cheng Y, Xie C-X, Wang Y-D, et al. Chatbots and health: Mental health. In: Ho E, Bylund C, van Weert J, Basnyat I, Bol N, Dean M, editors. The international encyclopedia of health communication. New York: Wiley; 2023.
47. Cheng Y, Jiang H. AI-powered mental health chatbots: examining users' motivations, active communicative action, and engagement after mass-shooting disasters. J Contingencies Crisis Manag. 2020;28:339–54. https://doi.org/10.1111/1468-5973.12319.
48. Cheng Y, Jiang H. How do AI-driven chatbots impact user experience? Examining gratifications, perceived privacy risk, satisfaction, loyalty, and continued use. J Broadcast Electron Med. 2020b;65(4):592–614. https://doi.org/10.1080/08838151.2020.1834296.
49. Fitzpatrick KK, Darcy A, Vierhile M. Delivering cognitive behavior therapy to young adults with symptoms of depression and anxiety using a fully automated conversational agent (Woebot): a randomized controlled trial. JMIR Mental Health. 2017;4(2):e19. https://doi.org/10.2196/mental.7785.
50. Kocaballi AB, Berkovsky S, Quiroz JC, et al. A comprehensive analysis of interactions between psychiatric patients and an AI-powered chatbot. NPJ Digit Med. 2019;2(1):1–12.
51. Inkster B, Sarda S, Subramanian V. An empathy-driven, conversational artificial intelligence agent (Wysa) for digital mental Well-being: real-world data evaluation mixed-methods study. JMIR Mhealth Uhealth. 2018;6(11):e12106. https://doi.org/10.2196/12106.
52. Ravizza A, De Maria C, Di Pietro L, et al. Comprehensive review on current and future regulatory requirements on wearable sensors in preclinical and clinical testing. Front Bioeng Biotech. 2019;7:313. https://doi.org/10.3389/fbioe.2019.00313.
53. Loncar-Turukalo T, Zdravevski E, Machado da Silva J, et al. Literature on wearable technology for connected health: scoping review of research trends, advances, and barriers. J Med Internet Res. 2019;21(9):e14017. https://doi.org/10.2196/14017.

54. Bauer M, Glenn T, Geddes J, et al. Smartphones in mental health: a critical review of background issues, current status and future concerns. Int J Bipolar Disord. 2020;8(1):2. Published 2020 Jan 10. https://doi.org/10.1186/s40345-019-0164-x.
55. Harrison R, Flood D, Duce D. Usability of mobile applications: Literature review and rationale for a new usability model. J Interact Sci. 2013;1(1):1–16.
56. Depp C, Torous J, Thompson W. Technology-based early warning systems for bipolar disorder: a conceptual framework. JMIR Ment Health. 2016;3(3):e42.
57. Torous J, Roberts LW. The ethical use of mobile health technology in clinical psychiatry. J Nerv Ment Dis. 2017;205(1):4–8. https://doi.org/10.1097/nmd.0000000000000596.
58. Luxton DD, Kayl RA, Mishkind MC. mHealth data security: the need for HIPAA-compliant standardization. Tel J E-Health. 2012;18:284–8.
59. Hilty DM, Torous J, Parish M, et al. A literature review comparing clinicians' approaches and skills to in-person, synchronous and asynchronous care: moving toward asynchronous competencies to ensure quality care. Telemed J E-Health. 2020;27:356. https://doi.org/10.1089/tmj.2020.0054.
60. Hilty DM, Unutzer J, Ko DK, et al. Approaches for departments, schools and health systems to better implement technologies used for clinical care and education. Acad Psychiatry. 2019;43(6):611–6.
61. Hilty DM, Chan S, Torous J, et al. A framework for competencies for the use of mobile technologies in psychiatry and medicine. JMIR Uhealth Mob Health. 2020;8(2):e12229. http://mhealth.jmir.org/2020/2/e12229/.
62. Gaglani SM, Topol EJ. iMedEd: the role of mobile health technologies in medical education. Acad Med. 2014;89(9):1207–9. https://doi.org/10.1097/ACM.0000000000000361.
63. DECIDE-AI Steering Group. DECIDE-AI: new reporting guidelines to bridge the development-to-implementation gap in clinical artificial intelligence. Nat Med. 2021;27(2):186–7. https://doi.org/10.1038/s41591-021-01229-5.
64. Proctor E, Silmere H, Raghavan R, et al. Outcomes for implementation research: conceptual distinctions, measurement challenges, and research agenda. Admin Pol Ment Health. 2010;38(2):65–76.
65. Gargon E, Gorst SL, Williamson PR. Choosing important health outcomes for comparative effectiveness research: 5th annual update to a systematic review of core outcome sets for research. PLoS One. 2019;14(12):e0225980. https://doi.org/10.1371/journal.pone.0225980.
66. World Health Organization. 2020. Mar 22, [2020-05-26]. Draft global strategy on digital health, 2020–2024. https://www.who.int/docs/default-source/documents/gs4dh-daa2a9f352b0445bafbc79ca799dce4d.pdf.
67. Ray G, Muhanna WA, Barney JB. Competing with IT: the role of shared IT-business understanding. Commun Assoc Comput Mach. 2007;50(12):87–91.
68. Hilty DM, Uno J, Chan S, et al. Role of technology in professional development. Psych Clin N Amer. 2019;42:493–512.
69. Cornet VP, Holden RJ. Systematic review of smartphone-based passive sensing for health and wellbeing. J Biomed Inform. 2018;77:120–32.
70. Torous J, Baker JT. Why psychiatry needs data science and data science needs psychiatry: connecting with technology. JAMA Psychiatry. 2016;73(1):3–4.
71. Chassagnon G, Dohan A. Artificial intelligence: from challenges to clinical implementation. Diagn Interv Imaging. 2020;101(12):763–4. https://doi.org/10.1016/j.diii.2020.10.007.
72. Hermens HJ, Vollenbroek-Hutten MM. Towards remote monitoring and remotely supervised training. J Electromyogr Kinesiol. 2008;18(6):908–19.
73. Kvedar J, Coye MJ, Everett W. Connected health: a review of technologies and strategies to improve patient care with telemedicine and telehealth. Health Aff (Millwood). 2014;33(2):194–9.
74. Angehrn Z, Sostar J, Nordon C, et al. Ethical and social implications of using predictive modeling for Alzheimer's disease prevention: a systematic literature review. J Alzheimers Dis. 2020;76(3):923–40. https://doi.org/10.3233/JAD-191159.

Cognitive Behavioral Therapy, and Cognitive Bias Modification in Internet-Based Interventions for Mood, Anxiety, and Substance Use Disorders

14

Matthijs Blankers, Elske Salemink, and Reinout W. Wiers

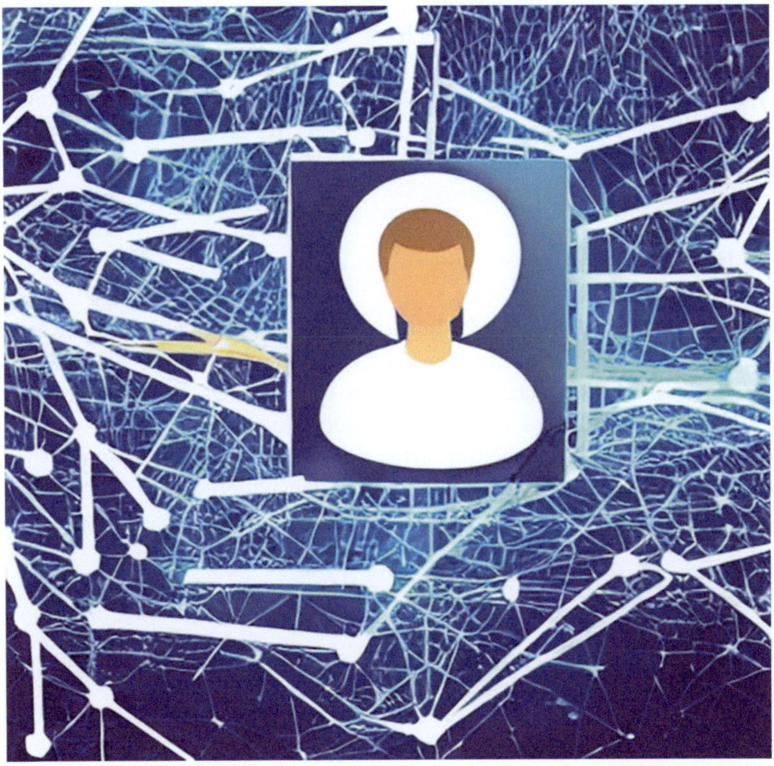

D. Mucić, D. M. Hilty (eds.), *Digital Mental Health*,
https://doi.org/10.1007/978-3-031-59936-1_14

Abstract

In this chapter, the theoretical background of (digital) cognitive behavioral therapy (CBT) is presented, along with cognitive bias modification (CBM), a novel set of interventions in which cognitive processes involved in a disorder are directly targeted. Next, the effectiveness of digital CBT and CBM for common mental health disorders (depression, anxiety disorders, and substance use disorders, SUDs) is evaluated based on recent meta-analyses and supplemented with recent studies. Based on the reviewed literature, there is a reasonably strong evidence base for the effectiveness of digital CBT interventions for depression, anxiety, and SUDs. The evidence base for CBM interventions depends on the type of intervention and disorder. There is accumulating evidence that CBM training targeting interpretations reduces anxiety, but there is less evidence for its effects on depression. The evidence for emotional symptom reduction after CBM targeting attention is inconsistent. In SUD, there is accumulating evidence for increased abstinence after supplementing CBT treatment for alcohol use disorder for one type of CBM: approach bias modification, and preliminary, less consistent evidence for other types. Therefore, it is concluded that based on the currently available evidence, CBM could be a useful add-on to digital CBT in the clinical treatment of common mental health disorders.

14.1 Introduction

The past 10 years have witnessed a huge growth in the utilization of the Internet to disseminate e-mental health interventions for common mental disorders such as mood disorders, harmful alcohol use, and other SUDs and anxiety disorders. Nowadays, a large variety of services and interventions are available, ranging from information provision to screening with tailored advice and unguided self-help modules to multisession-guided Internet-based psychotherapy interventions. The advantages are evident: Internet services are ubiquitously accessible, at any time,

M. Blankers (✉)
Trimbos Institute, Netherlands Institute of Mental Health and Addiction, Utrecht, The Netherlands

Department of Research, Arkin Mental Health Care, Amsterdam, The Netherlands
e-mail: mblankers@trimbos.nl

E. Salemink
Department of Clinical Psychology, Utrecht University, Utrecht, The Netherlands
e-mail: e.salemink@uu.nl

R. W. Wiers
Addiction Development and Psychopathology (ADAPT)-Lab, Department of Psychology, & Centre for Urban Mental Health, University of Amsterdam, Amsterdam, The Netherlands
e-mail: r.w.h.j.wiers@uva.nl

and costs are low. The possibility of using the services anonymously can be attractive for users as well, especially in the case of stigmatized disorders (e.g., SUDs). Internet services and interventions might therefore contribute to narrowing the treatment gap: the relatively large proportion of untreated persons with mental health disorders within a given population. For example, less than 10% of all persons with an alcohol use disorder are in treatment in Europe [1], while the economic costs of SUDs including alcohol use are among the highest of all mental and brain problems in Europe [2].

From this perspective, it is somewhat surprising that the implementation of Internet services has not been disseminated more widely yet, in particular in regions with suboptimal access to mental health facilities. This cannot be caused by a lack of evidence on the effectiveness of Internet interventions for common mental disorders. The development and implementation of Internet interventions have been accompanied by many randomized clinical trials (RCTs) and other research projects. The evidence for the effectiveness and cost-effectiveness of many interventions has been demonstrated in recent reviews and meta-analyses [3–9]—although effects are often of modest size. Still, given the high prevalence of common mental disorders and the relatively low marginal costs of providing Internet interventions to additional users, the potential economic gains are enormous [4, 9].

Many of the tested and implemented e-mental health interventions for common mental disorders are based on cognitive behavioral therapy (CBT) [10]. CBT has primarily been developed as a method to treat depression by Aaron Beck in the 1960s, while he was a psychiatrist at the University of Pennsylvania [11]. Since then, CBT has established itself as the therapeutic underpinning of many psychotherapy interventions and protocols, and more recently (digital) CBT has become one of the standard therapeutic orientations for Internet interventions. In general, we have mainly seen a process of assimilation in the developmental trajectory from traditional face-to-face interventions for common mental disorders to technology- and Internet-enabled interventions in the past decade. In analogy to Piaget's theory of cognitive development [12], new technology is currently incorporated in already existing cognitive schemas, without changing the overall schemas of treatment. In terms of Internet interventions, digital technology is often used to deliver the traditional, previously existing CBT intervention content that has already been delivered for years or even decades to address a variety of disorders. What this field may profit from, in the same analogy from cognitive development, would be accommodation. This would be a process of incorporating new developments by altering existing cognitive schemas in order to fit in these new developments. In terms of Internet interventions, this would encompass that the content of the interventions itself is enhanced, to optimally utilize technology. The guiding question should be: "What kinds of new interventions are now possible if we use new (Internet) technology?" instead of "How can we offer existing interventions using this new technology?"

Over the past two decades, many of the new findings in clinical psychology stem from cognitive, experimental psychopathology research. Findings have led to a number of new, experimental treatment modalities, including technology-enabled interventions such as cognitive bias modification (CBM) as an adjunct to (digital)

CBT [13]. In CBM, a cognitive process involved in the disorder is directly targeted in an intervention. For example, in SUDs, an attentional bias and an approach-bias to substance-related stimuli have been distinguished. Both can be directly targeted in a dedicated digital intervention, with promising first results (review: [14]). One question we address is whether the advent of technology- and Internet-based interventions proves to be an opportunity for the integration of more recent findings from (clinical) psychology into clinical practice.

In this chapter, the theoretical background of CBT will first be summarized. Next, the effectiveness of digital CBT for common mental disorders will be evaluated based on recent meta-analyses. Taking these findings into account, opportunities for accommodation of the current generation of Internet interventions will be explored. Hence, in the second part of this chapter, CBM, which is one of the promising means of accommodating CBT interventions to the technical opportunities provided by Internet technology, will be introduced. The evidence regarding the effectiveness of CBM as an adjunct to (digital) CBT will be evaluated and the advantages and disadvantages of CBM and practical applications of CBM will be discussed. The central theme of this chapter is: Will the advent of technology- and Internet-based interventions prove to be an opportunity to accommodate the clinical practice of common mental disorders to recent psychological research findings?

14.2 Theoretical Background of Digital CBT

14.2.1 Background of CBT

CBT is a structured, short-term psychotherapy, which aims at solving current problems through restructuring and modifying inaccurate or unhelpful thinking. The therapist tries to find ways to produce cognitive change, for example, through modifying a client's thinking and belief system, behavioral experiments, or exposure, in order to produce emotional and behavioral change. CBT was initially developed for depression but is nowadays being used for a variety of disorders, including anxiety disorders, substance use disorders, and eating disorders. The main constituents of a CBT intervention for depression include a focus on problem solving, behavioral activation, identifying, evaluating, and responding to depressed and negative thoughts, self-perception, and discussing the patient's future [10].

CBT builds upon previous research in the field of psychology and is based on various theories including those by Karen Horney, Alfred Adler, George Kelly, Albert Ellis, Richard Lazarus, and Albert Bandura. CBT itself is a source or predecessor for other therapeutic approaches. Those therapeutic approaches include problem-solving therapy, behavioral activation, cognitive behavior modification [10], and acceptance and commitment therapy [15]. Many outcome studies involving CBT have been performed and published, the first one already in 1977 [16]. Nowadays, more than 500 outcome studies report evidence on the efficacy of CBT for various psychiatric disorders, psychological problems, or psychological components of medical problems (e.g., pain in cancer patients). Positive results have been found in clinical settings, as well as in other settings such as community settings [17]. In more recent years, digital CBT interventions have been shown to be effective (e.g. [8, 18, 19]).

There are ten basic principles of CBT: [[10], p. 7–11].

1. Cognitive behavior therapy is based on an ever-evolving formulation of patients' problems and an individual conceptualization of each patient in cognitive terms.
2. Cognitive behavior therapy requires a sound therapeutic alliance.
3. Cognitive behavior therapy emphasizes collaboration and active participation.
4. Cognitive behavior therapy is goal-oriented and problem-focused.
5. Cognitive behavior therapy initially emphasizes the present.
6. Cognitive behavior therapy is educative, aims to teach the patient to be her own therapist, and emphasizes relapse prevention.
7. Cognitive behavior therapy aims to be time-limited.
8. Cognitive behavior therapy sessions are structured.
9. Cognitive behavior therapy teaches patients to identify, evaluate, and respond to their dysfunctional thoughts and beliefs.
10. Cognitive behavior therapy uses a variety of techniques to change thinking, mood, and behavior.

Although the basic principles apply to all patients, CBT can vary depending on the individual client, their problems or disorders, their age or life-stage, gender, intellectual level, and cultural background. Also, the goals the client set, their ability to build a strong therapeutic alliance, their motivation to bring about change, and earlier therapeutic experiences shape the contents of each individual therapy [10].

14.2.2 Background of Digital CBT

Over the past two decades, CBT has on an accumulating scale been offered using digital technology. There are several potential advantages of using digital CBT in treatment delivery. Two of the most important potential advantages are enhanced access to evidence-based psychotherapy and a reduction in therapy costs. By decreasing the amount of therapist time needed to achieve significant improvements in symptoms, a greater number of people can receive treatment by trained CBT therapists [20]. Another possible advantage of digital CBT could be that patients are reached who otherwise may not have accepted traditional therapy because of stigma or negative attitudes about treatment. The use of technology may also give patients more control and insight into the flow and progress of their therapy [20]. In recent years, both patients and professionals have tended to become more positive about the use of digital technology for mental health care [21]. The COVID-19 pandemic has functioned as a catalyst for the further implementation of digital CBT and telecare through videoconferencing in the mental health care practice, with similar outcomes as traditional in-person care [22]. Yet another potential advantage of using digital technology is to teach the basic principles of CBT or to provide learning opportunities in a way that is more efficient and self-guided than would be possible in traditional therapy [20]. For example, in a study on drug-free patients with major depressive disorder, [23] it was found that the digital CBT group showed a larger increase in CBT knowledge and a larger improvement in dysfunctional attitudes than the control group, which was provided standard CBT, while the total time spent with the therapist was reduced in the digital CBT group compared to the control group. As the digital psychoeducational intervention component in the digital CBT group was designed to educate patients and develop skills through multimedia interactions and interactive exercises, this may also have led to a more consistent and engaging educational component than would typically be the case in standard therapist-led CBT [20].

However, there are also concerns regarding the acceptability and potential adverse consequences of digital CBT in comparison with traditional CBT. In a review [24], barriers to the uptake of digital CBT were systematically evaluated. The authors focused on the acceptability, accessibility, and adverse consequences associated with digital CBT. Among the main results, the authors report that recruited patients have only a 38% chance of actually starting digital CBT, with little data on why this is. When patients do start therapy, personal circumstances still negatively influence adherence in many. Though travel is eliminated by (Internet-based) digital CBT, time to participate in the intervention is still a limiting factor. Some additional concerns are coined regarding the accessibility to the technology—it is not known how screen readers (for partially sighted users) cope with digital CBT interventions. Also, some patients might find digital therapy too demanding, patronizing, or fast-paced and might prefer face-to-face therapy [24]. In addition to the patients, therapists may not all be enthusiastic about the use of digital telecare such as video communication as an alternative to face-to-face care, depending on their patient population, based on an evaluation during the COVID-19 pandemic [25].

14.3 Effectiveness of Digital CBT

Over the past two decades, many RCTs and systematic reviews on the effectiveness of various forms of digital CBT have been performed. In this section, the results with regard to the effectiveness of digital CBT for mood disorders, anxiety disorders, and SUDs will briefly be reviewed.

14.3.1 Mood Disorders

There is compelling evidence that both guided (therapist or counselor supported) and unguided digital CBT interventions efficaciously reduce (subclinical) mood disorders. A recent individual patient data meta-analysis (IPDMA) [26] combined data from 39 RCTs and 9751 patients to assess the effectiveness of guided and unguided digital CBT interventions. Patients were recruited from community, clinical, workplace, or mixed samples. Studies were conducted across 12 countries in Europe, North America, and China. Comparisons were made post-treatment and at approximately 6 and 12 months post-randomization. At post-treatment and at six months post-randomization, both guided and unguided digital CBT interventions significantly outperformed the control conditions (treatment as usual or waitlist) in terms of effectiveness, measured using the Patient Health Questionnaire-9 or equivalent instruments. Only at post-treatment, guided interventions significantly outperformed the unguided interventions. Baseline depression scores were found to be an important moderator of this relative effectiveness of guided vs. unguided interventions at post-treatment: the higher the baseline severity, the larger the benefit of therapeutic guidance. Hence, in this IPDMA, both guided and unguided digital CBT interventions led to better outcomes than control conditions and guided digital CBT was associated with larger effects than unguided digital CBT at post-intervention, especially for individuals with moderate to severe depression. The findings of this IPDMA are generally in line with other systematic reviews on guided and unguided digital CBT interventions for depression (e.g [3, 19, 27]).

Probably among the best-known and best-studied digital CBT interventions for depression is MoodGYM. MoodGYM is an innovative, interactive Web program designed to prevent depression. It consists of five modules, an interactive game, anxiety and depression assessments, downloadable relaxation audio, a workbook, and a feedback assessment. MoodGYM was designed and developed by staff at the National Institute for Mental Health Research at The Australian National University, in collaboration with researchers, mental health experts, Web and graphic designers, and software engineers [28]. MoodGYM is available in Chinese, Dutch, English, Finnish and Norwegian. There is some evidence that MoodGYM is helpful for its users [29, 30]. A meta-analysis with comparisons from 11 MoodGYM studies indicated its effectiveness for depression symptoms post-intervention, although the pooled effect size was in the small range (g = 0.36, 95% confidence interval: 0.17–0.56) [31]. One trial also found that the effects are still observable after 12 months [32].

14.3.2 Anxiety Disorders

There are a number of systematic reviews and meta-analyses on digital interventions for anxiety disorders. The effects of therapist-supported digital CBT for anxiety disorders in adults were assessed in a Cochrane review [33]. The included RCTs assessed social phobia (11 trials), panic disorder with/without agoraphobia (8 trials), generalized anxiety disorder (5 trials), post-traumatic stress disorder (2 trials), obsessive-compulsive disorder (2 trials), specific phobia (2 trials), and eight other trials, which assessed a range of anxiety disorders. The included RCTs were from Sweden (18 trials), Australia (14 trials), Switzerland (3 trials), the Netherlands (2 trials), and the USA (1 trial). The authors concluded that therapist-supported digital CBT appears as an efficacious intervention for anxiety in adults. More specifically, findings suggest that these interventions are more efficacious than waiting lists or information, or online discussion group-only control options. Given the lack of data, it is unclear to what extent therapist-supported digital CBT is more effective than unguided CBT. The authors also indicated that the effects of therapist-supported digital CBT may be rather similar to those of face-to-face CBT in reducing anxiety. These findings were generally corroborated by other recent systematic reviews (e.g., [34, 35]).

The effectiveness of guided digital CBT interventions for affective disorders including anxiety disorders in routine care was assessed in a systematic review [36]. In this review, the acceptability, effectiveness, and any negative effects under routine care conditions were assessed. The 19 nonrandomized pre-post studies included in the analysis provide evidence for the acceptability and effectiveness of guided digital CBT interventions for the treatment of affective disorders including anxiety in routine care.

Over the last decade, a few reviews have addressed the cost-effectiveness of digital anxiety interventions, and these report preliminary positive results while they stipulate that more research is needed in this area [7, 9, 37].

With regard to the use of digital CBT interventions for anxiety disorders tailored to specific populations, there is accumulating evidence for its effectiveness among college students [38], limited evidence for its effectiveness among pregnant women [39], and among children and adolescents with long-term physical conditions [40]. A recent systematic review indicated that digital mental health interventions including those based on CBT are at least moderately effective in reducing depression and anxiety symptoms in low- and middle-income countries [41].

14.3.3 Substance Use Disorders

Most of the research on digital CBT interventions for SUDs has focused on interventions to reduce alcohol, tobacco, and cannabis use.

Based on an individual patient data meta-analysis (IPDMA), digital interventions have been shown to be effective in moderating adult problem drinking in diverse settings [8]. This IPDMA included patient-level data obtained from 19 RCTs and performed various moderator and effectiveness analyses on the pooled dataset. Many of the included RCTs had evaluated CBT-based digital interventions. Results indicated that digital alcohol interventions in both community and healthcare populations can be efficacious in reducing weekly alcohol consumption and in achieving adherence to low-risk drinking limits. It was also found that interventions focusing on normative feedback only were less effective than interventions using integrated therapeutic approaches, including CBT. Human-guided interventions led to better drinking outcomes than unguided interventions, although this finding may in part be impacted by the selected control conditions. A review of reviews published a year before the IPDMA reported findings that largely corroborate the results of the IPDMA, although it was highlighted that in some relevant areas, such as longer-term follow-up outcomes, or effectiveness in populations such as employees and cultural minority groups, evidence is lagging behind [42].

Digital interventions have also been found to be at least moderately effective for tobacco use cessation. A 2017 Cochrane review identified 67 RCTs with data from over 110,000 participants; they were able to pool data from 35,969 participants [43]. The evidence from RCTs among adults suggests that interactive and tailored digital interventions with or without additional behavioral support are moderately more effective than non-active controls at six months or longer, while no evidence was found that these interventions outperformed other active smoking treatments. A Cochrane review on mobile phone text messaging and app-based interventions for smoking cessation [44] concluded that there is moderate-certainty evidence that automated text message-based smoking cessation interventions lead to greater quit rates than minimal smoking cessation support, while the amount of evidence comparing smartphone apps with less intensive support was very limited. Whether specifically CBT-based interventions for smoking cessation are more or less effective than others is not clear from the reviewed literature.

With regard to cannabis, a systematic review on the short- and long-term effects of digital prevention and treatment interventions for cannabis use reduction [45] evaluated data from 10 prevention interventions targeting 8138 participants (aged 12–20) and 20 treatment interventions targeting 5195 Cannabis users (aged 16–40). They concluded that these interventions show small, significant reductions in cannabis use among various populations, compared to their controls at post-treatment short-term follow-ups. For prevention interventions only, the post-treatment effects were maintained at follow-up up to 12 months later.

With regard to opioids and stimulants, a 2017 systematic review synthesized the evidence and found some support for effectiveness to address opioid use but not to address stimulants use, while the amount and quality of evidence were rather limited [46].

Figure 14.1 provides a schematic representation of a CBT (and motivational interviewing) based digital substance use intervention.

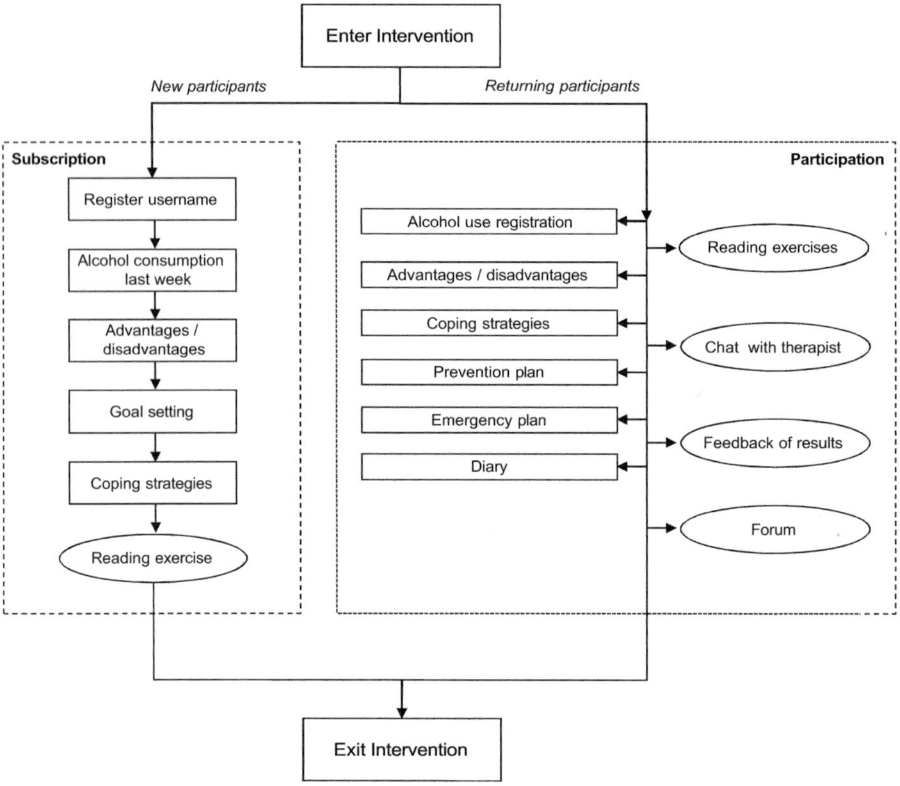

Fig. 14.1 Schematic representation of a CBT-based digital alcohol intervention. Note. Figure 14.1 presents the different modules and exercises of a CBT-based digital alcohol intervention (see [47, 48]). During the subscription procedure, the participant is first asked to report his or her alcohol use in the last week. Next, the advantages of quitting/moderation and the disadvantages of drinking are reviewed. Then a personal goal is set: to moderate alcohol use, or to abstain from drinking. After the personal drinking goals are set, attention is focused on how this goal can be achieved. To conclude the subscription procedure, a reading exercise is provided on how to cope with alcohol cravings. Only after the subscription is completed, participants can enter the participant area. Here, the six main treatment modules, four reading exercises, and a result feedback page are available. In the therapist-led version of the intervention, a chat module is available for the participant and the therapist to have one-on-one chat therapy contact. A forum provides opportunities for peer support or for reading previous posts of fellow intervention participants

14.4 Practical Applications of Digital CBT

Based on the current evidence base and practical experiences, several influential global professional organizations and treatment guidelines have recognized the effectiveness and potential of digital CBT interventions in mental health care (see e.g.: [49–52]). Digital CBT interventions are often recommended as an add-on to standard care, rather than as a replacement. Treatment guidelines emphasize the importance of using digital CBT interventions, which have been found to be effective, or at least based on evidence-based underpinnings. The importance of developing interventions that are user-friendly, accessible across different devices, and suitable for diverse populations is also emphasized. Digital CBT interventions should also aim to provide tailored or personalized treatment experiences as personalization can help to optimize engagement and outcomes. On the security side, digital interventions should adhere to relevant data protection laws such as the general data protection regulation (GDPR) in the EU. Some guidelines suggest integrating therapist support, for example, via messaging, virtual sessions, or check-ins to provide guidance and monitor progress. Last but not least, the need for ongoing evaluation and improvement of digital CBT interventions is underlined, e.g., by collecting user feedback, performing research, and refining the interventions based on this evidence and user experiences.

14.5 Theoretical Underpinning of Cognitive Bias Modification

Positive effects have been reported regarding digital CBT interventions, although further accommodation to what is possible when using computer technology would be desirable. A promising development in this regard could be to supplement digital CBT with CBM. In the following sections, the theoretical underpinning and the effectiveness and possibilities of interventions based on CBM (specifically attentional bias modification, interpretive bias modification, and action tendency bias modification) will therefore be discussed. Cognitive theories argue that biases in information processing (attentional bias, interpretive bias, and action tendency bias) play a crucial role in psychopathology [53, 54]. CBM started from the perspective of investigating the causal status of these cognitive processes in relation to a disorder.

14.5.1 Attentional Bias Modification

In their seminal first study, MacLeod and colleagues [55] selected students with a medium anxiety level, and randomly assigned them to one of two conditions: one in which their attention was trained toward threatening stimuli, and one in which their attention was trained away from threatening stimuli. They did this by modifying an assessment instrument (visual probe test). In the original test, the probe to which the participant reacts (e.g., an arrow pointing up or down) appears equally often in the location of a threat stimulus and a neutral stimulus. The attentional bias (AB) is then calculated by subtracting the reaction time on threat trials from the reaction time to non-threat trials. In a modification or training version of the task, a contingency is introduced, with the probe appearing more often on the location occupied by the threat stimulus (to induce a bias), or more often on the location occupied by the neutral stimulus (to reduce a bias) (see Fig. 14.2 for an example in the field of alcohol use). Results across two studies indicated that the attentional bias modification

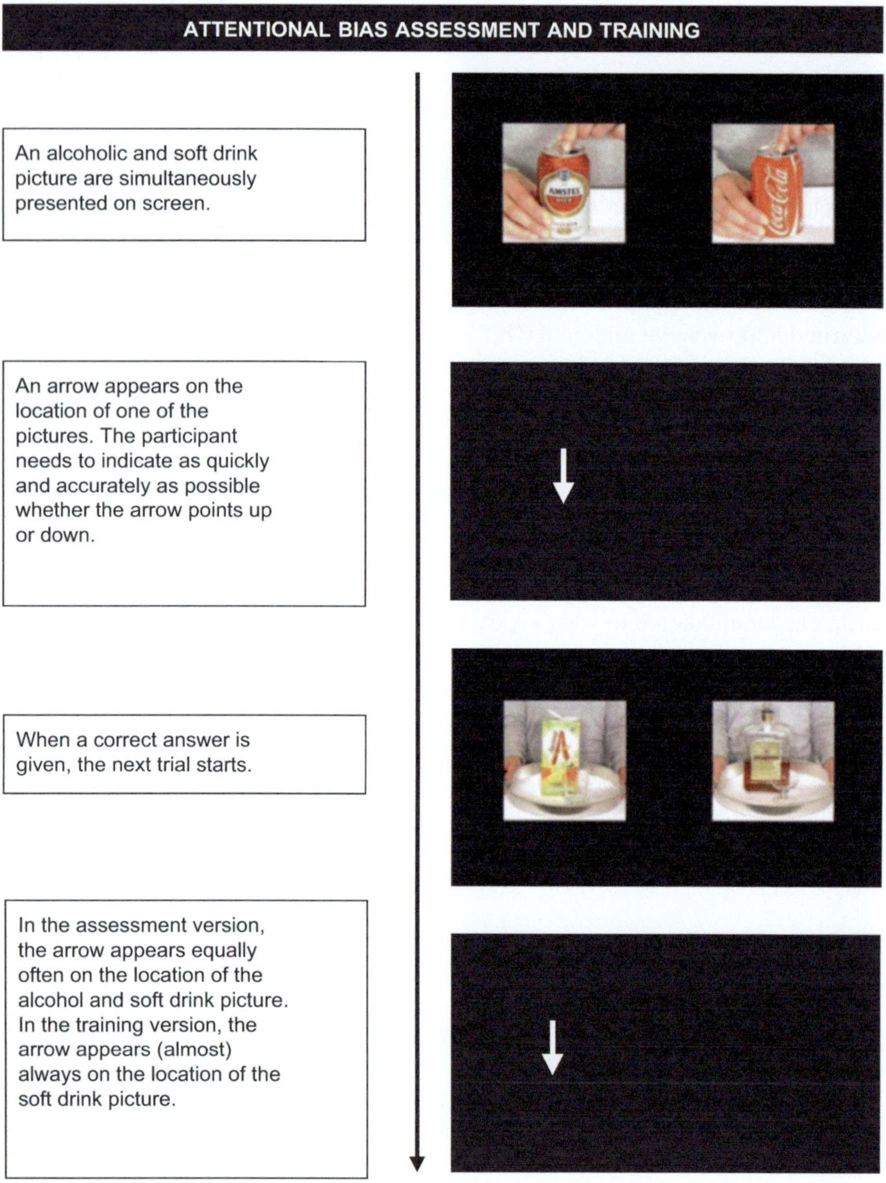

Fig. 14.2 Attentional bias assessment and training

had been successful, as assessed with different stimuli in the same task (close generalization), and further generalization was found in a subsequent stress-inducing task, with participants in the attend threat condition showing greater distress than participants in the attend neutral condition [55]. Subsequent research in this domain investigated clinical applications, typically with multiple training sessions. Initial studies in clinically anxious patient groups [56, 57], and in unselected and targeted prevention (respectively [58]; [59]) had promising findings. However, it should be noted that after initial successes, later large Internet studies on retraining attentional bias in patients with anxiety disorders showed more heterogeneity in effects on symptoms.

While studies examining attentional retraining in the field of anxiety have proliferated, testing the effects of this training on depression has lagged behind. Initial studies suggested that multiple sessions of attentional retraining in dysphoric students resulted in improvements in symptoms in students with mild depressive symptoms (and replicated, see [60]), but increased depressive symptoms in students with moderate to severe symptoms (Experiment 1; [61]). In a sample of depressed in- and outpatients (Experiment 2; [61]), the attentional retraining was unsuccessful in changing attentional bias and depressive symptoms. Generally, meta-analyses evaluating the clinical effectiveness of attentional retraining in anxiety and depression [62, 63] indicated that effects in anxiety have been stronger than in depression.

Subsequent research applied the same logic of attentional retraining in SUDs, with initial studies testing the effect of a single-session attentional bias manipulation (see Fig. 14.2). The effects of single-session training across studies and substances (alcohol, smoking) can be summarized as follows: like a threat-related attentional bias, a substance-related attentional bias can be manipulated in both directions [64], but the effects do not generalize to untrained stimuli, nor to behavior [65–67]. When added to the treatment of SUDs, results have been heterogeneous, with the largest study finding a positive effect (12% reduction in relapse one year later [68]), but a recent study in which a gamified version of attentional retraining was used, finding no add-on effects [69]. However, this study was much smaller and included patients treated for alcohol and cannabis use disorder, who either had an abstinence or moderation goal. Given the strong consistent evidence for an add-on effect to the abstinence-oriented treatment of alcohol use disorders for another variety of CBM, discussed below (approach bias modification), and the similar effects reported in this context for attentional retraining [68], this intervention still holds promise.

14.5.2 Cognitive Bias Modification of Interpretive Bias (CBM-I)

In a similar vein, another cognitive bias was addressed in manipulation studies: an interpretation bias. Mathews and Mackintosh [70] developed a scenario-based training to modify interpretations. Participants read ambiguous social scenarios, for which half of the participants were required to generate emotionally positive outcomes, and the remaining half negative outcomes. The scenarios were three lines of text in length and remained ambiguous in terms of their emotional meaning until the final word of the text. This last word was a word fragment, the completion of which produced either a positive or negative disambiguation/interpretation of the scenario. Because there was only one possible meaningful solution for each fragment, participants were forced to disambiguate the fragment in either a benign or a threatening way. Their studies with mid-range anxious students revealed that the training is capable of changing interpretations and subsequently affecting self-reported anxiety. The initial effects in anxiety have been replicated with the same type of scenario-based training [71], with other types of interpretive bias modification training [72], and extended to anxious non-clinical populations [73–75] and clinical populations [76–78]. Importantly, it has been shown that effects on anxiety were mediated by changes in interpretations [76, 79] and that effects are not restricted to self-report measures as effects have been observed on clinician-rated symptoms [80] and in heart rate response to a stressor [81]. In a review of multiple meta-analyses, Jones and Sharpe [82] showed that CBM-I training has a significant effect on changes in interpretation biases, and thus conclude that CBM-I training can reliably modify interpretation biases. With respect to transfer effects on anxiety symptoms, Jones and Sharpe [82] concluded that CBM training (combining the findings for CBM-I training with the findings for attentional bias modification (ABM), trainings designed to change attentional biases) consistently reduced anxiety symptoms. These effects on anxiety are consistent with the conclusions drawn in a recent network meta-analysis [63] where CBM-I training outperformed both waitlist and sham-training control conditions in reducing anxiety symptoms.

In the context of depression, interpretation retraining has been used in a more imagery-based format. Given the importance of mental images in emotions and affect, CBM-I training paradigms have been developed that use images and pictures instead of sentences as stimuli, with positive scenarios being presented auditorily (e.g., [83]). Several studies have shown positive effects on mood in healthy adults [84] and depressive symptoms in clinical populations [83, 85, 86]. Two sessions of interpretation retraining in individuals diagnosed with major depressive disorder resulted in participants reporting more positive interpretations, and more positive memory intrusions, and showing a smaller increase in heart rate in response to a stressor [87]. Though results have been inconsistent across studies, as also null findings have also been reported [88].

While there is some evidence that SUDs are associated with substance-related interpretive bias [89, 90], and attempts to apply this technique in SUDs have not had consistent effects on substance use [91, 92].

14.5.3 Action Tendency Bias Modification

In the field of SUDs, a third cognitive bias was addressed, an action tendency to approach disorder-related stimuli. This bias has been observed with different instruments, for different substances, including alcohol [93, 94], cannabis use [95, 96], cigarette smoking [97], and even for non-substance addiction gambling [98]. Applying the same logic as developed in attentional retraining, Wiers and colleagues developed a training version of the alcohol approach avoidance task [99]. This task started with an equal contingency. Half of the alcohol pictures and half of the non-alcohol pictures were to be responded to by pulling a joystick toward themselves, the other half were to be pushed away. Participants react to a feature of the

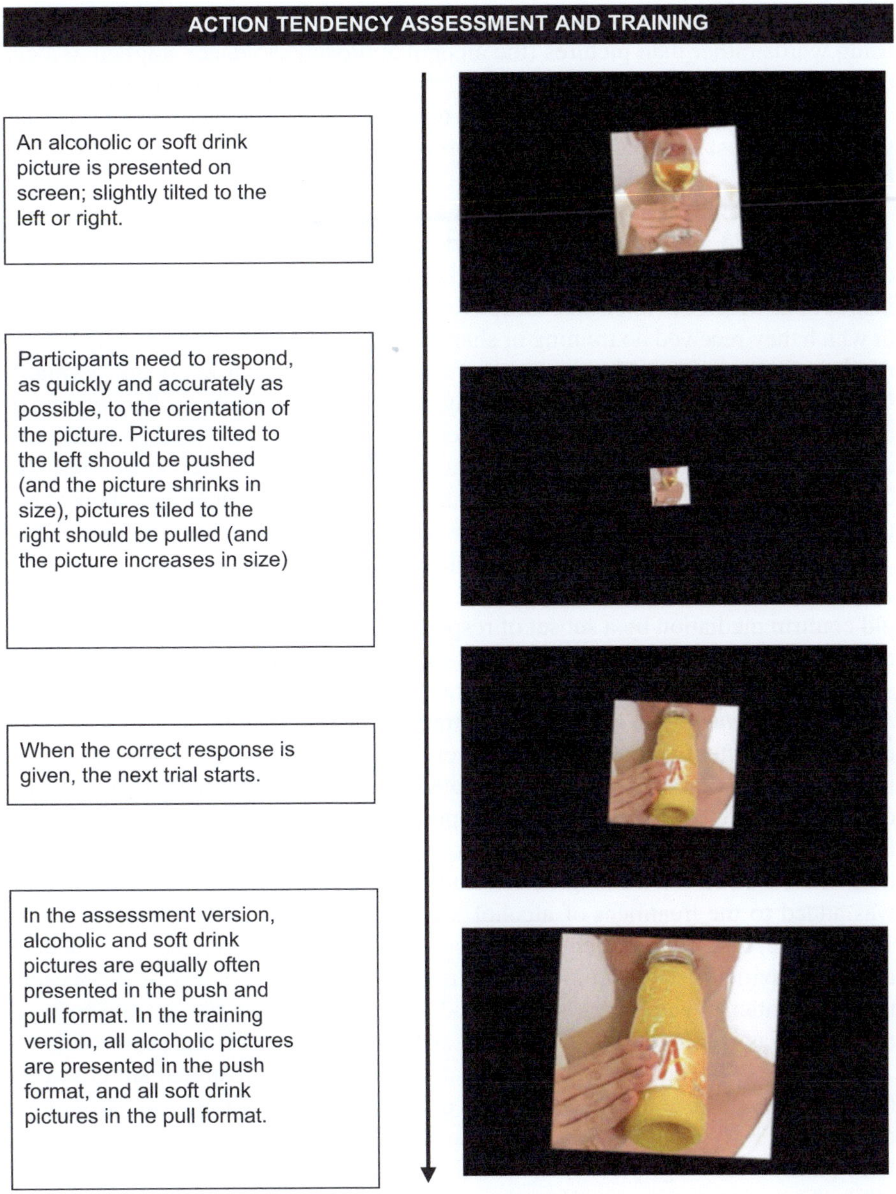

Fig. 14.3 Alcohol approach avoidance task

stimulus unrelated to the contents, for example, the format or a little tilt left or right (see Fig. 14.3). Without notification, the contingencies changed, so that half of the (socially drinking) students were pulling most of the alcohol pictures (approach alcohol condition), and the other half were pushing most of the alcohol pictures (avoid alcohol condition). This brief intervention resulted in generalized effects, both to untrained pictures in the same task and to a different test of associations using words rather than pictures (the alcohol approach/avoidance implicit association test—IAT, see [100]). Moreover, those heavier-drinking students whose approach bias was successfully retrained toward avoidance drank less beer in a subsequent taste test than those heavier-drinking students trained toward approaching beer [99].

In the first clinical application of this approach-bias retraining paradigm [101], 214 alcohol-dependent patients were randomly assigned to one of two experimental conditions, in which they were trained to avoid alcohol (with or without explicit instruction, which did not differ for the results), or to one of two control conditions, in which they received no training or sham training (which also did not differ for the results). Four sessions of training preceded regular inpatient treatment, primarily CBT. In the experimental conditions only, patients' approach bias changed into an avoidance bias for alcohol. This effect generalized to untrained pictures in the task used and to an IAT, in which alcohol and soft drink words were categorized with approach and avoidance words. Patients in the experimental conditions showed better treatment outcomes a year later (13% less relapse), which was significant after controlling for gender. The clinical effect was not significantly related to either the change of bias as assessed with the AAT or with the IAT, although further analyses did confirm mediation by a subset of responses in the approach/avoid IAT [102]. In a first replication study [13], 509 alcohol-dependent patients received either 12 sessions of approach-bias retraining or no training (sham training was left out because no difference was found between sham training and no training in [101]). Clinical effects 1 year after treatment discharge were again found (now 9% less relapse), and in this study mediation and moderation were both found: the effect on clinical outcome was mediated by a change in the approach bias for alcohol, and the strongest training effect was found for participants with the strongest approach bias for alcohol, who received the training. Later studies in which approach bias modification was added to the treatment of alcohol use disorders confirmed effectiveness [68, 103]. Interestingly, the latter study found a stronger add-on effect for alcohol-dependent patients with a comorbid internalizing disorder (anxiety or depression), than for patients without. Manning and colleagues tested the effectiveness of approach bias modification during detox and found positive effects [104–106].

While these effects of CBM as adjunct to clinical CBT treatment are promising (a small but consistent add-on effect), online-only studies found no differential effects of CBM (attentional retraining or approach-bias retraining) as compared with placebo training; participants in all conditions reduced their drinking [107, 108]. This suggests that a combination with CBT is necessary to obtain differential effects [14, 107]. For that reason, the combination of digital CBT and CBM appears promising. Recently, researchers have started investigating the potential of action tendency training in the field of anxiety with some initial promising results with respect to contamination fear [109] and social phobia [110, 111].

Based on proof-of-principle studies into the working mechanisms of approach bias modification, recently a new variety has been proposed, ABC-training [112], in which action tendencies are trained in reaction to personalized antecedents (A), for which a personally relevant behavioral alternative (B) is trained, in relation to the consequences (C) of the participant's own long-term goals. While no clinical studies have been performed yet, the first studies in volunteers indicate better effects than for regular CBM.

14.6 Effectiveness of Cognitive Bias Modification

14.6.1 Depression and Anxiety Disorders

In the context of CBM's effects on anxiety and depression; a review of multiple meta-analyses [82] and a network meta-analysis [63] were recently published. In the review of meta-analyses, it was concluded that CBM training (combining the findings for attentional and interpretation bias training) consistently reduced anxiety symptoms. With respect to potential differences between attention and interpretation training, they concluded that "CBM-I training may have more power as a paradigm in symptom reduction compared with action tendency bias modification." ([82]: p. 179). These effects on anxiety are consistent with the conclusions drawn in a recent network meta-analysis [63] where CBM-I training outperformed both waitlist and sham-training control conditions in reducing anxiety symptoms. While there is variability in the effects of CBM-I training on anxiety in individual studies, across all studies, there seems to be a promising effect on anxiety.

The CBM-I effects on depressive symptoms seem less compelling as Fodor et al. [63] concluded that CBM-I only outperformed waitlist control conditions (and not sham-training) in reducing depressive symptoms. Similarly, [82] indicated that CBM effects (again action tendency bias modification and CBM-I combined) on depressive symptoms are less robust and smaller than the effects on anxiety.

When taking together the recent meta-analyses, the findings for CBM-I as an anxiolytic intervention have been quite positive and underscore the conclusion formulated by Fodor et al. [63]: "CBM-I emerged as a promising treatment." (p. 507). For depression, there is insufficient evidence to draw conclusions.

14.6.2 Substance Use Disorders

A first meta-analysis on the effects of CBM in SUDs [113] concluded that CBM had an effect on the bias, but not on substance use and was therefore not clinically useful. However, this meta-analysis was criticized [114], because it combined many proof-of-principle studies in volunteers (typically students) who were not motivated to reduce or quit their drinking, but participated for course credit or free beer, with a few studies in which CBM was added to the treatment of SUDs, which all found positive effects. It is invalid to combine these, as they constitute different phases of the experimental medicine approach to treatment development [114, 115]. For example, in proof-of-principle studies, a cognitive bias is typically manipulated in two directions, either temporarily increased or decreased, in order to study effects on disorder-related behavior (e.g., stress in anxiety, [55]; alcohol-tasting in addictive behaviors [99]). In clinical RCTs, patients either receive the intervention that reduces the cognitive bias or no training or sham training (e.g., [68, 101]). A second meta-analysis [116] included only studies with a clinical purpose: participants were motivated to participate to moderate or quit their substance use (alcohol or cigarette smoking). As there were not many clinical studies yet, a Bayesian individual patient data approach was taken. It found evidence for CBM decreasing the targeted cognitive bias and for an effect on abstinence, but not for reduced use. The latter is likely related to the fact that the positive studies all added CBM to abstinence-oriented inpatient treatment, while the negative outcomes were mostly internet studies in which participants typically wanted to reduce their use. As noted above, this pattern of results has continued since, with positive outcomes in the context of add-ons to the abstinence-oriented treatment of alcohol use disorders [68, 104–106], and non-differential effects in online-only studies [107, 117]. Effects have been more mixed for smoking, with some positive effects in an online attentional retraining where abstinence was required [118], but also negative findings, even when CBM was added to CBT for smoking cessation [119].

In summary, the picture so far is that CBM is a useful add-on to CBT in the clinical treatment of alcohol use disorders, with improved clinical outcomes of about 10% less relapse one year after treatment discharge (a small effect but similar to the effect size of current medications). However, there is no evidence so far that it can work as a stand-alone intervention, and should rather be seen as a useful add-on to regular CBT and should be tested as an add-on to digital CBT.

14.7 Practical Applications of CBM

One advantage of CBM is that it can be offered online in a flexible way, with 24/7 access. In this way, it could be offered as a stand-alone intervention, and also as an adjunct to (digital) CBT. CBM might be used as a pre-treatment training completed for example during the time an individual is on a waitlist for treatment, or training could be offered in parallel to CBT treatment as an adjunct or be offered after treatment to prevent the return of fear, depression, or relapse. This may be particularly helpful for patients for whom CBT alone is not sufficient, because they have trouble acting on their higher-order goals (to remain abstinent), in the face of temptations. Indeed, there is a literature in non-SUD adolescents that in those individuals with relatively poor executive control, automatically activated cognitive processes are a more important predictor of substance use and problems than in adolescents with well-developed executive control functions [120–123]. This would suggest that CBM is especially useful for participants with relatively weak executive control functions (for an indication in anxiety, see [124]). However, this was not confirmed in the recent large trial [13], while better results were found for older participants (which could have suppressed the effects of executive control, the measure used was also not optimal). Second, adding CBM would seem especially useful for those with a strong bias (moderation). This has been confirmed in a large study [13], but it should be noted that the reliability of the attentional bias and action tendency bias measures is relatively poor (and better for interpretation bias measures), permitting no prediction yet at the individual level. However, new assessment methods are being developed with much better reliability (e.g., [125]).

Regarding disadvantages, one important caveat to the usefulness of CBM as an add-on to (digital) CBT is that many patients regard the training as boring and use less, especially attentional retraining using a variety of the visual probe test [126]. One way out is to increase motivation to train by providing information on the effects of automatically triggered processes in a motivational interviewing style, thus increasing motivation to train (see [127]). Another way is to develop more engaging playful varieties of training (e.g., [58, 128]) and/or to introduce game elements (anxiety: [129]; review SUDS: [130]) and/or combine with virtual reality [131]. However, while this may increase motivation to train, we believe it is also essential to link the training to further treatment goals, as activated in CBT. In fact, this is done in the new ABC training [112].

14.8 Discussion and Conclusions

In this chapter, the theoretical background and effectiveness of clinical applications of digital CBT and CBM have been discussed. Based on the reviewed literature, there is a reasonably strong evidence base for the effectiveness of digital CBT interventions for depression, anxiety, and substance use disorders. The evidence base for standalone CBM interventions is strong for interpretive bias modification for anxiety symptoms and more inconsistent for attentional bias modification and effects on depression. The evidence base for CBM as an adjunct to CBT interventions is accumulating with (in general) positive findings regarding the effectiveness in alcohol use disorders, although it should be noted that these positive findings are only found when CBM is added to face-to-face abstinence-oriented treatment for alcohol use disorders. A good test of the add-on effects of CBM to (guided) digital CBT is yet to be done. Recently, studies have evaluated the delivery of CBT and CBM interventions using mobile devices such as smartphones and tablets, which are now the most common platforms for newly developed digital health interventions. Among the therapeutic orientations present in the evaluated mobile interventions was CBT. Also, CBM could be administered using mobile devices. Interpretation bias training offered on a smartphone was shown to be successful in changing the bias and changing anxiety [132] and smoking cessation [133] the bias was successfully changed, but no effects on behavior could be reported. This was not surprising in the study on smoking, as these were smokers who did not intend to quit. Another promising future development is the optimization of the integration of CBM with digital CBT. To what extent can CBM and digital CBT create the synergy needed to interfere with dominant action tendencies in an emotional situation (e.g., negative mood, desire, cf., ABC training [112, 134])? All in all, attempts at answering this question will lead to advancement in the delivery of mental health interventions and progress in the accommodation of depression, anxiety, and SUDs to the possibilities of digital technology. Based on the currently available evidence, CBM is an interesting tool to study further as an add-on to digital CBT in the treatment of common mental health disorders.

References

1. Rehm J, Shield KD, Rehm MX, Gmel G, Frick U. Modelling the impact of alcohol dependence on mortality burden and the effect of available treatment interventions in the European Union. Eur Neuropsychopharmacol. 2013;23:89–97.
2. Effertz T, Mann K. The burden and cost of disorders of the brain in Europe with the inclusion of harmful alcohol use and nicotine addiction. Eur Neuropsychopharmacol. 2013;23(7):742–8.
3. Andrews G, Cuijpers P, Craske MG, McEvoy P, Titov N. Computer therapy for the anxiety and depressive disorders is effective, acceptable and practical health care: a meta-analysis. PLoS One. 2010;5(10):e13196.
4. Riper H, Blankers M, Hadiwijaya H, Cunningham J, Clarke S, Wiers R, Ebert D, Cuijpers P. Effectiveness of guided and unguided low-intensity internet interventions for adult alcohol misuse: a meta-analysis. PLoS One. 2014;9(6):e99912.
5. Civljak M, Stead LF, Hartmann-Boyce J, Sheikh A, Car J. Internet-based interventions for smoking cessation. Cochrane Database Syst Rev. 2013;7:CD007078.
6. Cuijpers P, Marks IM, van Straten A, Cavanagh K, Gega L, Andersson G. Computer-aided psychotherapy for anxiety disorders: a meta-analytic review. Cogn Behav Ther. 2009;38(2):66–82.
7. Hedman E, Ljótsson B, Lindefors N. Cognitive behavior therapy via the internet: a systematic review of applications, clinical efficacy and cost-effectiveness. Expert Rev Pharmacoecon Outcomes Res. 2012;12(6):745–64.
8. Riper H, Hoogendoorn A, Cuijpers P, Karyotaki E, Boumparis N, Mira A, Andersson G, Berman AH, Bertholet N, Bischof G, Blankers M, Boon B, Boß L, Brendryen H, Cunningham J, Ebert D, Hansen A, Hester R, Khadjesari Z, Kramer J, Murray E, Postel M, Schulz D, Sinadinovic K, Suffoletto B, Sundström C, de Vries H, Wallace P, Wiers RW, Smit JH. Effectiveness and treatment moderators of internet interventions for adult problem drinking: an individual patient data meta-analysis of 19 randomised controlled trials. PLoS Med. 2018;15(12):e1002714.
9. Kählke F, Buntrock C, Smit F, Ebert DD. Systematic review of economic evaluations for internet- and mobile-based interventions for mental health problems. NPJ Digit Med. 2022;5(1):175.
10. Beck JS. Cognitive behavior therapy: basics and beyond. 2nd ed. New York: The Guilford Press; 2011.
11. Beck Institute. History of cognitive therapy. https://archive today/MkHiX. Accessed 6 Feb 2015.
12. Piaget J, Cook MT. The origins of intelligence in children. New York: International University Press; 1952.
13. Eberl C, Wiers RW, Pawelczack S, Rinck M, Becker ES, Lindenmeyer J. Approach bias modification in alcohol dependence: do clinical effects replicate and for whom does it work best? Dev Cogn Neurosci. 2013;4:38–51.
14. Wiers RW, Gladwin TE, Hofmann W, Salemink E, Ridderinkhof KR. Cognitive bias modification and cognitive control training in addiction and related psychopathology mechanisms, clinical perspectives, and ways forward. Clin Psychol Sci. 2013;1(2):192–212.
15. Hayes SC, Levin ME, Plumb-Vilardaga J, Villatte JL, Pistorello J. Acceptance and commitment therapy and contextual behavioral science: examining the progress of a distinctive model of behavioral and cognitive therapy. Behav Ther. 2013;44(2):180–98.

16. Rush AJ, Beck AT, Kovacs M, Hollon SD. Comparative efficacy of cognitive therapy and pharmacotherapy in the treatment of depressed outpatients. Cogn Ther Res. 1977;1(1):7–37.
17. Stirman SW, Buchhofer R, McLaulin JB, Evans AC, Beck AT. The Beck initiative: a public academic collaborative partnership to implement cognitive therapy in a community behavioral health system. Psychiatr Serv. 2009;60:1302–4.
18. Khanna MS, Kendall PC. Computer-assisted cognitive behavioral therapy for child anxiety: results of a randomized clinical trial. J Consult Clin Psychol. 2010;78(5):737–45.
19. Massoudi B, Holvast F, Bockting CL, Burger H, Blanker MH. The effectiveness and cost-effectiveness of e-health interventions for depression and anxiety in primary care: a systematic review and meta-analysis. J Affect Disord. 2019;245:728–43.
20. Spurgeon JA, Wright JH. Computer-assisted cognitive-behavioral therapy. Curr Psychiatry Rep. 2010;12(6):547–52.
21. Mayer G, Gronewold N, Alvarez S, Bruns B, Hilbel T, Schultz JH. Acceptance and expectations of medical experts, students, and patients toward electronic mental health apps: cross-sectional quantitative and qualitative survey study. JMIR Ment Health. 2019;6(11):e14018.
22. de Beurs E, Blankers M, Peen J, Rademacher C, Podgorski A, Dekker J. Impact of COVID-19 social distancing measures on routine mental health care provision and treatment outcome for common mental disorders in The Netherlands. Clin Psychol Psychother. 2022;29(4):1342–54. https://doi.org/10.1002/cpp.2713.
23. Wright JH, Wright AS, Albano AM, et al. Computer-assisted cognitive therapy for depression: maintaining efficacy while reducing therapist time. Am J Psychiatry. 2005;162:1158–64.
24. Waller R, Gilbody S. Barriers to the uptake of computerized cognitive behavioural therapy: a systematic review of the quantitative and qualitative evidence. Psychol Med. 2009;39(5):705–12.
25. de Beurs E, Blankers M, Goudriaan AE, de Koning M, Dekker JJM. Zorgverlening in tijden van corona: ervaringen van behandelaars met zorg-op-afstand [Mental health care in times of corona: experiences of professionals with eHealth]. Tijdschr Psychiatr. 2021;63(4):242–9. Dutch
26. Karyotaki E, Efthimiou O, Miguel C, Bermpohl FMG, Furukawa TA, Cuijpers P, Individual Patient Data Meta-Analyses for Depression (IPDMA-DE) Collaboration, Riper H, Patel V, Mira A, Gemmil AW, Yeung AS, Lange A, Williams AD, Mackinnon A, Geraedts A, van Straten A, Meyer B, Björkelund C, Knaevelsrud C, Beevers CG, Botella C, Strunk DR, Mohr DC, Ebert DD, Kessler D, Richards D, Littlewood E, Forsell E, Feng F, Wang F, Andersson G, Hadjistavropoulos H, Christensen H, Ezawa ID, Choi I, Rosso IM, Klein JP, Shumake J, Garcia-Campayo J, Milgrom J, Smith J, Montero-Marin J, Newby JM, Bretón-López J, Schneider J, Vernmark K, Bücker L, Sheeber LB, Warmerdam L, Farrer L, Heinrich M, Huibers MJH, Kivi M, Kraepelien M, Forand NR, Pugh N, Lindefors N, Lintvedt O, Zagorscak P, Carlbring P, Phillips R, Johansson R, Kessler RC, Brabyn S, Perini S, Rauch SL, Gilbody S, Moritz S, Berger T, Pop V, Kaldo V, Spek V, Forsell Y. Internet-based cognitive behavioral therapy for depression: a systematic review and individual patient data network meta-analysis. JAMA Psychiatry. 2021;78(4):361–71.
27. Cuijpers P, Donker T, van Straten A, Li J, Andersson G. Is guided self-help as effective as face-to-face psychotherapy for depression and anxiety disorders? A systematic review and meta-analysis of comparative outcome studies. Psychol Med. 2010;40(12):1943–57.
28. National Institute for Mental Health Research. MoodGYM website, 2014. https://moodgym.anu.edu.au.
29. Christensen H, Griffiths KM, Jorm AF. Delivering interventions for depression by using the internet: randomised controlled trial. BMJ. 2004;328(7434):265.
30. Lintvedt OK, Griffiths KM, Sørensen K, Østvik AR, Wang CE, Eisemann M, Waterloo K. Evaluating the effectiveness and efficacy of unguided internet-based self-help intervention for the prevention of depression: a randomized controlled trial. Clin Psychol Psychother. 2013;20(1):10–27.

31. Twomey C, O'Reilly G. Effectiveness of a freely available computerised cognitive behavioural therapy programme (MoodGYM) for depression: meta-analysis. Aust N Z J Psychiatry. 2017;51(3):260–9.
32. Mackinnon A, Griffiths KM, Christensen H. Comparative randomised trial of online cognitive-behavioural therapy and an information website for depression: 12-month outcomes. Br J Psychiatry. 2008;192(2):130–4.
33. Olthuis JV, Watt MC, Bailey K, Hayden JA, Stewart SH. Therapist-supported internet cognitive behavioural therapy for anxiety disorders in adults. Cochrane Database Syst Rev. 2016;3(3):CD011565. https://doi.org/10.1002/14651858.CD011565.pub2. PMID: 26968204
34. Andrews G, Basu A, Cuijpers P, Craske MG, McEvoy P, English CL, Newby JM. Computer therapy for the anxiety and depression disorders is effective, acceptable and practical health care: an updated meta-analysis. J Anxiety Disord. 2018;55:70–8. https://doi.org/10.1016/j.janxdis.2018.01.001. Epub 2018 Feb 1
35. Andersson G, Carlbring P, Titov N, Lindefors N. Internet interventions for adults with anxiety and mood disorders: a narrative umbrella review of recent meta-analyses. Can J Psychiatr. 2019;64(7):465–70. https://doi.org/10.1177/0706743719839381. Epub 2019 May 16. PMID: 31096757
36. Etzelmueller A, Vis C, Karyotaki E, Baumeister H, Titov N, Berking M, Cuijpers P, Riper H, Ebert DD. Effects of internet-based cognitive behavioral therapy in routine Care for Adults in treatment for depression and anxiety: systematic review and Meta-analysis. J Med Internet Res. 2020;22(8):e18100. https://doi.org/10.2196/18100. PMID: 32865497
37. Arnberg FK, Linton SJ, Hultcrantz M, Heintz E, Jonsson U. Internet-delivered psychological treatments for mood and anxiety disorders: a systematic review of their efficacy, safety, and cost-effectiveness. PLoS One. 2014;9(5):e98118.
38. Lattie EG, Adkins EC, Winquist N, Stiles-Shields C, Wafford QE, Graham AK. Digital mental health interventions for depression, anxiety, and enhancement of psychological Well-being among college students: systematic review. J Med Internet Res. 2019;21(7):e12869.
39. Evans K, Rennick-Egglestone S, Cox S, Kuipers Y, Spiby H. Remotely delivered interventions to support women with symptoms of anxiety in pregnancy: mixed methods systematic review and meta-analysis. J Med Internet Res. 2022;24(2):e28093.
40. Thabrew H, Stasiak K, Hetrick SE, Wong S, Huss JH, Merry SN. E-health interventions for anxiety and depression in children and adolescents with long-term physical conditions. Cochrane Database Syst Rev. 2018;8(8):CD012489.
41. Kim J, Aryee LMD, Bang H, Prajogo S, Choi YK, Hoch JS, Prado EL. Effectiveness of digital mental health tools to reduce depressive and anxiety symptoms in low- and middle-income countries: systematic review and Meta-analysis. JMIR Ment Health. 2023;10:e43066.
42. Sundström C, Blankers M, Khadjesari Z. Computer-based interventions for problematic alcohol use: a review of systematic reviews. Int J Behav Med. 2017;24(5):646–58.
43. Taylor GMJ, Dalili MN, Semwal M, Civljak M, Sheikh A, Car J. Internet-based interventions for smoking cessation. Cochrane Database Syst Rev. 2017;9(9):CD007078.
44. Whittaker R, McRobbie H, Bullen C, Rodgers A, Gu Y, Dobson R. Mobile phone text messaging and app-based interventions for smoking cessation. Cochrane Database Syst Rev. 2019;10(10):CD006611.
45. Boumparis N, Loheide-Niesmann L, Blankers M, Ebert DD, Korf D, Schaub MP, Spijkerman R, Tait RJ, Riper H. Short- and long-term effects of digital prevention and treatment interventions for cannabis use reduction: a systematic review and meta-analysis. Drug Alcohol Depend. 2019;200:82–94.
46. Boumparis N, Karyotaki E, Schaub MP, Cuijpers P, Riper H. Internet interventions for adult illicit substance users: a meta-analysis. Addiction. 2017;112(9):1521–32.
47. Blankers M, Nabitz U, Smit F, Koeter MW, Schippers GM. Economic evaluation of internet-based interventions for harmful alcohol use alongside a pragmatic randomized controlled trial. J Med Internet Res. 2012;14(5):e134.

48. Blankers M, Koeter MW, Schippers GM. Internet therapy versus internet self-help versus no treatment for problematic alcohol use: a randomized controlled trial. J Consult Clin Psychol. 2011;79(3):330–41.
49. Joint Task Force for the Development of Telepsychology Guidelines for Psychologists. Guidelines for the practice of telepsychology. Am Psychol. 2013;68(9):791–800. https://doi.org/10.1037/a0035001.
50. Iacobucci G. NICE recommends online therapies to treat depression and anxiety in adults. BMJ. 2023;380:495. https://doi.org/10.1136/bmj.p495.
51. WHO guideline recommendations on digital interventions for health system strengthening. Geneva: World Health Organization; 2019. Available from: https://www.ncbi.nlm.nih.gov/books/NBK541902/
52. The eMEN Consortium. Transnational Policy for e-Mental Health: a guidance document for European policymakers and stakeholders. Düsseldorf/Cologne, March 2020 Available from: https://vb.nweurope.eu/media/10450/emen__transnational-policy-for-e-mental-health_guidance-document_3-2020.pdf
53. Mathews A, Mackintosh B. A cognitive model of selective processing in anxiety. Cogn Ther Res. 1998;22(6):539–60.
54. Wiers RW, Bartholow BD, van den Wildenberg E, Thush C, Engels RC, Sher KJ, Grenard J, Ames SL, Stacy AW. Automatic and controlled processes and the development of addictive behaviors in adolescents: a review and a model. Pharmacol Biochem Behav. 2007;86(2):263–83.
55. MacLeod C, Rutherford E, Campbell L, Ebsworthy G, Holker L. Selective attention and emotional vulnerability: assessing the causal basis of their association through the experimental manipulation of attentional bias. J Abnorm Psychol. 2002;111(1):107–23.
56. Amir N, Beard C, Burns M, Bomyea J. Attention modification program in individuals with generalized anxiety disorder. J Abnorm Psychol. 2009;118(1):28–33.
57. Schmidt NB, Richey JA, Buckner JD, Timpano KR. Attention training for generalized social anxiety disorder. J Abnorm Psychol. 2009;118(1):5–14.
58. De Voogd EL, Wiers RW, Prins PJ, Salemink E. Visual search attentional bias modification reduced social phobia in adolescents. J Behav Ther Exp Psychiatry. 2014;45(2):252–9.
59. See J, MacLeod C, Bridle R. The reduction of anxiety vulnerability through the modification of attentional bias: a real-world study using a home-based cognitive bias modification procedure. J Abnorm Psychol. 2009;118(1):65–75.
60. Wells TT, Beevers CG. Biased attention and dysphoria: manipulating selective attention reduces subsequent depressive symptoms. Cogn Emot. 2010;24(4):719–28.
61. Baert S, De Raedt R, Schacht R, Koster EH. Attentional bias training in depression: therapeutic effects depend on depression severity. J Behav Ther Exp Psychiatry. 2010;41(3):265–74.
62. Mogoaşe C, David D, Koster EH. Clinical efficacy of attentional bias modification procedures: an updated meta-analysis. J Clin Psychol. 2014;70(12):1133–57.
63. Fodor LA, Georgescu R, Cuijpers P, Szamoskozi Ş, David D, Furukawa TA, Cristea IA. Efficacy of cognitive bias modification interventions in anxiety and depressive disorders: a systematic review and network meta-analysis. Lancet Psychiatry. 2020;7(6):506–14.
64. Field M, Eastwood B. Experimental manipulation of attentional bias increases the motivation to drink alcohol. Psychopharmacology. 2005;183(3):350–7.
65. Field M, Duka T, Eastwood B, Child R, Santarcangelo M, Gayton M. Experimental manipulation of attentional biases in heavy drinkers: do the effects generalise? Psychopharmacology. 2007;192(4):593–608.
66. Attwood AS, O'Sullivan H, Leonards U, Mackintosh B, Munafò MR. Attentional bias training and cue reactivity in cigarette smokers. Addiction. 2008;103(11):1875–82.
67. Schoenmakers T, Wiers RW, Jones BT, Bruce G, Jansen AT. Attentional re-training decreases attentional bias in heavy drinkers without generalization. Addiction. 2007;102(3):399–405.
68. Rinck M, Wiers RW, Becker ES, Lindenmeyer J. Relapse prevention in abstinent alcoholics by cognitive bias modification: clinical effects of combining approach bias modification and attention bias modification. J Consult Clin Psychol. 2018;86(12):1005–16.

69. Heitmann J, van Hemel-Ruiter ME, Huisman M, Ostafin BD, Wiers RW, MacLeod C, et al. Effectiveness of attentional bias modification training as add-on to regular treatment in alcohol and cannabis use disorder: a multicenter randomized control trial. PLoS One. 2021;16(6):e0252494.
70. Mathews A, Mackintosh B. Induced emotional interpretation bias and anxiety. J Abnorm Psychol. 2000;109(4):602–15.
71. Salemink E, van den Hout M, Kindt M. Trained interpretive bias: validity and effects on anxiety. J Behav Ther Exp Psychiatry. 2007;38(2):212–24.
72. Wilson EJ, MacLeod C, Mathews A, Rutherford EM. The causal role of interpretive bias in anxiety reactivity. J Abnorm Psychol. 2006;115(1):103.
73. Mathews A, Ridgeway V, Cook E, Yiend J. Inducing a benign interpretational bias reduces trait anxiety. J Behav Ther Exp Psychiatry. 2007;38(2):225–36.
74. Salemink E, van den Hout M, Kindt M. Effects of positive interpretive bias modification in highly anxious individuals. J Anxiety Disord. 2009;23(5):676–83.
75. Steinman SA, Teachman BA. Modifying interpretations among individuals high in anxiety sensitivity. J Anxiety Disord. 2010;24(1):71–8.
76. Hayes S, Hirsch CR, Krebs G, Mathews A. The effects of modifying interpretation bias on worry in generalized anxiety disorder. Behav Res Ther. 2010;48(3):171–8.
77. Hirsch CR, Krahé C, Whyte J, Krzyzanowski H, Meeten F, Norton S, Mathews A. Internet-delivered interpretation training reduces worry and anxiety in individuals with generalized anxiety disorder: a randomized controlled experiment. J Consult Clin Psychol. 2021;89(7):575.
78. Amir N, Taylor CT. Interpretation training in individuals with generalized social anxiety disorder: a randomized controlled trial. J Consult Clin Psychol. 2012;80(3):497.
79. Salemink E, van den Hout M, Kindt M. How does cognitive bias modification affect anxiety? Mediation analyses and experimental data. Behav Cogn Psychother. 2010;38(1):59–66.
80. Wolters L, Hagen A, Op de Beek V, Dol P, de Haan E, Salemink E. Effectiveness of an online interpretation training as a pre-treatment for cognitive behavioral therapy for obsessive-compulsive disorder in youth: a randomized controlled trial. J Obsessive Compuls Relat Disord. 2021;29:100636. https://doi.org/10.1016/j.jocrd.2021.100636.
81. Van Bockstaele B, Clarke P, Notebaert L, MacLeod C, Salemink E. Effects of cognitive load during interpretation bias modification on interpretation bias and stress reactivity. J Behav Ther Exp Psychiatry. 2020;68:101561. https://doi.org/10.1016/j.jbtep.2020.101561.
82. Jones EB, Sharpe L. Cognitive bias modification: a review of meta-analyses. J Affect Disord. 2017;223:175–83. https://doi.org/10.1016/j.jad.2017.07.034.
83. Blackwell SE, Holmes EA. Modifying interpretation and imagination in clinical depression: a single case series using cognitive bias modification. Appl Cogn Psychol. 2010;24:338–50.
84. Rohrbacher H, Blackwell SE, Holmes EA, Reinecke A. Optimizing the ingredients for imagery-based interpretation bias modification for depressed mood: is self-generation more effective than imagination alone? J Affect Disord. 2014;152–154:212–8.
85. Williams AD, Blackwell SE, Mackenzie A, Holmes EA, Andrews G. Combining imagination and reason in the treatment of depression: a randomized controlled trial of internet-based cognitive-bias modification and internet-CBT for depression. J Consult Clin Psychol. 2013;81(5):793–9.
86. Hirsch CR, Krahé C, Whyte J, Loizou S, Bridge L, Norton S, Mathews A. Interpretation training to target repetitive negative thinking in generalized anxiety disorder and depression. J Consult Clin Psychol. 2018;86(12):1017–30.
87. Joormann J, Waugh CE, Gotlib IH. Cognitive bias modification for interpretation in major depression: effects on memory and stress reactivity. Clin Psychol Sci. 2015;3(1):126–39. https://doi.org/10.1177/2167702614560748.
88. Blackwell SE, Browning M, Mathews A, Pictet A, Welch J, Davies J, Holmes EA. Positive imagery-based cognitive bias modification as a web-based treatment tool for depressed adults: a randomized controlled trial. Clin Psychol Sci. 2015;3(1):91–111. https://doi.org/10.1177/2167702614560746.

89. Salemink E, Wiers RW. Alcohol-related memory associations in positive and negative affect situations: drinking motives, working memory capacity, and prospective drinking. Psychol Addict Behav. 2014;28(1):105–13.
90. Woud ML, Fitzgerald DA, Wiers RW, Rinck M, Becker ES. 'Getting into the spirit': alcohol-related interpretation bias in heavy-drinking students. Psychol Addict Behav. 2012;26(3):627–32.
91. Woud ML, Hutschemaekers MH, Rinck M, Becker ES. The manipulation of alcohol-related interpretation biases by means of cognitive bias modification–interpretation (CBM-I). J Behav Ther Exp Psychiatry 2015. pii: S0005-7916(15)00031-2.
92. Salemink E, Woud ML, Roos M, Wiers RW, Lindgren KP. Reducing alcohol-related interpretive bias in negative affect situations: using a scenario-based cognitive bias modification training paradigm. Addict Behav. 2019;88:106–13. https://doi.org/10.1016/j.addbeh.2018.07.023.
93. Field M, Kiernan A, Eastwood B, Child R. Rapid approach responses to alcohol cues in heavy drinkers. J Behav Ther Exp Psychiatry. 2008;39(3):209–18.
94. Wiers RW, Rinck M, Dictus M, van den Wildenberg E. Relatively strong automatic appetitive action-tendencies in male carriers of the OPRM1 G-allele. Genes Brain Behav. 2009;8(1):101–6.
95. Cousijn J, Goudriaan AE, Wiers RW. Reaching out towards cannabis: approach-bias in heavy cannabis users predicts changes in cannabis use. Addiction. 2011;106(9):1667–74.
96. Field M, Eastwood B, Bradley BP, Mogg K. Selective processing of cannabis cues in regular cannabis users. Drug Alcohol Depend. 2006;85:75–82.
97. Wiers CE, Kühn S, Javadi AH, Korucuoglu O, Wiers RW, Walter H, Gallinat J, Bermpohl F. Automatic approach bias towards smoking cues is present in smokers but not in ex-smokers. Psychopharmacology. 2013;229(1):187–97.
98. Boffo M, Smits R, Salmon JP, Cowie ME, de Jong DTHA, Salemink E, Collins P, Stewart SH, Wiers RW. Luck, come here! Automatic approach tendencies toward gambling cues in moderate-to-high risk gamblers. Addiction. 2018;113(2):289–98.
99. Wiers RW, Rinck M, Kordts R, Houben K, Strack F. Retraining automatic action-tendencies to approach alcohol in hazardous drinkers. Addiction. 2010;105(2):279–87.
100. Ostafin BD, Palfai TP. Compelled to consume: the Implicit Association Test and automatic alcohol motivation. Psychol Addict Behav. 2006;20(3):322–7.
101. Wiers RW, Eberl C, Rinck M, Becker ES, Lindenmeyer J. Retraining automatic action tendencies changes alcoholic patients' approach bias for alcohol and improves treatment outcome. Psychol Sci. 2011;22(4):490–7.
102. Gladwin TE, Rinck M, Eberl C, Becker ES, Lindenmeyer J, Wiers RW. Mediation of cognitive bias modification for alcohol addiction via stimulus-specific alcohol avoidance association. Alcohol Clin Exp Res. 2015;39(1):101–7.
103. Salemink E, Rinck M, Becker E, Wiers RW, Lindenmeyer J. Does comorbid anxiety or depression moderate effects of approach bias modification in the treatment of alcohol use disorders? Psychol Addict Behav. 2021;36(5):547–54. https://doi.org/10.1037/adb0000642.
104. Manning V, Staiger PK, Hall K, Garfield JB, Flaks G, Leung D, et al. Cognitive bias modification training during inpatient alcohol detoxification reduces early relapse: a randomized controlled trial. Alcohol Clin Exp Res. 2016;40(9):2011–9.
105. Manning V, Garfield JBB, Staiger PK, Lubman DI, Lum JAG, Reynolds J, Hall K, Bonomo Y, Lloyd-Jones M, Wiers RW, Piercy H, Jacka D, Verdejo-Garcia A. Effect of cognitive bias modification on early relapse among adults undergoing inpatient alcohol withdrawal treatment: a randomized clinical trial. JAMA Psychiatry. 2021;78(2):133–40. https://doi.org/10.1001/jamapsychiatry.2020.3446.
106. Manning V, Garfield JB, Reynolds J, Staiger PK, Piercy H, Bonomo Y, et al. Alcohol use in the year following approach bias modification during inpatient withdrawal: secondary outcomes from a double-blind, multi-site randomized controlled trial. Addiction. 2022;117(11):2837–46.
107. Wiers RW, Houben K, Fadardi JS, van Beek P, Rhemtulla M, Cox WM. Alcohol cognitive bias modification training for problem drinkers over the web. Addict Behav. 2015;40:21–6.

108. Jones A, McGrath E, Robinson E, Houben K, Nederkoorn C, Field M. A randomized controlled trial of inhibitory control training for the reduction of alcohol consumption in problem drinkers. J Consult Clin Psychol. 2018;86(12):991.
109. Amir N, Kuckertz JM, Najmi S. The effect of modifying automatic action tendencies on overt avoidance behaviors. Emotion. 2013;13(3):478–84.
110. Rinck M, Telli S, Kampmann IL, Woud ML, Kerstholt M, Te Velthuis S, Wittkowski M, Becker ES. Training approach-avoidance of smiling faces affects emotional vulnerability in socially anxious individuals. Front Hum Neurosci. 2013;7:481.
111. Taylor CT, Amir N. Modifying automatic approach action tendencies in individuals with elevated social anxiety symptoms. Behav Res Ther. 2012;50(9):529–36.
112. Wiers RW, Van Dessel P, Köpetz C. ABC training: a new theory-based form of cognitive-bias modification to foster automatization of alternative choices in the treatment of addiction and related disorders. Curr Dir Psychol Sci. 2020;29(5):499–505. https://doi.org/10.1177/0963721420949500.
113. Cristea IA, Kok RN, Cuijpers P. The effectiveness of cognitive bias modification interventions for substance addictions: a meta-analysis. PlosOne. 2016;11(9):e0162226. https://doi.org/10.1371/journal.pone.0162226.
114. Wiers RW, Boffo M, Field M. What's in a trial? On the importance of distinguishing between experimental lab studies and randomized controlled trials: the case of cognitive bias modification and alcohol use disorders. J Stud Alcohol Drugs. 2018;79(3):333–43.
115. Sheeran P, Klein WM, Rothman AJ. Health behavior change: moving from observation to intervention. Annu Rev Psychol. 2017;68:573–600.
116. Boffo M, Zerhouni O, van Beek RJJ, Gronaua QF, Nikolaou K, Marsman M, Wiers RW. Cognitive bias modification for behavior change in alcohol and smoking addiction: a Bayesian meta-analysis of individual participant data. Neuropsychol Rev. 2019;29(1):52–78.
117. Van Deursen D. WHERE IS THE BIAS? Measuring and retraining cognitive biases in problem drinkers. Unpublished Doctoral Dissertation. University of Amsterdam 2019.
118. Elfeddali I, de Vries H, Bolman C, Pronk T, Wiers RW. A randomized controlled trial of web-based attentional bias modification to help smokers quit. Health Psychol. 2016;35(8):870–80. https://doi.org/10.1037/hea0000346.
119. Wittekind CE, Reibert E, Takano K, Ehring T, Pogarell O, Rüther T. Approach-avoidance modification as an add-on in smoking cessation: a randomized-controlled study. Behav Res Ther. 2019;114:35–43.
120. Grenard JL, Ames SL, Wiers RW, Thush C, Sussman S, Stacy AW. Working memory capacity moderates the predictive effects of drug-related associations on substance use. Psychol Addict Behav. 2008;22(3):426–32.
121. Thush C, Wiers RW, Ames SL, Grenard JL, Sussman S, Stacy AW. Interactions between implicit and explicit cognition and working memory capacity in the prediction of alcohol use in at-risk adolescents. Drug Alcohol Depend. 2008;94(1–3):116–24.
122. Peeters M, Wiers RW, Monshouwer K, van de Schoot R, Janssen T, Vollebergh WA. Automatic processes in at-risk adolescents: the role of alcohol-approach tendencies and response inhibition in drinking behavior. Addiction. 2012;107(11):1939–46.
123. Peeters M, Monshouwer K, van de Schoot RA, Janssen T, Vollebergh WA, Wiers RW. Automatic processes and the drinking behavior in early adolescence: a prospective study. Alcohol Clin Exp Res. 2013;37(10):1737–44.
124. Salemink E, Wiers RW. Adolescent threat-related interpretive bias and its modification: the moderating role of regulatory control. Behav Res Ther. 2012;50(1):40–6.
125. Wiechert S, Grafton B, MacLeod C, Wiers RW. When alcohol adverts catch the eye: a psychometrically reliable dual-probe measure of attentional bias. Int J Environ Res Public Health. 2021;18(24):13263.
126. Beard C, Weisberg RB, Primack J. Socially anxious primary care patients' attitudes toward cognitive bias modification (CBM): a qualitative study. Behav Cogn Psychother. 2012;40(5):618–33.

127. Boffo M, Pronk T, Mannarini S, Wiers RW. Combining cognitive bias modification training with motivational support in alcohol dependent outpatients: study protocol for a randomised controlled trial. BMC Trials. 2015;16:63.
128. Notebaert L, Clarke PJ, Grafton B, MacLeod C. Validation of a novel attentional bias modification task: the future may be in the cards. Behav Res Ther. 2015;65:93–100.
129. Salemink E, de Jong SC, Notebaert L, MacLeod C, Van Bockstaele B. Gamification of cognitive bias modification for interpretations in anxiety increases training engagement and enjoyment. J Behav Ther Exp Psychiatry. 2022;76:101727. https://doi.org/10.1016/j.jbtep.2022.101727.
130. Boendermaker WJ, Prins PJ, Wiers RW. Cognitive bias modification for adolescents with substance use problems—can serious games help? J Behav Ther Exp Psychiatry. 2015. [Epub ahead of print];49:13.
131. Otkhmezuri B, Boffo M, Siriaraya P, Matsangidou M, Wiers RW, Mackintosh B, Ang CS, Salemink E. Believing is seeing: a proof-of-concept, semi-experimental study on using mobile virtual reality to boost the effects of interpretation bias modification for anxiety. JMIR Ment Health. 2019;6:e11517. https://doi.org/10.2196/11517.
132. Yang R, Cui L, Li F, Xiao J, Zhang Q, Oei TP. Effects of cognitive bias modification training via smartphones. Front Psychol. 2017;8:1370. https://doi.org/10.3389/fpsyg.2017.01370.
133. Kerst WF, Waters AJ. Attentional retraining administered in the field reduces smokers' attentional bias and craving. Health Psychol. 2014;33(10):1232–40.
134. Van Dessel P, Cummins J, Wiers RW. ABC-training as a new intervention for hazardous alcohol drinking: two proof-of-principle randomized pilot studies. Addiction. 2023;118:2141. In press

Internet-Delivered Psychodynamic Therapy in Psychiatric Disorders

15

Jakob Mechler and Karin Lindqvist

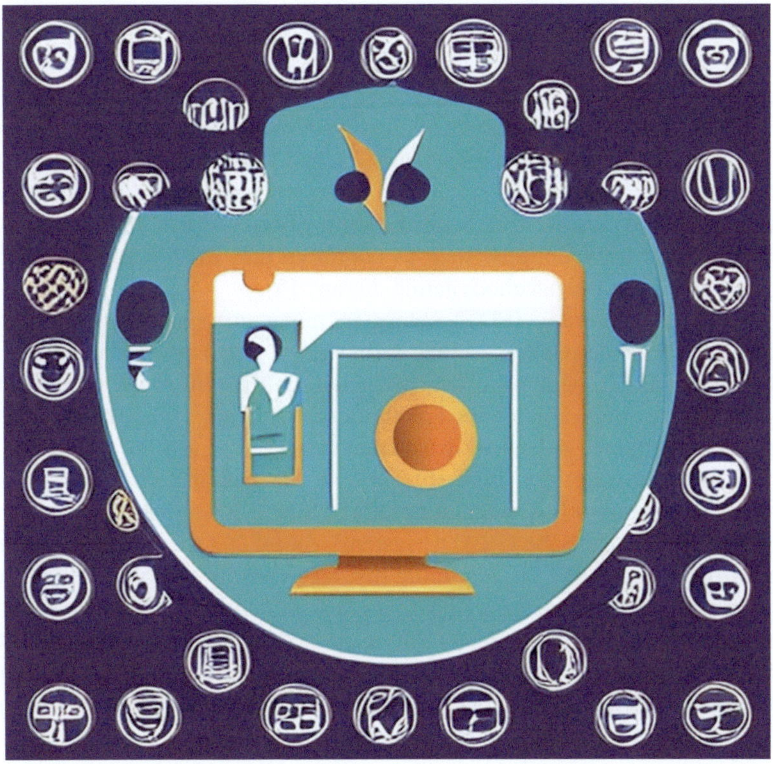

J. Mechler (✉)
Department of Psychology, Uppsala University, Uppsala, Sweden
e-mail: jakob.mechler@psyk.uu.se

K. Lindqvist
Department of Psychology, Stockholm University, Stockholm, Sweden
e-mail: karin.lindqvist@psychology.su.se

D. Mucić, D. M. Hilty (eds.), *Digital Mental Health*,
https://doi.org/10.1007/978-3-031-59936-1_15

Abstract

Internet-delivered psychodynamic treatments (IPDT) have a shorter history and smaller research base than those based on CBT, but the number of studies is rapidly growing. This chapter introduces the theoretical background and main principles of those IPDT treatments researched as of yet. Furthermore, it presents an overview of the research base for IPDT for different psychiatric disorders, where IPDT shows promising results for adult depression, adolescent depression, and several anxiety disorders in adulthood, as well as an adjunct treatment for inpatients with mixed disorders. Lastly, the chapter provides an illustrative case example of a treatment process in IPDT for adolescent depression.

15.1 Introduction

To date, Internet-delivered cognitive behavioral therapy (ICBT) is the most widely studied digital intervention targeting adult and youth psychopathology [1]. However, there is a large heterogeneity in response rates, and ICBT, much like CBT delivered face-to-face, is no panacea. This indicates an urgent need for treatment alternatives. Fortunately, a wide range of treatments have now been adapted and evaluated in the context of digital interventions, such as cognitive bias modification [2], interpersonal therapy [3, 4], and psychodynamic therapy [5].

Psychodynamic therapy (PDT) comes in many different forms. Historically, PDT has often been delivered as a long-term treatment [6] informed by the practice of psychoanalysis [7], which is often conducted multiple times per week stretching over years Today however, there is a plethora of different psychodynamic therapies that have been adapted to shorter time frames as well. Even though there is now some evidence for long-term PDT [6], most of the available studies are based on short-term treatments [8]. A recent umbrella review [9], summarizing the available evidence for PDT (using the GRADE system), found that there is high-quality evidence for the efficacy of PDT regarding disorder-specific symptoms and functioning compared to control groups in the treatment of depressive disorders and somatic symptom disorders, and moderate quality evidence for anxiety and personality disorders. Furthermore, the authors found that there are no meaningful differences in terms of efficacy when comparing PDT to other active therapies, and that the evidence for this is of moderate quality. The authors conclude that results suggest that a "strong" recommendation for PDT in the treatment of depressive, anxiety, personality, and somatic symptom disorders is warranted.

PDT has a long and rich history, stemming from Sigmund Freud, with new theoretical strands being introduced and elaborated on continuously. Blagys and Hilsenroth [10] reviewed studies comparing the processes and techniques of short-term PDT and CBT. They found seven interventions that distinguished therapy based on psychodynamic principles from therapy based on cognitive behavioral principles:

1. a focus on affect and the expression of patients' emotions
2. an exploration of patients' attempts to avoid topics or engage in activities that hinder the progress of therapy

3. the identification of patterns in patients' actions, thoughts, feelings, experiences, and relationships
4. an emphasis on past experiences
5. a focus on a patients' interpersonal experiences
6. an emphasis on the therapeutic relationship
7. an exploration of patients' wishes, dreams, or fantasies

Different forms of PDT emphasize different of thc above-mentioned principles. For instance, experiential dynamic (i.e., affect-focused) therapies [11] put a larger emphasis on in-session expression of emotions as compared to other short-term PDTs, while relational therapies such as brief relational therapy [12] would presumably emphasize the therapeutic relationship and use of the countertransference to a greater extent, and so on.

15.2 Background of Internet-Delivered Psychodynamic Therapy

The advantages of internet-delivered treatments are many and well known. Internet-delivered interventions address several barriers to seeking and receiving treatment. For instance, in children and adolescents, evidence suggests a complex set of factors responsible for untreated psychopathology. Perceived stigma, psychiatric symptoms not taken seriously, limited access to and availability of qualified mental health care as well as a wish to be a self-reliant are some of the suggested factors [13, 14]. Many of these obstacles can be lessened or removed using Internet-delivered interventions. Additionally, a recent meta-analysis suggests that ICBT is of similar efficacy as CBT delivered face-to-face [15].

It took a while for PDT to be developed and evaluated as a digital intervention. This may have been due to PDT's emphasis on the therapeutic relationship (i.e., the transference). Research indicates that clinicians practicing CBT are more positive toward computerized/digital interventions while practitioners of other therapy formats (among them PDT) are more concerned about the lack of therapist contact and therapeutic alliance and that it might render future treatment attempts (if needed) less effective [16]. Wangberg et al. [17] also found that psychodynamic therapists held more negative attitudes toward digitally delivered treatment. These may be contributing factors as to why research on digitally delivered interventions based on psychodynamic theory and practice has been lagging behind research on CBT-based interventions.

15.3 Research on Internet-Delivered Psychodynamic Therapy

As of yet, relatively few studies exist assessing the efficacy of IPDT in psychiatric disorders. A recent meta-analysis by Lindegaard et al. [18], based on seven primary studies, found IPDT to be significantly superior to inactive control conditions, showing small effects in overall outcome (g = 0.44 [95% CI 0.15, 0.72), adult depression ($g = 0.46$ [95% CI 0.17, 0.74]), anxiety ($g = 0.20$ [95% CI 0.07, 0.32]), and quality of life ($g = 0.40$ [95% CI 0.12, 0.67]). When one large study, aiming at supporting return to work rather than treating psychopathology, was removed, heterogeneity was reduced and the effect of IPDT was somewhat increased (overall effect $g = 0.52$ [95% CI 0.22, 0.82], depression $g = 0.55$ [95% CI 0.27, 0.83], anxiety 0.32, [95% CI 0.12, 0.52]). Gains made during treatment were maintained or increased at follow-up. However, it should be noted that the effect size for depression in the study by Lindegaard et al. [18] is based on a sample including studies with other target diagnoses than depression. This means that participants who were primarily treated for anxiety are used in the assessment of efficacy for depression, potentially rendering smaller treatment effects due to floor effects on the outcome measure. The same is true for the effects on anxiety. The meta-analysis also contains an assessment of study quality, where four out of seven studies were rated as being of high quality. The authors conclude that IPDT is a promising treatment alternative and that this is especially true for the treatment of depression.

15.4 Research on Internet-Delivered Psychodynamic Therapy for Depression

A handful of studies exist on IPDT for depression. The first study was published by Johansson et al. [19] where the treatment was based on an adapted version of a self-help book called *Make the leap* [20]. Ninety-two adult patients diagnosed with major depressive disorder were randomized to IPDT or an active control condition. IPDT consisted of nine treatment modules delivered over 10 weeks. The control condition was a structured support intervention, providing psychoeducation and basic support. Both conditions contained weekly text support from a therapist. The treatment was called SUBGAP, an acronym for (1) seeing unconscious patterns that contribute to emotional difficulties, (2) understanding these patterns, (3) breaking such unhelpful patterns, and (4) guarding against patterns and/or relapses [20]. The material was adapted to the treatment of depression by adding several examples of unconscious patterns that are theorised to be particularly relevant to depression. These case examples focused on unresolved grief, guilt about feelings of anger associated with key relationships, and persistent experiences of not feeling seen by others [21]. Participants in the control condition were provided with information on depression. In addition, they received scheduled weekly support from an assigned therapist who they were also able to contact whenever they wanted through asynchronous text-chat messages [19]. Results from this trial were highly promising. After 10 weeks of treatment, IPDT was superior to the control condition with a large between-group effect ($d = 1.11$ [95% CI 0.67, 1.56]) on the primary outcome measure (Beck's Depression Inventory–2 [22]). This effect was also evident in two secondary outcome measures on depression (MADRS-S [23]; $d = 0.86$ [95% CI 0.43, 1.30] and PHQ-9 [24]; $d = 0.95$ [95% CI 0.51, 1.39]). IPDT was also significantly superior to the control group in the treatment of comorbid anxiety (GAD-7 [25]; $d = 0.52$ [95% CI 0.09, 0.94]) and quality of life (QOLI [26], $d = 0.59$ [95% CI 0.16,

1.02]). However, IPDT failed to reach statistical significance on a second anxiety measure (BAI [27]; $d = 0.15$ [95% CI −0.27, 0.57]).

15.5 Internet-Delivered Psychodynamic Therapy for Adolescent Depression

Up until recently, all research on IPDT was conducted on adult populations. Overall, research on Internet-delivered therapies has mainly focused on adults, rendering a weaker evidence base for children and adolescents [28]. This is perhaps somewhat surprising, given young people's affinity with the Internet, as social media has increasingly become part of the day-to-day lives of adolescents [29]. Recently, an affect-focused psychodynamic intervention has been developed and evaluated in the treatment of adolescent depression. It was first evaluated in an RCT comparing IPDT to a minimal contact control condition. Seventy-six adolescents, aged 15–18, were randomized to either IPDT or control condition. Both conditions were 8 weeks long and IPDT consisted of eight weekly modules. Therapist support in IPDT contained weekly asynchronous messages and one 30 minutes synchronous text-chat session per week. The control condition had weekly asynchronous messages with an assigned therapist. No therapeutic interventions except for non-directive supportive interventions were used in the control condition. At post-treatment IPDT significantly outperformed the control condition regarding symptoms of depression (QIDS-A17-SR [30]; $d = 0.82$ [95% CI 0.35, 1.29]), generalized anxiety (GAD-7; $d = 0.78$ [95% CI 0.30, 1.26]), dysregulated emotions (DERS-16 [31]; $d = 0.97$ [95% CI 0.48, 1.46]) and self-compassion ([32]; $d = 0.65$ [95% CI 0.18, 1.12]). Furthermore, 56% of participants in IPDT responded to treatment compared to 21% in the control group, and 35% and 8% of patients were classified as in remission in IPDT and the control condition, respectively. At a six-month follow-up, treatment effects regarding depression and anxiety were largely maintained with no significant deterioration [33].

The same treatment program was then evaluated in a larger randomized controlled non-inferiority trial comparing IPDT to ICBT. The ICBT used had previously been evaluated in two RCTs on adolescent depression [34, 35]. A study protocol was published before recruitment completion, predefining key aspects of the study such as primary outcome measure, planned statistical analyses, and the non-inferiority margin [36]. The final outcome study [37] was based on 272 adolescents, aged 15–19, diagnosed with major depressive disorder according to DSM-5 [38]. Notably, almost 40% reported having been persistently depressed for a year or more, meaning that they fulfilled the criteria for persistent depressive disorder. Both treatments consisted of eight modules, delivered over 10 weeks. All patients were provided with a therapist guiding them throughout treatment through feedback on exercises via asynchronous text messages as well as synchronous text-chat sessions (30 minutes per week). Both treatments rendered large within-group effects (ICBT: $d = 1.75$ [95% CI 1.49, 2.01]; IPDT: $d = 1.93$ [95% CI 1.67, 2.20]). At end of treatment, the estimated difference in change between groups in depressive symptoms during treatment was $d = -0.18$ (90% CI −0.49, 0.13) in favor of IPDT. As the upper bound of the 90% CI was below the prespecified non-inferiority margin of $d = 0.30$, IPDT was deemed as non-inferior to ICBT regarding change in depressive symptoms. In ICBT, 49% ($n = 67$) were classified as responders (i.e., having achieved clinically significant improvements). The same was true for 48% ($n = 65$) in IPDT. Partial treatment response (i.e., achieving reliable change) was 12% ($n = 16$) in ICBT and 13% ($n = 18$) in IPDT. Remission rates were also highly similar, 38% ($n = 51$) in ICBT and 40% ($n = 54$) in IPDT. Furthermore, differences on secondary outcome measures were non-significant: comorbid anxiety (GAD-7; $d = -0.18$ [95% CI −0.44, 0.09]), emotion regulation (ERSQ-27 [39]; $d = 0.11$ [95% CI −0.21, 0.43]) and self-compassion (SCS-SF; $d = 0.03$ [95% CI −0.29, 0.36]). The only significant difference found was in the per protocol analyses, where IPDT was superior to ICBT in the treatment of comorbid anxiety with an estimated difference of $d = -0.29$, $p = 0.047$. All in all, results from this large non-inferiority trial seem to suggest that IPDT is non-inferior to ICBT and that few or no clinically important differences exist between the two treatments for adolescent depression. The trial was conducted just prior to, and during the COVID-19 pandemic. However, it is unclear if this in any way affected the results.

A smaller feasibility study on the same IPDT treatment was conducted in the United Kingdom in 2020. Due to the COVID-19 pandemic, access to treatment was limited, leaving many children and adolescents in distress. Midgley, Guerrero-Tates et al. [40] included 23 adolescents, 16–18 years old, suffering from MDD in a trial assessing the effects of IPDT. Included participants were offered IPDT over the course of 10 weeks. Within-group changes from pre- to post-treatment were significant ($d = 1.12$ [95% CI 0.39, 2.01]), and improvements were maintained at a three-month follow-up. Compared to trials conducted in Sweden [33, 37], results were not as pronounced regarding secondary outcome measures. Although emotion regulation did improve, the effects were not as strong as in previous trials [40]. Furthermore, patients did not improve significantly on comorbid anxiety ($d = 0.30$ [95% CI −0.49, 0.98]). A possible explanation for this could be the fact that this trial was conducted in the midst of the COVID-19 pandemic, meaning that participants might have been negatively affected by restrictions, such as repeated lockdowns, home-schooling, and social distancing. Also, therapists in the UK study had no prior clinical experience, unlike the students used as therapists in the Swedish studies.

15.6 Research on Internet-Delivered Psychodynamic Therapy for Anxiety Disorders

A few trials have also assessed IPDT in the treatment of anxiety. The first trial that was published [5] targeted generalized anxiety disorder (GAD) and utilized the same psychodynamic treatment as Johansson et al. [19] based on the self-help book by Silverberg [20]. Participants were randomized to IPDT, ICBT, or wait-list condition. Eighty-one patients were randomized (1:1:1) and treatments were delivered over 8 weeks. At treatment termination, there were no significant differences between any of the groups. However, at a three-month follow-up, both IPDT and ICBT demonstrated between-group effects compared to the control group, which were close to significance for IPDT on the primary outcome measure (Penn State Worry Questionnaire [41]), (d = 0.64 [95% CI –0.05, 1.30]) and significant for ICBT (d = 0.76 [95% CI 0.10, 1.33]). Gains were maintained at an 18-month follow-up, but at this point, the control group had received treatment and could thus not be included in the comparison. At the three-month follow-up, IPDT, but not ICBT, was significantly superior to the control condition on comorbid depression (d = 0.68; 95% CI: 0.01–1.34). However, at the 18-month follow-up, ICBT was significantly superior to IPDT regarding depressive symptoms. At posttreatment, 45.5% in IPDT still fulfilled the diagnosis of GAD, compared to 65.0% in the ICBT group and 84.0% in the control group. At the 18-month follow-up, by which time the control group had received treatment these numbers changed to 27.3%, 33.3%, and 38.1%.

A later RCT [37] investigated the effects of IPDT on patients suffering from social anxiety disorder (SAD). Participants in the study were randomized to either IPDT or a wait-list control condition. Treatment was based on the self-help book *Living Like You Mean It* [42], adapted to suit the format of guided self-help and to specifically target problems pertinent to patients suffering from SAD. Treatment principles build on experiential dynamic therapy (EDT; [11]). How these principles can be adapted and used in IPDT will be described more in detail below. This particular treatment program was adapted to SAD by adding a newly written module based on self-compassion and working with shame. Treatment was delivered over 10 weeks and treatment content was divided into nine modules. All participants were guided by a therapist through treatment. The treatment aimed at helping participants to mindfully approach feelings, regulate anxiety, and to notice and let go of their defenses. The nine modules addressed themes such as: introducing the affect phobia model, reducing shame and fostering the capacity for self-compassion, identifying and relinquishing defenses, anxiety regulation, noticing and accepting feelings through emotional mindfulness, affect expression, and restructuring sense of self [37]. At the end of treatment, IPDT was significantly superior to the wait-list condition, with an effect of d = 1.05 (95% CI 0.62, 1.53). Impressively, treatment gains were maintained and even improved over a two-year follow-up period with very little missing data. Significantly more patients in IPDT responded to treatment compared to patients in the control group (58.3% vs. 27.8%). In IPDT, 27.8% were classified as in remission, while this was true for 11.1% of patients in the control group. This difference almost reached statistical significance (p = 0.07). At post-treatment, significantly more patients in IPDT were classified as clinically improved compared to participants in the control condition (85.3% vs. 45.7%). Outcomes on secondary measures (depression and symptoms of generalized anxiety) were less pronounced. Moderate within-group effects were observed on the PHQ-9 and the GAD-7 in the treatment group. However, there were no significant differences when comparing the treatment group to patients allocated to the control group. Between-group effect sizes in favor of IPDT were small (d = 0.25 on depression and d = 0.10 on generalized anxiety). These findings were corroborated in a recent RCT where 181 adult patients suffering from SAD were randomised to 8 weeks guided IPDT, unguided IPDT or waitlist. Both guided and unguided IPDT were significantly superior to waitlist on symptoms of social anxiety (d = 1.07, 95% CI 0.72, 1.43 and d = 0.61, 95% CI 0.25, 0.98 respectively). Furthermore, guided IPDT was superior to unguided IPDT (d = 0.46, 95% CI 0.11, 0.80). At six and twelve-month follow-ups, results were maintained in guided IPDT and improved in unguided IPDT, meaning that there were no significant differences between guided and unguided IPDT [43].

15.7 Research on Internet-Delivered Psychodynamic Therapy as a Transdiagnostic Intervention

IPDT has also been tested as a transdiagnostic treatment. Johansson et al. [44] evaluated the same treatment as described above, based on *Living Like You Mean It* [42], in a sample of 100 adult patients suffering from mood and/or anxiety disorders. Patients were randomized to either IPDT or a wait-list condition. IPDT was delivered over a 10-week period and consisted of eight modules. Both IPDT and the wait-list condition included therapist contact/guidance. However, participants in the control group received no treatment material or therapeutic interventions. After 10 weeks of treatment, IPDT was superior to the control group both in the treatment of depression (d = 0.77 [95% CI: 0.37–1.18]) and anxiety (d = 0.48 [95% CI: 0.08–0.87]). During the seven-month follow-up, treatment gains were maintained for depression while further significant improvements were seen for anxiety. Results of IPDT also extended further than mere symptom reductions, as the capacity for emotional processing and mindfulness increased during treatment.

This same treatment was later used as an adjunct treatment to inpatient or day clinic psychotherapy [45]. A total of 82 adults receiving inpatient or day clinic psychotherapy were randomized (1:1) to either receiving guided IPDT or a wait-list condition. Following discharge from inpatient therapy, patients randomized to IPDT received access to the treatment material and therapist support for 10 weeks. Thirteen patients not providing any baseline measures were dropped from the study, rendering a total sample of 69 participants. The patient sample consisted of severely and chronically ill patients, diagnosed with multiple diagnoses. The most frequent diagnoses were depressive and anxiety disorders (84% and 68% respectively), followed by personality disorders (38%), and depersonalization-derealization disorder (22%). Although interest to partake in the trial and satisfaction with completed modules were high, adherence to treatment was rather low. Only 36% were active throughout treatment, defined as completing at least 50% of the modules. Still, in the intent-to-treat analysis, participants receiving treatment improved significantly more than the control condition with small to moderate effects regarding symptoms of depression (d = 0.60), quality of life (d = 0.53), and emotion regulation (d = 0.49). Naturally, among treatment completers, effects were more pronounced, with effects for depression (d = 1.33), quality of life (d = 0.83), and emotion regulation (d = 0.68). Among treatment completers, symptoms of general anxiety improved as well (d = 0.62).

15.8 Research on Internet-Delivered Psychodynamic Therapy for Somatic Symptom Disorder

Two trials have been conducted for Internet-delivered psychodynamic treatment for somatic symptom disorder in adults. The treatment is based on emotional awareness and expression therapy [EAET; [46]], an integrative treatment with roots in affective and pain neuroscience, psychodynamic, emotion-focused, and exposure-based treatments. One of the main ideas underlying EAET is that unresolved and difficult emotional experiences can cause and maintain somatic symptoms. The self-help material was based on a self-help book based on EAET, called *Unlearn your Pain* [47]. The nine modules addressed three main topics: (1) psychoeducation and awareness of pain, neuroscience, and connections between stressful life-events and pain; (2) recognition of defenses and regulation of anxiety; and (3) emotional exposure.

In a pilot trial [48] including a total of 52 adults with somatic symptom disorder with centralized symptoms, a nine-week-long therapist-guided I-EAET was associated with large within-group effects on somatic symptoms ($d = 1.13$ [95% CI 0.84, 1.47)]), which were maintained at follow-up 4 months later. Following this pilot trial, a larger RCT was conducted [49], including 74 patients randomized to 10 weeks I-EAET or waitlist control. I-EAET had significantly larger reductions in somatic symptoms than waitlist at post-treatment ($d = 0.44$ [95% CI 0.02, 0.87]) and follow-up ($d = 0.46$ [95% CI 0.06, 0.84]). Furthermore, at post-treatment, I-EAET showed significantly larger effects than waitlist on depressive symptoms ($d = 0.50$), insomnia ($d = 0.40$), and anxiety symptoms ($d = 0.47$), but not on disability, trauma symptoms, and sleepiness. At the four-month follow-up, there were no differences between the conditions on any of the secondary measures.

15.9 Research on Mechanisms of Change in Internet-Delivered Psychodynamic Therapy

Even though research on IPDT is still limited, some research has already been conducted shedding light on the processes and mechanisms of change in the treatment.

One proposed mechanism of change in IPDT is emotion regulation, and a study by Mechler et al. [50] showed that improvements in emotion regulation predicted outcome week by week in IPDT for adolescent depression. In other words, increased emotion regulation one week was related to decreased depressive symptoms the following week. These results have been corroborated in a later study utilizing a more sophisticated statistical methodology [51], where emotion regulation not only predicted outcome week by week but also mediated the relationship between therapeutic alliance and outcome. In this study, therapeutic alliance predicted the outcome in depressive symptoms week by week, and it was shown that therapeutic alliance predicted emotion regulation the following week, which in turn predicted outcome in depressive symptom the week after that. The same relationship was found in ICBT, with no differences between treatments.

Related to emotion regulation, Maroti et al. [52] measured emotional processing as a mediator for change in somatic symptoms in I-EAET. Using the Emotional Processing Scale-25 ([EPS-25; [53]], they found that the subscale "signs of unprocessed emotions", measuring intrusive, overwhelming, unwanted, and recurring emotions, mediated the effect of I-EAET on somatic symptoms. Furthermore, change in depressive symptoms was a significant mediator of change. These two mediators together accounted for 72% of the treatment effect.

One common question raised when discussing IPDT is whether it really is a psychodynamic treatment. This question was addressed in a study by Leibovich et al. [54], letting therapists in IPDT rate which techniques they used after synchronous chat sessions using the common factors, behavioral, cognitive, and psychodynamic scales of the multitheoretical list of therapeutic interventions [MULTI; [55]] rating instrument. Most prominent were common factors, and even though quite surprisingly, psychodynamic interventions were the least commonly rated ones, they were the only ones that significantly predicted outcome week by week on a within-person level. This lends support to the notion that psychodynamic interventions are responsible for the change achieved in treatment. On a between-patient level, common factors were also related to outcome, meaning that treatments with higher average use of common factors had better outcomes. However, between-patient analyses cannot (unlike the previously described within-person analysis) assess causality. This means that it is possible that there is a reversed causality, where more successful treatments lead to higher use of common factor interventions, or that there is another between-person confounder responsible for the relationship.

15.10 Internet-Delivered Psychodynamic Therapy: An Example

Common for all EDTs are Malan's [56] triangles: the triangle of conflict and the triangle of persons. The triangle of conflict illustrates Freud's second anxiety theory [57], that is, how unconscious feelings and/or impulses evoke anxiety, leading to experiential avoidance through the use of defenses. However, in the long run, excessive and rigid use of defenses will result in negative consequences, such as the development of symptoms of anxiety and/or depression. Furthermore, relationships will be negatively affected by the use of maladaptive defenses. Throughout treatment, participants are encouraged to observe and relinquish their defenses as well as identify and regulate anxiety while gradually experiencing anxiety-laden feelings. The triangle is presented in the self-help material and continuously used throughout the treatment as a model for understanding depressive and anxious reactions.

Malan's triangle of persons, addressing how inner conflicts emerge in past relationships, current relationships as well as in the relationship to the therapist, is not presented in the treatment material, since less emphasis is put on the transference relationship compared to psychodynamic therapy conducted face-to-face. However, the idea of recurrent maladaptive relationship patterns lies at the heart of the treatment. In IPDT, transference phenomena are mainly addressed when seen as

Table 15.1 IPDT intervention overview

Module	Content	Assignment/exercise
1	Theory on attachment and basic emotions. Affect phobias (i.e., the triangle of conflict).	Set goals, identify relationship dynamics contributing to depression.
2	Super-ego, shame and self-compassion.	Identify and challenge self-critical thoughts, develop an inner narrative of self-compassion.
3	Differentiation between optimal and too high levels of anxiety. Anxiety regulation.	Identify different levels of anxiety, increase self-observing capacity and anxiety regulation.
4	Identifying and understanding defensive patterns.	Identify patterns of maladaptive defenses and their long-term consequences.
5	Affect theory and the visceral experience of affect.	Identify the affects being activated, how they are experienced, and what impulses that come with them.
6	Mixed feelings: Anger, sadness, and guilt.	Exposure to mixed feelings through expressive writing.
7	Maladaptive relationship patterns: Togetherness and independence.	Identify whether key relationships are overly characterized by dependency or independence.
8	Communicating and expressing affects appropriately, identifying relationship ruptures, and repairing them.	How to communicate and express affects adaptively, identify relationship ruptures and repair them. Relapse prevention.

Previously published in Mechler [59]. Reprinted with permission from the author

important to treatment. Furthermore, there is a focus on communicating feelings in important relationships for the participant. The participant is also invited to reflect on the balance between dependence and independence in close relationships, according to the theory by Blatt [58].

The goals of IPDT are to (a) improve emotional awareness and decrease emotional avoidance through maladaptive defenses; (b) increase capacity for anxiety regulation through self-observation/mentalization; (c) decrease super-ego attacks and develop a more compassionate way of relating self and others; (d) gain insight into inner conflicts and maladaptive relationship patterns; and (e) improve capacity for emotion regulation and for expressing and communicating affects in key relationships. For details on the content of the treatment, see Table 15.1.

15.11 The Case of Felicity

Felicity[1] was 17 years old when she applied to be part of a research study on affect-focused IPDT. At the intake interview, Felicity reported being currently depressed and that this episode of depression had been ongoing for more than a year.

[1] Felicity is not a real participant from any of the studies. The case example is based on our experiences from multiple young people taking part in treatment, but the details in the case material are purely fictitious. Any similarities to a particular participant are completely coincidental.

Furthermore, she fulfilled the criteria for social anxiety disorder and had a history of self-harm behavior. At the moment of intake, Felicity did not report any specific thoughts of suicide, but she confirmed that she did indeed often think of death and that dying would in some ways feel like a relief.

Felicity's therapist Andrew presented himself in a welcome message at the same time as Felicity was given access to the first IPDT module. In this first module, where participants are introduced to the interplay between attachment and emotional needs—which can sometimes lead to the development of affect phobias, Felicity described that she recognized that she covered up her anger with tears, distanced herself from others when feeling sad or distressed, avoided conflicts by being vague and often put up a façade toward others to hide her feelings. She also described being raised to become very self-reliant and that her parents' divorce led to her mother moving away from the family. Around that time, her father started drinking heavily. Felicity linked these two events to her withdrawing from her parents, and shutting down emotionally. At the same time, Felicity described feelings of loneliness and distance in relationships, both with her parents and her friends. She was given prompt feedback by Andrew; he helped Felicity see how crying and withdrawing acted as defenses toward underlying feelings of anger and sadness. He also clarified how this covering up of emotions might contribute to the distance she experienced in relationships. Andrew further asked Felicity whether she could see any reasons for why she started covering up her emotions. She replied to him saying:" Thank you, this makes sense to me. It feels like we are starting to shed light on some key aspects of why I am constantly feeling low. As to your questions, I cannot say for sure, but I do think that my emotions were often neglected and I know that my father could become terribly angry with me as a child. I think that is why my mom left in the end, she could not take his temper tantrums anymore. But then she left me and my brother, to deal with it on our own." Later in that week Andrew and Felicity had a text-chat session of 30 min. She described feeling low, and that the first module had felt relevant but also challenging. Felicity described having felt anxious and that she ruminated a lot after completing some of the exercises. Andrew identified rumination as a defense and inquired into whether Felicity could describe any underlying emotions triggering anxiety. She described feelings of anxiety when thinking about her parents' divorce and her mom leaving. However, she could not get in contact with the underlying, primary feelings connected to this memory.

Later in treatment, in module 4, Felicity recognized that she employed various defense mechanisms. Primarily, she could see that she would often cover up emotions with shame (defensive affects) and that she would often times think that others would think badly of her (projection) and thus distance herself. This had recently become particularly problematic to her as she had started dating. The relationship was not moving forward, as Felicity would often withdraw when the boyfriend opened up for emotional intimacy. She described to Andrew that she felt certain that she would be abandoned if she really opened up and expressed her true feelings, and that she felt ashamed of her body. She was certain that she could not be experienced as attractive in any way. Andrew clarified the price of the defenses (self-loathing leading to feelings of depression, and shying away from emotional intimacy leading to distance in the relationship), but he also interpreted her fear of abandonment as possibly being connected to her mother leaving the family.

In the following module, Felicity was given exercises helping her noticing, exploring, and accepting her emotions. She described great difficulties in achieving this. Accepting her emotions was experienced as particularly difficult. She described having felt angry with her best friend, but this emotion was hard to accept and she almost immediately started feeling depressed and self-critical instead. Andrew responded by identifying the defense of self-directed anger. He clarified the function (protecting the relationship), but also the price (feelings of depression). Later in that week's chat session, Felicity reported having gained access to some of her anger after reading Andrew's response. She had also explored it further, trying to understand it and what she needed to do to act on it. In the end, she had addressed the conflict that had arisen with her friend by talking it through. Her friend had become sad, but was also understanding and had apologized.

In the next module, Felicity explored the anger and sadness associated with her mother leaving the family. She could access some anger toward the mother but described that it was hard being angry with her father. She described him as completely different now, since he stopped drinking and that she felt bad for even thinking about being angry with him. Felicity also reported feeling very sad after having completed the exercise. Andrew responded by validating her feelings. He also underlined how hard it seemed to be for Felicity to allow herself to feel mixed feelings of anger and love toward her father. "It seems to me like you are repressing your anger towards your dad by turning it onto yourself? Would that not make you more depressed? Today he is sober and you have a much better relationship, but then—when you really needed him—he was not up for the task. He was too distraught by the break up and he was not there for you. Can we allow you to be both angry and compassionate towards your dad, and make room for all those mixed feelings?"

In the final part of treatment, Felicity explored pervasive maladaptive relationship patterns in terms of dependency and/or self-criticism/self-reliance. She highly identified with the latter and described numerous relationships where she would withdraw from contact, and instead become self-critical and competitive. In the chat session with Andrew, Felicity further explored these relationship dynamics and made own connections to her upbringing with an absent mother and a father that could not be relied upon: "It is like I have always had to rely on myself." Andrew then asked what it had been like relying on him for help these last couple of weeks, and Felicity replied: "It has been fine, it felt hard at first, but then I noticed that I have kept all these emotions bottled up and when you encouraged me to share them with you, I felt this tension lifting. It has been a new experience to me." They continued discussing the therapeutic relationship and whether Felicity thought that it might be helpful to try to open up and rely on others more, even though this would come with the risk of being let down and hurt.

In the last module, Felicity got to describe gains from treatment and future goals to strive toward. She expressed a lot of gratitude toward Andrew and in the chat session they explored her feelings associated with treatment coming to an end.

Felicity reported feeling much better from the treatment, but also feelings of worry regarding how she would make it on her own. Given her history of abandonment, Andrew asked whether there might be a part of Felicity that felt abandoned by him as well. At first, she did not reply, but after a couple of minutes she wrote back: "I guess I do feel slightly angry with you for leaving me, but I feel like I have no right being cross with you." Since the chat session was coming to an end, Andrew replied that he understood her angry feelings, and again highlighted that feelings are often mixed—that perhaps she could allow herself to feel the positive feelings toward him for being there for her during treatment, together with the angry feelings as he was now to leave her. Later that week Felicity sent Andrew a message on the platform, saying that it was hard to end treatment, but that she also had felt stronger after the session: "You know, I have been really angry with you, but I have also felt like you are here with me in a sense. I will continue thinking of you, I am so grateful to you for listening to me. It really made a difference. Thank you, Andrew."

This vignette shows how principles from psychodynamic therapy are transferred into a text-based treatment where the patient and therapist never meet in person. Andrew applies techniques to address emotional avoidance through the use of defenses, links past experiences to present relationship patterns, and also uses the transference in order to explore mixed emotions. At the end of treatment, Felicity seems to be able to better contain mixed emotions and she is able to use new experiences made in the therapeutic relationship in order to improve key relationships in her everyday life.

15.12 Conclusions and Future Directions

More trials comparing active, bonafide Internet-delivered treatments are needed. Today, the evidence base for IPDT is small, but promising and growing. IPDT can be used as an alternative to ICBT, and should be further researched, preferably in trials with adequate sample size to detect also small differences of clinical importance. Future studies should also investigate potential predictors as well as moderators of change in IPDT and other active Internet-delivered treatments, and further potential mechanisms of change should be tested. Trials utilizing a cross-over design could potentially also be used to assess whether non-responders in IPDT would fare better in ICBT, or vice versa. Results suggesting this might be the case could potentially lead to a higher number of patients receiving effective care.

References

1. Andersson G, Titov N, Dear BF, Rozental A, Carlbring P. Internet-delivered psychological treatments: from innovation to implementation. World Psychiatry. 2019;18:20–8.
2. Zhang M, Ying J, Song G, Fung DSS, Smith H. Web-based cognitive bias modification interventions for psychiatric disorders: scoping review. JMIR Ment Health. 2019;6:e11841.
3. Dagöö J, Asplund RP, Bsenko HA, Hjerling S, Holmberg A, Westh S, et al. Cognitive behavior therapy versus interpersonal psychotherapy for social anxiety disorder delivered via smartphone and computer: a randomized controlled trial. J Anxiety Disord. 2014;28:410–7.

4. Donker T, Bennett K, Bennett A, Mackinnon A, Van Straten A, Cuijpers P, et al. Internet-delivered interpersonal psychotherapy versus internet-delivered cognitive behavioral therapy for adults with depressive symptoms: randomized controlled noninferiority trial. J Med Internet Res. 2013;15:e82.
5. Andersson G, Paxling B, Roch-Norlund P, Östman G, Norgren A, Almlöv J, et al. Internet-based psychodynamic versus cognitive behavioral guided self-help for generalized anxiety disorder: a randomized controlled trial. Psychother Psychosom. 2012;81:344–55.
6. Leichsenring F, Rabung S. Long-term psychodynamic psychotherapy in complex mental disorders: update of a meta-analysis. Br J Psychiatry. 2011;199:15–22.
7. De Maat S, De Jonghe F, De Kraker R, Leichsenring F, Abbass A, Luyten P, et al. The current state of the empirical evidence for psychoanalysis: a meta-analytic approach. Harv Rev Psychiatry. 2013;21:107–37.
8. Lilliengren P. A comprehensive overview of randomized controlled trials of psychodynamic psychotheraipes. Psychoanal Psychol. 2023;37(2):117–40. https://doi.org/10.1080/02668734.2023.2197617.
9. Leichsenring F, Abbass A, Heim N, Keefe JR, Kisely S, Luyten P, et al. The status of psychodynamic psychotherapy as an empirically supported treatment for common mental disorders—an umbrella review based on updated criteria. World Psychiatry. 2023;22:286–304.
10. Blagys MD, Hilsenroth MJ. Distinctive features of short-term psychodynamic-interpersonal psychotherapy: a review of the comparative psychotherapy process literature. Clin Psychol Sci Pract. 2000;7:167–88.
11. Lilliengren P, Johansson R, Lindqvist K, Mechler J, Andersson G. Efficacy of experiential dynamic therapy for psychiatric conditions: a meta-analysis of randomized controlled trials. Psychotherapy. 2016;53:90–104.
12. Safran JD. Brief relational psychoanalytic treatment. Psychoanal Dialogues. 2002;12:171–95.
13. Gulliver A, Griffiths KM, Christensen H. Perceived barriers and facilitators to mental health help-seeking in young people: a systematic review. BMC Psychiatry. 2010;113
14. Radez J, Reardon T, Creswell C, Lawrence PJ, Evdoka-Burton G, Waite P. Why do children and adolescents (not) seek and access professional help for their mental health problems? A systematic review of quantitative and qualitative studies. Eur Child Adolesc Psychiatry. 2021;30:183–211.
15. Hedman-Lagerlöf E, Carlbring P, Svärdman F, Riper H, Cuijpers P, Andersson G. Therapist-supported Internet-based cognitive behaviour therapy yields similar effects as face-to-face therapy for psychiatric and somatic disorders: an updated systematic review and meta-analysis. World Psychiatry. 2023;22:305–14.
16. Vigerland S, Ljótsson B, Bergdahl Gustafsson F, Hagert S, Thulin U, Andersson G, et al. Attitudes towards the use of computerized cognitive behavior therapy (cCBT) with children and adolescents: a survey among Swedish mental health professionals. Internet Interv. 2014;1:111–7.
17. Wangberg SC, Gammon D, Spitznogle K. In the eyes of the beholder: exploring psychologists' attitudes towards and use of e-therapy in Norway. Cyberpsychol Behav. 2007;10:418–23.
18. Lindegaard T, Berg M, Andersson G. Efficacy of internet-delivered psychodynamic therapy: systematic review and meta-analysis. Psychodyn Psychiatry. 2020;48:437–54.
19. Johansson R, Ekbladh S, Hebert A, Lindström M, Möller S, Petitt E, et al. Psychodynamic guided self-help for adult depression through the internet: a randomised controlled trial. Bruce A, editor. PLoS One. 2012;7:e38021.
20. Silverberg F. Make the leap: a practical guide to breaking the patterns that hold you back. New York: Marlowe & Co; 2005.
21. Johansson R. Internet-based psychodynamic psychotherapy. Contemporary Psychodynamic Psychotherapy [Internet]. Elsevier; 2019 [cited 2023 May 23]. p. 337–47. Available from: https://linkinghub.elsevier.com/retrieve/pii/B9780128133736000234
22. Beck AT, Steer RA, Brown G. Beck depression inventory–II [Internet]. 1996 [cited 2023 May 31]. Available from: http://doi.apa.org/getdoi.cfm?doi=10.1037/t00742-000
23. Svanborg P, Åsberg M. A new self-rating scale for depression and anxiety states based on the comprehensive psychopathological rating scale. Acta Psychiatr Scand. 1994;89:21–8.

24. Kroenke K, Spitzer RL, Williams JBW. The PHQ-9: validity of a brief depression severity measure. J Gen Intern Med. 2001;16:606–13.
25. Spitzer RL, Kroenke K, Williams JBW, Löwe B. A brief measure for assessing generalized anxiety disorder: the GAD-7. Arch Intern Med. 2006;166:1092.
26. Frisch MB, Cornell J, Villanueva M, Retzlaff PJ. Clinical validation of the quality of life inventory. A measure of life satisfaction for use in treatment planning and outcome assessment. Psychol Assess. 1992;4:92–101.
27. Beck AT, Epstein N, Brown G, Steer R. Beck anxiety inventory [internet]. 1988 [cited 2023 May 31]. Available from: http://doi.apa.org/getdoi.cfm?doi=10.1037/t02025-000
28. Vigerland S, Lenhard F, Bonnert M, Lalouni M, Hedman E, Ahlen J, et al. Internet-delivered cognitive behavior therapy for children and adolescents: a systematic review and meta-analysis. Clin Psychol Rev. 2016;50:1–10.
29. Boer M, Stevens GWJM, Finkenauer C, De Looze ME, Van Den Eijnden RJJM. Social media use intensity, social media use problems, and mental health among adolescents: investigating directionality and mediating processes. Comput Hum Behav. 2021;116:106645.
30. Bernstein IH, Rush AJ, Trivedi MH, Hughes CW, Macleod L, Witte BP, et al. Psychometric properties of the quick inventory of depressive symptomatology in adolescents: QIDS and adolescents. Int J Methods Psychiatr Res. 2010;19:185–94.
31. Bjureberg J, Ljótsson B, Tull MT, Hedman E, Sahlin H, Lundh L-G, et al. Development and validation of a brief version of the difficulties in emotion regulation scale: the DERS-16. J Psychopathol Behav Assess. 2016;38:284–96.
32. Raes F, Pommier E, Neff KD, Van Gucht D. Construction and factorial validation of a short form of the self-compassion scale. Clin Psychol Psychother. 2011;18:250–5.
33. Lindqvist K, Mechler J, Carlbring P, Lilliengren P, Falkenström F, Andersson G, et al. Affect-focused psychodynamic internet-based therapy for adolescent depression: randomized controlled trial. J Med Internet Res. 2020;22:e18047.
34. Topooco N, Berg M, Johansson S, Liljethörn L, Radvogin E, Vlaescu G, et al. Chat- and internet-based cognitive–behavioural therapy in treatment of adolescent depression: randomised controlled trial. BJPsych Open. 2018;4:199–207.
35. Topooco N, Byléhn S, Dahlström Nysäter E, Holmlund J, Lindegaard J, Johansson S, et al. Evaluating the efficacy of internet-delivered cognitive behavioral therapy blended with synchronous chat sessions to treat adolescent depression: randomized controlled trial. J Med Internet Res. 2019;21:e13393.
36. Mechler J, Lindqvist K, Carlbring P, Lilliengren P, Falkenström F, Andersson G, et al. Internet-based psychodynamic versus cognitive behaviour therapy for adolescents with depression: study protocol for a non-inferiority randomized controlled trial (the ERiCA study). Trials. 2020;21:587.
37. Johansson R, Hesslow T, Ljótsson B, Jansson A, Jonsson L, Färdig S, et al. Internet-based affect-focused psychodynamic therapy for social anxiety disorder: a randomized controlled trial with 2-year follow-up. Psychotherapy. 2017;54:351–60.
38. American Psychiatric Association. Diagnostic and statistical manual of mental disorders. 5th ed. Washington, DC: American Psychiatric Publishing; 2013.
39. Grant M, Salsman NL, Berking M. The assessment of successful emotion regulation skills use: development and validation of an English version of the emotion regulation skills questionnaire. Moitra E, editor. PLoS One. 2018;13:e0205095.
40. Midgley N, Guerrero-Tates B, Mortimer R, Edbrooke-Childs J, Mechler J, Lindqvist K, et al. The depression: online therapy study (D:OTS)—a pilot study of an internet-based psychodynamic treatment for adolescents with low mood in the UK, in the context of the COVID-19 pandemic. Int J Environ Res Public Health. 2021;18:12993.
41. Meyer TJ, Miller ML, Metzger RL, Borkovec TD. Development and validation of the penn state worry questionnaire. Behav Res Ther. 1990;28:487–95.
42. Frederick RJ. Living like you mean it: use the wisdom and power of your emotions to get the life you really want. 1st ed. San Francisco, CA: Jossey-Bass; 2009.
43. Mechler J, Lindqvist K, Magnusson K, Ringström A, Krafman JD, Alvinzi P, Kassius L, Sowa J, Andersson G, Carlbring P. Guided and unguided internet-delivered psychodynamic therapy

for social anxiety disorder: a randomized controlled trial. Npj Ment Health Res. 2024;3(1):21. https://doi.org/10.1038/s44184-024-00063-0.
44. Johansson R, Björklund M, Hornborg C, Karlsson S, Hesser H, Ljótsson B, et al. Affect-focused psychodynamic psychotherapy for depression and anxiety through the internet: a randomized controlled trial. PeerJ. 2013;1:e102.
45. Zwerenz R, Becker J, Johansson R, Frederick RJ, Andersson G, Beutel ME. Transdiagnostic, psychodynamic web-based self-help intervention following inpatient psychotherapy: results of a feasibility study and randomized controlled trial. JMIR Ment Health. 2017;4:e41.
46. Lumley MA, Schubiner H. Emotional awareness and expression therapy for chronic pain: rationale, principles and techniques, evidence, and critical review. Curr Rheumatol Rep. 2019;21:30.
47. Schubiner H, Betzold M. Unlearn your pain: a 28-day process to reprogram your brain. 2nd ed. Pleasant Ridge, MI: Mind Body Publishing; 2012.
48. Maroti D, Ek J, Widlund R-M, Schubiner H, Lumley MA, Lilliengren P, et al. Internet-administered emotional awareness and expression therapy for somatic symptom disorder with centralized symptoms: a preliminary efficacy trial. Front Psych. 2021;12:620359.
49. Maroti D, Lumley MA, Schubiner H, Lilliengren P, Bileviciute-Ljungar I, Ljótsson B, Johansson R. Internet-based emotional awareness and expression therapy for somatic symptom disorder: A randomized controlled trial. Journal of Psychosomatic Research 2022;163:111068. https://doi.org/10.1016/j.jpsychores.2022.111068.
50. Mechler J, Lindqvist K, Falkenström F, Carlbring P, Andersson G, Philips B. Emotion regulation as a time-invariant and time-varying covariate predicts outcome in an internet-based psychodynamic treatment targeting adolescent depression. Front Psych. 2020;11:671.
51. Lindqvist K, Mechler J, Falkenström F, Carlbring P, Andersson G, Philips B. Therapeutic alliance is calming and curing—the interplay between alliance and emotion regulation as predictors of outcome in internet-based treatments for adolescent depression. J Consult Clin Psychol. 2023;91:426–37.
52. Maroti D, Lumley MA, Schubiner H, Lilliengren P, Bileviciute-Ljungar I, Ljótsson B, et al. Internet-based emotional awareness and expression therapy for somatic symptom disorder: a randomized controlled trial. J Psychosom Res. 2022;163:111068.
53. Baker R, Thomas S, Thomas PW, Gower P, Santonastaso M, Whittlesea A. The emotional processing scale: scale refinement and abridgement (EPS-25). J Psychosom Res. 2010;68:83–8.
54. Leibovich L, Mechler J, Lindqvist K, Mortimer R, Edbrooke-Childs J, Midgley N. Unpacking the active ingredients of internet-based psychodynamic therapy for adolescents. Psychother Res. 2022;33:108–17.
55. McCarthy KS, Barber JP. The multitheoretical list of therapeutic interventions (MULTI): initial report. Psychother Res. 2009;19:96–113.
56. Malan DH. Individual psychotherapy and the science of psychodynamics. 2nd ed. London ; Boston: Butterworths; 1995.
57. Freud S. Inhibitions, symptoms, and anxiety. New York: Norton; 1936.
58. Blatt SJ. Polarities of experience: relatedness and self-definition in personality development, psychopathology, and the therapeutic process. [internet]. Washington: American Psychological Association; 2008. [cited 2022 Dec 21]. Available from: http://content.apa.org/books/11749-000
59. Mechler J. Beyond the blank screen: internet-delivered psychodynamic therapy for adolescent depression: evaluating non-inferiority, the role of emotion regulation, and sudden gains [Internet] [PhD dissertation]. Department of Psychology, Stockholm University; 2023. Available from: https://urn.kb.se/resolve?urn=urn:nbn:se:su:diva-218837

16 Psychiatric Apps: Patient Self-Assessment, Communication, and Potential Treatment Interventions

Nanik Ram, Aditya Vaidyam, Amrik Eadara, Carsten Langholm, and John Torous

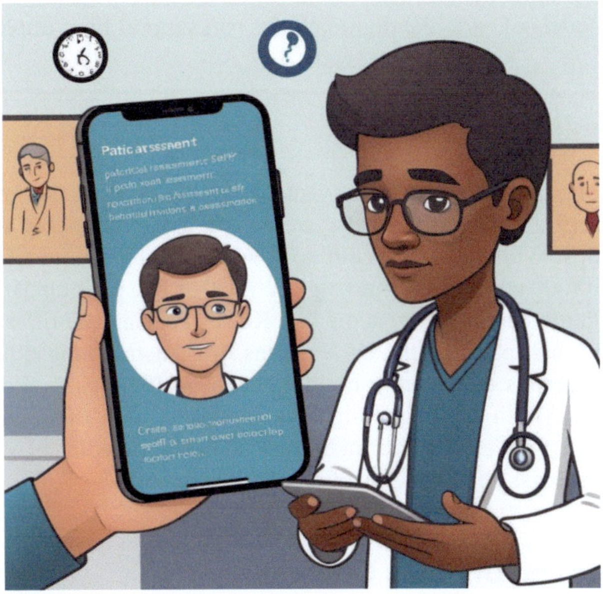

N. Ram (✉) · C. Langholm · J. Torous
Division of Digital Psychiatry, BIDMC, Harvard Medical School, Boston, MA, USA
e-mail: nram2@bidmc.harvard.edu; clanghol@bidmc.harvard.edu; jtorous@bidmc.harvard.edu

A. Vaidyam
Division of Digital Psychiatry, BIDMC, Harvard Medical School, Boston, MA, USA

Carle Illinois College of Medicine, Urbana, IL, USA

A. Eadara
Division of Digital Psychiatry, BIDMC, Harvard Medical School, Boston, MA, USA

Brown University, Providence, RI, USA
e-mail: amrik_eadara@brown.edu

D. Mucić, D. M. Hilty (eds.), *Digital Mental Health*,
https://doi.org/10.1007/978-3-031-59936-1_16

Abstract

Mobile device applications can complement traditional stages of mental health treatment by providing treatment monitoring, improved adherence to treatment plans, psychoeducation, symptom assessment, and clinical decision support. An increasing number of patients and clinicians have access to smartphones that can run interactive apps (applications). Spurred by coronavirus disease 2019 (COVID-19), rising interest and use cases of mobile apps in care underscore the potential of this approach to increase access to and quality of care. However, concomitant risks around privacy, safety, engagement, and clinical integration require the clinician to carefully consider the unique features of each app before integration into care. This chapter will provide an overview of these smartphone mental health apps with a review of their evidence, utility, and risks as well as how new models of care like digital clinics can support their implementation.

16.1 Introduction

While synchronous telehealth (video visits) expanded during coronavirus disease 2019 (COVID-19), there was a parallel expansion in asynchronous telehealth with smartphone apps. While mental health apps were popular before COVID-19, with an estimated 10,000 apps on the marketplace in 2017 [1], their uptake into care was lower. Today, large healthcare systems like Kaiser Permanente offer mental health apps directly to their patients, the US Veterans Administration is expanding its app library, and numerous employers provide mental health apps as a benefit to their employees [2–4]. With this widening use, combined with millions of dollars of direct-to-consumer advertising on traditional and social media [5], clinicians need to be aware of the risks and benefits of mental health apps.

16.2 Rapid and Ongoing Changes

The landscape of smartphone apps for mental health continues to rapidly change. These changes are not only limited to the technology and functionalities of apps themselves but also to the research methods used to assess them, the regulations used to govern them, and even the professional standards used to guide their role in care. Thus, any chapter on the topic must focus on broad themes as specific examples are likely to soon be out of date.

One area of rapid change and growth in smartphone apps is digital phenotyping. Defined in 2016 as "the moment-by-moment quantification of the individual-level human phenotype using from personal digital devices [6]," it refers to the ability of devices like smartphones to capture clinically relevant behavioral patterns such as exercise, sleep behavior, social media activity, and many others. Given 85% of the US population owns a smartphone today (nearly 100% among youth populations), digital phenotyping presents the opportunity for novel data capture at a population scale. Emerging research highlights how this form of smartphone sensing is not only acceptable to patients, including those with illnesses like schizophrenia [7]. Broad use cases include helping people understand responses to medication, predicting the risk of relapse, and even elucidating understanding of mechanisms of illness [8]. The potential of digital phenotyping continues to rise. Recently, Apple released a software package for digital phenotyping that provides robust and scalable approaches to capturing relevant smartphone and sensor data [9]. The ability of apps to soon be more aware of each person's unique mental health state means that a generation of more responsive apps able to support more personalized and even preventative care may soon be possible.

Research methods are also evolving. While the first generation of smartphone apps offering elements of CBT or mindfulness-based therapy often marketed themselves as effective, newer studies suggest a more nuanced picture [10]. The first generation of studies on the clinical efficacy of various apps often did not deploy a control group and so compared the change in one group using the app compared to another group using nothing. Needless to say, the adage that "something is better than nothing" proved true [11]. Newer studies are now employing digital control groups (e.g., another app but missing the active ingredient) and the results of this new generation of studies will likely inform the actual clinical role of smartphone apps as therapeutic tools [12]. This higher standard will also hopefully spur the innovation of more effective apps that deliver greater benefits to patients. With the recent breakthroughs in large language models, this next generation of apps will likely appear and react to user input very differently than those we often see today.

Likewise, regulation of the entire digital health space, and especially the digital mental health space, remains in flux [13]. In September 2022, the US Food and Drug Administration ended its pilot program for a new generation of regulation of digital tools like health apps, noting challenges with its goal to use real-world data to guide new approvals. In Europe, regulators are experimenting with new schemes such as DIGA in Germany and the results of these efforts will likely be informative for countries around the world [14]. A further sign of change around digital mental health is new regulators stepping into the space, such as in the US the Federal Trade Commission which has brought numerous lawsuits related to privacy violations of specific apps or online programs. The final outcome of new regulations and new regulators will have a profound role in shaping the future of the space.

The flux of new sensing and therapeutic potential for apps will quickly usher in a new generation of tools that will be subject to a new generation of regulation. While time will reveal the details, awareness of these changes is important for framing any discussion of apps today.

16.3 Assessing Apps Today: Practical and Informed Decision Making

Changes in the app space have not dampened interest in their use today. Clinicians need to be aware of the current generation of tools and how to guide a discussion around reasons why they recommend using (or not using) any app. Weighing the risks and benefits requires the same clinical judgment exercised today when selecting a therapy or medication. But knowing what those risks and benefits are takes extra consideration.

With 10,000 or more mental health-related apps on the marketplace, selecting one without a plan is dangerous. A randomly picked app without careful reason could be unhelpful and even dangerous. Metrics like downloads, stars, or higher page ranking will indicate which are more popular, but popularity is not associated with either privacy or effectiveness. The magazine Consumer Reports looked at the privacy practices of highly-ranked mental health apps in 2021 and found numerous concerns [15]. The Mozilla Foundation released reports in both 2022 and 2023 highlighting ongoing privacy concerns in popular mental health apps, suggesting the situation is not improving.

Another common trap in selecting mental health apps is scoring systems or those that present rankings such as the "top 10 apps for depression." Conceptually, the scoring of medications, therapists, or therapy programs has never worked in practice, and the same holds for apps. It is almost ridiculous, yet some services attempt to rate the aesthetics, engagement, and other factors that are unique to each person and the app they are considering [16]. Worse, these app rating websites are often out of date with their information not able to keep up with the rapidly updating and changing world of apps [17]. An analogy for these services may be a website that attempts to tell you how you will feel about the weather (without knowing anything about your preferences) in different cities based on climate data that is years out of date.

Thus, a different approach is necessary for clinicians to make informed decisions in selecting apps they may wish to use or avoid, for particular patients.

16.4 Mental Health App Evaluation

While there is not a simple answer to the single best app to use, it is possible to make more informed and educated decisions today. The American Psychiatric Association (APA) has created and supports a well-established app evaluation framework [18]. The framework has been created with input from patients, psychologists, nurses, social workers, students, administrators, and psychiatrists. It is designed to be used by anyone—not just psychiatrists [10]. The framework is simple in that it suggests one to evaluate apps in order of first accessibility, second privacy/harm, third efficacy/benefit, fourth engagement/ease of use, and final clinical integration/utility/therapeutic goal. If an app does not meet the standards at each level, the framework suggests looking for a new app (Fig. 16.1).

The reason for each of these five core levels is that they are designed to reflect the primary challenges around apps. While we have already discussed privacy and evidence challenges, issues around engagement and clinical integration are also important to consider.

In terms of engagement, it is impossible to know what person will find an app easy to use. But population data suggests that over 95% of people will stop using mental health apps within 10 days [19]. Even apps that offer superior privacy

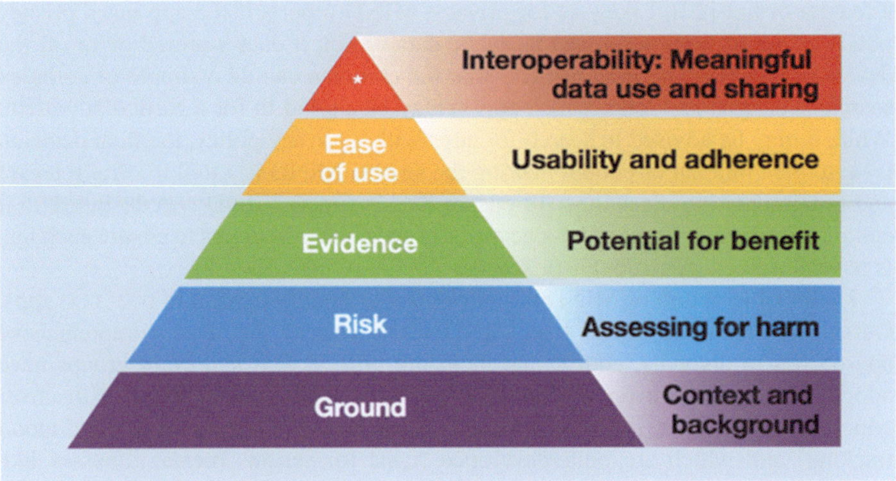

Fig. 16.1 APA app evaluation model

protections and are based on evidence (the first two layers of the APA framework) are not guaranteed to have high rates of engagement, with less than 2% of users sticking with one such app in a recent study [20]. While not everyone is looking to use an app long-term, the evidence for finding one that will keep users engaged is rather bleak. This is not to say that apps cannot be highly engaging, but rather that efforts to support engagement such as selecting appropriate apps are likely more important than often realized. Likewise, when apps are used in conjunction with clinical care and supported by a clinical team, engagement is often greatly improved. This finding makes sense as self-help around anything, for example, diet is often challenging, and "sticking with it" is easier when a person is involved.

It also relates to the final layer of the APA framework in selecting apps that support clinical integration. In essence, this equates to selecting apps that integrate smoothly into treatment plans and workflow rather than fragmenting care. While ideally, apps could share data with electronic medical records, at least in 2023 this is still so rare as to be notable when it does occur.

The APA framework represents principles that reflect best clinical practice, but few people have the time to apply these criteria to each app. Thus, a related approach to operationalizing the APA framework for app evaluation is exemplified in the M-Health Index and Navigation Database (MIND), which is freely available at https://mindapps.org/ [21]. MIND evaluates each app against 105 questions related to the principles already covered like privacy, evidence, engagement factors, clinical integration, and more. As noted above, it is impossible to know if any app will be engaging for any particular person. MIND's solution is to break engagement down into factors such as questions around whether the app offers music, video, texting, graphs, gamification, etc., and many other factors that people may want to drive engagement. MIND does not judge any app but simply reports if the app offers such a feature or not [22]. Likewise for privacy, MIND reports if the app has a privacy policy or not, if it allows a user to delete data or not, if data is stored on or off the device or not, etc. The final result is that the clinician can do a simple or complex search as desired and learn which app(s) may be a good fit for a particular patient. While it may be advised to search for apps with a privacy policy, the final decision is up to the clinician or patient making the search. MIND is a tool to offer relevant and timely data, not decisions. To ensure data is timely MIND was designed so it could be frequently updated by a network of staff and volunteers to ensure each app is re-reviewed every 6 months or sooner.

The flexible nature of MIND has allowed it to rapidly expand to over 600 apps. Outside research has found that MIND offers one of the most comprehensive approaches to diversity, equity, and inclusion criteria [23] and other groups have adopted it to evaluate even more apps [24]. Research has utilized MIND to discover which areas of the app marketplace are over-saturated [25] (mindfulness and mood tracking) and which are underdeveloped (apps for serious mental illnesses like schizophrenia and bipolar disorder).

16.5 Applying MIND to Find an App

Understanding how MIND is used is best demonstrated using a simple example of seeking an app for PTSD. In this fictional case, the desired app should be free of cost, keep patient data on the device (i.e., not send it to the cloud), and offer at least some supporting studies. By selecting "totally free" under the cost filter, "PTSD" under the supported conditions filter, "data stored on device" under the privacy filter, and "supporting studies" under the evidence & clinical foundations filter, around five potential apps emerge. The reader is encouraged to visit mindapps.org and try this exercise. Results may not be exactly the same as the apps update over time but seeing which apps match this criterion at any time is informative. Expanding the example to select apps based on the features patients may want or have reported is even more informative.

16.6 Implementing Apps into Care

While selecting apps is critical, being able to implement them into models of care is equally important. The challenges of both low engagement with apps and implementation into busy clinics may be solved via a new concept of digital clinics, a new type of clinic that fosters a collaborative approach to using technology as part of care.

Given the way many mental health clinics today are funded and structured in their workflow, there is a need to create a new clinical model that allows for the best of face-to-face clinical care to intersect with the best that digital mental health can offer [26]. This means ensuring that technology is not a barrier between a patient and clinician, but rather serves as a bridge to strengthen the therapeutic relationship between them. Figure 16.2 below suggests how an app could collect important

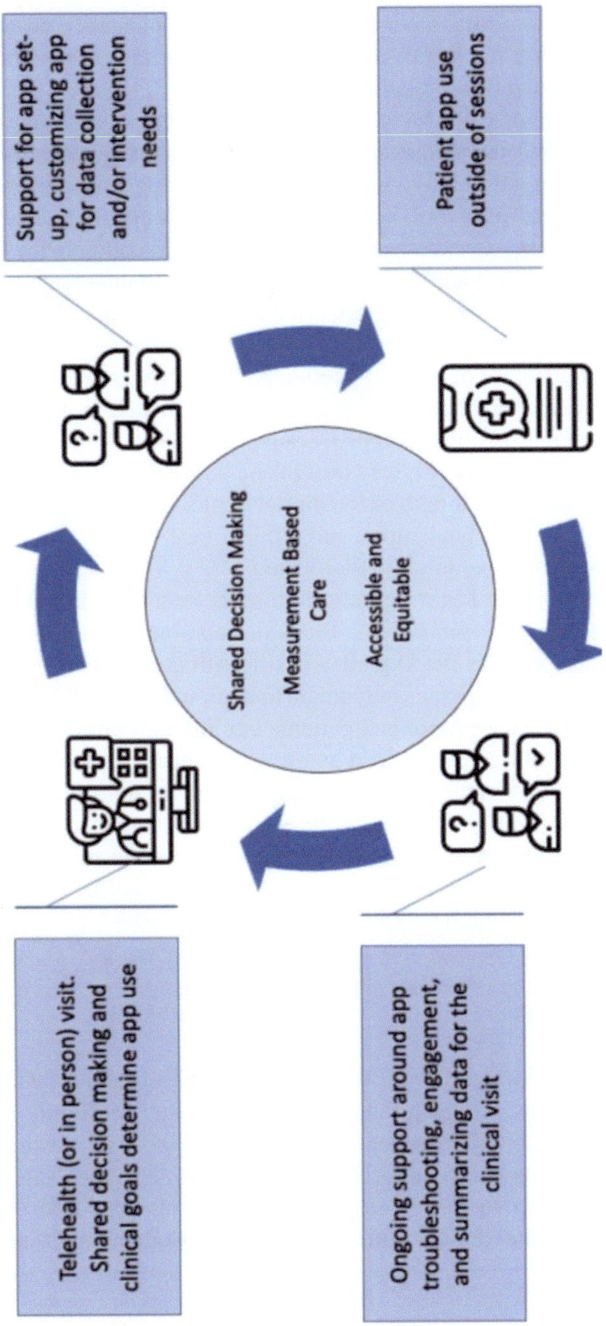

Fig. 16.2 Digital clinical model of care integrates telehealth/video visits with mobile health/apps

real-time data that could be automatically monitored with algorithms to identify critical risks (e.g., safety) but also interpreted by new members of the care team, digital clinical staff, or digital navigators, who serve as liaisons between clinicians and patients in learning the technical aspects of this digital tool and help translate app data into personalized care plans and [27].

This digital navigator would work with both the patient and clinician to ensure the digital care plan informs and enhances the traditional care plan and that the recommended tool(s) directly aligns with the patient's needs [28, 29]. In addition to collecting passive data, these tools would also allow patients to practice skills introduced during clinical sessions between visits and to build competency in managing their mental health independently. Because patients would understand how the recommended app is informing their clinical care and how it fits within their lives, engagement may be higher. A strategically structured support system with the presence of digital navigators encouraging active patient activity builds upon patients' investment into their own individualized care plans, which in turn retains more involved and dynamic use of the app. Because clinicians would be supported in effectively using apps through the very design and structure of the treatment setting, implementation is another strength of the digital clinic. Using an agile approach, the correct use of apps, digital navigators, and clinical face-to-face time, effective and robust clinical care could be quickly established.

Given that any app used in a digital clinic must be a tool that can support the needs of both patients and clinicians, a focus on relationships must also extend to the app. New scales such as the Digital Working Alliance Inventory [30] can help inform how patients and clinicians may relate to apps and ensure the next generation of tools is designed to support not just patients or clinicians but rather both.

Though mental health apps are used and implemented mainly in outpatient care currently, the potential scope is wide, expanding to other clinical settings including inpatient psychiatric units, integrated care, geriatric psychiatric units, and emergency/crisis settings among others. More research is needed in these settings and across varied patient populations to better determine the alignment of which app to use for which patient in which clinical setting.

16.7 Conclusions

Even though it is rapidly evolving, the future of digital mental health is bright. Today's myriad of apps and features already support app feasibility and the new generation of tools will support better data capture and more promising therapeutic interventions. Clinicians today can utilize tools like the APA app evaluation framework and mindapps.org to make informed decisions on apps and then consider applying aspects of the digital clinic model to implement and integrate apps into care.

References

1. Torous J, Roberts LW. Needed innovation in digital health and smartphone applications for mental health: transparency and trust. JAMA Psychiatry. 2017;74(5):437–8.
2. Mordecai D, Histon T, Neuwirth E, Heisler WS, Kraft A, Bang Y, Franchino K, Taillac C, Nixon JP. How Kaiser Permanente created a mental health and wellness digital ecosystem. NEJM Catal Innov Care Deliv. 2021;2:1.
3. Reger GM, Harned M, Stevens ES, Porter S, Nguyen J, Norr AM. Mobile applications may be the future of veteran mental health support but do veterans know yet? A survey of app knowledge and use. Psychol Serv. 2022;19(3):480.
4. Stratton E, Lampit A, Choi I, Malmberg Gavelin H, Aji M, Taylor J, Calvo RA, Harvey SB, Glozier N. Trends in effectiveness of organizational eHealth interventions in addressing employee mental health: systematic review and meta-analysis. J Med Internet Res. 2022;24(9):e37776.
5. https://medium.com/invisible-illness/how-effective-has-betterhelps-advertising-been-5be2b214ab39
6. Torous J, Kiang MV, Lorme J, Onnela JP. New tools for new research in psychiatry: a scalable and customizable platform to empower data driven smartphone research. JMIR Ment Health. 2016;3(2):e5165.
7. Torous J, Kwon S, Firth J, Joshi D. Accessibility and availability of smartphone apps for schizophrenia. Schizophrenia (Heidelb). 2022;8(1):98.
8. Torous J, Bucci S, Bell IH, Kessing LV, Faurholt-Jepsen M, Whelan P, Carvalho AF, Keshavan M, Linardon J, Firth J. The growing field of digital psychiatry: current evidence and the future of apps, social media, chatbots, and virtual reality. World Psychiatry. 2021;20(3):318–35.
9. Langholm C, Kowatsch T, Bucci S, Cipriani A, Torous J. Exploring the Potential of Apple SensorKit and Digital Phenotyping Data as New Digital Biomarkers for Mental Health Research. Digit Biomark. 2023;7(1):104–114.
10. Goldberg SB, Lam SU, Simonsson O, Torous J, Sun S. Mobile phone-based interventions for mental health: a systematic meta-review of 14 meta-analyses of randomized controlled trials. PLOS Digit Health. 2022;1(1):e0000002.
11. Cuijpers P, Cristea IA. How to prove that your therapy is effective, even when it is not: a guideline. Epidemiol Psychiatr Sci. 2016;25(5):428–35.
12. Ghaemi SN, Sverdlov O, van Dam J, Campellone T, Gerwien R. A smartphone-based intervention as an adjunct to standard-of-care treatment for schizophrenia: randomized controlled trial. JMIR Form Res. 2022;6(3):e29154.
13. Kahane K, François J, Torous J. PERSPECTIVE: the digital health app policy landscape: regulatory gaps and choices through the lens of mental health. J Ment Health Policy Econ. 2021;24(3):101–8.
14. Dahlhausen F, Zinner M, Bieske L, Ehlers JP, Boehme P, Fehring L. Physicians' attitudes toward prescribable mHealth apps and implications for adoption in Germany: mixed methods study. JMIR Mhealth Uhealth. 2021;9(11):e33012.
15. https://www.consumerreports.org/health-privacy/mental-health-apps-and-user-privacy-a7415198244/
16. Lagan S, Sandler L, Torous J. Evaluating evaluation frameworks: a scoping review of frameworks for assessing health apps. BMJ Open. 2021;11(3):e047001.
17. Lagan S, Aquino P, Emerson MR, Fortuna K, Walker R, Torous J. Actionable health app evaluation: translating expert frameworks into objective metrics. NPJ Digit Med. 2020;3(1):1–8.
18. King DR, Emerson MR, Tartaglia J, Nanda G, Tatro NA. Methods for navigating the mobile mental health app landscape for clinical use. Curr Treat Options Psychiatry. 2023;24:1–5.
19. Baumel A, Muench F, Edan S, Kane JM. Objective user engagement with mental health apps: systematic search and panel-based usage analysis. J Med Internet Res. 2019;21(9):e14567.

20. Jaworski BK, Taylor K, Ramsey KM, Heinz A, Steinmetz S, Pagano I, Moraja G, Owen JE. Exploring usage of COVID coach, a public mental health app designed for the COVID-19 pandemic: evaluation of analytics data. J Med Internet Res. 2021;23(3):e26559.
21. Camacho E, Cohen A, Torous J. Assessment of mental health services available through smartphone apps. JAMA Netw Open. 2022;5(12):e2248784.
22. Bold KW, Garrison KA, DeLucia A, Horvath M, Nguyen M, Camacho E, Torous J. Smartphone apps for smoking cessation: systematic framework for app review and analysis. J Med Internet Res. 2023;25:e45183.
23. Ramos G, Ponting C, Labao JP, Sobowale K. Considerations of diversity, equity, and inclusion in mental health apps: a scoping review of evaluation frameworks. Behav Res Ther. 2021;147:103990.
24. Spadaro B, Martin-Key NA, Funnell E, Bahn S. mHealth solutions for perinatal mental health: scoping review and appraisal following the mHealth index and navigation database framework. JMIR Mhealth Uhealth. 2022;10(1):e30724.
25. Lagan S, D'Mello R, Vaidyam A, Bilden R, Torous J. Assessing mental health apps marketplaces with objective metrics from 29,190 data points from 278 apps. Acta Psychiatr Scand. 2021;144(2):201–10.
26. Connolly SL, Hogan TP, Shimada SL, Miller CJ. Leveraging implementation science to understand factors influencing sustained use of mental health apps: a narrative review. J Technol Behav Sci. 2021;6:184–96.
27. Connolly SL, Kuhn E, Possemato K, Torous J. Digital clinics and mobile technology implementation for mental health care. Curr Psychiatry Rep. 2021;23(7):38.
28. Wisniewski H, Gorrindo T, Rauseo-Ricupero N, Hilty D, Torous J. The role of digital navigators in promoting clinical care and technology integration into practice. Digit Biomark. 2020;4(1):119–35.
29. Emerson MR, Dinkel D, Watanabe-Galloway S, Torous J, Johnson DJ. Adaptation of digital navigation training for integrated behavioral health providers: interview and survey study. Transl Behav Med. 2023;22:ibad016.
30. Goldberg SB, Baldwin SA, Riordan KM, Torous J, Dahl CJ, Davidson RJ, Hirshberg MJ. Alliance with an unguided smartphone app: validation of the digital working alliance inventory. Assessment. 2022;29(6):1331–45.

Part V

Perspectives on Technology, Healthcare and Life

Advancing Mental Health Care: Global Perspectives on Digital and Telepsychiatry Solutions

17

Davor Mucić, Donald M. Hilty, and Peter M. Yellowlees

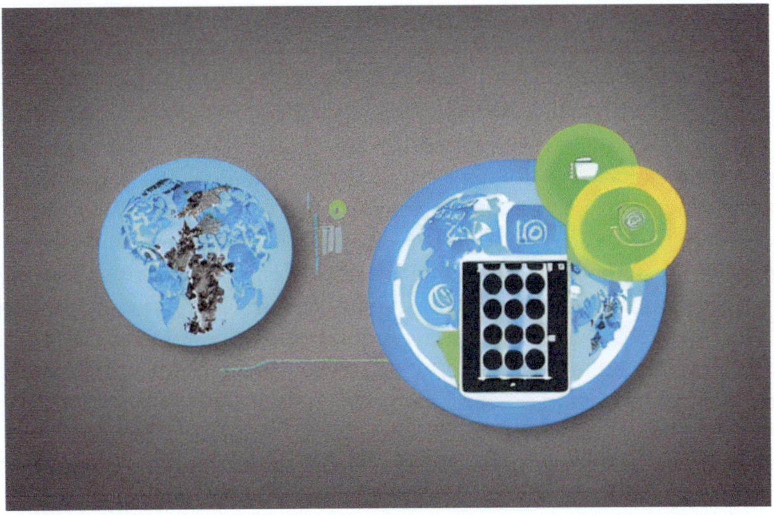

D. Mucić (✉)
The Little Prince Psychiatric Centre, Copenhagen, Denmark
e-mail: davor@denlilleprins.org

D. M. Hilty
Department of Psychiatry and Behavioral Sciences, Keck School of Medicine University of Southern California, Los Angeles, CA, USA
e-mail: donald.hilty@uhsinc.com; hilty@med.usc.edu

P. M. Yellowlees
Department of Psychiatry and Behavioral Sciences, UC Davis, Sacramento, CA, USA
e-mail: pmyellowlees@ucdavis.edu

D. Mucić, D. M. Hilty (eds.), *Digital Mental Health*,
https://doi.org/10.1007/978-3-031-59936-1_17

Abstract

Telemedicine and Internet-based clinical systems are already widely accessible and beginning to affect the dynamics between doctors and patients. Studies have demonstrated that online mental health interventions are just as beneficial as conventional in-person counseling for illnesses like anxiety and depression. We look into how new technologies and clinical procedures (e.g., like the employment of virtual patient advocates) are being incorporated into patient care and how it may be affecting the doctor–patient relationship. In order to better serve underprivileged people, especially those from varied cultural backgrounds, it is likely that clinical practices will change over time. New hybrid care models with synchronous and asynchronous technologies will emerge in creative ways. Research on user-centered design and implementation is important.

17.1 Introduction

Telemedicine and clinical systems enabled by the Internet are currently widely accessible and are beginning to affect the dynamics between doctors and patients, with this trend expected to continue in the future. Telemedicine consultations have become so ubiquitous that they are now routinely conducted via broadband Internet systems hosted in the cloud. This has enabled professionals from various fields within mental health (MH), including psychiatrists, psychologists, marriage and family therapists, and career counselors, to offer e-therapy services. Yellowlees and Nafiz [1] have described how MH resources and services available to patients at home or in the community may be provided through a multitude of Internet devices, ranging from computers to iPhones, including:

- Online/video/telephone-based patient support groups and websites for health information
- Telepsychiatry consultations and email/phone/instant messaging with physicians and other providers from fixed and mobile locations
- Multimedia educational materials developed by patients and providers for both patient and provider education
- Scheduling systems, personal electronic health records, and tools for self-directed decision support and chronic disease management

Mobile applications created expressly to assist people in managing their mental health are available in addition to the aforementioned resources. These apps might have functions like mood tracking, cognitive behavioral therapy (CBT) activities, relaxation and meditation approaches, and custom coping mechanisms.

Commercial websites that provide telepsychiatry services offer not only information about how telepsychiatry works but also a range of services, including mental health consultations for clients in both larger and smaller cities, as well as more remote communities, prisons, and clinics. These services have the potential to increase access to mental health care for underserved populations who may have difficulty accessing traditional in-person care. The patients who received telepsychiatry services reported high levels of satisfaction with the care they received, and that telepsychiatry was associated with lower costs and fewer missed appointments compared to in-person care [2]. Telepsychiatry consultations are now well established with guidelines existing for both adult and child psychiatry and have been demonstrated to be diagnostically valid and show substantial patient satisfaction [3, 4].

However, there are also concerns about the quality of care provided through telepsychiatry, particularly in cases where the patient and clinician have never met in person. Despite the fact that the quality of psychiatric evaluations conducted via telepsychiatry was not significantly different from in-person evaluations, the clinicians reported feeling less confident in their ability to diagnose and treat patients remotely [5]. According to a 2021 survey conducted by Pew Research Center, 85% of Americans now own smartphones, up from 81% in 2019. Additionally, the same survey found that 51% of adults have used their phone to look up health information, up from 35% in 2012 [6].

Mood-tracking applications for smartphones have become increasingly popular and numerous in recent years. These apps enable users to monitor their mood as well as other mental health-related symptoms and habits.

Some examples of mood-tracking applications for smartphones:

- Daylio: A mood-tracking app that allows users to log their daily activities and rate their mood. The app also includes a diary feature and the ability to set custom reminders.
- Moodfit: This app helps users track their mood over time, providing insights into patterns and triggers. It includes a mood journal, guided meditations, and personalized coping strategies.
- eMoods: Created especially for those with bipolar disorder, it enables the users to keep tabs on their symptoms, meds, and mood. The app also produces reports that may be distributed to health care professionals.
- MoodCast: This app uses artificial intelligence (AI) to analyze patterns in the user's mood data and provides personalized insights and recommendations. It also includes a journal feature and the ability to track daily habits.
- Mood tracker: A simple and intuitive app for tracking mood, emotions, and energy levels. Users can view their mood history and track progress over time. The app also includes customizable reminders and a daily mood quiz.

Research has shown that mood-tracking apps can provide objective measures of bipolar disorder symptoms and reduce depression and anxiety symptoms [7]. The app used in another study showed an improvement in self-awareness and emotional regulation in individuals with bipolar disorder, allowing users to track their mood, sleep, and medication adherence and providing personalized feedback and coping strategies [8]. Smartphone sensors could be used to monitor the behavior and mental health, paving the way for next-generation psychiatric assessment [9]. Apps that track mood can also help depressed people better manage their mental health and promote self-management. Users could monitor their mood, sleep, and physical activity on the study's app, which also included tools for establishing goals and individualized feedback [10]. However, there are also concerns about the quality and effectiveness of some mood-tracking apps. Therefore it is essential to choose an app that is evidence-based, user-friendly, and aligned with individual needs and goals while some apps may be helpful for individuals with bipolar disorder, there is a lack of evidence-based research on the effectiveness of many mood-tracking apps [11].

Free self-help websites include advice, support, and a range of tools, such as reading lists, quizzes, and evidence-based therapy techniques. The National Institute for Mental Health Research at the Australian National University developed the free self-help website MoodGYM. CBT techniques are used by the MoodGYM interactive online application to help people manage their anxiety and depression symptoms.

Self-help websites can be useful resources for treating mental condition symptoms. Internet-based CBT (iCBT) interventions were effective in reducing symptoms of depression and anxiety, and that the effects were sustained over time [12]. A guided self-help program for social anxiety disorder delivered via a website was effective in reducing symptoms of social anxiety [13]. Online mental health interventions can be a successful substitute by offering people with mental health illnesses convenient and accessible help. Online cognitive behavioral therapy (iCBT) has equal effects as the in-person approach on treating conditions including panic disorder and agoraphobia [14]. Further, both online CBT and psychoeducation are effective in reducing symptoms of depression [12].

This chapter will help the reader review trends in international Digital Mental Health (DMH) care: (1) the best of what is being done now with new technologies, (2) the application of new technologies to patient care (e.g., virtual patient advocates [VPAs]), and (3) how we will move forward with changes in clinical processes, models of care (e.g., hybrids), applying new developments to the underserved (e.g., cross-cultural populations), and sizing up even newer technologies over the next decade or two.

17.2 Impact on the Doctor–Patient Relationship

The doctor–patient connection is crucial to the therapeutic process. Michael Balint described the doctor–patient relationship as a three-stage process in his book *The Doctor, His Patient, and the Illness*. These stages are the gathering of symptoms from the patient (including physical and mental state exams), diagnostic evaluation, and attempting to reach a mutual understanding of a management plan [15].

Balint's study of the doctor–patient relationship has been extremely beneficial to the fields of many mental health care professions including psychiatry. His approach emphasizes the importance of communication, empathy, and collaboration between the doctor and the patient in promoting healing and achieving positive outcomes. Ever since there were many studies that have investigated the importance of the doctor–patient relationship on treatment outcomes, and have shown that a strong relationship can lead to better outcomes, improved patient satisfaction, and better adherence to treatment [16, 17]. Due to provider shortages and limited access to care, there is a need to be creative, i.e., "think out of the box," and utilize technology on a larger scale. Digital mental health treatments (DMHTs) utilize widely available devices such as smartphones, tablets, and computers to provide treatment, education, and support for self-management skills related to mental health [18]. Numerous randomized controlled trials (RCTs) have repeatedly shown that DMH therapies are successful in treating depression and anxiety [19–21]. According to studies, it is possible to create a fruitful therapeutic relationship when using a variety of different technology-based depression interventions [22]. However, DMHTs that are self-guided may provide only modest benefits [12]. On the contrary, studies have shown that when a DMHT is supported by a human coach or care manager, the effect sizes can be similar to those seen for psychotherapy [23, 24].

E-therapy, also known as online therapy, teletherapy, or virtual therapy, provides mental health support from any location. Some forms of online therapy include texts, emails, phone calls, and video services [25].

E-therapy offers flexibility, accessibility, and affordability to patients who may otherwise struggle to access mental health services. The use of email in therapy can create a "zone of reflection" that allows clients to slow down and pay closer attention to their thoughts and feelings during therapy sessions. This can lead to a deeper exploration of issues and may facilitate the therapeutic process. The use of email as an adjunct to therapy has both costs and benefits. While it appears to have a positive impact on treatment efficacy, it requires an additional expenditure of therapist time [26].

Another advantage of email therapy is that it allows clients to express themselves in writing, which may be particularly beneficial for those who struggle to communicate verbally. There were no significant differences found in patients' perceptions of effective communication when using IT-mediated communication compared to in-person communication with their physicians [27].

While the benefits of emails in enhancing communication were recognized by both patients and providers, concerns about confidentiality and security were also expressed [28].

Note that not all patients or diseases are candidates for email therapy, though.

To ensure effective e-therapy, it is crucial that both practitioners and clients appreciate the limitations of this medium. Therefore, practitioners need to:

- Assess if the client is suitable for online treatment, taking into consideration if the client is in immediate crisis, is engaged in active suicidal ideation, or if there are other serious concerns such as domestic violence or severe drug use.
- Have backup resources in place to address urgent issues.
- Educate clients and provide informed consent.
- Assess the suitability of clients and work within ethical parameters.

One of the numerous benefits of e-therapy is the convenience of obtaining care in the privacy of your own home rather than having to travel to a mental health care expert. It makes mental health care accessible to people with limited mobility or those who reside in rural places by removing time and geographic constraints. Clients may feel less inhibited when receiving counseling online than they would in an in-person situation, making them more comfortable discussing difficult issues. Clients claimed that Internet counseling was more comfortable than in-person counseling for discussing delicate subjects [29].

One issue with online therapy is the artificial distance created between the doctor and the client, and researchers have argued that this can have both positive and negative consequences. The clinical limitations of distance involve a lack of visual and auditory cues, body language, and spontaneous clarification (if communication is via email or text), which can be very important in some instances in therapy. However, with treatments of disorders that have a potential element of shame, stigma, or embarrassment, such as post-traumatic stress disorder (PTSD), eating disorders, or for those struggling with social anxiety, the prospect of receiving treatment from a distance can be appealing [30].

Moreover, the use of videoconferencing, i.e., telepsychiatry, both synchronous and asynchronous (i.e., store-and-forward), has been widely adopted, particularly during the coronavirus disease-2019 (COVID-19) pandemic [31]. When clinical, technical, and practical preconditions were met, video consultations appeared safe and were popular with some patients and staff. Compared with in-person consultations for similar conditions, video consultations were very slightly shorter, patients did slightly more talking, and both parties sometimes needed to make explicit things that typically remained implicit in a traditional encounter. Video consultations appeared to work better when the clinician and patient already knew and trusted each other [32].

While telepsychiatry has potential benefits, there are also limitations and challenges, such as technical issues and concerns about technology and privacy in rural areas [33]. Children and adolescents are now receiving more mental health care because of telepsychiatry. Telepsychiatry has the benefit of assisting young people in getting the mental health care they need by removing obstacles like distance or transportation problems. Due to shorter wait periods for child and adolescent mental health treatments in rural locations, research has revealed that telepsychiatry is efficient in delivering timely care. Another advantage of telepsychiatry is that it can provide comfortable and familiar setting for the patient. Telepsychiatry is a feasible and acceptable approach to providing psychiatric services to youths in underserved communities. However, sustainability of telepsychiatry is challenged by infrastructure costs and low reimbursement by public payers [34]. Telepsychiatry has been used sparingly, but it is crucial to emphasize. More research is required to determine which conditions and patients are most suitable for telepsychiatry [35]. Chapter 9 provides a detailed exploration of telepsychiatry.

Given the information presented so far, it is reasonable to question how technology affects the patient–doctor relationship. With the advent of DMH technologies, the relationship of the doctor–patient has undoubtedly changed. However, as Andersson has written, "Emerging evidence across trials clearly suggests that the computer cannot totally replace human contact" [30].

Health care professionals can connect with patients at a distance due to the extensive use of telemedicine and other digital health technology. Consequently, it could alter the dynamics of the conventional in-person doctor–patient relationship. Technology can enhance access to treatment, and patient-centered services by making them more affordable and convenient. However, the patient–provider connection could be faced with new obstacles, such as a struggle in building rapport, problems with maintaining privacy and confidentiality, and a potential loss of significant nonverbal cues [36–38]. That is why in-person consultations will probably remain the core of most psychiatrist–patient relationships. Initially, patients may have a traditional in-person visit but this might be followed with video visits such as online therapy and psychoeducation with in-person visits occurring as needed so that increasing numbers of patients and doctors now have a "hybrid relationship."

A key consideration is to determine whether digital communication will supplement or replace traditional modes of health care delivery. With digital communication becoming more prevalent in society, replacing certain aspects of traditional clinical communication with digital methods may be crucial in ensuring access to health care services for those who prefer digital means. However, it is important to find a balance and guarantee that patients may access more conventional health care delivery methods as well.

Further, the role of digital communication technology in overcoming barriers to health care access for marginalized groups cannot be overlooked. Practical access issues, negative experiences with health care providers, and stigmatizing reactions from staff and other patients are some of the main challenges. This technology can provide anonymity and benefits to patients who require an interpreter, thereby reducing patient-related barriers. However, it cannot overcome all barriers, such as the inability to communicate with health care professionals or lack of candidacy. It is also important to note that digital communication technology may work best in the context of an existing clinician–patient relationship [39]. The ability for people to track and monitor their own health data via digital devices also transfers part of the duties and decision-making authority from doctors to patients. As patients become increasingly active in their own care, established roles and responsibilities must change to reflect this. Additionally, doctors must learn to evaluate and use this new data in their clinical decision-making processes [40].

The integration of technology in medicine has brought significant advancements and breakthroughs. To balance technology and patient-centered treatment, however, is essential. Prioritizing patient needs and ensuring that technology enhances rather than replaces the human touch in health care are two things that medical practitioners must do [41, 42].

New technologies are continually being created to enhance the delivery and efficacy of mental health care as the area of DMH continues to advance. As a subset of artificial intelligence, machine learning, for instance, may be a helpful tool for determining which patients may benefit from a specific therapeutic strategy. Additionally, it may lead to more accurate mental health diagnoses and more customized treatment regimens, which would eventually benefit patients [43].

However, Chap. 11 provides more information on the impact of AI on mental health.

There are still discrepancies in access despite the favorable response that telemedicine has received from many patients and health care professionals. Older patients, non-white individuals, those living in rural areas, and those from lower socioeconomic groups continue to use telemedicine at lower rates. One of the causes of this inequality is uneven access to technology, but more investigation is necessary to completely comprehend and solve the problem [44]. As mental health care moves toward using the Internet routinely, ethical and legal concerns arise. These include the use of email in doctor–patient relationships, state licensing and credentialing, confidentiality and privacy, and the right of providers to have a work–life balance. The locus of power in health care is shifting as we move to this future of increasing amounts of care delivered online in one form or another. Instead of the doctor having full control of the patient's needs, a consumerist model has emerged in which patients and their doctors are partners in managing the patient's care. In this new digital age, the relationships between health care practitioners and their patients are increasingly developing into collaborative partnerships as patients have more control over their health care needs than ever before.

Telemedicine will continue to grow as demands for real-time remote delivery systems grow across the health care spectrum. The mental health care field needs to seize this opportunity, as this is clearly where the future of health care is headed.

We have described how mental health care is changing and moving forward in most clinical environments, certainly in Western Countries, and how it is becoming more patient-centric and consumer-focused. But what about the role of those who support patients, i.e., their families, friends, and anyone else who might be what has typically been described in the past as a patient advocate—someone who works with patients to ensure that they receive the best possible care, understands the decisions they have to make, and frequently guides patients through our sometimes highly complicated health system.

Recent technological developments have led to the emergence of novel forms of e-therapy, including virtual reality (VR), which is further discussed in Chap. 10. However, below we will discuss a specific use of VR as a tool for patient advocacy.

17.3 Patient Advocacy in the Present and Future

The role of patient advocates is becoming more crucial as health care systems develop and grow more complex in order to guarantee that patients receive high-quality care. Patients frequently struggle to grasp their medical illnesses and treatments as well as the health care system. Frequently, in situations when they need to make qualified decisions about their health, individuals need the assistance of a patient advocate. Patient advocates can also assist with scheduling appointments and medical tests, and help patients access financial, legal, and social resources. The attributes of patient advocacy are safeguarding (tracking medical errors, and protecting patients from incompetency or misconduct of co-workers and other members of health care team), apprising (providing information about the patient's diagnosis, treatment, and prognosis, suggesting alternatives of health care, and providing information about the discharge program), valuing (maintaining self-control, enabling patients to make decisions freely, maintaining individualization and humanity, maintaining patient privacy, and acting according to the patient's values, culture, beliefs, and preferences), mediating (liaison between patients, families, and health care professionals, being patients' voice, and communicating patient preferences and cultural values to members of the health care team), and championing social justice in the provision of health care (confronting inappropriate policies or rules in the health care system, identifying and correcting inequalities in delivery of health services, and facilitating access to community health services and health resources) [45].

An encouraging advancement in technology, the Virtual Patient Advocate (VPA) is a computerized, animated character designed to integrate best practices from provider–patient communication theory. The VPA emulates the in-person conversational behavior of an empathic clinician, including nonverbal communicative behavior such as gaze, posture, and hand gestures, to deliver patient education messages tailored to individual needs, assess patient comprehension, and record progress. It also allows for sophisticated levels of tailoring of information [46, 47]. VPAs are ideal for delivering Patient Centred Care (PCC) because they can potentially reach a large number of patients, alleviate clinician time restraints, and control costs while simultaneously having high patient acceptability through culturally appropriate content and information appropriate to those with low health literacy [48, 49].

The authors have described a study using a VPA called the Gabby System, which showed that some of the study participants preferred talking to the VPA rather than interacting with a real person [50]. One explanation for this could be that the study demographic was comprised of young women who were "digital natives" and had never known a world without the Internet. A recent study shows that "Gabby" enables end-users to be knowledgeable about their health risks in advance of a staff–client or patient–provider interaction and to be better informed in their separate and collaborative health decision-making. In essence, "Gabby" empowers end-users to be active participants during conversations with their providers [51]. Additional studies on how older populations of patients feel about using avatars as patient advocates are necessary because there may be less enthusiasm for this form of support among patients not familiar with virtual reality (VR) environments.

"Louise" is another VPA system designed to improve and re-engineer hospital discharges while improving patient safety and reducing readmissions [52]. Louise is designed to work with people who have limited computer skills. While it does take some initial nursing time to set up the use of this software program, it has been shown to reduce hospital utilization (readmission and emergency visits). An advantage of using a VPA is that the program avatar can potentially be accessed at the convenience of the patient from wherever he or she may be located and yet it can seem quite real, as if the patient is talking to an actual person.

The use of VPAs for children would be an interesting area of study. Children might find that interacting with a "virtual friend" is less threatening than dealing with an adult, especially if the avatar is also a child. Many children are accustomed to cartoon characters as well as avatars in video games so it might be a very natural transition from those characters to a VPA. The VPA could be tailored to explain things at the level of understanding that is appropriate for the child [53]. The SimCoach project was developed to create virtual human support agents that can act as online guides and therapists and was designed to attract and engage military service members, veterans, and their significant others who might not be inclined to seek help from a live health care provider [54].

SimSensei is a fully automatic system designed to create an engaging in-person interaction with a user. It is an intelligent virtual human designed to "listen" to and analyze the speech and nonverbal cues of a person to make determinations about their emotional state. It was developed as a clinical decision support tool that would complement existing self-assessment questionnaires by giving health care providers quantifiable measures of the user behaviors that are correlated with psychological distress [55].

The virtual therapist model as developed for the SimCoach and SimSensei projects could also be applied to the patient navigator role in future and opens up a whole new style of potentially automated clinical practice, and one where machine-based translation and interpretation programs, used across different languages, could potentially open up a global market. Robotic assistance is expected to provide potential relief in various application areas. At the same time, there was a great need for measures that support professionals in their responsibility for the care process and consider the professional values of care in the interpersonal relationship [56]. Most likely is that the current role of in-person patient advocates will be taken over or supplemented by virtual patient advocates that use natural language processing and artificial intelligence to provide patient assistance. While it may be unlikely that a robot could be programmed with full human wisdom, there are some examples of partial programming, such as robotic social workers and physical therapists that have been deployed in nursing homes [57, 58], social robots for loneliness, and those providing cognitive assistance to older adults [59]. The potential negative impacts of technology on mental health care are balanced by the potential benefits such as developing behavior-based digital biomarkers, facilitating earlier detection of mental illnesses, and personalized approaches to diagnosis and treatment. It is important to consider ways to develop artificial intelligence to support mental health care while addressing concerns around transparency, trust, and wisdom. Achieving sustainability, implementation, and clinician and patient acceptance will be crucial for the success of these efforts [60].

Although robotic caregiver use is still in its infancy, studies indicate that this technology has the potential to enhance the quality of life for vulnerable groups. However, it is crucial to take into account the moral ramifications of using robots to provide care, including concerns about privacy, autonomy, and human respect. Professional stakeholders have various ethical concerns related to the use of intelligent assistive technology (IAT) in health care. Robots and AI are viewed to be lacking specific essential elements fundamental to the therapeutic patient–nurse relationship, such as empathy [61, 62], friendship [63], mutual trust and human contact [64], insufficient time, and social connection [65]. Finally, the concerns include issues related to autonomy and informed consent, privacy and confidentiality, safety and reliability, and the potential for IAT to reinforce or exacerbate existing inequalities and discrimination [64].

The use of computer-based technologies and processes, such as VPAs and robots, will be encouraged as the future of health care delivery develops. However, there are situations when providing patient care and assistance in-person is the preferable option. This is where a hybrid model of the patient advocate role may prove useful. When accompanying a patient to provider appointments or facilitating the relationship of the patient to the health care provider, being physically present is important. Using fixed and mobile devices as a tool to be "virtually physically present" may allow the patient advocate to become more versatile and to become accessible to remotely located patients. The role of patient advocate and the form that role takes—be it in-person, digital/online, avatar, or some hybrid model of these technologies—should be expressly tied to the patient population for which the role is employed.

17.4 VR Systems: Future Directions

Virtual reality (VR) has drawn a lot of interest as a potentially useful tool for clinical and educational purposes in mental health care. A variety of mental health issues, including PTSD, depression, and anxiety disorders, can be effectively treated by the use of VR [66, 67].

Virtual reality (VR) has become an increasingly popular tool in various professional fields, such as education, marketing, and health care. VR is an effective tool for enhancing student engagement and improving learning outcomes in higher education [68]. The use of VR in health care for patient communication, treatment, and medical training has been highlighted [69]. In addition to training mental health care providers, VR can also be used as an educational tool for patients. VR simulations can be used to help patients learn about their mental health conditions, practice coping skills, and prepare for exposure therapy sessions.

One of the pioneer VR applications is Second Life (www.secondlife.com). It is a VR platform that is open to the public and can be accessed free of charge. Every user is given an avatar that can be customized to reflect one's own physical appearance or character. Avatars can walk, run, or fly from one island to another. Some can go shopping, visit museums, or even go on a date. It all depends on the user's preference and liking. However, Second Life is no longer considered to be one of the leading or more popular VR applications. In recent years, there have been significant advances in VR technology and a range of new VR applications have emerged for mental health care and other purposes. Examples of more popular and widely used VR applications in mental health care include AppliedVR, Brain Power, BraveMind, HealthTech, KindVR, Limbix, Oncomfort, Psious, SnowWorld, Verapy, Virtual Reality Medical Center, and Virtually Better. Augmented/VR-based interventions could potentially improve knowledge, attitudes, and empathy and decrease stigma regarding people with mental illness [70].

Another type of VR platform is a fully immersive system. It offers a "like-being-there" experience as the user is fully surrounded by the simulated environment providing a highly realistic and interactive experience. Fully immersive VR systems are being utilized more frequently in mental health care for a range of functions, including exposure treatment, stress management, and cognitive training [69]. As an illustration, completely immersive VR systems have been used to create simulations of social scenarios that can assist people with social anxiety in practicing and developing their social skills in a secure setting.

Overall, VR has the potential to revolutionize the way mental health care education and training is conducted, offering a safe and effective alternative to traditional methods. Health educators can target many audiences and ethnic groups to promote health awareness, and games, billboards, and videos are simple approaches that can target big audiences. Health care providers can also use these virtual environments to educate their patients about diseases or conditions they may acquire. Instead of flipping through a brochure or going through web pages, VR can offer important and beneficial sources of information with more appealing visual aids, especially in mobile environments.

Before VR can be extensively used in mental health care, there are still issues like cost, accessibility, and ethical concerns that need to be resolved despite its advantages. VR in mental health care is expected to become more popular as technology advances and costs come down.

17.5 Hybrid Care Models Through the Use of Multiple Technologies

In addition to increasing efficacy and efficiency in the delivery of mental health care, hybrid approaches to care have the potential to increase access to mental health care for underserved groups. Virtual hybrid provider–patient connections in digital mental health provide various benefits, including enhanced access to care, comfort and flexibility, increased privacy, cost savings, and increased access to specialist care. By utilizing these technologies, mental health care can be made more easily available, reasonably priced, and efficient for both patients and practitioners.

One example of a successful hybrid approach is the Seattle-based project run by Meyers and her colleagues. They have developed a program that uses a combination of in-person and technological approaches to provide evidence-based assessment and treatment to children with ADHD (attention deficit/hyperactivity disorder) living in several states in the North West USA. In this project, child psychiatrists provide both direct care and education online, patients see physicians, behaviorists, and psychiatrists online and in person, and the whole delivery platform for care and monitoring is online, but focused on primary care clinics, from where all therapy sessions are coordinated. The program uses telepsychiatry to provide remote evaluations, followed by in-person visits with local providers to deliver treatment. It demonstrated the effectiveness of a "remote service" model to treat ADHD in communities with limited access to specialty mental health services [71].

We know that most mental health care takes part in primary care across the world and that most patients with psychiatric disorders never see or are never evaluated by a psychiatrist; such versatile telehealth models help remedy this problem. Myers project has affirmed the contemporary view that psychiatrists may use technology to disseminate their skills (consulting, training, supervision) and develop innovative treatment programs that an interdisciplinary team (primary care providers, behavior therapists, community partners like teachers, family, care coordinators, and psychiatrists) may efficiently deliver.

Other examples of hybrid approaches to care include the use of advanced technology platforms and mobile applications to support mental health treatment and the integration of online therapy sessions into traditional treatment plans. Some platforms are incorporating remote- tracking tools, like wearables and mobile health sensors, to gather patient data in real time and give doctors insights. To improve data security and privacy, these companies are also investigating the use of blockchain technology. AI-powered chatbots, virtual reality therapy, and smartphone apps that use machine learning to personalize treatment plans based on user data can all offer remote, instant support and interventions for mental health problems. However, reliance on conversational assistants for actionable medical information represents a safety risk for patients and consumers. Patients should be cautioned to not use these technologies for answers to medical questions they intend to act on without further consultation from a health care provider [72].

Nevertheless, harnessing machine learning technologies to process big data in health care will allow health care providers and other users to create and contribute to personalized content. These insights may be leveraged to facilitate patient activation and enable patients to make healthy choices, ultimately improving outcomes [73]. The swift advancement of digital technology has facilitated the establishment of a new level of health care provision.

However, while virtual hybrid provider–patient relationships offer many benefits, there are also some potential disadvantages, including technical difficulties (e.g., poor video or audio quality, network connectivity challenges), limited nonverbal cues, limited physical exams, security and privacy risks, digital divide (as virtual platforms may not be accessible to all patients), and lack of personal connection.

Asynchronous telepsychiatry (ATP) encourages *sustainable* integration of technology in the three core components of a traditional doctor–patient interaction: (1) the history and physical exam, (2) assessment and diagnosis, and (3) creation of a treatment plan. ATP, however, has received much less research attention than synchronous telepsychiatry (STP). Yellowlees et al. reported the clinical outcomes of a 2-year randomized controlled clinical trial of STP vs ATP in primary care performed from 2014 to 2018, which showed positive outcomes for both groups, without major differences in efficacy [74–82]. This is the first such study examining the two telepsychiatry modalities from the perspective of both patients and providers. Patients expressed overall satisfaction with both STP and ATP, although ATP reported more concerns due to a slower feedback response than after an STP consultation [83]. Patients have been more satisfied with the delivery of care [84] in addition to the ATP workflow, which allows for more flexible scheduling than STP for both patients and providers [75]. If ATP were to become a regular clinical service, clinician recommendations could go from a 2-week to a 24-h turn-around time [84].

To accelerate the necessary attitudinal changes and minimize the occurrence of the above-mentioned disadvantages, the use of hybrid models of care should be taught in all psychiatric residency programs as well as within other disciplines and at medical and nursing schools. Then we will be able to work on quality improvement, sustainability, new approaches to collecting clinical outcome evidence that are not purely dependent on traditional randomized controlled trials, and the further integration of technology into daily practice to provide the context and the infrastructure for continuing discoveries in science and in psychiatry. In our own MH disciplines, we see the next steps being the further integration and implementation of algorithmically and evidence-driven care within this hybrid model and how we can learn to effectively use mobile technologies.

So, while all of this is exciting and interesting, how does it fit in with global MH services and the provision of cross-cultural internationalized care?

17.6 Applying Technology to Underserved Populations: Cross-Cultural DMH and Trends in International Care

This key section aims to build on the innovations described above and explore how Digital Mental Health (DMH) can improve the quality of care for ethnic minorities worldwide. One of the benefits of DMH is that it has the potential to reduce stigma (which is often culturally conditioned) and increase access to mental health services in this population via digital platforms and mobile applications [85]. Additionally, this section seeks to identify potential obstacles and suggest solutions for the development of both national and international cross-cultural DMH services.

Telemental health is useful in reducing barriers to mental health care access for traditionally marginalized communities, such as those living in remote locations, migrants, refugees, and asylum seekers. Because of the near-ubiquity of smartphones and other Internet-enabled devices, telemental health can cater to the needs of such populations [86].

Although telepsychiatry has been utilized in various forms for several decades, there are still relatively few published reports specifically focused on the use of telepsychiatry to provide MH care to cross-cultural patients [87–89]. As awareness of the need for culturally sensitive care continues to grow, efforts are underway to develop and evaluate telepsychiatry interventions that are tailored to meet the unique needs of diverse patient populations. This includes identifying critical factors to guide the development of culturally informed telehealth services, with a particular focus on meeting the needs of ethnic minorities and promoting equitable access to care and positive health outcomes [90].

Some telepsychiatry studies have focused on transcultural aspects of care, such as providing culturally sensitive care to refugees and immigrants finding that telepsychiatry interventions could be an effective mode of delivery for MH services to this population [91]. Telehealth-delivered care for racial/ethnic minorities offers promise across a range of conditions and outcomes, particularly when delivered in the patient's preferred language. However, telehealth may be problematic for some due to cost and limited digital and health literacy [92].

The term "cross-cultural telepsychiatry" covers the delivery of culturally appropriate MH care from a distance in "real time" by the use of videoconferencing, i.e., "synchronous telepsychiatry" and/or "asynchronous telepsychiatry" ("store and forward" model, where we speak about a transmission of recorded clinical-related material, i.e., assessment, psychiatric interview/consultation between referring physicians and specialist). This approach allows for MH care to be delivered remotely, which can be particularly important for patients who live in areas with limited access to MH services or who may face barriers to accessing care due to cultural or linguistic differences [35].

Chapter 8 provides a detailed elaboration on the issues related to ethnic minorities within mental health care systems worldwide.

Equal access to MH services is a human right for both domestic and immigrant population in modern communities worldwide. However, due to geographical distances and other barriers, e.g., cultural, religious, and linguistic, cross-cultural patient population face difficulties in access to MH professionals in a desired way. Cross-cultural patient treatment within MH care demands a high standard of communication between the patient and the care provider, since linguistic, cultural, or even racial barriers may affect patient satisfaction. Cultural differences and language difficulties result in communication gaps where important nuances are either obscured or missed. In such a situation, both patients and professionals are often exposed to the "lost-in-translation syndrome." Several studies have found that language barriers are associated with lower rates of patient satisfaction and poor care delivery in comparison with care received by patients who speak the language of the care provider [93, 94].

Telemedicine provides operational and logistical efficiencies that enable medical interpreters to be more readily accessible to health care providers and is increasingly being used in hospitals and clinics via mobile carts, tablets, or smartphones. Compared with phone interpretation, videoconferencing enables interpreters to observe and interpret nonverbal cues for the provider [95], making interpreters more available with no need to travel between consultations. The use of videoconferencing for interpretation services has been demonstrated to increase efficiency and decrease costs in various health care settings [96].

An alternative equally innovative, disruptive approach to providing international cross-cultural care is the use of language translation smartphone apps. The neural Machine Translation (MT) model utilizes artificial intelligence to acquire linguistic skills and continuously enhance its understanding, in a manner similar to neural networks in the human brain. Once trained, it is faster, more precise, and simpler to incorporate new languages. It is currently the most commonly employed form of machine translation. The technology used in neural (MT) models can also be applied to speech-to-speech translation, which is commonly known as simultaneous interpretation. This involves translating spoken language in real time, allowing individuals who speak different languages to communicate with each other effectively.

The same underlying principles of neural MT, involving artificial intelligence and machine learning, are used in developing speech-to-speech translation technology.

Tougas et al. [97] have identified that patients with Limited English Proficiency (LEP) frequently receive substandard health care and proposed that the addition of automated speech recognition (ASR) and automated machine translation (AMT) technologies to asynchronous telepsychiatry (ATP) may be a viable artificial intelligence (AI)-language interpretation option. They measured the frequency and accuracy of translation of figurative language devices (FLDs—such as similes and metaphors), and the patient word count per minute in a subset of psychiatric interviews from a larger trial, as an approximation to patient speech complexity and quantity in clinical encounters requiring interpretation. Six patients were selected from the original trial, where they had undergone two assessments, once by an English-speaking psychiatrist through a Spanish-speaking human interpreter and once in Spanish by a trained mental health interviewer-researcher with AI-interpretation. Three patients were interviewed via videoconferencing because of the COVID-19 pandemic. Interview transcripts were created by ASR with manual corrections for *transcriptional* accuracy and assessment for *translational* accuracy of FLDs. Both human and AI-interpreted FLDs were frequently translated inaccurately, while human-interpreted interviews were found to have a significant reduction in the use of FLDs and the patient word count per minute; FLD translation was more accurate on videoconferencing. The authors concluded that AI-interpretation is not sufficiently accurate at this time for use in clinical settings. However, this study suggests that alternatives to human interpretation are needed to circumvent modifications to patients' speech. While AI-interpretation technologies are being further developed using ChatGPT and similar approaches, using videoconferencing for human interpreting may be more accurate than in-person interpreting.

There are several apps that use speech-to-speech translation technology, some of which include:

1. Google Translate: This popular translation app provides speech-to-speech translation for more than 100 languages. It can translate spoken words and phrases in real time.
2. iTranslate: This app offers speech-to-speech translation for more than 100 languages, as well as text translation and voice recognition.
3. SayHi Translate: SayHi Translate provides speech-to-speech translation for more than 90 languages, with the ability to save commonly used phrases for future use.
4. Microsoft Translator: This app supports speech-to-speech translation for more than 60 languages, as well as text translation and image translation.
5. TripLingo: This app provides speech-to-speech translation for several languages, along with features such as local dialects, cultural information, and a built-in phrasebook.

Accordingly, automated speech recognition and MT technologies can be used to facilitate cross-cultural communication in health care settings. DMH applications offer new possibilities for reducing disparities in access to relevant mental health care to the most vulnerable patient groups, such as refugees, migrants, and asylum seekers worldwide. The use of technology services/applications described in this book has the potential to provide efficient and cost-effective opportunities to reach individuals and groups with poor service access despite geographical distances and/or national borders.

However, when it comes to remote real-time DMH consultations via video conferencing, there are only a few studies describing international, cross-border studies and none involve developing countries [98]. A consulting psychiatrist was licensed in Australia, but living in New Zealand, provided care for two patients in a facility in Australia; one of the cases was a new consultation and the other was a follow-up [99]. A 6-month trial of telepsychiatry tertiary care from South London to the Island of Jersey reported five teleconsultations of a single second opinion and four case reviews [100]. International tele-education for Swedish medical students about cross-cultural issues in refugees with MH problems was conducted between Sweden, the USA, and Australia. There was one real patient at the American site and one simulated patient at the Australian site, with patient interviews by experts while medical students were observed via videoconference and participated in the discussion [101]. Videoconferencing provided psychoanalytic clinical care and training to psychoanalytic candidates in China by US psychoanalysts, and this involved 40 psychoanalytic and 30 psychodynamic psychotherapies [102].

The most comprehensive international telepsychiatry service in the world was established in Denmark in mid-2006 as a part of cross-cultural telepsychiatry pilot-project launched by The Little Prince Psychiatric Centre located in Copenhagen [103, 104]. Due to lack of bilingual clinicians in Denmark, psychiatrists who spoke Arabic, Polish, Kurdish, and ex-Yugoslavian languages, but were physically located in Sweden, were employed to provide care due to their cross-cultural skills. Furthermore, bilingual psychiatrists not only have the selected skills but also a detailed knowledge of the MH system in Scandinavia as well as knowledge about health systems in the patients' home countries. Over a period of 18 months, 31 patients (i.e., refugees, migrants, and asylum seekers) were assessed and treated via video conferencing by providers who spoke the patients' own language. Videoconferencing equipment connected the Swedish Department of the Little Prince Psychiatric Centre with two hospitals, one asylum seekers' center and one social institution in Denmark. The distances from the Swedish station located in Malmö to the Danish telepsychiatry stations were from 140 to 300 km. Overall, high patient satisfaction was reported and minor disadvantages were offset by the fact that the doctors and the patients linguistically and culturally matched. The use of bilingual clinicians with a similar ethnic and cultural background to their patients compensates for the distance and lack of physical presence.

Experiences from projects over the last decade—described above and in Chap. 8—may pave the way for development of an International DMH Network within the European Union (EU). The initiative can be taken for various reasons.

The misdiagnosis of mental disorders is a significant issue that happens in primary and secondary care mental health settings as well as in general practitioner (GP) settings. Mental health professionals misdiagnose 69% of patients with bipolar disorder [105]. On average, patients remain misdiagnosed for 5.0–7.5 years [106]. Only 47.3% of patients with depression are correctly diagnosed by GPs [107].

As a consequence, the global gap between the need for treatment and its provision is large. Regardless of the severity of the symptoms, receiving an initial psychiatric assessment and following medical care typically takes 7–30 days in the majority of EU countries [108]. However, in low- and middle-income countries, between 76% and 85% of people with severe mental disorders receive no treatment. For high-income countries, the corresponding range is also wide (between 35% and 50%) [109]. Furthermore, untreated medical conditions are prevalent among individuals with psychiatric illnesses [110].

Based on all of the above, the idea of better national but no less international cooperation and exchange of expertise across national borders sounds logical [111]. Clinical and scientific objectives and goals of such international DMH service are to:

1. Improve the mental health care across national boundaries by providing psychiatric consultations between countries within the EU
2. Develop international treatment teams with select skills (e.g., sign language and many foreign languages staff)
3. Provide acute psychiatric assessments at a distance
4. Establish a second opinion service and shared care service between MH professionals and general practitioners
5. Improve discharge planning by involvement of clinicians with specialized skills and expertise
6. Develop subsequent follow-up service via videoconferencing
7. Increase access to child, adult, geriatric, forensic, and deaf services specialty staff
8. Provide distance supervision and staff consultation
9. Provide psychoeducation to patients' family members
10. Improve distance learning via case conferencing and best practice demonstration across the national boundaries
11. Create a database over cross-cultural and other select skills professionals within the EU

The potential outcomes of the above are many:

1. Increased access to specialized expertise (e.g., sign language and many foreign languages staff)
2. Increased speed and accuracy of diagnosis and treatment that otherwise will be provided by translators
3. Increased access to child, adult, geriatric, forensic, and deaf services specialty staff
4. Increased continuity of care and professional contact

5. Improved education of the stuff and psychoeducation of the patients and their family members
6. Increased efficiency and effectiveness through improved performance
7. Cost benefits as a result of reduced staff and translator costs: travel time, staff time, decreased use of translators
8. Reduced waiting time/waiting lists for the treatment due to increased access to respective resources
9. Decrease in the number of inappropriate admissions and readmissions into the acute sector

Finally, the international digital mental health network established in 2019 consists of top clinicians, regulatory and information and communications technology (ICT) experts, genetic scientists, and support organizations with long-standing experience and highly recognized expertise in mental health, e-health infrastructures, and decision support systems. The current international consortium aims to implement Integrated Proactive Approach (i-PROACH) principles into everyday practice within a range of geographically and socioeconomically diverse countries in order to improve identification, management, and prevention of mental disorders via digitized and personalized approaches, and to contribute to overall improvements in mental health services [112]. Perhaps this is the first step in establishing more extensive international cooperation in accordance with the above-suggested International DMH Network.

International collaboration and policy development are critical for the effective implementation and advancement of digital mental health services. That is why it is important to mention a collaborative effort across Europe to develop and implement digital mental health services within the eMEN ("e-mental health innovation and transnational implementation platform, North-West Europe") project. It is a six-country project aiming to increase the implementation of high-quality DMH lunched in May 2016 [113]. Within eMEN, the project partners from Belgium, France, Germany, Ireland, the Netherlands, and the United Kingdom carry out a unique combination of activities in research, product development, policy guidance development, and communications, and initiate a transnational cooperation platform for DMH stakeholders. One of the key outcomes of the project is the development of a Transnational Policy, which outlines the framework for the implementation and scaling up of digital mental health services in different countries [114].

And while digitalization in developed countries enables better access to care, at the same time lack of access to technology creates increased disparities. For underserved groups like non-Indigenous racial and ethnic minorities who already experience health disparities, there is a risk that care quality could be compromised and new access obstacles may arise [115].

Despite the rise in telemedicine use during the COVID-19 pandemic, there are still sizable gaps that need to be filled before widespread usage can occur. Some of the major issues that need to be addressed include: (1) establishing adequate policies to legislate telemedicine, license health care operators, protect patients' privacy, and implement reimbursement plans; (2) creating and disseminating practical guidelines for the routine clinical use of telemedicine in different contexts; (3) increasing the level of integration of telemedicine with traditional health care services; (4) improving health care professionals' and patients' awareness of and willingness to use telemedicine; and (5) overcoming inequalities among countries and population subgroups due to technological, infrastructural, and economic barriers. If all these requirements are met in the near future, remote management of patients will become an indispensable resource for health care systems worldwide and will ultimately improve the management of patients and the quality of care [31].

As technology advances, it becomes increasingly clear that differences in access to technology can lead to differences in access to care. This is particularly true for refugees, who may face additional barriers to accessing health care services, including language barriers and a lack of familiarity with the health care system in their new country. For underserved groups who already experience health disparities, there is a risk that new access obstacles may arise. Even though many people's access to care may be improved by new technologies, those without dependable Internet or mobile connectivity risk falling behind, e.g., refugees, who face financial constraints and limited access to technology. Furthermore, language barriers can make it difficult for refugees to access digital health platforms that may not be available in their native language. This can be particularly problematic in mental health care, where cultural and linguistic barriers already create additional challenges.

Health care disparities can be exacerbated by the use of technology. Recognizing its potential is crucial for health care providers and policymakers in order to address these inequalities. This may involve developing multilingual platforms, providing refugees with access to affordable technology, and providing education and training to help refugees navigate the health care system.

There are three key areas related to standards in design and development related to technology, health, and cultural literacy: usability testing and evaluation; post-deployment monitoring; and patient safety user-centered design (UCD) and system implementation [116, 117]. Challenges to assessing technology usability include the complexity of the technology. For example, with the electronic health record, it is important to consider interaction with the full socio-technical context in which it is used, the professional roles of the intended users, the peculiarities of the clinical collaboration patterns, and the difficulty in measuring the influence that systems have on downstream processes.

17.7 Conclusions

The field of mental health care is changing due to digital mental health advancements. While the COVID-19 pandemic has led to some of these changes, many were already underway and are likely to continue and grow in the coming years. The use of DMH will transform mental health care, making it more "user-friendly," flexible, productive, and responsive to patients' needs. Like with any new technology, it is crucial to thoroughly consider privacy, security, confidentiality, and cultural sensitivity concerns.

The creation of international telepsychiatry services that will permit the exchange of professional expertise and the evaluation and treatment of patients from a distance is anticipated as a result of the development of new technological devices and telecommunication technologies. These services allow patients to receive care in their native tongues rather than through interpreters, thereby facilitating cross-cultural care. This will not only enhance patient outcomes and satisfaction but also assist in lowering linguistic barriers, which can result in less effective health care.

However, there are several prerequisites to achieving the establishment of international services for telemedicine and telepsychiatry to provide care in patients' respective mother tongues. One of these is the creation and application of trustworthy and accurate language translation technologies. Another is the standardization and control of telemedicine procedures across various nations and areas. Additionally, ensuring the privacy and security of patient information across borders and addressing legal and ethical concerns related to providing health care services across international borders are also important factors to consider. The adoption and implementation of these technologies and services require improved patient and health care professional education and training, as well as general awareness of them.

References

1. Yellowlees PM, Nafiz N. The psychiatrist-patient relationship of the future: anytime, anywhere? Rev Psychiatry. 2010;18(2):96–102.
2. Fortney JC, Pyne JM, Turner EE, Farris KM, Normoyle TM, Avery MD, Hilty DM, Unützer J. Telepsychiatry integration of mental health services into rural primary care settings. Int Rev Psychiatry. 2015;27(6):525–39. https://doi.org/10.3109/09540261.2015.1085838. Epub 2015 Dec 4.
3. Mackinnon A, Griffiths KM, Christensen H. Comparative randomised trial of online cognitive-behavioural therapy and an information website for depression: 12-months outcomes. Br J Psychiatry. 2008;192(2):130–4.
4. Neufeld JD, Bourgeois JA, Hilty DM, et al. The e-Mental Health Consult Service: providing enhanced primary care mental health services through telemedicine. Psychosomatics. 2007;48:135–41.
5. Shore JH, Schneck CD, Mishkind MC. Telepsychiatry and the coronavirus disease 2019 pandemic-current and future outcomes of the rapid virtualization of psychiatric care. JAMA Psychiatry. 2020;77(12):1211–2. https://doi.org/10.1001/jamapsychiatry.2020.1643.
6. Pew Research Center. Mobile fact sheet. 2021. https://www.pewresearch.org/internet/fact-sheet/mobile/.
7. Faurholt-Jepsen M, Vinberg M, Christensen EM, Frost M, Bardram JE, Kessing LV. Daily electronic self-monitoring in bipolar disorder using smartphones—the MONARCA I trial: a randomized, placebo-controlled, single-blind, parallel group trial. J Med Internet Res. 2015;17(7):e193. https://doi.org/10.2196/jmir.4205.
8. Nicholas J, Fogarty AS, Boydell K, Christensen H. The reviews are in: a qualitative content analysis of consumer perspectives on apps for bipolar disorder. J Affect Disord. 2017;227:716–24. https://doi.org/10.1016/j.jad.2017.11.058.
9. Ben-Zeev D, Scherer EA, Wang R, Xie H, Campbell AT. Next-generation psychiatric assessment: using smartphone sensors to monitor behavior and mental health. Psychiatr Rehabil J. 2015;38(3):218–26. https://doi.org/10.1037/prj0000130.

10. Faurholt-Jepsen M, Frost M, Martiny K, Tuxen N, Rosenberg N, Busk J, et al. Reducing the rate and duration of Re-Admissions among patients with unipolar disorder and bipolar disorder using smartphone-based monitoring and treatment—The RADMIS trials. J Technol Behav Sci. 2015;1(3):96–104. https://doi.org/10.1007/s41347-016-0002-x.
11. Torous J, Roberts LW, Joyce M. The problem with mobile apps for bipolar disorder. JAMA Psychiatry. 2017;74(9):895–6. https://doi.org/10.1001/jamapsychiatry.2017.1112.
12. Karyotaki E, Riper H, Twisk J, Hoogendoorn A, Kleiboer A, Mira A, Mackinnon A, Meyer B, Botella C, Littlewood E, Andersson G, Christensen H, Klein JP, Schröder J, Bretón-López J, Scheider J, Griffiths K, Farrer L, Huibers MJ, Phillips R, Gilbody S, Moritz S, Berger T, Pop V, Spek V, Cuijpers P. Efficacy of self-guided internet-based cognitive behavioral therapy in the treatment of depressive symptoms: a meta-analysis of individual participant data. JAMA Psychiatry. 2017;74(4):351–9. https://doi.org/10.1001/jamapsychiatry.2017.0044.
13. Titov N, Dear BF, Staples LG, Terides MD, Karin E, Sheehan J, Johnston L, Gandy M, Fogliati VJ, Wootton BM, McEvoy PM. Disorder-specific versus transdiagnostic and clinician-guided versus self-guided treatment for major depressive disorder and comorbid anxiety disorders: a randomized controlled trial. J Anxiety Disord. 2015;35:88–102. https://doi.org/10.1016/j.janxdis.2015.08.002.
14. Andersson G, Carlbring P, Berger T, Almlöv J, Cuijpers P. What makes internet therapy work? Cogn Behav Ther. 2009;38(1):55–60. https://doi.org/10.1080/16506070902916400.
15. Balint M. The doctor, his patient, and the illness. Madison: International Universities Press; 1957.
16. DiMatteo MR. Variations in patients' adherence to medical recommendations: a quantitative review of 50 years of research. Med Care. 2004;42(3):200–9. https://doi.org/10.1097/01.mlr.0000114908.90348.f9.
17. Beach MC, Roter DL, Wang NY, Duggan PS, Cooper LA. Are physicians' attitudes of respect accurately perceived by patients and associated with more positive communication behaviors? Patient Educ Couns. 2006;62(3):347–54. https://doi.org/10.1016/j.pec.2006.06.004.
18. Mohr DC, Azocar F, Bertagnolli A, Choudhury T, Chrisp P, Frank R, Harbin H, Histon T, Kaysen D, Nebeker C, Richards D, Schueller SM, Titov N, Torous J, Arean PA, Banbury Forum on Digital Mental. Banbury forum consensus statement on the path forward for digital mental health treatment. Psychiatr Serv. 2021;72(6):677–83. https://doi.org/10.1176/appi.ps.202000561.
19. Linardon J, Cuijpers P, Carlbring P, Messer M, Fuller-Tyszkiewicz M. The efficacy of app-supported smartphone interventions for mental health problems: a meta-analysis of randomized controlled trials. World Psychiatry. 2019;18:325–36. https://doi.org/10.1002/wps.
20. Andrews G, Basu A, Cuijpers P, Craske MG, McEvoy P, English CL, Newby JM. Computer therapy for the anxiety and depression disorders is effective, acceptable and practical health care: an updated meta-analysis. J Anxiety Disord. 2018;55:70–8.
21. Weisel KK, Fuhrmann LM, Berking M, Baumeister H, Cuijpers P, Ebert DD. Standalone smartphone apps for mental health-a systematic review and meta-analysis. NPJ Digit Med. 2019;2:118.
22. Wehmann E, Köhnen M, Härter M, Liebherz S. Therapeutic alliance in technology-based interventions for the treatment of depression: systematic review. J Med Internet Res. 2020;22(6):e17195.
23. Andersson G, Topooco N, Havik O, Nordgreen T. Internet-supported versus face-to-face cognitive behavior therapy for depression. Expert Rev Neurother. 2016;16:55–60.
24. Nicholas J, Knapp AA, Vergara JL, Graham AK, Gray EL, Lattie EG, Kwasny MJ, Mohr DC. An exploratory brief head-to-head non-inferiority comparison of an internet-based and a telephone-delivered CBT intervention for adults with depression. J Affect Disord. 2021;281:673–7.
25. Maheu MM, Pulier ML, Wilhelm FH, McMenamin JP, Brown-Connolly NE. The mental health professional and the new technologies: a handbook for practice today. 1st ed. London: Routledge; 2004. https://doi.org/10.4324/9781410611444.

26. Murdoch JW, Connor-Greene PA. Enhancing therapeutic impact and therapeutic alliance through electronic mail homework assignments. J Psychother Pract Res. 2000;9(4):232–7.
27. Mirzaei T, Kashian N. Revisiting effective communication between patients and physicians: cross-sectional questionnaire study comparing text-based electronic versus face-to-face communication. J Med Internet Res. 2020;22(5):e16965. https://doi.org/10.2196/16965.
28. Ye J, Rust G, Fry-Johnson Y, Strothers H. E-mail in patient-provider communication: a systematic review. Patient Educ Couns. 2010;80(2):266–73. https://doi.org/10.1016/j.pec.2009.09.038.
29. Richardson LK, Frueh BC, Grubaugh AL, Egede L, Elhai JD. Current directions in videoconferencing tele-mental health research. Clin Psychol. 2014;21(3):223–38.
30. Andersson G, Carlbring P, Holmstrom A, et al. Internet-based self-help with therapist feedback and in vivo group exposure for social phobia: a randomized controlled trial. J Consult Clin Psychol. 2006;74(4):677–86.
31. Omboni S, Padwal RS, Alessa T, Benczúr B, Green BB, Hubbard I, Kario K, Khan NA, Konradi A, Logan AG, Lu Y, Mars M, McManus RJ, Melville S, Neumann CL, Parati G, Renna NF, Ryvlin P, Saner H, Schutte AE, Wang J. The worldwide impact of telemedicine during COVID-19: current evidence and recommendations for the future. Connected Health. 2022;1(1):7–35.
32. Greenhalgh T, Shaw S, Wherton J, Vijayaraghavan S, Morris J, Bhattacharya S, Hanson P, Campbell-Richards D, Ramoutar S, Collard A, Hodkinson I. Real-world implementation of video outpatient consultations at macro, meso, and micro levels: mixed-method study. J Med Internet Res. 2018;20(4):e150.
33. Barnett ML, Ray KN, Souza J, Mehrotra A. Trends in telemedicine use in a large commercially insured population, 2005-2017. JAMA. 2018;320(20):2147–9.
34. Myers KM, Valentine JM, Melzer SM. Feasibility, acceptability, and sustainability of telepsychiatry for children and adolescents. Psychiatr Serv. 2007;58(11):1493–6.
35. Hilty DM, Ferrer DC, Counsel SR, Parish MB, Johnston B, Callahan EJ, Yellowlees PM. The effectiveness of telemental health: a 2013 review. J Med Internet Res. 2013;19(2):e45.
36. Powell KR. Patient-perceived facilitators of and barriers to electronic portal use: a systematic review. Comput Inform Nurs. 2017;35(11):565–73.
37. Gesulga JM, Berjame A, Moquiala KS, Galido A. Barriers to electronic health record system implementation and information systems resources: a structured review. In: Proceedings of the 4th Information Systems International Conference; Bali, Indonesia, 2017, p. 544–551.
38. Entzeridou E, Markopoulou E, Mollaki V. Public and physician's expectations and ethical concerns about electronic health record: benefits outweigh risks except for information security. Int J Med Inform. 2018;110:98–107.
39. Huxley CJ, Atherton H, Watkins JA, Griffiths F. Digital communication between clinician and patient and the impact on marginalised groups: a realist review in general practice. Br J Gen Pract. 2015;65(641):e813–21.
40. Jongsma KR, Bekker MN, Haitjema S, Bredenoord AL. How digital health affects the patient-physician relationship: an empirical-ethics study into the perspectives and experiences in obstetric care. Pregnancy Hypertens. 2021;25:81–6.
41. Powell RE, Doty A, Casten RJ, Rovner BW, Rising KL. A qualitative analysis of interprofessional healthcare team members' perceptions of patient barriers to healthcare engagement. BMC Health Serv Res. 2016;16:493. https://doi.org/10.1186/s12913-016-1751-5.
42. Maheu MM, Pulier ML, McMenamin JP, Posen L. Future of telepsychology, telehealth, and various technologies in psychological research and practice. Prof Psychol Res Pract. 2012;43:613–21. https://doi.org/10.1037/a0029357.
43. Chekroud AM, Zotti RJ, Shehzad Z, Gueorguieva R, Johnson MK, Trivedi MH, Cannon TD, Krystal JH, Corlett PR. Cross-trial prediction of treatment outcome in depression: a machine learning approach. Lancet Psychiatry. 2016;3:243–50. https://doi.org/10.1016/S2215-0366(15)00471-X.
44. Shaver J. The state of telehealth before and after the COVID-19 pandemic. Prim Care. 2022;49(4):517–30. https://doi.org/10.1016/j.pop.2022.04.002.

45. Abbasinia M, Ahmadi F, Kazemnejad A. Patient advocacy in nursing: a concept analysis. Nurs Ethics. 2020;27(1):141–51. https://doi.org/10.1177/0969733019832950.
46. Bickmore T, Gruber A, Picard R. Establishing the computer-patient working alliance in automated health behavior change interventions. Patient Educ Couns. 2005;59:21–30.
47. Bickmore T, Giorgino T. Health dialog systems for patients and consumers. J Biomed Inform. 2006;39:556–71.
48. Bickmore T, Pfeifer L, Jack B. Taking the time to care: empowering low health literacy hospital patients with virtual nurse agents. Comp Med. 2009;10:1265–74.
49. Bickmore TW, Pfeifer LM, Byron D, et al. Usability of conversational agents by patients with inadequate health literacy: evidence from two clinical trials. J Health Commun. 2010;15(2):197–210.
50. Gardiner P, Hempstead MB, Ring L, et al. Reaching women through health information technology: the Gabby preconception care system. Am J Health Promot. 2013;27(3):S11–20. https://doi.org/10.4278/ajhp.1200113-QUAN-18.
51. Walter AW, Julce C, Sidduri N, et al. Study protocol for the implementation of the Gabby Preconception Care System - an evidence-based, health information technology intervention for Black and African American women. BMC Health Serv Res. 2020;20(1):889. https://doi.org/10.1186/s12913-020-05726-0.
52. Jack BW, Bickmore TW. Analysis of patient satisfaction with virtual patient advocate for hospital discharge. 2012. Unpublished raw data.
53. Parsons TD, Rizzo AA, Rogers S, York P. Virtual reality in paediatric rehabilitation: a review. Dev Neurorehabil. 2009;12(4):224–38. https://doi.org/10.1080/17518420902991719.
54. Rizzo A, et al. Virtual realty applications to address the wounds of war. Psychiatr Ann. 2013;43(3):123–38.
55. De Vault R, Artstein G, Benn T, Dey E, Fast A, Gainer K, Georgila J, Gratch A, Hartholt M, Lhommet G, Lucas S, Marsella F, Morbini A, Nazarian S, Scherer G, Stratou A, Suri D, Traum R, Wood Y, Xu A, Rizzo L-P. Morency. SimSensei Kiosk: a virtual human interviewer for healthcare decision support. In Proceedings of AAMAS; 2014.
56. Klebbe R, Klüber K, Dahms R, Onnasch L. Caregivers' perspectives on human–robot collaboration in inpatient elderly care settings. Machines. 2023;11:34. https://doi.org/10.3390/machines11010034.
57. Šabanović S, Chang W-L, Bennett CC, Piatt JA, Hakken D. A robot of my own: participatory design of socially assistive robots for independently living older adults diagnosed with depression. International Conference on Human Aspects of It for the Aged Population; 2015, p. 104–114.
58. Hebesberger D, Koertner T, Gisinger C, Pripfl J, Dondrup C. Lessons learned from the deployment of a long-term autonomous robot as companion in physical therapy for older adults with dementia a mixed methods study. 11th ACM/IEEE International Conference on Human-Robot-Interaction (HRI); 2016, p. 27–34.
59. Graham SA, Lee EE, Jeste DV, Van Patten R, Twamley EW, Nebeker C, et al. Artificial intelligence approaches to predicting and detecting cognitive decline in older adults: a conceptual review. Psychiatry Res. 2020;284:112732.
60. Torous J, Keshavan M, Gutheil T. Promise and perils of using technology to assess and treat mental health problems. Am J Psychiatry Residents J. 2014;9(2):1–5.
61. Metzler TA, Barnes SJ. Three dialogues concerning robots in elder care. Nurs Philos. 2014;15(1):4–13. https://doi.org/10.1111/nup.12027.
62. Luxton DD. Recommendations for the ethical use and design of artificial intelligent care providers. Artif Intell Med. 2014;62(1):1–10. https://doi.org/10.1016/j.artmed.2014.06.004.
63. de Graaf MMA. An ethical evaluation of human-robot relationships. Int J Soc Robot. 2016;8(4):589–98. https://doi.org/10.1007/s12369-016-0368-5.
64. Wangmo T, Lipps M, Kressig RW, Ienca M. Ethical concerns with the use of intelligent assistive technology: findings from a qualitative study with professional stakeholders. BMC Med Ethics. 2019;20(1):98. https://doi.org/10.1186/s12910-019-0437-z.

65. Liang H, Wu K, Weng C, Hsieh H. Nurses' views on the potential use of robots in the pediatric unit. J Pediatr Nurs. 2019;47:e58–64.
66. Carl E, Stein AT, Levihn-Coon A, Pogue JR, Rothbaum B, Emmelkamp P, Asmundson GJG, Carlbring P, Powers MB. Virtual reality exposure therapy for anxiety and related disorders: a meta-analysis of randomized controlled trials. J Anxiety Disord. 2019;61:27–36.
67. Maples-Keller JL, Bunnell BE, Kim S-J, Rothbaum BO. The use of virtual reality technology in the treatment of anxiety and other psychiatric disorders. Harv Rev Psychiatry. 2017;25(3):103–13.
68. Sattar MU, Palaniappan S, Lokman A, Hassan A, Shah N, Riaz Z. Effects of virtual reality training on medical students' learning motivation and competency. Pak J Med Sci. 2019;35(3):852.
69. Freeman D, Reeve S, Robinson A, Ehlers A, Clark D, Spanlang B, Slater M. Virtual reality in the assessment, understanding, and treatment of mental health disorders. Psychol Med. 2017;47(14):2393–400. https://doi.org/10.1017/S003329171700040X.
70. Tay JL, Xie H, Sim K. Effectiveness of augmented and virtual reality-based interventions in improving knowledge, attitudes, empathy and stigma regarding people with mental illnesses—a scoping review. J Pers Med. 2023;13:112. https://doi.org/10.3390/jpm13010112.
71. Myers K, Vander Stoep A, Zhou C, McCarty CA, Katon W. Effectiveness of a telehealth service delivery model for treating attention-deficit/hyperactivity disorder: a community-based randomized controlled trial. J Am Acad Child Adolesc Psychiatry. 2015;54(4):263–74. https://doi.org/10.1016/j.jaac.2015.01.009. Epub 2015 Jan 29. PMID: 25791143; PMCID: PMC4406418.
72. Bickmore TW, Trinh H, Olafsson S, O'Leary TK, Asadi R, Rickles NM, Cruz R. Patient and consumer safety risks when using conversational assistants for medical information: an observational study of Siri, Alexa, and Google Assistant. J Med Internet Res. 2018;20(9):e11510. https://doi.org/10.2196/11510. PMID: 30181110; PMCID: PMC6231817.
73. Guni A, Normahani P, Davies A, Jaffer U. Harnessing machine learning to personalize web-based health care content. J Med Internet Res. 2021;23(10):e25497. https://doi.org/10.2196/25497.
74. Lieng MK, Aurora MS, Kang Y, Kim JM, Marcin JP, Chan SR, Mouzoon JL, et al. Primary care physician adherence to telepsychiatry recommendations: intermediate outcomes from a randomized clinical trial. Telemed J E Health. 2022;28(6):838–46.
75. O'Keefe M, White K, Jennings JC. Asynchronous telepsychiatry: a systematic review. J Telemed Telecare. 2021;27(3):137–45. https://doi.org/10.1177/1357633X19867189. Epub 2019 Jul 29.
76. Yellowlees PM, Parish MB, Gonzalez AD, Chan SR, Hilty DM, Yoo BK, Leigh JP, McCarron RM, Scher LM, Sciolla AF, Shore J, Xiong G, Soltero KM, Fisher A, Fine JR, Bannister J, Iosif AM. Clinical outcomes of asynchronous versus synchronous telepsychiatry in primary care: randomized controlled trial. J Med Internet Res. 2021;23(7):e24047. https://doi.org/10.2196/24047. PMID: 33993104; PMCID: PMC8335606.
77. Parish MB, Gonzalez A, Hilty D, Chan S, Xiong G, Scher L, Liu D, Sciolla A, Shore J, McCarron R, Kahn D, Iosif AM, Yellowlees P. asynchronous telepsychiatry interviewer training recommendations: a model for interdisciplinary, integrated behavioral health care. Telemed J E Health. 2021;27(9):982–8. https://doi.org/10.1089/tmj.2020.0076. Epub 2021 Jan 12. PMID: 33434453; PMCID: PMC8558058.
78. Hilty DM, Torous J, Parish MB, Chan SR, Xiong G, Scher L, Yellowlees PM. A literature review comparing clinicians' approaches and skills to in-person, synchronous, and asynchronous care: moving toward competencies to ensure quality care. Telemed J E Health. 2021;27(4):356–73. https://doi.org/10.1089/tmj.2020.0054. Epub 2020 May 15.
79. Sivakumar PT, Mukku SSR, Kar N, Manjunatha N, Phutane VH, Sinha P, Kumar CN, Math SB. Geriatric telepsychiatry: promoting access to geriatric mental health care beyond the physical barriers. Indian J Psychol Med. 2020;42(5 Suppl):41S–6S. https://doi.org/10.1177/0253717620958380. PMID: 33354062; PMCID: PMC7736734.

80. Yellowlees P, Shore JH. Telepsychiatry and health technologies: a guide for mental health professionals. 1st ed. Washington: American Psychiatric Association Publishing; 2018.
81. Xiong GL, Iosif AM, Godwin HT, Khan M, Parish MB, Yellowlees P, Kahn D. A pilot randomized trial of asynchronous and synchronous telepsychiatry in skilled nursing facilities. J Am Med Dir Assoc. 2018;19(5):461–2. https://doi.org/10.1016/j.jamda.2018.02.007.
82. Yellowlees P, Burke Parish M, González Á, Chan S, Hilty D, Iosif AM, McCarron R, Odor A, Scher L, Sciolla A, Shore J, Xiong G. Asynchronous telepsychiatry: a component of stepped integrated care. Telemed J E Health. 2018;24(5):375–8. https://doi.org/10.1089/tmj.2017.0103. Epub 2017 Oct 12. PMID: 29024612; PMCID: PMC5953215.
83. Yellowlees PM, et al. Patient and provider satisfaction with asynchronous versus synchronous telepsychiatry in primary care: a mixed methods study nested within a randomized controlled trial. In press.
84. Shore JH, Yellowlees P, Caudill R, Johnston B, Turvey C, Mishkind M, Krupinski E, Myers K, Shore P, Kaftarian E, Hilty D. Best practices in videoconferencing-based telemental health April 2018. Telemed J E Health. 2018;24(11):827–32. https://doi.org/10.1089/tmj.2018.0237. Epub 2018 Oct 24.
85. Hassan G, Kirmayer LJ, Mekki-Berrada A, Quosh C, el Chammay R, Deville-Stoetzel JB, Youssef A, Jefee-Bahloul H, Barkeel-Oteo A, Coutts A, Song S, Ventevogel P. Culture, context and the mental health and psychosocial wellbeing of Syrians: a review for mental health and psychosocial support staff working with Syrians affected by armed conflict. Geneva: UNHCR; 2015.
86. Myers CR. Using telehealth to remediate rural mental health and healthcare disparities. Issues Ment Health Nurs. 2019;40:233–9. https://doi.org/10.1080/01612840.2018.1499157.
87. Yellowlees PM, Odor A, Burke MM, et al. A feasibility study of asynchronous telepsychiatry for psychiatric consultations. Psychiatr Serv. 2010;61(8):838–40.
88. Sherrill WW, Crew L, Mayo RM, et al. Educational and health services innovation to improve care for rural Hispanic communities in the US. Educ Health. 2005;18:356–67.
89. Shore J, Kaufmann LJ, Brooks E, et al. Review of American Indian veteran telemental health. Tel e-Health. 2012;18(2):87–94.
90. Moecke DP, Holyk T, Beckett M, et al. Scoping review of telehealth use by Indigenous populations from Australia, Canada, New Zealand, and the United States. J Telemed Telecare. 2023;30(9):1398–416. https://doi.org/10.1177/1357633X211100338.
91. Hassan A, Sharif K. Efficacy of telepsychiatry in refugee populations: a systematic review of the evidence. Cureus. 2019;11(1):e3984. https://doi.org/10.7759/cureus.3984.
92. Truong M, Yeganeh L, Cook O, Crawford K, Wong P, Allen J. Using telehealth consultations for healthcare provision to patients from non-Indigenous racial/ethnic minorities: a systematic review. J Am Med Inform Assoc. 2022;29(5):970–82. https://doi.org/10.1093/jamia/ocac015.
93. Karliner LS, Jacobs EA, Chen AH, Mutha S. Do professional interpreters improve clinical care for patients with limited English proficiency? A systematic review of the literature. Health Serv Res. 2007;42(2):727–54. https://doi.org/10.1111/j.1475-6773.2006.00629.x. PMID: 17362215; PMCID: PMC1955368.
94. Jacobs EA, Lauderdale DS, Meltzer D, Shorey JM, Levinson W, Thisted RA. Impact of interpreter services on delivery of health care to limited-English-proficient patients. J Gen Intern Med. 2001;16(7):468–74. https://doi.org/10.1046/j.1525-1497.2001.016007468.x. PMID: 11520385; PMCID: PMC1495243.
95. Nápoles AM, Santoyo-Olsson J, Karliner LS, O'Brien H, Gregorich SE, Pérez-Stable EJ. Clinician ratings of interpreter mediated visits in underserved primary care settings with ad hoc, in-person professional, and video conferencing modes. J Health Care Poor Underserved. 2010;21(1):301–17.
96. O'Neill DD, Anthony S, Laws M. Every language now. In: Berkowitz L, McCarthy C, editors. Innovation with information technologies in healthcare. London: Springer; 2013. p. 167–77.

97. Tougas H, Chan S, Shahrvini T, Gonzalez A, Chun Reyes R, Burke Parish M, Yellowlees P. The use of automated machine translation to translate figurative language in a clinical setting: analysis of a convenience sample of patients drawn from a randomized controlled trial. JMIR Ment Health. 2022;9(9):e39556. https://doi.org/10.2196/39556. PMID: 36066959; PMCID: PMC9490520.
98. Jefee-Bahloul H, et al. Pilot assessment and survey of Syrian refugees' psychological stress and openness to referral for telepsychiatry (PASSPORT Study). Telemed J E Health. 2014;20(10):977 9.
99. Samuels A. International telepsychiatry: a link between New Zealand and Australia. Aust N Z J Psychiatry. 1999;33:284–6.
100. Harley J. Economic evaluation of a tertiary telepsychiatry service to an island. J Telemed Telecare. 2006;12(7):354–7.
101. Ekblad S, Manicavasagar V, Silove D, et al. The use of international videoconferencing as a strategy for teaching medical students about transcultural psychiatry. Transcult Psychiatry. 2004;41:120–9.
102. Fishkin R, Fishkin L, Leli U, et al. Psychodynamic treatment, training, and supervision using internet-based technologies. J Am Acad Psychoanal Dyn Psychiatry. 2011;39:155–68.
103. Mucic D. International telepsychiatry: a study of patient acceptability. J Telemed Telecare. 2008;14:241–3.
104. www.denlilleprins.org.
105. Singh T, Rajput M. Misdiagnosis of bipolar disorder. Psychiatry. 2006;3(10):57–63.
106. Morselli PL, Elgie R, GAMIAN Europe. GAMIANEurope/BEAM survey I—global analysis of a patient questionnaire circulated to 3450 members of 12 European advocacy groups operating in the field of mood disorders. Bipolar Disord. 2003;5:265–78.
107. Mitchell AJ, Vaze A, Rao S. Clinicaldiagnosis of depression in primary care: a meta-analysis. Lancet. 2009;374:609–19.
108. Barbato A, Vallarino M, Rapisarda F, et al. Access to mental health care in Europe. https://ec.europa.eu/health/sites/health/files/mental_health/docs/ev_20161006_co02_en.pdf.
109. World Health Organization. Mental health action plan 2013–2020. Geneva: World Health Organization; 2013.
110. de Hert M, Correll CU, Bobes J, et al. Physical illness in patients with severe mental disorders. I. Prevalence, impact of medications and disparities in health care. World Psychiatry. 2011;10(1):52–77.
111. Mucic D, Hilty DM. e-Mental health. Cham: Springer; 2016. p. 246–7.
112. Maron E, Baldwin DS, Balõtšev R, et al. Manifesto for an international digital mental health network. Dig Psychiatry. 2019;2(1):14–24. https://doi.org/10.1080/2575517X.2019.1617575.
113. www.nweurope.eu/emen.
114. Gaebel W, Trost N, Diekmann S, et al. Transnational Policy for e-Mental health: a guidance document for European policymakers and stakeholders. Düsseldorf: Interreg North-West Europe; 2020.
115. Chunara R, Zhao Y, Chen J, Lawrence K, Testa PA, Nov O, Mann DM. Telemedicine and healthcare disparities: a cohort study in a large healthcare system in New York City during COVID-19. J Am Med Inform Assoc. 2021;28(1):33–41. https://doi.org/10.1093/jamia/ocaa217. PMID: 32866264; PMCID: PMC7499631.
116. Middleton B, Bloomrosen M, Dente MA, et al. Enhancing patient safety and quality of care by improving the usability of electronic health record systems: recommendations from AMIA. J Am Med Inform Assoc. 2013;20(e1):e2–8. https://doi.org/10.1136/amiajnl-2012-001458.
117. Hilty DM, Crawford A, Teshima J, et al. Mobile health and cultural competencies as a foundation for telehealth care: scoping review. J Tech Behav Sci. 2021;6:197–230.

How Does the Internet Influence the Doctor–Patient Relationship?

18

Mark Agius, Michaela Agius, Rashid Zaman, and Helen Stangeland

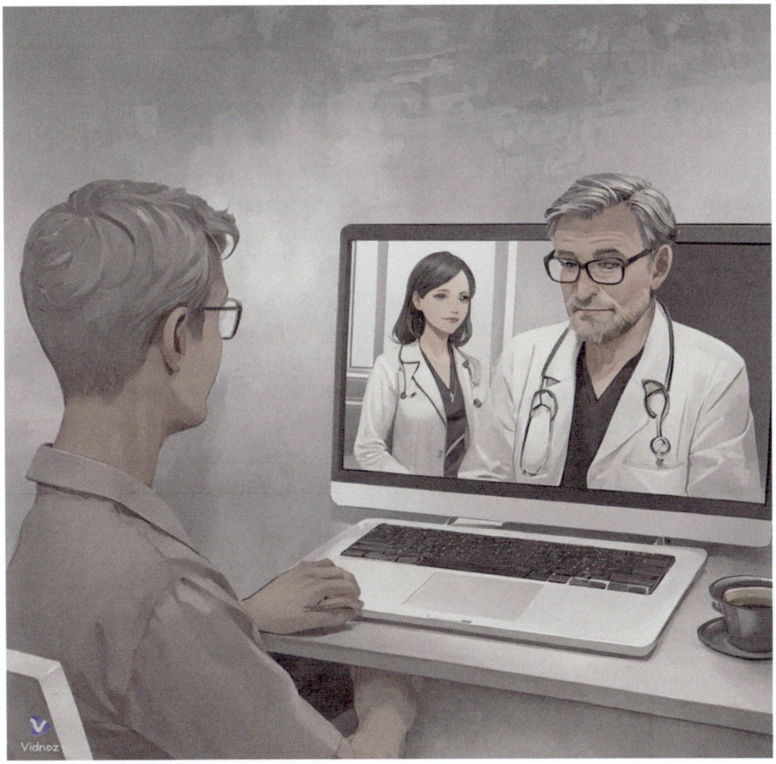

D. Mucić, D. M. Hilty (eds.), *Digital Mental Health*,
https://doi.org/10.1007/978-3-031-59936-1_18

Abstract

In this chapter, we consider the doctor–patient relationship as classically described. We then consider the impact of the Internet on the doctor–patient relationship in two ways. One way is the consequence of the use of the Internet for videoconferencing; the other is the availability of medical information on the Internet in various forms, so that patients are able to easily access information before or after the consultation, while various websites may even be recommended during the consultation itself. The doctor–patient relationship continues to be central to the practice of medicine; however, the Internet influences it in a number of ways, and it is important that clinicians are aware of these so as to optimize the help given to the patient.

18.1 Introduction

Over the last few years, with the Internet becoming widely available, concerns have been raised that the doctor–patient relationship may be in some way changed or even compromised by the ease of availability of information, which patients may glean from the Internet. There has been concern that by removing the position of the doctor as the sole source of medical information, there will be change in the balance of the relationship between doctor and patient to the detriment of one or other party [1, 2].

The aim of this chapter is to examine these concerns, firstly by examining the nature of the doctor–patient relationship, then by examining the reasons for these concerns, and subsequently by discussing the data presently available as to how the doctor–patient relationship has in fact been affected by the Internet. Finally, we shall produce some suggestions, based in fact on the literature about the relationship itself and our understanding of it as to how the use of the Internet can in fact be seen as potentially enhancing, rather than harming the doctor–patient relationship [3–5].

M. Agius
Centro Studi Psichiatrici, Iseo, Italy

Charles University, Prague, Czech Republic
Clare College, University of Cambridge, Cambridge, UK
South Essex Partnership Trust, Grays, UK

M. Agius (✉)
University of Malta, Msida, Malta
e-mail: michaela.agius.18@um.edu.mt

R. Zaman
Hertfordshire Partnership Foundation Trust, St Albans, UK

University of Cambridge, Cambridge, UK
e-mail: rz218@cam.ac.uk

H. Stangeland
Haukeland University Hospital, Bergen, Norway

18.2 The Doctor–Patient Relationship

In the UK, both General Practice and Psychiatry have made the idea of the doctor–patient relationship the central tenet of medical practice [6].

The key concept of the doctor–patient relationship is the consultation, which has been described by Sir James Spence as "The occasion when, in the intimacy of the consulting room, a person who is ill, or believes himself to be ill, seeks the advice of a doctor whom he trusts" [7]. It is this consultation that is the central moment in the relationship between two persons; one of whom may have a problem, but also much life experience, while the other, who also has had years of life experience and study of the art of medicine, is believed by the first to have the knowledge and skills to help find a solution [6].

18.2.1 Trust

Trust between the two persons concerned is essential to a successful outcome, but it can only be achieved by the two, doctor and patient, valuing each other as individual persons, each with their own knowledge, experiences, and frailties. There is the need for each of the two to accept the other: for the doctor to accept that the patient genuinely needs help but has intellect and willingness to understand what may be offered and make appropriate choices and for the patient to understand that the doctor may indeed have the knowledge to help solve his situation, but at the same time also has his/her human frailties and weaknesses, and indeed is not infallible, though well intentioned [6].

18.2.2 Holistic Approach

However, the doctor's approach must take many considerations into account; it must be holistic. Sir James continued "Before explanation and advice can be given to a patient, three diagnoses must be made: the diagnosis of the disease, of the concept or fears of the disease in the mind of the patient and of the patient's capacity to understand the explanation" [7]. A patient's illness may take on many different aspects, depending on what the patient understands about the doctor's explanation of the disease and what the patient fears or is concerned about, and the doctor's advice must take this into account [6].

Ian McWhinney has said, "This is not a matter of rejecting the reductive (disease) theory, but enlarging its scope to overcome its limitations" [8]. The holistic approach recognizes that illness is closely related to the personality and experience of the patient and that man cannot be understood in isolation from his environment. The holistic view acknowledges that every illness is different and that the physician himself is an important aspect of the healing process. The function of the doctor and his communication skills in the healing process is of great importance [9].

Brown and Freeling have stated: "The doctor's function is to understand the whole of his patient's communication so that he could assess the whole person and be able to consider the effect of any intervention in an illness on the whole life of his patient" [9].

Trust is essential. Francis Peabody as early as 1927 pointed out "Do you see what an opportunity you have? The foundation of your whole relation with the patient is laid in those first few minutes of contact. Here is a worried, lonely, suffering man, and if you begin by approaching him with sympathy, tact and consideration, you get his confidence and he becomes your patient" [9].

18.2.3 The Standard Pathway to Care

It should be remembered that patients consult doctors after a great deal of consideration on their part. Tuckett, in 1976, pointed out that, "Individuals have symptoms much of the time, and that dealing with them, particularly by self-medication, is a day-to-day activity; that individuals visit the doctor on average for only one of about ten symptoms that they suffer; that when they do go these symptoms have not necessarily got worse; that their motives for going and what they want from the doctor, may often have more to do with some change in their social circumstances than with any change in symptoms" [10].

The fact that patients tend to consider a great deal before consulting the doctor and that they usually think very hard, discuss with family and friends, even look up in books, or consult pharmacists or other mental health professionals they have access to, before seeing the doctor, is the "health seeking behavior," which has been described by Goldberg and Huxley as a "first filter" in their pathway to care [11–14]. This is very relevant to the issue of the use of the Internet by patients; the Internet is in fact one more source that the patient might use in attempting to clarify his/her thoughts and achieve some understanding of his/her situation before going to see the doctor. Hence, it is analogous to all the other sources of information the patient may have access to, even though it is a very accessible and powerful one [15, 16].

18.2.4 The Therapeutic Effect of Doctors

There is the need that both patient and doctor recognize the other as a unique person, as all human persons are indeed unique, and therefore in themselves have a value that is inestimable, because there shall never be another person like the one who is before them.

Michael Balint, in 1964, listed the doctor's tasks as "listening," "understanding," and "using" the understanding so that it should have a therapeutic effect [17]. Balint had pioneered "Balint Groups," which were in fact psychotherapeutic groups for doctors who could discuss within the group the difficulties that they encountered in relating to individual patients. This is how doctors work with patients in order to help them recover. The therapeutic effect of the doctor himself should never be underestimated. One of us (MA) was privileged in his general practitioner (GP) training to have met a doctor who was one of the original members of the first Balint Group. This doctor always quoted Balint as repeating "Remember that the first thing a doctor prescribes to a patient is himself."

18.2.5 The Relationship of Evidence-Based Medicine to the Doctor–Patient Relationship

It is all too easy in a medical system that is dominated by evidence-based treatment algorithms that prescribe "best practice" and that are dependent on biologically developed medication to fall into the trap of treating the disease identified only by science rather than attempting to help the patient. Such a mechanistic approach, which pays little heed to the patient's needs, fails to recognize the patient as a person. It is necessary that doctors "think laterally," in order that they may identify aspects of the patient's condition apart from the primary illness, which in themselves require treatment. One of us (MA) frequently recounts to students a mistake he once made as a General Practitioner, when he treated a patient with severe rheumatoid arthritis, who was severely distressed, without recognizing that the patient was actually also suffering from depression secondary to her arthritic condition. As a result, important needs of the patient remained unaddressed.

18.2.6 Consultation Analysis

What we have so far argued depends very much on the concept of viewing both the doctor and the patient as unique individuals who have their own understanding, experience, and knowledge, which may have been gleaned from many sources, one of which is the Internet but others are books, friends, and acquaintances with whom they have discussed their symptoms and which will have influenced how they each enter the consultation. It is the task of the doctor to ensure that the consultation is managed appropriately, so that both doctor and patient can understand each other, share their knowledge, apply it to a common problem, which is the one that the patient has brought, and then come up with a common solution [3–5].

Consultation analysis has developed as part of doctor's training in order to emphasize how this mutual understanding can be brought about in the consultation [18].

Roger Neighbour describes the phases of a consultation in his book *The Inner Consultation* as a five-stage mode [19]. The doctor first connects with the patient and develops rapport and empathy. He then "summarizes" with the patient their reasons for attending, including their feelings, concerns, and expectations from the consultation. Having made a diagnosis, he then "hands over" or shares with the patient an agreed management plan that hands back control to the patient. He then "safety-nets" or makes contingency plans with the patient in case the clinician is wrong or something unexpected happens. Finally, once the patient has left, the doctor "housekeeps" or takes measures to ensure the clinician stays in good shape for the next patient.

Another excellent model for the consultation is Silverman's Calgary Cambridge method of analyzing consultations [20], which is now used by a large number of medical schools in the UK. This method is based on previous work by Pendleton et al. [21] and is an evidence-based approach to integration of the "tasks" of the consultation and improving skills for effective communication. Silverman divides the consultation into: Firstly, initiating the session by establishing rapport and then establishing the reasons for the patient consulting. From this develops a shared agenda between doctor and patient. Next, information is gathered; the patient tells his/her story. The doctor uses open-ended questions initially, only using closed questions later to get additional information. The doctor identifies verbal and non-verbal cues given by the patient. Next, the doctor builds the relationship further—developing rapport, recording notes, accepting the patient's views and feelings, and demonstrating empathy and support. Then the doctor provides explanation and develops a treatment plan with the patient by giving digestible, understandable information and explanation. Finally, he closes the session by summarizing and clarifying the agreed plan.

The emphasis throughout is on mutuality and sharing of both the doctor's and patient's prior knowledge, fears and concerns, the doctor's acceptance of these with empathy, and the development of a mutual plan between doctor and patient [18].

Some of this knowledge, as well as fears and concerns, may have been gleaned by the patient from the Internet [15, 16]. Hence, the doctor must work together with the patient to clarify, using his medical training and understanding, what the patient has understood from many sources including Internet sources to place this knowledge in the context of the patient's real situation and develop a plan together with the patient in order to best manage the situation.

During the consultation, one must accept that the doctor and patient may see the consultation as having different aims. For the doctor, the history, examination, and investigation results in a differential diagnosis, while for the patient, expression of his ideas, expectations, and feelings results in an understanding of the patient's beliefs and concerns by the doctor. An integration of both these viewpoints is necessary in the consultation in order that a joint plan of action can be developed [18].

18.2.7 Consultation Style

The doctor's consultation style is important. A patient-centered consultation style is less authoritarian: It encourages the patient to express their own feelings and concerns and uses open questioning, because of the doctor's interest in the psychosocial aspect of illness, before going to closed questions to clinch the diagnosis [18].

Thus, an integrated approach to information gathering, seeking to identify physical, psychological, and social factors, is likely to produce a better outcome [18].

Body language is important in establishing rapport and empathy. Even how the doctor sits affects how he projects himself. If the patient is across the desk and the doctor sits like a headmaster, then the consultation becomes more authoritarian, while if the patient and doctor are not separated by a desk, then the consultation is held on a more equal footing [18].

Therefore, the doctor–patient relationship is very dependent on the adoption of a consultation style, which leads to an open discussion between doctor and patient, which leads to the sharing of information by both parties, so as to come to a common mutually agreed solution to the problem that the patient has presented for discussion, which is to be implemented by a mutually agreed plan [18]. Some but not necessarily all of this information may have been provided by the Internet [15, 16].

18.3 Applying Our Knowledge About the Consultation to Telemedicine

Up to now we have discussed the doctor–patient relationship in general terms. It should be added here that in the opinion of the present authors what has been said is equally applicable when the consultation is carried out not in a room, as is conventional, but across a televised screen, with the doctor and patient in different localities.

It is possible that telepsychiatry using two-way, interactive video instead of traditional face-to-face interactions may mean that the nature of these interactions may be different [22].

Telepsychiatry offers us new methods of human communication, enabling us to establish social connections between different communities, cultures, and continents [23]. When it became impossible to continue person-to-person, face-to-face consultations because of the lockdowns caused by the coronavirus disease-2019 (COVID-19) pandemic, we were all obliged to use telepsychiatry in order to give mental health care to our patients [24].

As well as literature regarding doctor–patient diagnostic consultations regarding telepsychiatry, there is literature about delivering psychological therapy over the Internet using videoconferencing [25, 26].

Telepsychiatry can be provided in various forms. These include telephone consultations, video consultations, as well as email or text communications between doctor/therapist and patient [22].

A number of studies have compared telephone consultations with face-to-face consultations. Such studies have reported that, patients' assessments of therapists' helpfulness and empathy were comparable in both groups [27–29]. In the same way, several studies have shown that patient satisfaction and ratings on the quality of relationships were similar for video consultations and in-person consultations [30–32].

In order for the psychiatrist to be able to diagnose and treat mental health disorders effectively, psychiatry has always depended on there being a strong patient–provider alliance that facilitates communication and enables the psychiatrist to recognize any changes in behavior or signs of mental health distress. These changes will suggest a diagnosis or give an indication of the development of the illness. Patients who need psychiatric care require this care to be individualized, and so this strong patient–provider alliance is needed in order for the patient to optimally benefit from treatment. This is so whether the consultation is in-person, or via telepsychiatry, and whether individual, family, or group-based therapy is being provided. Therefore, such a strong patient–provider alliance has always been the standard for mental health care [33].

Some professionals expressed the concern that the absence of in-person communication in telepsychiatry could prevent or modify the formation of a strong therapeutic alliance. This alliance is often described as the emotional connection between the patient and the therapist and their mutual cooperation and agreement on the objectives and tasks of the therapy [34].

Mutual engagement between doctor and patient may be affected by the technology used in telepsychiatry, but even low-cost equipment used in telepsychiatry can facilitate the possibility that the participants can share a virtual space, can get to know each other, and can discuss complex issues [35].

In order to create the strong therapeutic relationship necessary for effective telepsychiatry consultations, a number of prerequisites must be met.

Appointments must be regular, and of fixed duration, in order to create a positive environment and a therapeutic framework that promotes security, trust, and confidentiality to explore and discuss anything. As with in-person consultation, telepsychiatric care requires a clinical environment that is private, professional, and welcoming. There needs to be good seating for the doctor, adequate lighting (e.g., for facial illumination during the video work), soundproofing, and security from interruption. All the sites that the clinician uses need to be of similar specification in design, including the clinician's home, if that is used. If the clinician's home is used, planning in order to avoid interruptions, ensure silence, and avoid disruption is necessary. It is better to cancel appointments than to provide them in an unfavorable setting, which might lead to disruption.

Telepsychiatry may be used in many varied settings and to provide different types of care. The patients may vary in their personalities, disorders, ages, cultures, languages, as well as their psychosocial histories. The health care settings in which telepsychiatry is offered differ, and might include primary care, mental health clinics, emergency rooms, group homes, nursing homes, shelters, hospices, schools, forensic units, prisons, workplaces, public health centers, academic institutions, and the patient's own homes, depending on the service being provided. Different services may evaluate, triage, assess, and offer care and management in different ways [36].

It is clear that even in a televised consultation the doctor and patient must use an open consultation style, including appropriate body language, which develops an appropriate rapport, and empathy, and thus leads to the development of a mutually agreed plan. In studies of the outcome of telepsychiatry consultations, there is a consistent moderate relationship between positive therapeutic alliance and successful treatment outcomes [37].

Evidence is developing that this can be achieved in telepsychiatry.

Perhaps the best evidence for this is the fact that in British Clinical Schools and General Practice training programs, the common method of training doctors in the consultation skills mentioned above is in fact the videoing of consultations (real or simulated) and their consequent analysis for the aspects of a good consultation that we have mentioned above [38–40].

Studies of the doctor–patient communication in telepsychiatry include post-encounter surveys of participants in telepsychiatry consultations as well as qualitative investigations that involve observation, patient interviews, case reports, questionnaires, and analysis of the content of telepsychiatry consultations [41].

It has been shown that it is possible to train persons, in particular, younger and middle-aged adults to identify emotions by interpreting nonverbal behavior in audiovisual interviews after providing a short audiovisual emotion recognition training program [42].

Because many patients and mental health care professionals have gained experience with video consultations during the restrictions caused by the COVID-19 pandemic, they have developed videoconferencing-specific communication skills [24]. The skills they have acquired will help both patients and doctors better express their emotions even when experiencing video consultations, thus enabling them to act in a way that is more approximate to face-to-face consultations [24]. Therapists have reported that once they have acquired experience of video consultation, it became simpler for them to interact with their patients [24].

Data on telepsychiatry carried out in this way are well summarized by Hilty et al. [43]; it appears that there are no major impediments to the development of the doctor–patient relationship in terms of communication and satisfaction. Hilty rightly points out that many factors affect perception of the telemedicine visit and communication by those taking part. Disclosure may be affected by the presence of others in the room, belief of being videotaped, and concerns about stigma. Furthermore, patients who have not used telemedicine before may feel anxious, may be distracted by the equipment, or may be self-conscious about seeing himself/herself on a screen [43].

"Richness" is used to describe how telepsychiatry interviews facilitate the transfer of information. "Richness" is based on four factors: feedback, numerous cues, a range of languages, and individual focus. It is generally thought that oral and synchronous media—in other words, direct consultation in real time between two persons as in a telepsychiatry interview—are richer than asynchronous media, such as consulting via email or using the Internet for information rather than speaking with a person in real time [44].

Technology, including telepsychiatry consultations, can impact the clarity, responsiveness, and comfort of communication, which is essential to the transmission of ideas, emotions, and information between individuals [44].

During all medical consultations, medical practitioners use techniques including questioning, investigating fundamental concerns, spotting inconsistencies, and using reflection to explain issues and order fundamental values. The doctor always evaluates and gives priority to the patient's wishes, requirements, and preferences. The clinician's aim is always to establish supportive therapeutic engagement and emotional well-being for everybody involved [44]. When telepsychiatry by video or text is used, it is used to elicit the same experiences related to feelings, perception, images, and interaction as face-to-face consultations, therefore it is important that the differences between these different forms of consultation are considered [44]. This analysis will determine where the use of technologies such as video link or text will be useful [44].

It has been shown that the therapeutic alliance formed during psychotherapy provided via videoconferencing does not appear to affect treatment outcomes, so long as there is clear agreement on the therapeutic tasks and goals to be achieved [44]. The consequence of this is that even though many patients may feel that the psychotherapy sessions may feel less personal, they can still be professional and effective [44].

It is true however that patients may feel a more powerful therapeutic bond with the therapist during in-person sessions. Expectations of patients will vary, depending on whether patients have previously visited their psychiatrist in person or whether all appointments, including the initial evaluation, have taken place virtually. Furthermore, patients who have little familiarity with videoconferencing technology (for example, elderly patients or patients from culturally isolated populations) might prefer in-person consultations and could even find telepsychiatry stressful [36]. By contrast, it has been reported that patients from groups who are socially and geographically isolated report great benefits from telepsychiatry, with 90% of patients being comfortable with their telepsychiatry treatment and 84.5% believing it was as helpful as an in-person psychiatric interview [45]. This may well be that this is because such patients are able, through telepsychiatry, to be able to access care that otherwise they could not access. One can speculate that the same experience would have been reported by all patients during the recent lockdowns during the pandemic, when video consultations became the only source of psychiatric care available to the community.

From the point of view of diagnosis, it does not appear that the differences in therapeutic alliance between telepsychiatry and in-person consultations caused any differences in diagnosis [46].

Although patients do perceive video as similar to in-person care, the patients also highlight in several reports, several technological issues associated with video [47].

The free flow of the consultation may be interrupted by signal delay [48], so that a turn-taking conversation occurs rather than the free-flowing conversation indicative of a high-rapport interaction [49], and if parties speak at the same time, they may perceive the other as interrupting [25]. However, no differences with the development of rapport were found in a small cohort that experienced brief signal delays [48]. Patients tend to respond in a "conservative" or "stilted" way when audio delay occurs with videoconferencing [50].

The therapeutic relationship and the participants' ability to demonstrate empathy may be negatively affected by difficulties in hearing and interpreting the other person's speech [51–53].

The breaking up of the audio signal may be limiting, in particular, when a sensitive conversation is taking place. It has been pointed out that broken audio can be as disruptive as loud building work outside a clinic room in real life [54].

Poor audio quality may impact the psychiatrist–patient interaction. It has been shown in studies that audiovisual telepsychiatry services did not provide emotional support, and patients' satisfaction with the consultations was limited by low audiovisual quality [55].

It appears that patients usually tolerate occasional technological disturbances but do not tolerate pervasive disturbances [56]. This is worth considering when developing new telepsychiatry services. Since patients are more willing to accept video consultations when they know their therapist, it may be helpful to start a new telepsychiatry service first of all with patients who are well used to their therapist until the service is properly integrated and all the technological issues have been solved [56].

The environment of a telepsychiatry consultation is different from that of a face-to-face consultation, and as a result several cues, for example gait, are missing [57]; however, at present, it is assumed that the videoconferencing provides an appropriate physical environment for good decision-making [43]. Cukor et al. have reported that telepsychiatry enables a "social presence" to be established, which enables both doctor and patient to share a virtual space, get to know one another, and discuss complex issues [58].

Nonverbal communication is of great importance in establishing mutual connections and understanding. This it does through eye contact, gestures, posture, fidgeting, nods, grins, smiles, frowns, and lip reading [51]. Decoding these nonverbal clues is of great importance to better interpersonal outcomes [23]. It is reported that decreased ability to detect nonverbal cues occurs during videoconferencing for patient interviews [59]. This has been described as the "cuelessness" phenomena [60]. A task-oriented focus with a depersonalized content may occur as a consequence of this during telepsychiatry consultations.

Telepsychiatry using videoconferencing technology can allow access to verbal cues, but they can limit the ability of participants to engage in mutual eye gaze and to perceive body movements and gestures, thus limiting nonverbal cues and communication [61]. As a consequence, it has been noted that higher levels of mutual gaze were recorded in telepsychiatry [62], which was higher than usual interpersonal interactions [63]. This may help understanding between the two participants [43].

It appears that patients have reported lower levels of anxiety in telepsychiatry during the consultation, while physicians reported increased anxiety [43]. Patients also reported some sense of not having been understood [43].

An in-person conversation takes less time than videoconferencing [64, 65].

Issues have been raised regarding the privacy of consultations carried out by telepsychiatry. Telepsychiatry interactions could potentially have significant ethical and legal ramifications. Patients often worry about their privacy and security, in particular with regard to unauthorized access to computerized medical records [66]. As well as informational privacy, that is, the disclosure of personal files and data, privacy also includes psychological privacy, that is, the disclosure of private attitudes, beliefs, and feelings; social privacy, that is, the control over social contacts;

as well as physical privacy, which is the control over physical accessibility [67]. All these issues need to be taken into account when planning telepsychiatry services.

Patients have often reported that they feel comfortable when communicating via real-time video link and that they felt that the sessions were private in the sense that the information they gave to the therapist would be kept private [68].

The safety of the patient must always be the prime consideration when deciding what service is to be offered. This is so when there is a choice between a phone consultation and a video consultation, and the patient opts for phone consultation [69]. It is possible that without video, some important signs might be missed.

Therefore, factors including the type of service being offered (psychotherapy, medication management, or case management) and the specific mental and medical health issues of the patient (including good practice standards for prescription of such medications, as opioids or benzodiazepines), rather than patient preference, should all inform a provider's decision on whether to use phone or video for the consultation [69].

In general, it appears that telepsychiatry does not significantly interfere with the development of a therapeutic alliance [70]. It is still therefore possible for doctor and patient to have an effective interaction across the videoconferencing system, despite them being separated by distance.

To conclude, we have reviewed the consequences of the use of telepsychiatry utilizing the Internet here because it is important to be aware of the impact of the Internet, with the great amount of information of varying quality contained therein, when performing a diagnostic consultation over the Internet.

18.4 Has the Doctor–Patient Relationship in Fact Been Affected by the Internet?

Doctors have expressed concern that Internet access results in a more time-consuming consultation, because patients become more demanding and have more complex questions or may have misinterpreted the information they have acquired on the Internet [71].

However, rather than disrupting the doctor–patient relationship, the availability of information gleaned from the Internet appears to enhance to a degree the discussion between the patient and the doctor [1, 71–73]. Because of information gleaned from the Internet, patients appear better informed about their condition and better able therefore to help develop a jointly agreed treatment plan [71, 74].

It is nowadays a very frequent occurrence that patients seek information on the Internet before consulting the doctor, often without informing the doctor of that fact; however, fortunately, patients tend to value their doctor's opinion more highly than the information which they have found on the Internet [75]. Often, patients might also simply want the physician to explain, contextualize, or just give their professional opinion about the information they bring to the consultation [4].

If the doctor has not fully explained the situation to the patient, some patients seem to consider the Internet as a low-cost extension of their doctors' guidance, seeking information that the doctor had not made clear during the consultation [54, 73, 76]. On the other hand, anxiety and lack of trust in the physician can be the drive for individuals to use the Internet [54]. Given the wide availability of the Internet, it is useful for doctors to give the patients recommended Internet sites that they can use as supplementary sources of psychoeducation for the patient to reinforce the knowledge imparted in the consultation.

18.5 How the Internet Affects the Doctor–Patient Relationship: The Research Data

We can now review in some more detail the data published so far regarding the impact of the Internet on the doctor–patient relationship.

18.5.1 A Better-Informed Patient Equals Better Overall Health

Over the past several years, the Internet has given a broader access to health-related information and patients seem to use this possibility frequently [15, 16]. It is suggested that this factor actually improves the overall health to the individual patient by "*making subsequent health-related behavioural changes*" [77]. Several patients report changing their thinking about their health after exposure to health-related information on the Internet [78, 79]. It appears that patients seem to consider the Internet as a low-cost extension of their doctors' guidance, using it to seek information that the doctor had not made clear during the consultation [54, 73, 76]. Because of this, it would appear logical that the doctor should, during the consultation, offer some sites that he considers useful for the patient to consult. Internet support forums can be beneficial in giving patients psychological support [74].

18.5.2 Disparities Between Patient Groups

Socioeconomic factors can play a role regarding the propensity of patients to seek information on the Internet. Several factors are involved in lowering the threshold for searching the Internet for information. These include age, sex, education, household income, and work positions. Education seems to weigh most out of these factors. In general, the younger and higher educated people, especially women, seem to educate themselves about their health [3, 4, 54, 72, 75, 77, 80–82]. However, the outcome of consultations does not seem to be changed by the use of the Internet because the patients still regarded the doctors' opinion as having the highest value [75].

The elderly have a lower tendency to seek health-associated information and tend to maintain the traditional paternalistic relationship to their physician [83]. This has a strong connection to their generally lower computer skills [83]. Still, demographic and situational variables may play an important role here as well [83].

Sometimes, anxiety and lack of trust in the physician can be the drive for individuals to use the Internet [54].

18.5.3 The Active Patient

It has been reported that the use of information that the patient has abstracted from the Internet has led to a shift from the traditional paternalistic physician–patient relationship toward a more dynamic relationship based on partnership [1, 71–73]. The patients who discuss the health-related information they have retrieved from Internet seem to be more confident and active instead of being a passive recipient. Hence, patients who have used the Internet to seek information may feel that they have a better sense of control over their situation. This can especially be true for the long-term (chronic) patients who must manage their disease for a long period of time and visit the doctor more frequently than the average person. Since a chronic disease, such as diabetes, must be controlled at all times, the patient becomes more familiar with his/her body and how it responds to different treatments. These patients seem to educate themselves to a higher degree about their disease and treatment options on the Internet, and they then discuss these options with their physician [73]. In general, the patients seem to communicate better due to their increased understanding of their situation and so they are more able to participate in the decision-making regarding their treatment [71, 74]. Often, patients might also simply want the physician to explain, contextualize, or just give their professional opinion about the information they bring to the consultation [4]. This is particularly important, since there is evidence that the patients still regard the doctors' opinion as having the highest value, as compared to the Internet [75].

18.5.4 Time and Effectiveness

The informed patient can decrease the time spent in consultation with the doctor, making the diagnosing more smooth and effective [1, 16].

Internet information can help patients evaluate the importance of their complaints before the consultation, in order to get the best use of the limited time with the doctor [4].

The doctor might also benefit from the quick access to health-related information during consultations [82, 84]. On the other hand, some doctors have claimed that Internet access results in a more time-consuming consultation, because patients become more demanding and have more complex questions or may have misinterpreted the information they have acquired on the Internet [71].

18.5.5 Patient's Ability to Critically Review Internet Information

Whereas there are many excellent sites on the Internet, unfortunately, the quality of the Internet information is poorly controlled, and since patients lack the theoretical knowledge, they are unable to filter and critically review the information [75]. This along with other misinterpretations can lead to unnecessary fear and anxiety for the patient [71]. Support forums also give the opportunity for patients to exchange experiences and opinions about their disease. This is regarded as positive but it can become problematic when the forum users encourage others to demand instead of asking the physicians about their diagnosis and treatment [73]. Although most doctors seem to be positive toward the Internet-educated patients, some doctors fear that the number of patients with more specific demands or other inappropriate requests will increase [1].

18.5.6 Bringing Health Information from the Internet into the Doctors' Office

Some patients seem to experience hesitation to discuss information from the Internet with the doctor. They do not want to offend or seem challenging toward the doctor [85]. Not all patients share information with their doctor [5]. Patients who have checked the Internet for answers before going to the doctor may have higher anxiety levels compared with those who did not check the Internet [4, 54]. Others do not hesitate to bring information to the doctor and feel that if they show the doctor that they have invested time, then the doctor will take their problems more seriously. Other motives include *making the most* out of the consultation, clarifying their information, and developing a more equal relationship with their GP [4, 71]. On the other hand, patients can become overconfident and give less value to their doctor's opinion [2, 71, 73]. These patients may use the health information from the Internet to verify the doctors' competence [73, 85]. This can cause some problems and damage the doctor–patient relationship if the doctor's communication skills are not adequate.

18.5.7 Change to the Patient–Doctor Relationship

The shift in roles and dynamics between the doctor and the patient has raised the question of whether access to Internet information improves or worsens the doctor–patient relationship [1, 2]. In most instances, adequate communication skills will ensure that Internet information will lead to a positive improvement of the relationship [3–5]. As long as the doctor has the ability to listen and use good communication skills to show interest in what the patient wishes to tell, the relationship seems to improve. The feeling of being heard and taken seriously is very important for the patients and can increase trust considerably [4]. Even though most physicians feel that the Internet might have a positive effect on their relationship to their patients [71], some doctors report that they have difficulties dealing with Internet information, either because they lack communication skills or because they are not adequately updated on what information there actually is on the Internet [86]. If the doctor feels that his/her authority is being challenged and reacts by acting in a superior or condescending way, the relationship can worsen or possibly be destroyed [4].

This is not so true for patient groups who are in managed care or have other disadvantages [75]. Good communication skills seem to result in greatly improved relationships even though the doctor does not necessarily agree with the information that the patient brings. Faster diagnosis and better use of consultation time can also contribute to a better relationship [84].

18.5.8 Internet Skills and Guidance

Traditionally, doctors have been the only source of information for patients. The Internet has changed this dramatically and information now flows freely and in an uncontrolled way. Since patients have different predispositions to understand, evaluate, and filter information, there are suggestions that health staff should keep themselves updated regarding what the patients might find on the Internet and know where to direct and guide the patients to the best sites of the web. As the Internet influences patients more and more, this would be beneficial for both the doctor and the patients [1, 2, 5, 72, 73, 75, 87].

Until now, giving Internet recommendations and guidance from doctors and other health staff has not been normal procedure for doctors and other health staff [73, 88].

The Internet can prove to be an effective tool not only for education of the patient's current disease but also for prevention. This is especially true for the younger patient group [80]. The elderly do not always have the same adequate computer skills [89] and educating them in using the Internet to make better choices regarding their health has been attempted. However, there is no documentation that educating the elderly in computer skills actually makes a difference in their usage of this information source [83].

18.6 Conclusions and Recommendations Going Forward

There is no question that the Internet is here to stay with us for the foreseeable future. While it is true that the Internet is extremely widely available, and therefore is very frequently used, there is no reason to believe that its impact on the consultation is in any way really different from the other sources of patient information (family, friends, books, articles, etc.) that have been available for much longer. These have been described earlier as the "first filter" in the patient's "pathway to care" [11–14]. Hence the model of the consultation that we have already described [19–21] should be very effective in responding to the needs of the patient, including his/her questions about what he has read on the Internet. Such a consultation model includes empathy and a patient-centered consultation style, which is less authoritarian and which encourages the patient to express their own feelings and concerns and uses open questioning before going to closed questions to clinch the diagnosis. It also includes a collaborative approach to planning interventions to which the patient contributes, now putting to good use the information he had extracted from the

Internet and the questions that he had wanted to raise with the doctor. This will lead to a successful consultation [19–21]. Such a model is not "Internet specific," but the presence of information from the Internet can be used to enhance it.

18.6.1 Recommendations

Indeed, since both doctor and patient will be aware that information on the Internet is of varying quality, doctors should have available to themselves a series of useful websites that they can refer patients to for supplementary information regarding the problem they are dealing with. There are available a number of excellent sites based in the UK, such as the NICE (National Institute for Health and Care Excellence) site, which is excellent for information on the recommended National Health Treatment Pathways for all major conditions, and also sites of nongovernmental organizations (NGOs) that advocate for and support patients with specific conditions; Parkinson's UK, British Diabetic Association, Epilepsy Society, Depression Alliance, Manic Depression Fellowship are a few among many such NGOs. There also exist sites for some specific psychotherapies such as cognitive therapies that doctors can judiciously recommend to appropriate patients. Some examples of these are "Living Life to the Full" or "Beating the Blues" [90].

Thus, doctors can, by recommending appropriate sites on the Internet to patients as part of their joint plan to solve the problem, enhance the patient's knowledge and increase the patient's resilience.

18.6.2 Some Possible Problems

However, there may be some problems with Internet use linked with the nature of the Internet itself. All should be easily solved by the application of the consultation skills described above. Here we briefly discuss some such problems.

18.6.2.1 Discussion Boards

It is worth commenting on the issue of discussion boards, support forums, and blogs. Internet support forums can be beneficial in giving patients psychological support [74]. Support forums also give the opportunity for patients to exchange experiences and opinions about their disease. However, a risk has been observed that forum users might encourage others to demand instead of asking the physicians about their diagnosis and treatment [73]. It is wise for doctors to point out to patients that blogs and support forums contain subjective information that applies to the individual writers but not necessarily to all patients or indeed to the individual viewer. Therefore, information obtained from these sources needs to be particularly discussed with health professionals to establish appropriate guidance for the individual patient.

18.6.2.2 Misleading Information on the Internet

Another issue that can arise is that of websites that give misleading information, which could seriously affect the patient's chance of recovery. These misleading websites are often found within the Mental Health Field. One example of such a group of websites are the "pro-anorexia" websites [91–94]. Dealing with information from these sites will be particularly challenging, but again, the use of the consultation skills we have described should be sufficient to overcome the difficulties.

18.6.2.3 Social Media

A comment should be made about another possible use of the Internet for consultation purposes. This is the use of Social Media such as Facebook or Twitter. The General Medical Council has recently issued guidance regarding this [95]. Essentially, the issue is that confidentiality cannot be ensured on social media sites; therefore, consultations, discussion of patient's condition, and prescription cannot be carried out on these sites.

18.6.3 Conclusion

It is the present authors' view that appropriate training for doctors in consultation skills and the use of patient-centered consultation methods will enable doctors to consult effectively with patients who access the Internet for health care advice. The present evidence suggests that this is true, and that, on balance, access to the Internet can in fact enhance the impact of the consultation.

References

1. Moick M, Terlutter R. Physicians' motives for professional internet use and differences in attitudes toward the internet-informed patient, physician-patient communication, and prescribing behavior. Medicine. 2012;1(2):e2.
2. Al Ghamdi KM, Moussa NA. Internet use by the public to search for health-related information. Int J Med Inform. 2012;81(6):363–73.
3. Rider T, Malik M, Chevassut T. Haematology patients and the internet – the use of on-line health information and the impact on the patient-doctor relationship. Patient Educ Couns. 2014;97(2):223–38.
4. Bowes P, Stevenson F, Ahluwalia S, Murray E. 'I need her to be a doctor': patients' experiences of presenting health information from the internet in GP consultations. Br J Gen Pract. 2012;62(604):e732–8.
5. Russ H, Giveon SM, Catarivas MG, Yaphe J. The effect of the Internet on the patient-doctor relationship from the patient's perspective: a survey from primary care. Isr Med Assoc J. 2011;13(4):220–4.
6. Agius M, Micallef C. On patient centred psychiatry. Psychiatr Danub. 2008;20(3):339–41.
7. Spence J. The purpose and practice of medicine. London: OUP; 1960.
8. McWhinney I. An introduction to family medicine. London: OUP; 1981.
9. Brown K, Freeling P. The doctor-patient relationship. Edinburgh: Churchill-Livingstone; 1976.
10. Tuckett D. An introduction to medical sociology. London: Tavistock; 1976.

11. Goldberg D. Epidemiology of mental disorders in primary care settings. Epidemiol Rev. 1995;17:182–90.
12. Goldberg D, Huxley P. Common mental disorders: a bio-social model. London: Routledge; 1991.
13. Goldberg D, Huxley P. Mental illness in the community: the pathway to psychiatric care (International Behavioural and Social Sciences Library). London: Routledge; 2001.
14. Verhaak P. Determinants of the health-seaking process: Goldberg and Huxley's first level and first filter. Psychol Med. 1995;25:95–104.
15. Iverson SA, Howard KB, Penney BK. Impact of internet use on health-related behaviors and the patient-physician relationship: a survey-based study and review. J Am Osteopath Assoc. 2008;108(12):699–711.
16. Wald HS, Dube CE, Anthony DC. Untangling the web—the impact of Internet use on health care and the physician-patient relationship. Patient Educ Couns. 2007;68(3):218–24.
17. Balint M. The doctor, his patient, and the illness. London: Churchill Livingstone; 1964.
18. Agius M. The medical consultation and the human person. Psychiatr Danub. 2014;26(Suppl 1):15–8.
19. Neighbour R. The inner consultation. MTP: Lancaster; 1987.
20. Silverman J, Kurtz S, Draper J. Skills for communicating with patients. 3rd ed. Oxford: Radcliffe; 2013.
21. Pendleton D, Schofield T, Tate P, Havelock P. The new consultation: developing doctor-patient communication. Interact Comput. 1996;8:177–92.
22. Zeavin H. The distance cure: a history of teletherapy. Cambridge: The MIT Press; 2021.
23. Hall JA, Andrzejewski SA, Yopchick JE. Psychosocial correlates of interpersonal sensitivity: a meta-analysis. J Nonverbal Behav. 2009;33:149–80.
24. Gullslett MK, Kristiansen E, Nilsen ER. Therapists' experiences of video consultation in specialized mental health services during the COVID-19 pandemic: qualitative interview study. JMIR Hum Factors. 2021;8:e23150.
25. Postel M, de Haan H, De Jong C. E-therapy for mental health problems: a systematic review. Telemed e-Health. 2008;14(7):707–14.
26. Nelson E, Duncan A, Lillis T. Special considerations for conducting psychotherapy over videoconferencing. In: Myers K, Turvey C, editors. Telemental health: clinical, technical, and administrative foundations for evidence-based practice. London: Elsevier Insights; 2012.
27. Fann JR, Bombardier CH, Vannoy S, Dyer J, Ludman E, Dikmen S, et al. Telephone and in-person cognitive behavioral therapy for major depression after traumatic brain injury: a randomized controlled trial. J Neurotrauma. 2015;32(1):45–57.
28. Dobkin RD, Mann SL, Gara MA, Interian A, Rodriguez KM, Menza M. Telephone-based cognitive behavioral therapy for depression in Parkinson disease: a randomized controlled trial. Neurology. 2020;94(16):e1764–73.
29. Stiles-Shields C, Kwasny MJ, Cai X, Mohr DC. Therapeutic alliance in face-to-face and telephone-administered cognitive behavioral therapy. J Consult Clin Psychol. 2014;82(2):349–54.
30. Egede LE, Acierno R, Knapp RG, Walker RJ, Payne EH, Frueh BC. Psychotherapy for depression in older veterans via telemedicine: effect on quality of life, satisfaction, treatment credibility, and service delivery perception. J Clin Psychiatry. 2016;77(12):16304.
31. Luxton DD, Pruitt LD, Wagner A, Smolenski DJ, Jenkins-Guarnieri MA, Gahm G. Home-based telebehavioral health for US military personnel and veterans with depression: a randomized controlled trial. J Consult Clin Psychol. 2016;84(11):923.
32. Watts S, Marchand A, Bouchard S, Gosselin P, Langlois F, Belleville G, et al. Telepsychotherapy for generalized anxiety disorder: Impact on the working alliance. J Psychother Integr. 2020;30(2):208.
33. Zilcha-Mano S, Dinger U, McCarthy KS, Barber JP. Does alliance predict symptoms throughout treatment, or is it the other way around? J Consult Clin Psychol. 2014;82(6):931.
34. Lopez A, Schwenk S, Schneck CD, Griffin RJ, Mishkind MC. Technology-based mental health treatment and the impact on the therapeutic alliance. Curr Psychiatry Rep. 2019;21(8):76.

35. Kaigwa LC, Njenga F, Ongeri L, Nguithi A, Mugane M, Mbugua GM, Anundo J, Kimari MZ, Onono M. Implementation of telepsychiatry in Kenya: acceptability study. BJPsych Open. 2022;8(3):e85.
36. Borders CB. Realizing the promises of telepsychiatry in special populations. Ment Illn. 2017;9(1):7135.
37. Ardito RB, Rabellino D. Therapeutic alliance and outcome of psychotherapy: historical excursus, measurements, and prospects for research. Front Psychol. 2011;2:270.
38. Cahill P, Papageorgiou A. Video analysis of communication in paediatric consultations in primary care. Br J Gen Pract. 2007;57(544):866–71.
39. Salisbury C, et al. The content of general practice consultations: cross-sectional study based on video recordings. Br J Gen Pract. 2013;63(616):e751–9.
40. Pringle M, Stewart-Evans C. Does awareness of being video recorded affect doctors' consultation behaviour? Br J Gen Pract. 1990;40(340):455–8.
41. Wootton R, Yellowlees P, McLaren P, editors. Telepsychiatry and e-Mental health. New York: Taylor & Francis; 2003.
42. Schlegel K, Vicaria IM, Isaacowitz DM, Hall JA. Effectiveness of a short audiovisual emotion recognition training program in adults. Motiv Emot. 2017;41:646–60.
43. Hilty DM, et al. How telepsychiatry affects the doctor–patient relationship: communication, satisfaction, and additional clinically relevant issues. Primary Psychiatry. 2002;9:29–34.
44. Marcotte-Beaumier G, Bouchard S, Gosselin P, et al. The role of intolerance of uncertainty and working alliance in the outcome of cognitive behavioral therapy for generalized anxiety disorder delivered by videoconference: mediation analysis. JMIR Ment Health. 2021;8:e24541.
45. Campbell R, O'Gorman J, Cernovsky ZZ. Reactions of psychiatric patients to telepsychiatry. Ment Illn. 2015;7:54–5.
46. Morgan RD, Patrick AR, Magaletta PR. Does the use of telemental health alter the treatment experience? Inmates' perceptions of telemental health versus face-to-face treatment modalities. J Consult Clin Psychol. 2008;76(1):158.
47. Slightam C, Gregory AJ, Hu J, Jacobs J, Gurmessa T, Kimerling R, et al. Patient perceptions of video visits using veterans affairs telehealth tablets: survey study. J Med Internet Res. 2020;22(4):e15682.
48. Manning TR, Goetz ET, Street RL. Signal delay effects on rapport in telepsychiatry. CyberPsychol Behav. 2000;3:119–27.
49. Tickle-Degnen L, Rosenthal R. The nature of rapport and its nonverbal correlates. Psychol Inq. 1990;1:285–93.
50. Hilty DM, Ferrer DC, Burke Parish M, Johnston B, Callahan EJ, Yellowlees PM. The effectiveness of telemental health: a 2013 review. Telemed J E Health. 2013;19(6):444–54.
51. Fussell SR, Benimoff NI. Social and cognitive processes in interpersonal communication: implications for advanced telecommunications technologies. Hum Factors. 1995;37:228–50.
52. Whitten P, Kuwahara E. A multi-phase telepsychiatry programme in Michigan: organizational factors affecting utilization and user perceptions. J Telemed Telecare. 2004;10:254–61.
53. Shulman M, John M, Kane JM. Home-based outpatient telepsychiatry to improve adherence with treatment appointments: a pilot study. Psychiatr Serv. 2017;68:743–6.
54. D'Agostino TA, et al. Toward a greater understanding of breast cancer patients' decisions to discuss cancer-related internet information with their doctors: an exploratory study. Patient Educ Couns. 2012;89(1):109–15.
55. Orlando JF, Beard M, Kumar S. Systematic review of patient and caregivers' satisfaction with telehealth videoconferencing as a mode of service delivery in managing patients' health. PLoS One. 2019;14(8):e0221848.
56. Møller AM, Christensen LF, Hansen JP, Andersen PT. Patients' acceptance of video consultations in the mental health services – a systematic review and synthesis of qualitative research. Digital Health. 2022;8:20552076221075148. https://doi.org/10.1177/20552076221075148.
57. Kim T, Biocca F. Telepresence via television: two dimensions of telepresence may have different connections to memory and persuasion. J Comput-Mediat Commun. 1997;3:325.

58. Cukor P, Baer L, Willis BS, et al. Use of videophones and low-cost standard telephone lines to provide a social presence in telepsychiatry. Telemed J. 1998;4:313–21.
59. McLaren P, Ball CJ, Summerfield AB, Watson JP, Lipsedge M. An evaluation of the use of interactive television in an acute psychiatric service. J Telemed Telecare. 1995;1:79–85.
60. Rutter DR. Looking and seeing: the role of visual communication in social interaction. New York: Wiley; 1984.
61. Neureiter K, Fuchsberger V, Murer M, Tscheligi M. Hands and eyes: how eye contact is linked to gestures in video conferencing. In: Mackay WE, Brewster SA, Bødker S, editors. Proceedings of the CHI '13 extended abstracts on human factors in computing systems. New York: Association for Computing Machinery; 2013. p. 127–32.
62. Ball CJ, McLaren PM, Summerfield AB, Lipsedge MS, Watson JP. A comparison of communication modes in adult psychiatry. J Telemed Telecare. 1995;1:22–6.
63. Argyle M. Bodily communication. London: Methuen; 1975.
64. Ochsman RB, Chapanis A. The effects of 10 communication modes on the behavior of teams during co-operative problem-solving. Int J Man-Machine Stud. 1974;6:579–619.
65. O'Malley C, Langston S, Anderson A, et al. Comparison of face-to-face and videomediated. Interact Comput. 2018;8:177–92.
66. Starr P. Health and the right to privacy. Am J Law Med. 1999;25:193–201.
67. Parrot R, Burgoon JK, Burgoon M, LePoire BA. Privacy between physicians and patients: more than a matter of confidentiality. Soc Sci Med. 1989;29:1381–5.
68. Jenkins-Guarnieri MA, Pruitt LD, Luxton DD, Johnson K. Patient perceptions of telemental health: systematic review of direct comparisons to in-person psy- chotherapeutic treatments. Telemed J E Health. 2015;21:652–60.
69. Chen PV, Helm A, Caloudas SG, Ecker A, Day G, Hogan J, Lindsay J. Evidence of phone vs video-conferencing for mental health treatments: a review of the literature. Curr Psychiatry Rep. 2022;24(10):529–39.
70. Manchanda M, McLaren P. Cognitive behaviour therapy via interactive video. J Telemed Telecare. 1998;4:53–5.
71. Uden-Kraan CF, Drossaert CH, Taal E, Smit WM, Seydel ER, van de Laar MA. Experiences and attitudes of Dutch rheumatologists and oncologists with regard to their patients' health-related internet use. Clin Rheumatol. 2010;29(11):1229–36.
72. McMullan M. Patients using the Internet to obtain health information: how this affects the patient-health professional relationship. Patient Educ Couns. 2006;63(1–2):24–8.
73. Hewitt-Taylor J, Bond CS. What e-patients want from the doctor-patient relationship: content analysis of posts on discussion boards. J Med Internet Res. 2012;14(6):e155.
74. Valero-Aguilera B, Bermúdez-Tamayo C, García-Gutiérrez JF, Jiménez-Pernett J, Vázquez-Alonso F, Suárez-Charneco A, Guerrero-Tejada R, Cózar-Olmo JM. Factors related to use of the Internet as a source of health information by urological cancer patients. Support Care Cancer. 2012;20(12):3087–94.
75. Murray E, Lo B, et al. The impact of health information on the internet on the physician-patient relationship: patient perceptions. Arch Intern Med. 2003;163(14):1727–34.
76. Armstrong N, Powell J. Patient perspectives on health advice posted on Internet discussion boards: a qualitative study. Health Expect. 2009;12(3):313–20.
77. Al Ghamdi KM, Almohideb MA. Internet use by dermatology outpatients to search for health information. Int J Dermatol. 2011;50(3):292–9.
78. Cooley DL, Mancuso AM, Weiss LB, Coren JS. Health-related Internet use among patients of osteopathic physicians. J Am Osteopath Assoc. 2011;111(8):473–82.
79. Marin-Torres V, et al. Internet as an information source for health in primary care patients and its influence on the physician-patient relationship. Aten Primaria. 2013;45(1):46–53.
80. Beck F, et al. Use of the internet as a health information resource among French young adults: results from a nationally representative survey. J Med Internet Res. 2014;16(5):e128.
81. Houston TK, Allison JJ. Users of internet health information: differences by health status. J Med Internet Res. 2002;4(2):E7.

82. Bernard E, et al. Internet use for information seeking in clinical practice: a cross-sectional survey among French general practitioners. Int J Med Inform. 2012;81(7):493–9.
83. Campbell RJ, Nolfi DA. Teaching elderly adults to use the internet to access health care information: before-after study. J Med Internet Res. 2005;7(2):e19.
84. Purcarea VL, Petrescu DG, Gheorghe IR, Petrescu CM. Optimizing the technological and informational relationship of the health care process and of the communication between physician and patient—factors that have an impact on the process of diagnosis from the physician's and the patient's perspectives. J Med Life. 2011;4(2):198–206.
85. Chiu YC. Probing, impelling, but not offending doctors: the role of the internet as an information source for patients' interactions with doctors. Qual Health Res. 2011;21(12):1658–66.
86. Jacob J. Consumer access to health care information: its effect on the physician-patient relationship. Alaska Med. 2002;44(4):75–82.
87. Tonsaker T, Bartlett G, Trpkov C. Health information on the internet: gold mine or minefield? Can Fam Physician. 2014;60(5):407–8.
88. Dominguez M, Sapina L. Pediatric cancer and the internet: exploring the gap in doctor-parents communication. J Cancer Educ. 2015;30(1):145–51.
89. Lin X, et al. Health literacy, computer skills and quality of patient-physician communication in Chinese patients with cataract. PLoS One. 2014;9(9):e107615.
90. Chadwick S. Some useful web resources for depression and bipolar disorder. Cutting Edge Psychiatr Pract. 2013;3:359–60.
91. Tierney S. The dangers and draw of online communication: pro-anorexia websites and their implications for users, practitioners, and researchers. Eat Disord. 2006;14(3):181–90.
92. Abbate Daga G, Gramaglia C, Pierò A, Fassino S. Eating disorders and the internet: cure and curse. Eat Weight Disord. 2006;11(2):e68–71.
93. Harshbarger JL, Ahlers-Schmidt CR, Mayans L, Mayans D, Hawkins JH. Pro-anorexia websites: what a clinician should know. Int J Eat Disord. 2009;42(4):367–70.
94. Christodoulou M. Pro-anorexia websites pose public health challenge. Lancet. 2012;379(9811):110.
95. General Medical Council Doctor's use of Social Media. 2013.

Lessons Learned or Forgotten? Future Direction of Global Digital Mental Health Care

19

Davor Mucić, Jay Shore, Donald M. Hilty, Marek Krzystanek, and Krzysztof Krysta

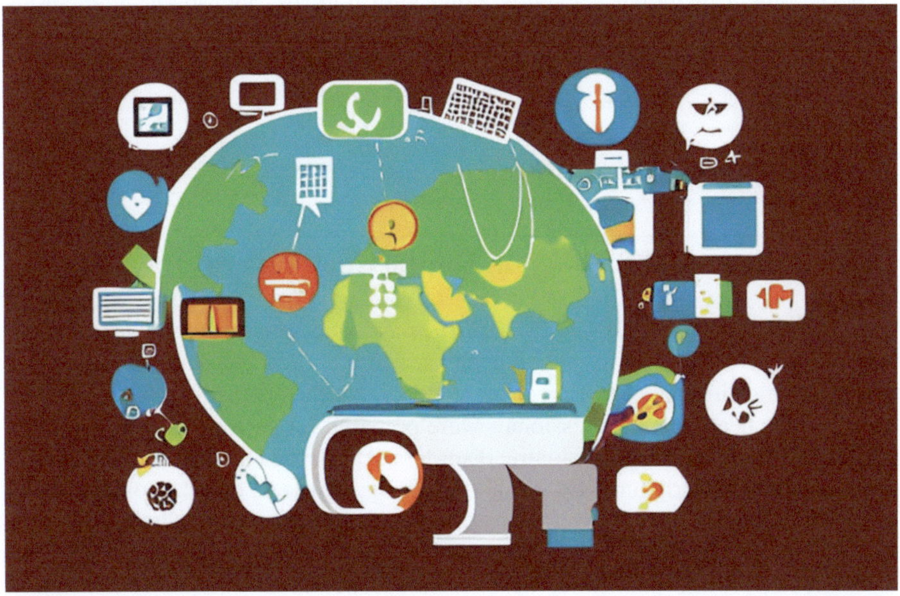

D. Mucić
The Little Prince Psychiatric Centre, Copenhagen, Denmark
e-mail: davor@denlilleprins.org

J. Shore
Psychiatry and Public Health, University of Colorado, Anschutz, Aurora, CO, USA
e-mail: jay.shore@cuanschutz.edu

D. M. Hilty
Department of Psychiatry and Behavioral Sciences, Keck School of Medicine University of Southern California, Los Angeles, CA, USA
e-mail: donald.hilty@uhsinc.com; hilty@med.usc.edu

D. Mucić, D. M. Hilty (eds.), *Digital Mental Health*,
https://doi.org/10.1007/978-3-031-59936-1_19

Abstract

The coronavirus disease-2019 (COVID-19) pandemic was an "eye opener" when it comes to limitations of the (mental) health systems that we have known for decades. It has impacted lives globally, posing unique challenges to mental health services exposing vulnerability and limitations within these systems. During the course of the pandemic, digital mental health (DMH) care have served a critical role in psychiatric care. It is important to understand and remember the lessons learned about DMH care and their implications for global mental health systems both during and after the pandemic. There are significant regulatory, policy, and evaluation challenges for global DMH impacting patients, clinicians, health systems, and decision-makers. These include complex regulatory issues, difficulties of providing care across boundaries, and keeping pace with the implementation of new technologies in behavioral health. The collaborative development of global standards along with policies, appropriate regulations, and developing new models of research and development opens the possibility of improved access to care across national boundaries.

Before anything else, preparation is the key to success. (A. Bell)

19.1 Impact of COVID-19 on Mental Health (Care)

The coronavirus disease-2019 (COVID-19) pandemic has impacted lives globally, posing unique challenges to mental health services around the globe exposing vulnerability and limitations within these systems. Neither governments, health care systems, nor health care professionals were prepared for such a scenario. Globally, patients with pre-existing psychiatric disorders experienced an exacerbation of psychiatric symptoms triggered by social distancing, isolation, and the loss or fear of losing their jobs [1]. They became more anxious, angry, stressed, agitated, and withdrawn during the pandemic outbreak or in quarantine [2]. The general public was also affected by the pandemic, with lower psychological well-being and higher scores of anxiety and depression among them [1]. In the first year of the COVID-19 pandemic, global prevalence of anxiety and depression increased by a massive 25%, according to a scientific brief released by the World Health Organization (WHO) in March 2022 [3]. Numerous reports concluded that the pandemic caused massive increases in anxiety and depression [4–8]. Participants reported various mental

M. Krzystanek (✉) K. Krysta
Department and Clinic of Psychiatric Rehabilitation, Faculty of Medical Sciences in Katowice, Medical University in Katowice, Katowice, Poland
e-mail: m.krzystanek@sum.edu.pl; krysta@mp.pl

health symptoms and experiences due to COVID-19, including increased feelings of boredom, loneliness, increased worry and stress, and increased suicidal ideation [9]. The COVID-19 pandemic period was characterized by changing drug availability, increased overdose risk, and other drug-related harms faced by people who use drugs in rural areas [10].

A systematic review of data from both scientific and nonscientific sources in several languages from 28 countries found numerous reports of deteriorations in symptoms, impacts of loneliness and social isolation, and lack of access to services and resources [11]. On the other hand, they also observed examples of resilience, effective self-management, and peer support (ibid.). In a study performed among 23 European experts in the early phase of the pandemic, it was found that some measures implemented by state authorities led to elevated stress levels, depression, domestic violence, and suicide among the inhabitants of involved countries [12].

Changes in the functioning of mental health services were also observed. Health care providers postponed several routines, elective care, and outpatient services [13, 14].

Face-to-face consultations were disrupted because of hesitation in consulting doctors in a hospital setting. As per a WHO survey conducted in 155 countries, the majority of countries reported partial or complete disruption of health care services for non-COVID-19 diseases [15]. Due to the pandemic, only the most affected patients, i.e., suicidal, psychotic, or delirious, accessed public health facilities through emergency wards as the activity of many outpatient clinics was discontinued [12]. The pandemic led to a drastic reduction in levels of care in community mental health centers and general hospital psychiatric wards [16], including treatment refusal by the patients, difficulty complying with safety precautions due to psychosis, agitated behavior, and problems with staff psychological well-being [17]. Schizophrenia is a prototypical severe mental illness in which the insufficiency of the existing medical care system can be traced. It is known that patients with schizophrenia are at a higher risk of developing respiratory diseases, including more severe forms of COVID-19 [18]. Accordingly, people with this diagnosis during a pandemic should have received more care and attention. Unfortunately, it did not happen. Patients had difficulty getting in touch with a doctor let alone accessing better care and prevention [19].

The COVID-19 pandemic has put health care professionals across the world in an unprecedented situation, having to make difficult decisions, e.g., how to allocate scant resources to equally needy patients, how to balance their own physical and mental health care needs with those of patients, how to align their desire and duty to patients with those to family and friends, and how to provide care for all severely unwell patients with constrained or inadequate resources [20]. Accordingly, health care professionals reported increased depressive symptoms, anxiety, mental illness, and poor sleep quality [1]. Health care professionals were confronted by unprecedented traumatic experiences during the COVID-19 pandemic, especially in countries that had not experienced similar epidemic outbreaks in several years prior to

COVID-19 outbreak [21]. The psychological pressure on health care workers, who were on the front lines of efforts to contain the spread, was enormous [22, 23]. A study among health care professionals in a tertiary infectious disease hospital for COVID-19 in China, revealed a high incidence of anxiety and stress disorders among frontline medical staff, with nurses having a higher incidence of anxiety than doctors [24]. Younger adults, racial/ethnic minorities, essential workers, and unpaid adult caregivers reported having experienced disproportionately worse mental health outcomes, increased substance use, and elevated suicidal ideation. In response to growing mental health concerns among youth, integration of mental health services in school-based settings became a priority [5].

The epidemic has had an uneven impact on young people's mental health. Some groups were particularly at risk. For instance, it was more challenging for young people with pre-existing mental health conditions to access support services, and they more severely experienced the pandemic's psychological effects [25]. During COVID-19, young people from the lesbian, gay, bisexual, transgender, queer, intersex, and asexual plus (LGBTQIA+) population were more likely to experience mental health problems, particularly if they were raised in a challenging home setting. Lockdowns also prohibited many from taking part in community events, which was a significant barrier preventing LGBTQIA+ youth from experiencing the psychological pain brought on by prejudice [25].

The studies on the impact of the COVID-19 pandemic on mental health are still ongoing [26, 27]. A profound understanding of the impact of the pandemic could facilitate an optimized governmental, social, and individual health preparedness during future pandemics and/or natural disasters. It may lead to coordinated actions through multi-level guideline development with the aim to improve mental health outcomes globally.

During the course of the pandemic, telecommunications technologies, telemedicine, have played a critical role in the provision of medical care in general and psychiatric care specifically as both widespread and sporadic quarantines and lockdowns in response to COVID-19 limited access to in-person care. The pandemic led to a wave of rapid adoption of telehealth services by the health care organizations, a sector that has been slow to adopt new technologies [28].

The use of video telehealth sessions, i.e., Telepsychiatry (TP), was welcomed by mental health professionals worldwide, who also expressed high levels of satisfaction with the treatment they received and a strong desire to keep using this modality as a substantial part of their clinical work [29].

TP has proved to be beneficial, efficient, and satisfactory for patients and providers across various disease types, unless the need for physical examination becomes imperative [30]. For example, the New York-Presbyterian/Weill Cornell Medical Center reported an increase of 8729% in the use of video visits during the COVID-19 period as compared with the pre-COVID-19 period [31], and increase seen across both individual providers, organizations, and systems. In psychiatry, an American Psychiatric Association (APA) survey conducted at the beginning of the pandemic reported that most psychiatrists (64%) were not using telehealth prior to the pandemic with a shift to 85% seeing more than 75% of their patients via telehealth in 2 months.

A review that focused on access, quality, patient outcomes, feasibility, effectiveness, outcomes, and cost showed that studies with cost-effectiveness, cost–benefit, and other analytic models are more common with telehealth than telepsychiatric studies [32].

A standard framework for economic cost analysis should include, if at all possible: an economist for planning; implementation and evaluation; a toolkit or guideline framework; comprehensive analysis (e.g., cost-effectiveness or cost–benefit) with an incremental cost-effectiveness ratio; measures for population health, quality of life, and utility outcomes; methods to convert outcomes into economic benefits (e.g., monetary, quality of adjusted life year); a broad perspective (e.g., societal perspective rather than a clinic perspective); sensitivity analysis for uncertainty in modeling; and adjustments for differential timing (e.g., discounting and future costs).

Telehealth has played a crucial role in Australia's largely effective response to COVID-19 in the area of mental health. Accurately assessing changes in psychiatric practice is made possible by the public availability of Medicare Benefits Schedule (MBS) data. MBS is a list of medical services and procedures subsidized by the Australian Government through the Medicare system. MBS data refers to the information collected from claims submitted by medical practitioners, including psychiatrists, for services covered by the schedule. The Australian Federal Government pays a patient refund for each consultation for MBS telepsychiatry care, demonstrating how quickly extra care may be provided by government-funded programs. Australia's quick and extensive adoption of telepsychiatry suggests that it could replace or supplement in-person care in the event of future pandemics and natural disaster [33].

Numerous reports have been published describing lessons learned from psychiatric organizations' rapid virtualization and conversion to telehealth operations emphasizing how telehealth was a critical lifeline in maintaining services and access to care during the pandemic [34–36]. It is important to understand the trends in telecommunications technologies leading up to and impacting their widespread use in the pandemic, current lessons learned, and implications for global mental health systems emerging both during the pandemic and after the pandemic has ended. This information with particular attention to impacts on policy issues is critical in shaping the future direction of global mental health care.

This chapter will help the reader review trends in current digital mental health (DMH) synthesizing the policy implications and recommendations for mental health providers and organizations. The reader will gain insight into: current needs related to DMH clinical practice, such as education and competencies; benefits for both patients and providers achieved within virtual hybrid provider–patient relationships; and future directions of global mental health care seen in the light of globalization.

19.2 Digital Mental Health

Digital mental health (DMH), a.k.a. e-mental health, digital psychiatry, e-psychiatry, etc., refers to the use of telecommunication technologies for the treatment or prevention of mental health disorders [37]. The use of digital psychiatry is supported by evidence as a practicable, user-acceptable, and successful platform for enhancing outcomes and quality of life in a range of mental disorders [38]. Thus, psychosis is underrepresented in literature, which focuses mostly on mood and anxiety disorders [38].

Telepsychiatry (TP), i.e., live interactive videoconferencing, is the longest known and best evidence-documented DMH application. With proof demonstrating its parity with in-person care in terms of therapeutic alliance and patient satisfaction, TP has continued to advance over the past 20 years [39, 40]. Moreover, evidence from systematic reviews and meta-analyses has shown that treatment effects achieved via TP are largely comparable with in-person approaches [41, 42]. Unfortunately, prior to the pandemic, mental health professionals did not widely adopt TP (or any other DMH tools) in daily clinical routines. Legislative issues, and the concerns of professionals related to the quality of care and patient safety, have kept TP from broader adoption. However, the American Telemedicine Association (ATA) and the American Psychiatric Association have developed best practice guidelines on the use of videoconferencing for the provision of care [43].

Despite six decades of TPs existence, at the outbreak of the COVID-19 pandemic, the vast majority of mental health professionals had little to no experience with TP. This posed significant challenges to mental health care delivery, as the need for remote services increased due to social distancing and lockdown measures. Mental health professionals were forced to quickly adapt to the use of TP to continue providing care to their patients. To address these challenges, the World Psychiatric Association (WPA) developed "Telepsychiatry Global Guidelines." The guidelines were developed with a universal approach to support all countries with intent to specifically assist low- and middle-income countries (LAMICs) in adopting and establishing TP services amid the COVID-19 outbreak.

Experiences reported during the COVID-19 time, describes not only a huge potential of DMH (primarily TP) to change how health care is delivered, but also many obstacles to its adoption and more optimal acceptance niveau. In outpatient settings, the COVID-19 epidemic has raised awareness of TP; nevertheless, hospital-based settings have received less attention. Hospital-based telepsychiatry has different difficulties than outpatient telepsychiatry, which necessitates further research and wider use of these technologies [44].

Studying the ways in which TP use may be associated with specific changes in practices (e.g., consultation rates, psychotropic prescribing, use of restraints) is crucial [44]. Modifying and promoting the development of remote services requires evaluating how patients, clinicians, administrators, politicians, and other stakeholders view hospital-based TP. One strategy is to ask participants about the advantages and downsides of hospital-based telepsychiatry in comparison to standard care [45]. Future research should look at how TP influences interactions between on-site and off-site employees as well as communication channels like routine team teleconferences. These research findings could help develop inpatient-specific training modules that would prepare personnel for new telepsychiatry-related tasks. Moreover, research is required to determine whether on-site direct supervision of trainees providing hospital-based psychiatric care is feasible compared to off-site remote supervision, in part because supervisors may be concerned about the effects of TP on teaching, medico-legal liability, and other issues [46].

Now, let us take a look at the challenges reported during the implementation of the remote services (mostly outpatient, i.e., Home-TP services) due to COVID-19 restrictions. Communication challenges that patients and providers faced during video consultations have been analyzed and an outline of the technologies developed to make such communication possible is proposed [47]. During video consultations, many people express difficulty developing relationships of trust [48–51].

Due to the hampered nonverbal communication [52], absence of physical contact, and overall sense of loss felt on both sides of the screen, trust is indeed challenging in the setting of video consultations [53]. Accordingly, it is challenging to forge a strong relationship given the physical distance between patients and physicians [54]. Building relationships between providers and patients is also impacted by changes in sensory data collecting during visits. For instance, both verbal and nonverbal communication are required to carry out the customary handshake greeting that initiates or maintains a trusting connection during face-to-face consulting [48]. As a result, health care professionals lose their capacity to interact with patients in a way that earns their trust. Collaboration talks are weakened by video consultations, which reduces confidence [55].

Despite the fact that patients and providers can interact verbally and visually, the interaction is less intimate in this situation [56]. Because patients and clinicians utilize their senses differently, developing a relationship, a type of proximity, at a distance is consequently more difficult [49]. The physician's interpretation of what the patient is attempting to express is altered when the provider cannot read the patient's body language [48]. It is not easy to rely on the physical cues generally used during consultations, such as eye contact and body language, when the meeting is conducted virtually. Both patients and doctors expressed their desire to meet in person before remote consultation [52]. They believed that trust is difficult to establish if they did not meet in person before the TP consultation [52, 56, 57].

In accordance with the above, the video conference between patient and therapist was of better quality when they already knew each other [57]. Accordingly, it is more difficult to establish a new relationship during video consultations than to maintain an existing one [47]. Moreover, it has been reported that confidence in clinical assessment and embodied engagement were not optimal. Both patients and providers find it difficult to perceive the assessment as accurate when the virtual consultation requires a physical examination [48, 49, 53, 58–60]. Patients worry about medical errors when a visit necessitates completing a physical examination because they are concerned about the lack of physical inspections, especially when they are symptomatic [49].

The absence of interpersonal ties and physical contact weakens customary practices that are meant to improve patient–provider relationships [53]. Yet, video consultations are preferred over telephone consultations since they allow the patients to see the provider [61], and receive care without having to visit a clinic [62].

Thus, patients encounter difficulties related to: the complexity of scheduling appointments [48], technical issues like time lag that can result in some talking over and affect the consultation [57], and limited access to technology or a lack of technical skills [51, 58, 63].

Patients complain that doctors do not show up for appointments or call them after the scheduled time, and that consultations are not long enough [58]. They notice that the professionals are under time constraints. They experience providers, who mostly regulate the pace of talk, as rushing them [50]. Patients regret not always having enough time to talk about all their concerns. Accordingly, decreased patient participation can lead to patient disengagement [49, 64]. Yet, health care professionals claim that because people talk less and/or generally speak more quickly, consultations are shorter [58]. Technology disadvantages some populations, raising the possibility of access to care inequities even as it makes it easier for those who find it difficult to travel. Some vulnerable patient populations lack the technology needed to participate in telemedicine visits or are unable to use it [53]. They include people who are older, have a low socioeconomic status, or have trouble hearing or speaking a foreign language [51, 55, 58]. Moreover, patients from racial/ethnic minority backgrounds face barriers and challenges related to the cost of equipment, limited understanding of the use of technology, limited health literacy, and challenges in navigating mainstream health care systems [65–67], which may hinder access to remote services.

Based on all mentioned above, it has been concluded that TP appears to be more advantageous for consultations involving mental health and chronic illnesses, managing test findings, or reviewing medications where a physical examination is not necessary [57]. Moreover, suggestions were also given on how to improve the quality of remote communication/care. In order to build trust with the patient, the practitioner needs to develop a strong website manner, put in extra effort to engage with the patient on a regular basis, make sure the right equipment are available (such as a headset and an Internet connection), arrange the environment, "dressing for success," inspect the technology, pay attention to all movements, and be mindful of eye movement. It is advised to start talks with small chat, encourage the patient to ask questions, use vocal empathetic comments to supplement what is communicated through body language and facial expressions, avoid overly enthusiastic body language that may be distracting, and increase your use of verbal empathic remarks [68].

Above outlined findings suggest that remote communicating via TP is not just learning how to use the technology, but includes the added challenges of coordinating visits with a less flexible schedule, relearning how to collect information about physical findings, and recognizing how sensory differences in the technology-mediated medical interaction change providers' practices and influence doctor–patient relationship [48].

However, many of the above-mentioned obstacles and barriers also apply when it comes to in-person care of ethnic minorities through translators. Language barriers are likely to affect patients' trust in their providers. Patients who do not speak the language of respective care providers have reported feelings of being discriminated against in clinical settings, whereas communicating with health professionals in a common language is associated with increased trust and confidence [69]. But, when patient and therapist speak the same language, e.g., within TP cross-cultural ethnic matching settings, then physical distance is not perceived as a barrier because of the closeness achieved through shared language and culture and no translators involved [70].

While remote consultations may be challenging for certain patient populations, the same approach obviously increases trust, confidence, and ultimately quality of care for other patient populations. Therefore, the choice of the DMH tool is a matter of triage, knowledge, competence, flexibility, and creativity of (mental) health service providers. All of these prerequisites must be met before we praise or condemn, accept or reject the use of the DMH applications described in this book. Digital technology training and education are certainly the key to overcoming most of the above-mentioned difficulties. This includes teaching future doctors how to perform a physical exam remotely and how to adapt their communication style for this situation. To allow physicians to experience multiple teleconsultation settings and learn to modify their clinical practice, using simulation as a teaching approach may be a direction to pursue [47]. The World Psychiatric Association (WPA) launched the first online Continuing Medical Education (CME) course on its educational platform in conjunction with the release of the Global Guidelines for Telepsychiatry in February 2021 [71]. Furthermore, in-person CME courses addressing DMH literacy, core competencies, and skills will hopefully become a default offering for participants at regional as well as global WPA conferences.

19.3 Benefits of Global Crises or How Adversity Can Lead to Success

COVID-19 pandemic seems to be a turning point for TP as well as for the DMH in general [72, 73]. Since the pandemic outbreak, the global impact of TP's precipitous rise was palpable. In light of the COVID-19 pandemic, many alleged obstacles to the global adoption of virtual care have been removed, despite the fact that TP has encountered a number of implementation challenges [74, 75]. Although the Royal College of Psychiatrists had previously issued warning advice, the National Health Service in the UK enabled the fast expansion of virtual psychiatric care [76]. By the COVID-19 emergency, millions of Americans were introduced to telehealth services, which offered significant advantages to patients, including but not limited to those who reside in rural locations with restricted access to health care [77]. A number of administrative steps, such as changes to coverage and reimbursement policies, have been taken by the U.S. Department of Health and Human Services to accelerate the adoption and awareness of telehealth during the pandemic. Some of these telehealth flexibilities have been made permanent while others are temporary [78].

Medicare, a provider of health care services in Australia, moved to support telehealth initiatives so that mental health services could continue to serve the population without interruption in spite of geographical limitations [79]. Medicare started financing telemental health in mid-March of 2020, and in the 6 weeks since then until April, 35 million Australian dollars were spent on these services [80]. Israeli, Singaporean, Korean, and Taiwanese governments responded quickly to the COVID-19 pandemic and extensively relied on technology [81]. Although TP has increased in low- and middle-income countries (LAMICs) as well, the complete benefits of using virtual platforms in these countries have not yet been fully realized [82]. Most LAMICs lag behind in the creation and application of data governance frameworks that strike a balance between innovation and privacy and protection of personal information. Digital technology training and education are essential, but few LAMICs have included digital skills in their health worker training [83]. There is a need to spread public knowledge/awareness of digital health issues through media and social media channels. Public–private partnerships are used to deliver digital health in high-income countries; LAMICs can also use this paradigm. Enhancing access to smartphones and the Internet is also necessary [82].

COVID-19 was eye-opener not only for TP but also for a wide range of other DMH tools, e.g., Internet-based interventions that have been shown to be effective in the treatment of various mental disorders compared with care-as-usual, i.e., face-to-face treatment, and waiting list control groups [84]. Internet-based cognitive behavioral therapy (iCBT) is the most commonly used intervention method in digital mental health studies [38]. It can be unguided or guided, with the instruction often coming from qualified volunteers or certified health professionals. Generally speaking, guided therapies outperform unguided ones in terms of clinical efficacy [85–87]. Although the idea of treatment adherence as a working mechanism has been put out, human support increases adherence [88]. However, in terms of effectiveness, it is still unclear how exactly human support accounts for the difference. The superiority of guided approaches is most likely explained by the interaction between the participant and the person providing guidance, i.e., by the quality of the interpersonal relationship. Although iCBT programs train participants in a wide range of cognitive and behavioral skills using a variety of delivery techniques, it is yet unknown which of these components is most effective and for whom. Combining human and automated encouragement reduced dropouts from treatment [89]. Guided iCBT was associated with more effectiveness than unguided iCBT for individuals with depression while benefits were more substantial in individuals with moderate to severe depression. Unguided iCBT was associated with similar effectiveness among individuals with symptoms of mild/subthreshold depression [90]. A specially developed web app can facilitate shared decision-making by therapists and patients in choosing their preferred iCBT package by including beneficial components and excluding ones that are potentially detrimental [89]. Moreover, interesting research is emerging regarding the use of Embodied Conversational Agents (ECA) in terms of improving the clinical results of iCBT by bridging the gap between guided and unguided therapies [91]. ECA can be defined as "more or less autonomous and intelligent software entities with an embodiment used to communicate with the user" [92]. Interactive video game characters and virtual characters that help consumers in online retailing are examples of ECAs in the real world. Technologically advanced ECA applications are very interesting and show promising results, but their complex nature makes it difficult for now to prove that they are effective and safe to use in clinical practice including iCBT guidance [91]. Mobile health (mHealth) and other technology-based services facilitate mental health service delivery and may also be considered part of a DMH spectrum of care [93]. Virtual reality applications are used in the treatment of Post Traumatic Stress Disorder (PTSD), specific phobias, anorexia, autism spectrum disorders, and schizophrenia [94, 95]. In 2019, researchers identified 1435 mobile apps for treating anxiety disorders, depression, schizophrenia, self-harm, and substance abuse, although the number is increasing every year [95]. Smartphone-based mobile apps have contributed significantly to the development of personalized psychiatry. New technologies associated with artificial intelligence (AI) are machine learning (ML) and deep learning in a form of convolutional neural networks (CNNs). ML and CNNs allow for an earlier and more precise diagnosis of the patient, the determination of the risk of deterioration or suicidal behavior, and the prediction of the therapeutic effect based on the analysis of the earlier effectiveness of drugs in patients with similar symptom clusters as well as the prediction of long-term effects such as relapse, side effects, or health complications [96–98]. In the future, AI may become a technology that supports physicians in diagnosis, drug selection, and prediction of improvement outcome. The possibilities that AI offers, based on the analysis of the collected records, are unpredictable and limitless (for more on AI please see Chap. 12).

In the case of mentally ill individuals, however, the COVID-19 pandemic was a turning point for primarily TP, while various DMH applications followed in addition to either personal contact with the professionals, i.e., hybrid care models (i.e., in-person and/or technology combinations), or "remote" consultation or as a part of self-directed assessment and care. On a spectrum of low to high engagement and technology requirements, participants use website information, support and chat groups, social media, resources for self-directed assessment and care, asynchronous patient–clinician communication (i.e., mobile health app, text, or email), video, and hybrid care models [99, 100]. While it is enjoyable and helpful to be spontaneous in using technology, it is helpful to consider the source used (e.g., Internet, social media, e-consultation, video), the user's goal/aim, liabilities, and approaches to make this meaningful and prudent (Table 19.1). For example, easy-to-use options like chat rooms or social media may vary in quality, yet largely offer a positive form of support for a patient, spouse, or caregiver, though more meaningful change may require an in-depth evaluation and clinical relationship via video.

Table 19.1 e-Behavioral health continuum of interventions for patients and families in behavioral health

Tier	Source	User goals/aims	Liabilities	Suggestions
1.	Website information	Gain perspective, obtain standard and updated health information Good for somatic symptom disorders	Quality of information and lack of regulation Ease of access	Refer to sites by psychiatric and medical organizations Keep information simple
2.	Support/chat groups	Patient: education and perspective Caregivers: tips and support on coping	Peer compatibility Information quality	Verify quality and those with a professional facilitator
3.	Social media (SM) passive and active	Patient: education and perspective Caregivers: tips and support on coping	Privacy Little time for clinicians	Active participation is more therapeutic than passive surfing
4.	Education program for self-assessment	Person/patient: education, tips Caregiver: education, support, and advice	Some learners prefer in-person Ease of access Quality of information	Give assignments Clarify if knowledge vs. skill development
5.	Consult with e-services clinician for self-care decisions	Person/patient/caregiver: additional options, perspective, context Clinician: helps independent learners and requires less time with patient	Complexity: not often as simple as do A or do B Scope of practice questions	Link with social work, hotline, and/or clinic, if needed Context with input from own clinician is better
6.	Assisted self-care assessment and decision making	Person/patient/caregiver: empowering as customized and supported Clinician: effective to distribute skills	Asynchronous communication has limitations Context for decisions is lacking	Use clinicians in health system Integrate in electronic health record (EHR) and care team
7.	eConsult between primary care provider (PCP) and specialist in EHR	PCP (geriatrician, family medicine): timely to visit and sent 'in time' Specialist: simple questions (e.g., facts, steps to do) can be answered	May not work for difficult patient cases that require integration Time to clarify question, review chart and communicate plan	Monitor timeliness, follow up and quality; build into care workflow and culture of care Use video: effective and easier

(continued)

Table 19.1 (continued)

Tier	Source	User goals/aims	Liabilities	Suggestions
8.	Asynchronous, between-session, patient clinician contact (e.g., wearable, app text)	Person/patient/ caregiver has minor question or needs a detail e-mail/text; tracking symptoms app Clinician: e-mail/ text for quick, simple advice; apps good for monitoring	Align 1–2 apps with 1–2 purposes to focus Errors, miscommunications Time, documentation, and privacy issues	Training for faculty and team Integrate into EHR for clinical decision support Use evidence-based app and evidence-based approach
9.	Synchronous, telepsychiatry (TP)	Person/patient: effective and is much more convenient Clinician: if patients like it, it is good	Has to be scheduled (and paid for) Workflow sometimes a little more demanding on clinician/team	Have technology, clerical and administrative support Training on clinical skills
10.	Hybrid care: in-person and e-option (TP and e-option)	Person/patient: options to connect Clinician: preferred if gives options and workflow not cumbersome	Systems vary in quality, training, prioritization, and quality improvement; time and $ costs	Develop integrated workflow for clinicians and administrators Facilitate positive e-culture

19.4 Shifts in Moving to Care with Asynchronous Technologies

In-person clinical care, care provided by TP, and care provided through asynchronous technologies have significant commonalities, but there are also differences [101, 102]. There are namely paradigm shifts happening with technology-based care. One shift is moving from structural (e.g., office visit) to functional "in time" clinical care. New research is focusing on how technology affects the therapeutic frame, communication, boundaries, and trust by applying neuroscience, communication, business, and augmented and virtual reality literature to psychiatry [103]. Correspondence via technology outside the office visit creates a new, previously impossible, sense of continuity, connection, and ease of communication (ibid.). Another shift is "in-time" data collection with wearables and sensors, for heart rate, steps/activity, and other parameters in older adults, which is known as ecological momentary assessment (EMA) that yields more valid, reliable, and meaningful data [104], which empowers clinician decision-making (e.g., mood and medication management). To use that data, though, mobile health, video, social media, and other technologies have to be integrated into the clinical workflow—this requires administrative planning, training, and faculty development [105]. Currently, DMH concentrates on creating machine learning (ML) and artificial intelligence (AI) methods for evaluating, diagnosing, and treating mental health issues in order to improve mental health outcomes with digital technologies [106]. According to a global survey, psychiatrists were somewhat dubious that AI could take the place of human empathy, but many predicted that "man and machine" would work together more to make clinical decisions. Psychiatrists were also hopeful that AI might increase efficiency, increase access to mental health services, and lower costs [107]. Clinical objectives such as diagnosis, prognosis, treatment, and readmission can be used to classify most ML applications in psychiatry. Traditional diagnoses in psychiatry, which are still limited to observable indications and subjective symptoms in contrast to most medical specialties, necessitate a paradigm shift. To obtain automated and more objective assessments for diverse psychiatric illnesses, ML offers a new paradigm [108].

However, in order to implement, accept, and maximize the benefits of the abovementioned paradigms, it is necessary first of all to be well prepared, i.e., educated, trained, and experienced, in the use of digital technologies. And that is exactly what the next section of this chapter deals with.

19.5 Competencies for Video and Other Technologies

As new generations adapt smartphones, social media, and other technologies, they have more personal technology experience than their teachers [105]. Many professionals may not consider asynchronous or store-and-forward technologies like mobile health and social media as a part of care, but patients do [101]. To keep up with society's use of technology and to ensure quality care, clinicians need skills (i.e., competencies), knowledge, and attitudes for synchronous and asynchronous technologies [102, 109]. Competency-based education focuses on clinical skill development in addition to knowledge acquisition. Competencies dovetail with lifelong learning as a part of ongoing practice, but clinicians are pushed toward quality care for many other reasons. Clinical experience—propelled forward by COVID-19—appears to predict interest and level of concerns. Perhaps, conservatively a dose of 1–5 h is needed to debunk preliminary questions/concerns or 6–10+ h to gain skills [110].

Competencies for video and other technologies have been organized into the six Accreditation Council of Graduate Medical Education (ACGME) domains [111], which are Patient Care, Medical Knowledge, System-Based Practice, Professionalism, Practice-Based Learning and Improvement, and Interpersonal and Communication Skills. Fortunately, mobile health [112, 113], social media [101, 114], wearable sensor [115], and broader asynchronous technologies for adults [32] and children [116] have been developed.

For example, using the ACGME domains but in the specific area of mobile health, the *Patient Care* competency mainly includes history taking, engagement and interpersonal skills, assessment, and management. It also includes administration, documentation, and medico-legal issues such as privacy, confidentiality, safety, data protection/integrity, and security. In general, clinicians should help patients and trainees reflect on the pros/cons of mobile phones, apps, and other DMH applications. A competent/proficient clinician selects the DMH option based on patient preference, skill, and need (i.e., purpose) so that patient and clinician decisions in-time are enhanced. It is helpful to know if the patient uses, e.g., videoconferencing, apps, or texts for personal life, health care, and/or behavioral health care, and if the patient is aware of risks (e.g., privacy, security).

Even though many medical specializations and health care services have gone digital, there is a lack of shared DMH competencies among the various fields of psychiatry/medicine, psychology, social work, counseling, marriage/family, behavioral analysis, and other behavioral sciences. The scope of professional guidelines and standards about technology is broad (e.g., practice of telepsychology; Internet and social media use in social work practice), to mid-range (e.g., American Telemedicine Association [ATA], American Counseling Association [ACA]), to narrow (e.g., preliminary "guidelines" for asynchronous communication such as email and texts) [117].

There is only one set of competencies for TP, which discusses skills, training, and evaluation. These competencies suggested (1) novice/advanced beginner, competent/proficient, and expert levels; (2) domains of patient care, communications, system-based practice, professionalism, practice-based improvement, knowledge, and technological know-how; and (3) pedagogical methods to teach and evaluate skills. Revisions to this framework and technology-specific competencies with additional domains may be needed. A challenge to competencies across disciplines may be finding consensus, due to varying scopes of practice, training differences, and faculty development priorities. Disciplines and organizations involved with Telebehavioral Health (TBH) need to consider certification/accreditation and ensure quality care [117].

In this new age, providers must deal with slightly different workflows and care processes whether using DMH care to supplement in-person care or in place of it. The following fundamental considerations are relevant to remote care and associated education:

- What is the best method to match a technology to meet the unique demands of any given client or patient?
- How can clients/patients and providers be empowered, reflect, and weigh the pros and cons of available options in order to learn new behaviors and evaluate outcomes?
- How can one encourage trainees and other clinicians to learn this spectrum of care and develop skills?
- How do we ensure clients/patients prevent and/or avoid untoward bad outcomes (e.g., posting on social media that one has suicidal thoughts instead of calling a crisis line and/or setting up an appointment)?

Wider understanding and the use of the new technologies allow many mentally ill individuals to receive high-quality treatment and care that otherwise remain inaccessible. DMH improves access, reduces costs, and compliments other care options.

However, the spread of DMH may be constrained by the absence of theoretical and practical knowledge during the academic years. Therefore, it is advisable to promote the creation of a toolbox of essential DMH competencies and their integration into *education and clinical practice both during medical school and psychiatry training programs* [118].

To summarize, the need for competency training, global TP guidelines, and regulatory and statutory changes, e.g., unified licensure regulations, etc., are crucial for modernizing mental health care delivery, successful adoption/implementation of DMH, and preparation for future unprecedented events.

19.6 Virtual Hybrid Provider–Patient Relationships in Digital Mental Health

The concept of hybrid partnerships between a psychiatrist and a provider or patient has gained popularity during the past decade [119]. With the increasing use of technology in medicine and psychiatry, the provider–patient relationship is now managed across multiple settings and platforms including in-person, videoconferencing, patient portals, mobile devices, websites, and social networks. Technology's rise has fundamentally changed how patients and doctors connect and communicate, hence it is essential for physicians to be flexible and proficient in using new platforms. Providers need to be able to effectively work with an individual patient across these settings with an appreciation of the strengths, challenges, nuances, and need for adapting clinical styles and processes to best fit an individual patient's circumstances, problems, and environment [120]. The trend to work with patients in hybrid manners was greatly accelerated by the COVID pandemic, necessitating individual providers to increase their mastery of hybrid relationships as well as provide an impetus for the field to gain a deeper understanding of the utility and impact on provider–patient relationships of commonly used technology. Virtual hybrid provider–patient relationships in digital mental health offer several advantages for both patients and providers:

- Greater access to care is one of the main benefits of virtual hybrid provider–patient partnerships. Patients can still receive treatment using virtual platforms even if they reside in rural or remote places, have limited mobility, or may find it difficult to leave their homes or office for sessions. This can greatly increase their ability to get the care and assist them in getting the support they require.
- Convenience and flexibility, as scheduling visits is made easier and more flexible with virtual hybrid provider–patient partnerships.
- Increased privacy, as some patients may feel more comfortable discussing sensitive topics in the privacy of their own homes or office. Virtual platforms can offer increased privacy and reduce the stigma sometimes associated with seeking mental health treatment.
- Cost savings, as virtual hybrid provider–patient relationships can be more cost-effective for both patients and providers. Patients save on travel and parking expenses, and providers can save on overhead costs associated with maintaining a physical office.

- Greater access to specialized care via online platforms that connect patients with expert health care professionals who may not be nearby. This could raise the standard of service and result in improved therapeutic outcomes.

While virtual hybrid provider–patient relationships offer many benefits, there are also some potential disadvantages to consider:

- Technical issues: The virtual platform's technical issues can be a significant drawback. Communication between patients and physicians may be hampered by poor video or audio quality, network connectivity challenges, and other technological concerns.
- Limited nonverbal cues: Using virtual platforms may make it more difficult for patients and health care professionals to read nonverbal cues such as body language, facial expressions, and voice tone. As a result, it could be more challenging to recognize and address emotional and mental health requirements.
- Limited physical exam: In-person visits allow providers to conduct a physical exam, which can be essential for diagnosis and treatment. With virtual platforms, this is not possible, which can limit the effectiveness of treatment.
- Security and privacy risks: There are security and privacy risks associated with transmitting sensitive patient information over the Internet. Providers must ensure that virtual platforms meet Health Insurance Portability and Accountability Act (HIPAA) requirements to protect patient confidentiality.
- Digital divide: Virtual platforms may not be accessible to all patients, particularly those who do not have reliable Internet access or the necessary technology. Unfair access to mental health services could come from this.
- Lack of personal connection: Some patients may feel a lack of personal connection with their providers when using virtual platforms. This can negatively impact the therapeutic relationship and the effectiveness of treatment.

Technology may change the nature of interaction for participants and communication related to the exchange of information, clarity, responsiveness, and comfort [105]. The goal with technology is to simulate real-time experiences related to feelings, perception, images, and interaction. TP, practiced via standardized, remote control, i.e., pan-tilt-zoom video equipment, is closest to the "golden standard" for personal consultations. Even low-cost, video-platform-based TP facilitates engagement and a "social presence." Ultimately, the goal via any modality is to create an environment that facilitates the therapeutic engagement and emotional well-being for all parties [109].

19.7 Telemedicine Psychiatric Systems

Deinstitutionalization is the procedure of shifting the care and support from long-stay psychiatric hospitals to community mental health services for patients diagnosed with severe mental disorders [121]. The changes that led to lack of space within the public mental health systems, as well as changes to the institutionalization process, have made it impossible for people with severe mental illness to find appropriate care and shelter, resulting in homelessness or "housing" in the criminal justice system's jails and prisons [122]. It is estimated that 10–20% of jail inmates and 25% of prison inmates have a serious mental illness; the proportion of affected jail inmates is estimated to be three to six times the rate in the general population. A significant percentage of these individuals are not receiving the psychiatric care they need and deserve [123]. After the initial treatment in state hospitals, severe mentally ill individuals will still be in need of long-term treatment. More housing with various degrees of supervision and facilities with a full-range of services must be brought back into the mental health system, along with revised laws for access to those services, to appropriately care for this population [124].

The integration of psychiatry with somatic medicine and the development of a community psychiatry require the organization and creation of a complex and coordinated care system, including primary care, specialized mental health care, crisis management services, housing programs, inpatient units, and centers running a specialized treatment program, and supervising this system and consulting them as clinical academic centers [19]. This creates great opportunities to introduce innovative technologies in the form of telemedicine systems coordinating the operation of a multi-module care system. Such a telemedicine system may include other mobile medical applications that enable screening diagnosis, early diagnosis, cognitive training, video education, and digital forms of treatment with the use of virtual reality, augmented reality, and applications for relaxation or phonotherapy [125, 126]. Such systems can automatically accelerate patient care by monitoring symptoms and processing them through algorithms that prioritize patients with more severe mental health problems [19, 127].

19.8 Digital Mental Health Care and Future Directions of Global Mental Health Care

With the widespread workforce shortage of psychiatrists and mental health providers prior to COVID-19, it is imperative to discuss how the mental health care systems will manage future unprecedented events. One way that mental health care providers can accommodate an increasing demand for mental health services is through the increased use of DMH within and across national borders. Increasing the use and availability of DMH applications and online resources is one way in which we can prepare for the growing demand for psychiatric services during and after the pandemic. As 45% of the world's population has access to 1 psychiatrist for every 100,000 people, and 50% of the population has a smartphone, the potential of providing psychiatric care through mobile applications is significant, especially with an emphasis on population health-based approaches [128]. Increased adoption, competencies, and investments in digital health today lay the groundwork of increased access and use of mental health care of the future [129].

However, there are still areas where DMH has not been utilized. One of them is natural disasters, which commonly result in distress reactions, increased health risk behaviors, and exacerbation or manifestation of psychiatric disorders [130].

Despite its enormous potential, telemedicine has not yet been utilized in the management of disasters. Establishing telemedicine programs in disaster-prone areas is urgently needed so that when disasters happen, existing telemedicine networks can be utilized rather than attempting to implement solutions in the midst of a chaotic scenario thereafter.

Along with developing and testing DMH applications, spending money on new technology development is also necessary to support the delivery of digital health. Numerous factors must be taken into account while choosing apps and mobile technology. While using consumer or well-known apps is handy, it is more crucial to make sure the app is evidence-based, or built on research. Additionally useful is the ease with which it (and its data) may be incorporated into workflow, such as the Electronic Health Record. Furthermore, we must take into account improving and reusing current infrastructure, such as phone booths with integrated tablets that would enable participation from people without access to digital platforms. Initiatives that provide mobile devices to those without the means to buy them could also contribute to the parity of treatment. It is also possible to create "virtual walk-in centers" by designating areas in hospitals and walk-in clinics for patients to use certain laptops or tablet devices. To lessen the discrepancy in access to digital care, digital health literacy must be improved through focused educational interventions. In the near future, when digital platforms are probably going to play a big role in how health care is delivered, these initiatives would improve digital inclusion and perhaps solve health disparity [131]. Clinicians, academics, funders, developers, and policymakers must work together to provide the evidence foundation for real-world pragmatic effectiveness trials of virtual care platforms, e-therapies, applications, wearable technology, and actigraphy[1] in order for digital health care to advance. Future paths for research include clinical trials that compare virtual care with in-person care and include a range of mental health presentations and service settings, as well as rigorous and robust clinical effectiveness trials. Additionally, more study is required on the implementation of AI and mobile applications. Mobile applications powered by AI have the potential to offer individualized real-time intervention and give quick attention to the patient's changing requirements. We have attained Digital Psychiatry 1.0, enabling us to communicate with our patients more effectively (virtual care vs in-person). Digital Psychiatry 2.0 must advance past connections and patient empowerment through remote mental health monitoring and in-the-moment clinical interventions [133].

In this exciting era of innovation and the adoption of new technologies in mental health care, many tensions have arisen including those of innovation vs

[1] Actigraphy is a procedure that records and integrates the occurrence and degree of limb movement activity over time. Actigraphic devices can be worn on the wrist, ankle, or waist, relatively unobtrusively over a period of days to weeks. For sleep applications, the devices are typically worn on the wrist or ankle [132].

regulation, access vs evidence, monetization vs privacy, and pragmatism vs rigor. COVID-19 has resulted in a loosening of regulations impacting digital mental health, which has allowed easier access to care. These rules often well-intentioned can create barriers and limit access to care. Overall, the benefits of access outweigh many of the concerns of technology in mental health care that the regulations have attempted to address. Patients, providers, and many health systems for sure do not want to go back to pre-COVID-19 circumstances but it is unclear what the right balance between in-person and digital mental health treatment is and what the optimal balance of hybrid relationships is. Ultimately, the solution is one that prioritizes the individual patient's needs taking into account the context of their environment and treatment systems. The following actors play a crucial for the future of DMH care:

1. *Patients* are the ones who have the most stake in the tools used for their treatments and have individual mediated levels of comfort and access with technologies that impact their ability to engage in digital mental health.
2. *Clinicians* are the ones who use the technology and require a good understanding of available technology's capabilities and the relevant *competencies* to use these in treatment.
3. *Health systems* provide the structure and environments for clinical engagement and drive the decision on which tools are used and require appropriate information (e.g., evidence, Release of Information (ROI)) to make systemwide decisions.
4. *Decision-makers* need to coordinate at the national and global levels to facilitate implementation, collaboration, and engagement in DMH (e.g., exchange of expertise and resources across national borders).

The increased need for just-in-time information about the technical aspects, implementation, and effectiveness of digital mental health is vital in helping the key actors make appropriate decisions and planning for digital mental health. Our current models of research and development and information dissemination were not keeping pace and were not designed for an era of rapid technological change that has accelerated even more during the COVID-19 pandemic. Only about half of evidence-based practice ever achieve widespread dissemination in health care taking an average of 17 years to be incorporated into routine practice [134]. There is an urgent need to develop new research and development models that can more rapidly evaluate DMH applications and services including critical lessons currently being learned during the COVID pandemic.

Addressing these regulatory, policy, and evaluation challenges could have significant benefits for global DMH for:

1. Patients: The ability to reach out to providers in other countries who have more availability and cultural understanding of their backgrounds reduces waiting times and travel. For those patients who work, study, or travel abroad, the opportunity to maintain continuity in care despite distance will be greatly appreciated. The current EU refugee crisis is perfectly positioned to benefit from an interna-

tional network of bilingual experts aimed at assessing and/or treating refugees and migrants via TP without the use of interpreters, i.e., via mother tongue.
2. Clinicians: Availability of timely qualified "second opinion" from colleagues with a relevant cultural and linguistic background regarding assessment and/or treatment of ethnic minorities with limited language proficiency. Furthermore, international expertise may be brought via TP to local health workers as a part of education, supervision, and scientific collaboration.
3. Health systems: Increase their quality of care and address greater potential health through improving access to care in mental health systems.
4. For decision-makers: Raise the quality of national health care, be better prepared to respond to future "unprecedented events," and widen participation in the global community.

19.9 Globalization of DMH

Digitalization is an important component of (mental) health services and infrastructures. It may ensure continuity of care in (mental) health services that could be abruptly discontinued due to the crisis/emergency situation. Accordingly, digitalization may represent a protective factor against the recrudescence of mental health conditions. In order to prepare for future unprecedented events (i.e., pandemics and/or natural disasters), one of the main goals now should be to create national as well as international, multilingual medical platforms and processes that facilitate access to medical services [135]. This requires consideration of telemedicine as an integral part of the health care system and the creation of telemedicine systems that integrate different medical specialties and provide interoperability to their users—both health care professionals and patients.

DMH is unfortunately still an underrepresented topic globally and plays a minor to moderate role in (national) mental health policies. Globally, the main limiting factors on the sustainable implementation of telemedicine are infrastructure, costs, lack of digital literacy, and staff resistance to change [54, 135]. Health professionals have mixed attitudes toward the implementation of DMH interventions in mental health care. On the one hand, many professionals recognize the potential benefits, e.g., increased access to care, improved efficiency, and reduced stigma. On the other hand, professionals identified a number of challenges to implementing DMH interventions, including concerns about patient engagement, privacy and security, and the need for additional training and support [136].

Moreover, there are current significant barriers to global collaboration, which include the global regulation of the use of various DMH applications not only within national borders but largely across national borders. The analysis of the current development of DMH in the world indicates the need to create an international framework and uniform standards for telemedicine that are currently lacking. "Transnational Policy for Digital Mental Health," a guidance document, aimed to foster the potential for adoption and implementation of DMH solutions throughout Europe [137].

There has been a steady increase in global migration and immigration as people are now moving further, faster, and in greater numbers than ever before propelled on by a number of interacting and complex factors including conflict, economics, and education [138]. Many of migrants and immigrants who have a potential need for mental health assistance can benefit from technology that knows no borders [139]. Unfortunately, current local licensure regulations are still an obstacle to international collaboration and expansion of the scope of digital services. Concerns related to, e.g., TP are primarily based on rules regarding the patient's location and the professional's, respectively. It is common that the patient cannot be treated if not located within the same country boundaries as the professional. The World Psychiatric Association (WPA) took specific steps in support of "telepsychiatry globalization" publishing the first global guidelines, aimed at promoting and facilitating TP services capable of providing remote consultations across national borders [140].

The WPA guidelines provide recommendations for:

1. *Video equipment producers*, to improve data and patient safety features of currently unsafe but widely adopted applications. The video tools' interoperability and inter-compatibility are crucial suggested/needed enhancements. Cross-brand and cross-category video equipment communication barriers will be eliminated via improved interoperability.
2. *Policy makers*, who are encouraged to start the work of creating uniform licensing rules, first regional and then global.
3. *Clinicians*, who must obtain the pertinent skills and competencies required to perform assessments and treatments using these tools since there are many distinct types of video conferencing technology, each with a unique feature and associated advantages and disadvantages. The clinicians' top focus is competency training in digital mental health as a result.

19.10 Conclusions

The delivery of mental health care will likely become more digitalized in the near future. With technological improvements, the incorporation of digital mental health care is providing creative solutions to address the burden of mental disease in the world. Digitalization of mental health care can offer benefits like better patient outcomes, enhanced effectiveness, lower costs, and better access to care. There is a significant gap in the availability of mental health treatment facilities and funding relative to the burden of mental disorders. There is hope that DMH will close this gap, enhancing patients' access to care and therefore their outcomes; however, these solutions may have unintended consequences for health equity [141]. Poverty, lack of access to digital health, poor engagement with digital health for some communities, and barriers to digital health literacy are some factors that can contribute to poor health outcomes. A Digital Health Equity Framework can be used to consider health equity factors—with a focus on person-centered care, and health provider training and support at the individual, institutional, and social levels.

Since the COVID-19 pandemic breakout, the technology enabled provision of traditional treatments with modern approaches. As clinicians tried to treat their patients at home instead of sending them to an office or hospital where they might risk exposure to the novel coronavirus or risk infecting others, patients have more frequently resorted to digital health platforms, tools, and services to consult with caregivers as a result of regulatory and statutory changes. The increased accessibility to DMH applications, like TP, has been crucial in controlling the spread by keeping individuals at home.

Global COVID-19-caused crisis offers the opportunity to advance our understanding of how to develop models of "traditional services with modern approaches" through digital technologies. Regulatory constraints, however, still pose significant barriers to the broader adoption of DMH within and across country borders. The collaborative development of global standards along with policies and appropriate regulations opens the possibility of improved access to care, including the free choice of health care providers, even across national boundaries. For these reasons, it is important to make a start in developing a global perspective for this work in the field of DMH. It is partially dependent on policymakers' insight and willingness to act promptly. Efforts such as the WPA's "Telepsychiatry Global Guidelines" along with "Transnational Policy for Digital Mental Health" can pave the way for improved international cooperation. National and international psychiatric associations can play a crucial role in promoting and providing education and training in core competencies in DMH. This includes disseminating guidelines, providing training and support, and advocating for policies that support the integration of DMH into mental health care delivery. By taking a leadership role in this area, psychiatric associations can help to ensure that mental health professionals have the knowledge and skills necessary to provide safe, effective, and culturally responsive remote services to patients. Above-mentioned documents can provide an example for decision-makers to inspire steps toward unifying rules and global regulations for the entire DMH spectrum in order to break down the barriers of accessibility. Reaching a common understanding of the appropriate standards, policies, and medico-legal requirements for the use of DMH, while considering its constant technological and methodological upgrading, is likely to make a crucial contribution to reducing global disparity in access to care. Additional obstacles related to lack of expertise and/or a lack of clinical experience can be addressed by making sure clinicians and systems have the tools and information with appropriate training and guidance related to the selection of video tools as well as their proper use.

The substantial mental health divide in low- and middle-income countries (LAMICs) can be closed with the help of DMH. However, the lack of relevant infrastructure, national DMH policies, and data governance frameworks sometimes hinder the growth of DMH in these circumstances. DMH can help LAMICs address the more traditional barriers to care by removing them, such as stigma, discrimination, a staffing shortage, and physical resource constraints. The majority of mental health care providers are concentrated in big cities in many LAMICs, hence employing digital technologies can be essential in bridging this gap. Progressively declining costs of mobile devices and widespread acceptance of mobile health interventions offer a practical solution to addressing the mental health treatment gap in these countries. Future DMH care should enable patient-centered access to affordable, clinically beneficial, and readily available real-time interventions regardless the income levels across the globe. Limitation drives innovation. Identifying the problem is the first step toward the solution. The Global Community must act more aggressively to improve access to qualified care for all.

References

1. Vindegaard N, Benros ME. COVID-19 pandemic and mental health consequences: systematic review of the current evidence. Brain Behav Immun. 2020;89:531–42. https://doi.org/10.1016/j.bbi.2020.05.048.
2. Torales J, O'Higgins M, Castaldelli-Maia JM, et al. The outbreak of COVID-19 coronavirus and its impact on global mental health. Int J Soc Psychiatry. 2020;66(4):317–20. https://doi.org/10.1177/0020764020915212.
3. https://www.who.int/news/item/02-03-2022-covid-19-pandemic-triggers-25-increase-in-prevalence-of-anxiety-and-depression-worldwide.
4. Twenge JM, Joiner TE. Mental distress among U.S. adults during the COVID-19 pandemic. J Clin Psychol. 2020;76(12):2170–82. https://doi.org/10.1002/jclp.23064.
5. Czeisler MÉ, Lane RI, Petrosky E, et al. Mental health, substance use, and suicidal ideation during the COVID-19 pandemic—United States, June 24-30, 2020. MMWR Morb Mortal Wkly Rep. 2020;69(32):1049–57.
6. Daly M, Sutin AR, Robinson E. Depression reported by US adults in 2017-2018 and March and April 2020. J Affect Disord. 2021;278:131–5.
7. Ettman CK, Abdalla SM, Cohen GH, Sampson L, Vivier PM, Galea S. Prevalence of depression symptoms in US adults before and during the COVID-19 pandemic. JAMA Netw Open. 2020;3(9):e2019686.
8. McGinty EE, Presskreischer R, Han H, Barry CL. Psychological distress and loneliness reported by US adults in 2018 and April 2020. JAMA. 2020;324(1):93–4.
9. Stack E, Leichtling G, Larsen JE, Gray M, Pope J, Leahy JM, Gelberg L, Seaman A, Korthuis PT. The impacts of COVID-19 on mental health, substance use, and overdose concerns of people who use drugs in rural communities. J Addict Med. 2021;15(5):383–9. https://doi.org/10.1097/ADM.0000000000000770.
10. Bolinski RS, Walters S, Salisbury-Afshar E, Ouellet LJ, Jenkins WD, Almirol E, Van Ham B, Fletcher S, Johnson C, Schneider JA, Ompad D, Pho MT. The impact of the COVID-19 pandemic on drug use behaviors, fentanyl exposure, and harm reduction service support among people who use drugs in rural settings. Int J Environ Res Public Health. 2022;19(4):2230. https://doi.org/10.3390/ijerph19042230.
11. Sheridan Rains L, Johnson S, Barnett P, et al. Early impacts of the COVID-19 pandemic on mental health care and on people with mental health conditions: framework synthesis of international experiences and responses. Soc Psychiatry Psychiatr Epidemiol. 2021;56(1):13–24. https://doi.org/10.1007/s00127-020-01924-7.
12. Thome J, Deloyer J, Coogan AN, et al. The impact of the early phase of the COVID-19 pandemic on mental-health services in Europe. World J Biol Psychiatry. 2020;23:1–10. https://doi.org/10.1080/15622975.2020.1844290.
13. World Health Organization. COVID-19: operational guidance for maintaining essential health services during an outbreak: interim guidance. 2020. https://apps.who.int/iris/handle/10665/331561.
14. World Health Organization. Weekly operational update on COVID-19. 2020. https://www.who.int/docs/default-source/coronaviruse/situation-reports/wou-4-september-2020-approved.pdf?sfvrsn=91215c78_2.

15. World Health Organization (WHO). COVID-19 significantly impacts health services for noncommunicable diseases. 2020. https://www.who.int/news/item/01-06-2020-covid-19-significantly-impacts-health-services-for-noncommunicable-diseases.
16. Carpiniello B, Tusconi M, Zanalda E, et al. Psychiatry during the Covid-19 pandemic: a survey on mental health departments in Italy. BMC Psychiatry. 2020;20(1):593. https://doi.org/10.1186/s12888-020-02997-z.
17. Mahgoub N, Agarkar S, Radosta M, et al. Inpatient psychiatry unit devoted to COVID-19 patients. Compr Psychiatry. 2021;9(107):152237. https://doi.org/10.1016/j.comppsych.2021.152237.
18. Fonseca L, Diniz E, Mendonça G, Malinowski F, Mari J, Gadelha A. Schizophrenia and COVID-19: risks and recommendations. Braz J Psychiatry. 2020;42(3):236–8. https://doi.org/10.1590/1516-4446-2020-0010.
19. Mari JJ, Gadelha A, Kieling C, Ferri CP, Kapczinski F, Nardi AE, Almeida-Filho N, Sanchez ZM, Salum GA. Translating science into policy: mental health challenges during the COVID-19 pandemic. Braz J Psychiatry. 2021;12:S1516–44462021005004200. https://doi.org/10.1590/1516-4446-2020-1577.
20. Esterwood E, Saeed SA. Past epidemics, natural disasters, COVID19, and mental health: learning from history as we deal with the present and prepare for the future. Psychiatry Q. 2020;91:1121–33. https://doi.org/10.1007/s11126-020-09808-4.
21. Braquehais MD, Vargas-Cáceres S, Gómez-Durán E, Nieva G, Valero S, Casas M, Bruguera E. The impact of the COVID-19 pandemic on the mental health of healthcare professionals. QJM. 2020. https://doi.org/10.1093/qjmed/hcaa207.
22. Tsamakis K, Rizos E, Manolis AJ, Chaidou S, Kympouropoulos S, Spartalis E, Spandidos DA, Tsiptsios D, Triantafyllis AS. COVID-19 pandemic and its impact on mental health of healthcare professionals. Exp Ther Med. 2020;19(6):3451–3. https://doi.org/10.3892/etm.2020.8646.
23. Greenbaum Z. Psychologist leads innovative approach to tackle psychological toll of COVID-19. Washington: APA; 2020. https://www.apa.org/news/apa/2020/03/psychologist-covid-19.
24. Huang JZ, Han MF, Luo TD, Ren AK, Zhou XP. Mental health survey of medical staff in a tertiary infectious disease hospital for COVID-19. Zhonghua Lao Dong Wei Sheng Zhi Ye Bing Za Zhi. 2020;38(3):192–5. https://doi.org/10.3760/cma.j.cn121094-20200219-00063.
25. https://ampeu.hr/files/COVID-Youth-mental-health.pdf.
26. Agorastos A, Tsamakis K, Solmi M, Correll CU, Bozikas VP. The need for holistic, longitudinal and comparable, real-time assessment of the emotional, behavioral and societal impact of the COVID-19 pandemic across nations. Psychiatrike. 2021. https://doi.org/10.22365/jpsych.2021.010.
27. Knolle F, Ronan L, Murray GK. The impact of the COVID-19 pandemic on mental health in the general population: a comparison between Germany and the UK. BMC Psychol. 2021;9:60. https://doi.org/10.1186/s40359-021-00565-y.
28. Lin CCC, Dievler A, Robbins C, Sripipatana A, Quinn M, Nair S. Telehealth in health centers: key adoption factors, barriers, and opportunities. Health Aff. 2018;37:1967–74.
29. Gentry MT, Puspitasari AJ, McKean AJ, Williams MD, Breitinger S, Geske JR, Clark MM, Moore KM, Frye MA, Hilty DM. Clinician satisfaction with rapid adoption and implementation of telehealth services during the COVID-19 pandemic. Telemed J E Health. 2021;27(12):1385–92. https://doi.org/10.1089/tmj.2020.0575.
30. Nanda M, Sharma R. A review of patient satisfaction and experience with telemedicine: a virtual solution during and beyond COVID-19 pandemic. Telemed J E Health. 2021. https://doi.org/10.1089/tmj.2020.0570.
31. Ramaswamy A, Yu M, Drangsholt S, et al. Patient satisfaction with telemedicine during the COVID-19 pandemic: retrospective cohort study. J Med Internet Res. 2020;22:e20786.
32. Hilty DM, Torous J, Parish M, et al. A literature review comparing clinicians' approaches and skills to in-person, synchronous and asynchronous care: moving toward asynchronous competencies to ensure quality care. Telemed J E-Health. 2021;27(4):356–73.

33. Looi JC, Bastiampillai T, Pring W, Reay RE, Kisely SR, Allison S. Lessons from billed telepsychiatry in Australia during the COVID-19 pandemic: rapid adaptation to increase specialist psychiatric care. Public Health Res Pract. 2022;32(4):3242238. https://doi.org/10.17061/phrp3242238.
34. Connolly SL, Stolzmann KL, Heyworth L, Weaver KR, Bauer MS, Miller CJ. Rapid increase in telemental health within the Department of Veterans Affairs during the COVID-19 pandemic. Telemed e-Health. 2021;27(4):454–8.
35. Mishkind MC, Shore JH, Bishop K, D'Amato K, Brame A, Thomas M, Schneck CD. Rapid conversion to telemental health services in response to COVID-19: experiences of two outpatient mental health clinics. Telemed J E Health. 2020;27(7):778–84.
36. Yellowlees P, Nakagawa K, Pakyurek M, Hanson A, Elder J, Kales HC. Rapid conversion of an outpatient psychiatric clinic to a 100% virtual telepsychiatry clinic in response to COVID -19. Psychiatr Serv. 2020;71(7):749–52.
37. Mucic D, Hilty DM, editors. e-Mental health. Cham: Springer; 2016.
38. Bashshur RL, Shannon GW, Bashshur N, Yellowlees PM. The empirical evidence for telemedicine interventions in mental disorders. Telemed J E Health. 2016;22:87–113. https://doi.org/10.1089/tmj.2015.0206.
39. Hilty DM, Ferrer DC, Parish MB, Johnston B, Callahan EJ, Yellowlees PM. The effectiveness of telemental health: a 2013 review. Telemed J E Health. 2013;19:444–54. https://doi.org/10.1089/tmj.2013.0075.
40. Parish MB, Fazio S, Chan S, Yellowlees PM. Managing psychiatrist-patient relationships in the digital age: a summary review of the impact of technology-enabled care on clinical processes and rapport. Curr Psychiatry Rep. 2017;19:90. https://doi.org/10.1007/s11920-017-0839-x.
41. Batastini AB, Paprzycki P, Jones ACT, MacLean N. Are video conferenced mental and behavioral health services just as good as in-person? A meta-analysis of a fast-growing practice. Clin Psychol Rev. 2020;83:101944. https://doi.org/10.1016/j.cpr.2020.1019.
42. Langarizadeh M, Tabatabaei MS, Tavakol K, Naghipour M, Rostami A, Moghbeli F. Telemental health care, an effective alternative to conventional mental care: a systematic review. Acta Inform Med. 2017;25:240–6. https://doi.org/10.5455/aim.2017.25.240-246.
43. Shore JH, Yellowlees P, Caudill R, Johnston B, Turvey C, Mishkind M, et al. Best practices in videoconferencing-based telemental health April 2018. Telemed J E Health. 2018;24:827–32. https://doi.org/10.1089/tmj.2018.023.
44. Morris NP, Hirschtritt ME. Telepsychiatry, hospitals, and the COVID-19 Pandemic. Psychiatr Serv. 2020;71:12.
45. Salmoiraghi A, Hussain S. A systematic review of the use of tele-psychiatry in acute settings. J Psychiatr Pract. 2015;21:389–39.
46. Szeftel R, Hakak R, Meyer S, et al. Training psychiatric residents and fellows in a telepsychiatry clinic: a supervision model. Acad Psychiatry. 2008;32:393–9.
47. Antoine MD, Cherba M, Grosjean S, Boet S, Waldolf R. How to support patient-provider communication during telemedicine consultations? A scoping review of challenges and existing tools. UOJM. 2023;12(1):6320.
48. Gopal RK, et al. Provider, staff, and patient perspectives on medical visits using clinical video telehealth: a foundation for educational initiatives to improve medical care in telehealth. J Nurse Pract. 2021;17:582–7.
49. Gordon HS, Solanki P, Bokhour BG, Gopal RK. "I'm not feeling like I'm part of the conversation" patients' perspectives on communicating in clinical video telehealth visits. J Gen Intern Med. 2020;35:1751–8.
50. Frankel RM, Beckman H. "Won't you be my doctor?" Four keys to a satisfying relationship in an increasingly virtual world. J Patient Exp. 2020;7:851–5.
51. Dahiya M, Olayinka L, Kaplan GG, Reeb L, Ma C, Panaccione R, Kroeker KI. The impact of the COVID-19 pandemic on IBD care in Alberta: patient and provider perspectives. J Can Assoc Gastroenterol. 2022;6(1):42–9.

52. Christensen LF, Wilson R, Hansen JP, Nelsen CT, Gildberg FA. A qualitative study of patients' and providers' experiences with the use of videoconferences by older adults with depression. Int J Ment Health Nurs. 2021;30:427–39.
53. Gomez T, Anaya YB, Shih KJ, Tarn DM. A qualitative study of primary care physicians' experiences with telemedicine during COVID-19. J Am Board Fam Med. 2021;34:S61–70.
54. Sagaro GG, Battineni G, Amenta F. Barriers to sustainable tele-medicine implementation in Ethiopia: a systematic review. Telemed Rep. 2020;1(1):8–15. https://doi.org/10.1089/tmr.2020.0002.
55. Howells B. Virtual consultations – the challenges for good communication with our patients. 2020.
56. Moeller AM, et al. Patients' acceptance of video consultations in the mental health services: a systematic review and synthesis of qualitative research. Digital Health. 2022;8:1–16.
57. Donaghy, et al. Acceptability, benefits, and challenges of video consulting: a qualitative study in primary care. Br J Gen Pract. 2019;69:e586–94.
58. Verma P, Robert K. Patients' and physicians' experiences with remote consultations in primary care, during the covid-19 pandemic: a multi-method rapid review of the literature. BJGP Open. 2022;6:192.
59. Matthews JC, Matthew DE, Mathur S, John NS, Nayak S, Bothra V. 411 patient perspectives regarding online consultations during the COVID-19 pandemic. BMJ J. 2021;5(Suppl 1):A1–A132.
60. Kieran R, Murphy C, Maher E, Buchalter J, Sukor S, Alken S. A permanent legacy of the pandemic? Outcomes of and staff views on the introduction of virtual clinics to an Irish oncology service. Ir J Med Sci. 2022;192(1):33–40.
61. Gleeson HB, Kalsi AS. Remote clinical consultations in restorative dentistry—A survey. J Dent. 2022;117:103914.
62. Byrne E, Watkinson S. Patient and clinician satisfaction with video consultations during the COVID-19 pandemic: an opportunity for a new way of working. J Orthod. 2020;48(1):64–73.
63. Canadian Medical Association. Virtual care guide for patients. 2020. https://www.cma.ca/sites/default/files/pdf/Patient-Virtual-Care-Guide-E.pdf.
64. Modic MB, Neuendorf K, Windover AK. Enhancing your webside manner: optimizing opportunities for relationship-centered care in virtual visits. J Patience Exp. 2020;7(6):869–77.
65. Truong M, Yeganeh L, Cook O, Crawford K, Wong P, Allen J. Using telehealth consultations for healthcare provision to patients from non-Indigenous racial/ethnic minorities: a systematic review. J Am Med Inform Assoc. 2022;29(5):970–82.
66. Kerrigan V, McGrath SY, Majoni SW, et al. From "stuck" to satisfied: aboriginal people's experience of culturally safe care with interpreters in a Northern Territory hospital. BMC Health Serv Res. 2021;21(1):1–13.
67. Ortega G, Rodriguez JA, Maurer LR, et al. Telemedicine, COVID-19, and disparities: policy implications. Health Policy Technol. 2020;9(3):368–71.
68. Dermer M. Virtual care playbook. Ottawa: Canadian Medical Association; 2021. p. 1–16.
69. Freeman GK, Rai H, Walker JJ, et al. Non-English speakers consulting with the GP in their own language: a cross-sectional survey. Br J Gen Pract. 2002;52:36–8.
70. Mucic D. Transcultural telepsychiatry and its impact on patient satisfaction. J Telemed Telecare. 2010;16:237–42.
71. https://3ba346de-fde6-473f-b1da-536498661f9c.filesusr.com/ugd/e172f3_19ce700c2a1f484b98efdcaf02c3c6ff.pdf.
72. O'Brien M, McNicholas F. The use of telepsychiatry during-COVID-19 and beyond. Ir J Psychol Med. 2020;37(4):250–5. https://doi.org/10.1017/ipm.2020.54.
73. Haxhihamza K, Arsova S, Bajraktarov S, et al. Patient satisfaction with use of telemedicine in university clinic of psychiatry: Skopje, North Macedonia during COVID-19 pandemic. Telemed J E Health. 2020. https://doi.org/10.1089/tmj.2020.0256.
74. Mann DM, Chen J, Chunara R, Testa PA, Nov O. COVID-19 transforms health care through telemedicine: evidence from the field. J Am Med Inform Assoc. 2020;27:1132–5.

75. Perez SP, et al. Turning the crisis into an opportunity: digital health strategies deployed during the COVID-19 outbreak. JMIR Public Health Surveill. 2020;6:e19106.
76. Dave S, Abraham S, Ramkisson R, Matheiken S, Pillai AS, Reza H, Bamrah JS, Tracy DK. Digital psychiatry and COVID-19: the Big Bang effect for the NHS? BJPsych Bull. 2021;45(5):259–63. https://doi.org/10.1192/bjb.2020.114.
77. Hoffman DA. Increasing access to care: telehealth during COVID-19. J Law Biosci. 2020;7(1):43. https://doi.org/10.1093/jlb/lsaa043.
78. Van der Werf M, Bernard J, Barta DT, et al. Pandemic action plan policy and regulatory summary telehealth policy and regulatory considerations during a pandemic. Telemed e-Health. 2022;28(4):457–66.
79. Davenport TA, Cheng VWS, Iorfino F, Hamilton B, Castaldi E, Burton A, et al. Flip the clinic: a digital health approach to youth mental health service delivery. JMIR Ment Health. 2020;7:e24578.
80. Rosenberg S, Mendoza J, Tabatabaei-Jafari H, Salvador-Carulla L. International experiences of the active period of COVID-19 - mental health care. Health Policy Technol. 2020;9:503–9. https://doi.org/10.1016/j.hlpt.2020.08.016.
81. Salvador-Carulla L, Rosenberg S, Mendoza J, Tabatabaei-Jafari H, Pandemic-Mental Health International N. Rapid response to crisis: health system lessons from the active period of COVID-19. Health Policy Technol. 2020;9:578–86.
82. Naeem F, Husain MO, Husain MI, Javed A. Digital psychiatry in low- and middle-income countries post-COVID-19: opportunities, challenges, and solutions. Indian J Psychiatry. 2020;62(Suppl 3):S380–2. https://doi.org/10.4103/psychiatry.IndianJPsychiatry_843_20.
83. Cory N, Stevens P. Building a global framework for digital health services in the era of COVID-19. Washington: Information Technology and Innovation Foundation; 2020.
84. Andrews G, Cuijpers P, Craske MG, McEvoy P, Titov N. Computer therapy for the anxiety and depressive disorders is effective, acceptable and practical health care: a meta-analysis. PLoS One. 2010;5(10):e13196.
85. Richards D, Richardson T. Computer-based psychological treatments for depression: a systematic review and meta-analysis. Clin Psychol Rev. 2012;32(4):329–42. https://doi.org/10.1016/j.cpr.2012.02.004.
86. Spek V, Cuijpers P, Nyklícek I, Riper H, Keyzer J, Pop V. Internet-based cognitive behaviour therapy for symptoms of depression and anxiety: a meta-analysis. Psychol Med. 2007;37(3):319–28. https://doi.org/10.1017/S0033291706008944.
87. Johansson R, Andersson G. Internet-based psychological treatments for depression. Expert Rev Neurother. 2012;12(7):861–70. https://doi.org/10.1586/ern.12.63.
88. Mohr DC, Cuijpers P, Lehman K. Supportive accountability: a model for providing human support to enhance adherence to eHealth interventions. J Med Internet Res. 2011;13(1):e30. https://doi.org/10.2196/jmir.1602.
89. Furukawa TA, et al. Dismantling, optimizing, and personalizing Internet cognitive behavioural therapy for depression: a systematic review and component network meta-analysis using individual participant data. Lancet Psychiatry. 2021;8(6):500–11.
90. Karyotaki E, et al. Internet-based cognitive behavioral therapy for depression: a systematic review and individual patient data network meta-analysis. JAMA Psychiatry. 2021;78(4):361–71.
91. Provoost S, Lau HM, Ruwaard J, Riper H. Embodied conversational agents in clinical psychology: a scoping review. J Med Internet Res. 2017;19(5):e151. https://doi.org/10.2196/jmir.6553.
92. Isbister K, Doyle P. The blind men and the elephant revisited evaluating interdisciplinary ECA research. In: Ruttkay Z, Pelachaud C, editors. From brows to trust evaluating embodied conversational agents. Dordrecht: Springer; 2004. p. 3–26.
93. Hilty DM, Chan S, Hwang T, Wong A, Bauer AM. Advances in mobile mental health: opportunities and implications for the spectrum of e-mental health services. Focus. 2018;16(3):314–27.

94. Park MJ, Kim DJ, Lee U, Na EJ, Jeon HJ. A literature overview of virtual reality (VR) in treatment of psychiatric disorders: recent advances and limitations. Front Psych. 2019;19(10):505. https://doi.org/10.3389/fpsyt.2019.00505.
95. Larsen ME, Huckvale K, Nicholas J, Torous J, Birrell L, Li E, Reda B. Using science to sell apps: evaluation of mental health app store quality claims. NPJ Digit Med. 2019;22(2):18. https://doi.org/10.1038/s41746-019-0093-1.
96. Ibrahim FA, Pahuja E, Dinakaran D, Manjunatha N, Kumar CN, Math SB. The future of telepsychiatry in India. Indian J Psychol Med. 2020;42(5 Suppl):112S–7S. https://doi.org/10.1177/0253717620959255.
97. Bzdok D, Meyer-Lindenberg A. Machine learning for precision psychiatry: opportunities and challenges. Biol Psychiatry Cogn Neurosci Neuroimaging. 2018;3(3):223–30. https://doi.org/10.1016/j.bpsc.2017.11.007.
98. Rajkomar A, Oren E, Chen K, et al. Scalable and accurate deep learning with electronic health records. NPJ Digit Med. 2018;8(1):18. https://doi.org/10.1038/s41746-018-0029-1.
99. Hilty DM, Chan S, Torous J, et al. New frontiers in healthcare and technology: Internet- and web-based mental options emerge to complement in-person and telepsychiatric care options. J Health Med Inform. 2015;6(4):1–14.
100. Chan S, Godwin H, Gonzalez A, et al. Review of use and integration of mobile apps into psychiatric treatments. Curr Psychiatry Rep. 2017;19(12):96. https://doi.org/10.1007/s11920-017-0848-9.
101. Zalpuri I, Liu H, Stubbe D, et al. A competency-based framework for social media for trainees, faculty and others. Acad Psychiatry. 2018;42(6):808–17.
102. Hilty DM, Uno J, Chan S, et al. Role of technology in professional development. Psychiatr Clin N Am. 2019;42:493–512.
103. Hilty DM, Randhawa K, Maheu MM, et al. A review of telepresence, virtual reality and augmented reality applied to clinical care. J Tech Behav Sci. 2020. https://doi.org/10.1007/s41347-020-00126-x.
104. Hilty DM, Armstrong CM, Luxton DD, et al. A framework of sensor, wearable and remote patient monitoring competencies for clinical care and training: scoping review. J Tech Behav Sci. 2021. https://doi.org/10.1007/s41347-020-00190-3.
105. Hilty DM, Torous J, Parish M, et al. A literature review comparing clinicians' approaches and skills to in-person, synchronous and asynchronous care: moving toward asynchronous competencies to ensure quality care. Telemed J E-Health. 2020. https://doi.org/10.1089/tmj.2020.0054.
106. Burr C, Morley J, Taddeo M, Floridi L. Digital psychiatry: risks and opportunities for public health and wellbeing. IEEE Trans Technol Soc. 2020;1:21–33.
107. Doraiswamy PM, Blease C, Bodner K. Artificial intelligence and the future of psychiatry: insights from a global physician survey. Artif Intell Med. 2020;102:101753.
108. Chen ZS, Kulkarni PP, Galatzer-Levy IR, Bigio B, Nasca C, Zhang Y. Modern views of machine learning for precision psychiatry. Patterns. 2022;3(11):100602. https://doi.org/10.1016/j.patter.2022.100602.
109. Maheu M, Drude K, Hertlein K, et al. An interdisciplinary frame-work for telebehavioral health competencies. J Tech Behav Sci. 2019;3(2):108–40.
110. Cruz C, Orchard K, Shoemaker EZ, Hilty DM. A survey of residents/fellows, program directors and faculty about telepsychiatry: clinical experience, interest, views and misconceptions. J Tech Behav Sci. 2021. https://doi.org/10.1007/s41347-021-00201-x.
111. Accreditation Council on Graduate Medical Education. Common program requirements. 2013. https://www.acgme.org/acgmeweb/Portals/0/PFAssets/ProgramRequirements/CPRs2013.pdf.
112. Hilty DM, Chan S, Torous J, et al. A telehealth framework for mobile health, smartphones and apps: competencies, training and faculty development. J Tech Behav Sci. 2019;4(2):106–23.
113. Hilty DM, Chan S, Torous J, et al. A framework for competencies for the use of mobile technologies in psychiatry and medicine. JMIR Uhealth Mob Health. 2020;8(2):e12229.

114. Hilty DM, Zalpuri I, Stubbe D, et al. Social media/networking as part of e-behavioral health and psychiatric education: competencies, teaching methods, and implications. J Tech Behav Sci. 2018;3(4):268–93.
115. Hilty DM, Armstrong CM, Stewart A, Luxton DD, Gentry M, Krupinski E. A framework of sensor, wearable and remote patient monitoring competencies for clinical care and training: scoping review. J Tech Behav Sci. 2021;6:252–77.
116. Hilty DM, Zalpuri I, Torous J, E-L. Nelson: child and adolescent asynchronous technology competencies for clinical care and training: scoping review. Fam Syst Health. 2021;39(1):121–52. https://doi.org/10.1037/fsh0000536.
117. Hilty DM, Maheu MM, Drude KP, et al. Telebehavioral health, telemental health, e-therapy and e-health competencies: the need for an interprofessional framework. J Technol Behav Sci. 2017;2:171–89. https://doi.org/10.1007/s41347-017-0036-0.
118. Orsolini L, et al. A preliminary Italian cross-sectional study on the level of digital psychiatry training, knowledge, beliefs and experiences among medical students, psychiatry trainees and professionals. Healthcare. 2022;10(2):390. https://doi.org/10.3390/healthcare10020390.
119. Yellowlees P, Shore JH. Telepsychiatry and health technologies: a guide for mental health professionals. Washington: APA; 2018.
120. Shore JH. Managing virtual hybrid psychiatrist-patient relationships in a digital world. JAMA Psychiat. 2020;77(5):541–2.
121. Fakhoury W, Priebe S. Deinstitutionalization and reinstitutionalization: major changes in the provision of mental healthcare. Psychiatry. 2007;6:313–6.
122. Lamb RH, Weinberger LE. The shift of psychiatric inpatient care from hospitals to jails and prisons. J Am Acad Psychiatry Law. 2005;33(4):529–34.
123. Matthew E, Hirschtritt, Renée L, Binder. Interrupting the mental illness-incarceration-recidivism cycle. JAMA. 2017;317(7):695–6. https://doi.org/10.1001/JAMA.2016.20992.
124. Yohanna D. Deinstitutionalization of people with mental illness: causes and consequences. Virtual Mentor. 2013;15(10):886–91. https://doi.org/10.1001/virtualmentor.2013.15.10.mhst1-1310.
125. Krzystanek M, Krysta K, Borkowski M, et al. The effect of smart-phone-based cognitive training on the functional/cognitive markers of schizophrenia: a one-year randomized study. J Clin Med. 2020;9(11):3681. https://doi.org/10.3390/jcm9113681.
126. Schuster I, Romańczyk M, Surma S, Krzystanek M. Phonotherapy – a new biological treatment proposal for the augmentation of pharmacotherapy in psychiatry and neurology. Adv Psychiatry Neurol. 2020;29(4):224–33. https://doi.org/10.5114/ppn.2020.103634.
127. Miyoshi NSB, Azevedo-Marques JM, Alves D, Azevedo-Marques PM. An eHealth platform for the support of a Brazilian Regional Network of Mental Health Care (eHealth-Interop): development of an interoperability platform for Mental Care Integration. JMIR Ment Health. 2018;5(4):e10129. https://doi.org/10.2196/10129.
128. Lovejoy CA, Buch V, Maruthappu M. Technology and mental health: the role of artificial intelligence. Eur Psychiatry. 2019;55:1–3. https://doi.org/10.1016/j.eurpsy.2018.08.004.
129. Torous J, Jän Myrick K, Rauseo-Ricupero N, Firth J. Digital mental health and COVID-19: using technology today to accelerate the curve on access and quality tomorrow. JMIR Ment Health. 2020;7(3):e18848. https://doi.org/10.2196/18848.
130. Morganstein JC, Ursano RJ. Ecological disasters and mental health: causes, consequences, and interventions. Front Psych. 2020;11:1. https://doi.org/10.3389/fpsyt.2020.00001.
131. Farooq S, Taylor CD, Gire N, Riley M, Caton N, Husain N. Digital inclusion: the concept and strategies for people with mental health difficulties. Aust N Z J Psychiatry. 2015;49:772–3. https://doi.org/10.1177/0004867415591827.
132. Smith MT, McCrae CS, Cheung J, Martin JL, Harrod CG, Heald JL, Carden KA. Use of actigraphy for the evaluation of sleep disorders and circadian rhythm sleep-wake disorders: an American Academy of Sleep Medicine systematic review, meta-analysis, and GRADE assessment. J Clin Sleep Med. 2018;14(7):1209–30. https://doi.org/10.5664/jcsm.7228.

133. Torous J, Wykes T. Opportunities from the coronavirus disease 2019 pandemic for transforming psychiatric care with telehealth. JAMA Psychiatry. 2020;77(12):1205–6. https://doi.org/10.1001/jamapsychiatry.2020.1640.
134. Bauer MS, Damschroder L, Hagedorn H, Smith J, Kilbourne AM. An introduction to implementation science for the non-specialist. BMC Psychol. 2015;3(1):1–2.
135. Scott Kruse C, Karem P, Shifflett K, Vegi L, Ravi K, Brooks M. Evaluating barriers to adopting telemedicine worldwide: a systematic review. J Telemed Telecare. 2018;24(1):4–12. https://doi.org/10.1177/1357633X16674087.
136. Riper H, Kleiboer A, van Ballegooijen W, Kramer J, Bosmans J, Cuijpers P. Implementing eHealth interventions in mental health care: a systematic review of health professionals' perspectives. Mhealth. 2017;3:51.
137. Gaebel W, et al. Transnational policy for e-mental health. 2020. https://www.nweurope.eu/media/10450/emen_transnational-policy-for-e-mental-health_guidance-document_3-2020.pdf.
138. Rousseau C. Addressing mental health needs of refugees. Can J Psychiatry. 2018;63(5):287–9.
139. Reinhardt I, Gouzoulis-Mayfrank E, Zielasek J. Use of telepsychiatry in emergency and crisis intervention: current evidence. Curr Psychiatry Rep. 2019;21(8):1–8.
140. WPA Telepsychiatry Global Guidelines. 2021. https://3ba346de-fde6-473f-b1da-536498661f9c.filesusr.com/ugd/e172f3_19ce700c2a1f484b98efdcaf02c3c6ff.pdf.
141. Crawford A, Serhal E. Digital health equity and COVID-19: the innovation curve cannot reinforce the social gradient of health. J Med Internet Res. 2020;22(6):e19361. https://doi.org/10.2196/19361.

MIX
Papier aus verantwortungsvollen Quellen
Paper from responsible sources
FSC® C105338

If you have any concerns about our products,
you can contact us on
ProductSafety@springernature.com

In case Publisher is established outside the EU,
the EU authorized representative is:
Springer Nature Customer Service Center GmbH
Europaplatz 3, 69115 Heidelberg, Germany

Printed by Libri Plureos GmbH
in Hamburg, Germany